PRACTICAL VASCULAR SURGERY

PRACTICAL VASCULAR SURGERY

Edited by

James S. T. Yao, MD, PhD
Magerstadt Professor of Surgery
Northwestern University Medical School
Acting Chair, Department of Surgery
Northwestern Memorial Hospital
Chicago, Illinois

William H. Pearce, MD
Professor of Surgery
Northwestern University Medical School
Chief, Division of Vascular Surgery
Northwestern Memorial Hospital
Chicago, Illinois

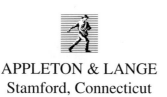

APPLETON & LANGE
Stamford, Connecticut

Notice: The authors and the publisher of this volume have taken care to make certain that the doses of drugs and schedules of treatment are correct and compatible with the standards generally accepted at the time of publication. Nevertheless, as new information becomes available, changes in treatment and in the use of drugs become necessary. The reader is advised to carefully consult the instruction and information material included in the package insert of each drug or therapeutic agent before administration. This advice is especially important when using, administering, or recommending new or infrequently used drugs. The authors and publisher disclaim all responsibility for any liability, loss, injury, or damage incurred as a consequence, directly or indirectly, of the use and application of any of the contents of this volume.

Copyright © 1999 by Appleton & Lange
A Simon & Schuster Company

www.appletonlange.com

99 00 01 02 03 / 10 9 8 7 6 5 4 3 2 1

Prentice Hall International (UK) Limited, *London*
Prentice Hall of Australia Pty. Limited, *Sydney*
Prentice Hall Canada, Inc., *Toronto*
Prentice Hall Hispanoamericana, S.A., *Mexico*
Prentice Hall of India Private Limited, *New Delhi*
Prentice Hall of Japan, Inc., *Tokyo*
Simon & Schuster Asia Pte. Ltd., *Singapore*
Editora Prentice Hall do Brasil Ltda., *Rio de Janeiro*
Prentice Hall, *Upper Saddle River, New Jersey*

Library of Congress Cataloging-in-Publication Data

Practical vascular surgery / edited by James S. T. Yao, William H. Pearce.
    p. cm.
  ISBN 0-8385-8164-1 (case : alk. paper)
  1. Blood-vessels--Surgery.   I. Yao, James S. T.   II. Pearce. William H.
  [DNLM: 1. Vascular Surgical Procedures.   WG 170 P895 1999]
RD598.5.P685 1999
617.4'13059—dc21
DNLM/DLC
for Library of Congress
         98-43442
         CIP

ISBN 0-8385-8164-1

90000

9 780838 581643

Acquisitions Editor: Michael P. Medina
Production Service: Spectrum Publisher Services
Designer: Janice Bielawa

PRINTED IN THE UNITED STATES OF AMERICA

Contents

Contributors

J. Dennis Baker, MD
Professor of Surgery
UCLA School of Medicine
Chief, Vascular Surgery Section
West Los Angeles VA Medical Center
Los Angeles, California

William H. Baker, MD
Professor of Surgery
Section of Peripheral Vascular Surgery
Department of Surgery
Loyola University Medical School,
  Stritch School of Medicine
Maywood, Illinois

Dennis F. Bandyk, MD
Professor of Surgery
Director, Division of Vascular Surgery
University of South Florida College of
  Medicine
Tampa, Florida

Thomas Bilfinger, MD
Associate Professor of Clinical Surgery
State University of New York at Stony
  Brook
University Hospital, State University of
  New York at Stony Brook
Stony Brook, New York

John D. Birkmeyer, MD
Assistant Professor of Surgery and
  Community and Family Medicine

Center for the Evaluative Clinical
  Sciences
Dartmouth-Hitchcock Medical Center
Lebanon, New Hampshire

**Andrew W. Bradbury, BSc, MD,
  FRCSEd**
Senior Lecturer in Surgery
Edinburgh University
Consultant Vascular Surgeon
Edinburgh Royal Infirmary
Edinburgh, Scotland

Brian G. Brazzo, MD
Assistant Attending Surgeon,
  Department of Ophthalmology
Manhattan Eye, Ear and Throat
  Hospital
New York, New York

David C. Brewster, MD
Clinical Professor of Surgery
Harvard Medical School
Massachusetts General Hospital
Boston, Massachusetts

Richard P. Cambria, MD
Associate Professor of Surgery
Harvard Medical School
Visiting Surgeon
Massachusetts General Hospital
Boston, Massachusetts

Sandra C. Carr, MD
Assistant Professor
University of Wisconsin Medical School
Madison, Wisconsin

Douglas A. Coe, MD
Vascular Fellow
Medical College of Wisconsin
Milwaukee, Wisconsin

Anthony J. Comerota, MD, FACS
Professor of Surgery
Temple University Medical School
Chief, Vascular Surgery/Director, Center
  for Vascular Diseases
Temple University Hospital
Philadelphia, Pennsylvania

Jack L. Cronenwett, MD
Professor of Surgery
Dartmouth-Hitchcock Medical Center
Lebanon, New Hampshire

Michael C. Dalsing, MD
Professor of Surgery
Indiana University School of Medicine
Indianapolis, Indiana
Director, Division of Vascular Surgery
Indiana University Hospital
Wishard, Indiana
Memorial Hospital
Indianapolis, Indiana

Julie S. Droste, BSN, RN
Vascular Surgery Nurse Coordinator
Evanston Northwestern Healthcare
Evanston, Illinois

Vincent Falanga, MD, FACP
Professor of Dermatology
Boston University
Chairman of Department of
  Dermatology and Skin Surgery
Roger Williams Medical Center
Providence, Rhode Island

David V. Feliciano, MD
Professor of Surgery
Emory University School of Medicine

Chief of Surgery
Grady Memorial Hospital
Atlanta, Georgia

John F. Golan, MD
Assistant Professor of Surgery
Northwestern University Medical School
Evanston Northwestern Healthcare
Evanston, Illinois

David Green, MD, PhD
Professor of Medicine
Northwestern University Medical School
Chicago, Illinois

Lazar J. Greenfield, MD
Frederick A. Coller Distinguished
  Professor and Chairman
Department of Surgery
University of Michigan
Ann Arbor, Michigan

John W. Hallett, Jr., MD
Professor of Surgery
Associate Dean for Faculty Affairs
Mayo Clinic and Mayo Medical School
Rochester, Minnesota

Roger Higgins, PhD
Director
Somerset Noninvasive Vascular
  Laboratory
Troy, Michigan

Robert W. Hobson II, MD
Professor of Surgery and Physiology
University of Medicine and Dentistry of
  New Jersey, New Jersey Medical School
Chief, Division of Vascular Surgery
Newark, New Jersey

Kaj Johansen, MD, PhD
Professor of Surgery
University of Washington School of
  Medicine
Director of Surgical Education
Providence Seattle Medical Center
Seattle, Washington

Steven S. Kang, MD
Assistant Professor of Surgery
Loyola University Chicago
Maywood, Illinois

Richard R. Keen, MD
Department of Surgery
Division of Vascular Surgery
Cook County Hospital
Chicago, Illinois

K. Craig Kent, MD
Professor of Surgery
Cornell University Medical College
Chief, Division of Vascular Surgery
New York Hospital-Cornell Medical
  Center
New York, New York

Nicos Labropoulos, PhD
Research Assistant Professor
Stritch School of Medicine
Loyola University Chicago
Maywood, Illinois

Michael D. Malone, MD
Instructor of Surgery
Temple University School of Medicine
Senior Vascular Surgery Fellow
Temple University Hospital
Philadelphia, Pennsylvania

M. Ashraf Mansour, MD
Assistant Professor of Surgery
Section of Peripheral Vascular Surgery
Department of Surgery
Loyola University Medical School,
  Stritch School of Medicine
Maywood, Illinois

Bernardo D. Martinez, MD
Endovascular Surgery Fellow
Stanford University Medical Center
Stanford, California

Mark A. Mattos, MD
Assistant Professor of Surgery
Southern Illinois University School of
  Medicine
Springfield, Illinois

Kenneth L. Mattox, MD
Professor and Vice Chairman of Surgery
Baylor College of Medicine
Chief of Staff, Chief of Surgery
Ben Taub General Hospital
Houston, Texas

Walter J. McCarthy III, MD
Associate Professor, Department of
  Cardiovascular–Thoracic Surgery
Chief, Section of Vascular Surgery
Rush-Presbyterian-St. Luke's Medical
  Center
Chairman, Division of Vascular Surgery,
  Cook County Hospital
Chicago, Illinois

William D. McMillan, MD
Vascular Surgeon
Minnesota Thoracic Associates
Minneapolis, Minnesota

Mark H. Meissner, MD
Assistant Professor of Surgery
University of Washington School of
  Medicine
Seattle, Washington

Mark W. Mewissen, MD
Professor of Radiology
Chief of Vascular and Interventional
  Radiology
Medical College of Wisconsin
Milwaukee, Wisconsin

Gregory L. Moneta, MD
Professor of Surgery
Division of Vascular Surgery
Department of Surgery
Oregon Health Sciences University
Portland, Oregon

Frank A. Nesi, MD
Associate Clinical Professor of
  Ophthalmology and Otolaryngology
Kresge Eye Institute, Wayne State
  University
Detroit, Michigan

Takao Ohki, MD
Assistant Professor of Surgery
Division of Vascular Surgery
Department of Surgery
The University Hospital for the Albert
  Einstein College of Medicine
Montefiore Medical Center
New York, New York

Frank T. Padberg, Jr., MD
Professor of Surgery
University of Medicine and Dentistry of
  New Jersey, New Jersey Medical School
Chief, Section of Vascular Surgery
New Jersey Veterans Health Care
  System
Newark, New Jersey

Peter J. Pappas, MD
Assistant Professor of Surgery
University of Medicine and Dentistry of
  New Jersey, New Jersey Medical School
Newark, New Jersey

Sheela T. Patel, MD
Vascular Surgery Fellow
New York Hospital-Cornell Medical
  Center
New York, New York

William H. Pearce, MD
Professor of Surgery
Northwestern University Medical School
Chief, Division of Vascular Surgery
Northwestern Memorial Hospital
Chicago, Illinois

Michael Petersen, MD
Assistant Professor
State University of New York at Stony
  Brook
Chief, Vascular Surgery
VA Medical Center
Stony Brook, New York

John R. Pfeifer, MD
Associate Clinical Professor of Surgery
Wayne State University School of
  Medicine
Detroit, Michigan

John M. Porter, MD
Professor of Surgery
Head, Division of Vascular Surgery
Department of Surgery
Oregon Health Sciences University
Portland, Oregon

Mary C. Proctor, MS
Senior Research Associate
Department of Surgery
University of Michigan
Ann Arbor, Michigan

John J. Ricotta, MD, FACS
Professor of Surgery
State University of New York at Stony
  Brook
Chairman, Department of Surgery
University Hospital, State University of
  New York at Stony Brook
Stony Brook, New York

C. Vaughan Ruckley, ChM, FRCSEd
Professor of Vascular Surgery
Edinburgh University
Consultant Vascular Surgeon
Edinburgh Royal Infirmary
Edinburgh, Scotland

Alvin H. Schmaier, MD
Professor of Internal Medicine and
  Pathology
University of Michigan
Departments of Internal Medicine and
  Pathology
Ann Arbor, Michigan

Joseph R. Schneider, MD, PhD
Associate Professor of Surgery
Northwestern University Medical School
Evanston Northwestern Healthcare
Evanston, Illinois

John H. Scurr, BSc, MBBS, FRCS
Senior Lecturer
Consultant Surgeon
Middlesex and University College
  Hospitals
London, England

Michael B. Silva, Jr., MD
Assistant Professor of Surgery
Chief, Division of Endovascular Surgery
University of Medicine and Dentistry of
  New Jersey, New Jersey Medical School
Newark, New Jersey

Donald Silver, MD
Department of Surgery
University of Missouri-Columbia
Columbia, Missouri

James C. Stanley, MD
Professor of Surgery
Head, Section of Vascular Surgery
Department of Surgery
University of Michigan
Ann Arbor, Michigan

D. E. Strandness, Jr., MD
Professor of Surgery
University of Washington School of
  Medicine
Seattle, Washington

David S. Sumner, MD
Distinguished Professor Emeritus of
  Surgery
Southern Illinois University School of
  Medicine
Springfield, Illinois

Lloyd M. Taylor, Jr., MD
Professor of Surgery
Division of Vascular Surgery
Department of Surgery
Oregon Health Sciences University
Portland, Oregon

Jonathan B. Towne, MD
Chair, Vascular Surgery
Froedtert Memorial Lutheran Hospital
Professor of Surgery
Medical College of Wisconsin
Milwaukee, Wisconsin

Hugh H. Trout III, MD, FACS
Clinical Professor of Surgery
George Washington University School of
  Medicine
Bethesda, Maryland

William D. Turnipseed, MD
Professor, Department of Surgery
Section of Vascular Surgery
University of Wisconsin Hospital and
  Clinics
Madison, Wisconsin

Frank J. Veith, MD
Montefiore Medical Center
Albert Einstein College of Medicine
Bronx, New York

Robert L. Vogelzang, MD
Professor of Radiology
Northwestern University Medical
  School
Chief of Vascular and Interventional
  Radiology
Northwestern Memorial Hospital
Chicago, Illinois

Thomas W. Wakefield, MD
Professor of Surgery
University of Michigan
Section of Vascular Surgery
Department of Surgery
Ann Arbor, Michigan

Anthony D. Whittemore, MD
Professor of Surgery
Harvard Medical School
Chief, Vascular Surgery
Brigham and Women's Hospital
Boston, Massachusetts

James S. T. Yao, MD, PhD
Magerstadt Professor of Surgery
Northwestern University Medical
  School
Acting Chair, Department of Surgery
Northwestern Memorial Hospital
Chicago, Illinois

Christopher K. Zarins, MD
Division of Vascular Surgery
Stanford University Medical Center
Stanford, California

Preface

In recent years vascular surgeons have been caught up in the enthusiasm over new technology. This new technology has provided minimally invasive approaches for treating a wide variety of vascular diseases. Unfortunately, this new technology is untried, and long-term results are scant. Although it is important to stay abreast of new developments, it is also important to review traditional techniques for treating vascular disease. These techniques have provided us with sound, durable treatments. The purpose of this book is to focus on the practical aspects of vascular surgery encompassing office practice, critical care, critical pathways, simplified operative approaches, and standard surgical procedures. In the current economic environment, it is important that our treatments be efficient, cost-effective, and durable. By critically reducing excesses in diagnostic modalities and limiting long-term follow-up protocols, standard vascular surgical procedures will compete satisfactorily with the newer endovascular techniques that may be more appealing on the surface, but may be less durable.

James S.T. Yao, MD, PhD
William H. Pearce, MD

I

Practice of Vascular Surgery in a Changing Environment

1

Medicare, Present and Future

Forces for Change

Hugh H. Trout III, MD, FACS

INTRODUCTION

Shortly after assuming office, President Clinton risked, and indeed spent, considerable and precious political capital on trying to change (euphemistically called "reform") the health care system in the United States. Political scientists and historians will no doubt debate why a young and untested president should take such a risk so early in his first term. Interestingly, perhaps an even more profound question is why he ventured into this health care morass at all. The answer is no doubt complex and filled with Byzantine intrigue but, at its core, it probably reflects that the president foresaw an impending national crisis and made a courageous, if flawed, attempt to address the fundamental problems so as to reduce the long-term adverse impact of enhanced technology and an aging population on our health care system. Although the "reform" effort failed, the future crisis that the president presciently perceived remains.

Medicare payment policies have, to a significant extent, become the *de facto* payment policy standard for most insurance companies—that is, the insurance companies base their payment schedules on some percentage of the Medicare payment. Accordingly, Medicare policies are of critical concern for most physicians. Moreover, the Medicare system has come under intense pressure to constrain costs and the changes now taking place are almost all related to these financial limitations. Trying to predict what changes in Medicare will take place in the early part of the 21st century is futile, but it is possible to describe the forces that mandate change. Although understanding these forces may not make physicians any happier, it may be helpful in reducing the belief that an ill-defined "they" are capriciously or duplicitously trying to wreck a perfectly good and efficient health care system. Accordingly, this chapter discusses the pressures requiring change and describes some of the changes that will occur in the beginning of the 21st century.

Some of the fundamental problems are a limited amount of money available for health care; an aging population; expanded technology, an oversupply of physicians (primary care physicians as well as specialists); a medico/legal system that is inefficient in addressing inappropriate medical practice; an appalling willingness of politicians and the public to accept conventional wisdom ("politically correct") rather than policy based on experimental evidence; lack of a system that provides appropriate incentives for the delivery of health care; and an ethos that does not include an understanding of how efficiently and at what cost the medical profession can prolong the process of dying. These problems are not unique to this country; indeed, they afflict all industrialized nations. Moreover, they cannot be "solved" (the only "solution" for most health care problems is death), but can only be managed.

Some of what follows is based on the author's opinion gleaned from living in Washington, DC, the home of policy mavens, as well as serving as the Chair of the Society for Vascular Surgery/International Society for Cardiovascular Surgery (SVS/ISCVS) Government Relations Committee. Each topic could serve as the basis for a book or a doctorate degree and much has been written about each. Accordingly, I have not attempted to use references for my statements as access to federal documents is not readily available to the medical profession, and much of what I have included comes from secondary sources, equally difficult to access. If any reader wishes to have additional information about a particular topic and has difficulty gathering it, they should contact me and I will try to help.

FORCES FOR CHANGE

Limited Money for Health Care

The percentage of the gross domestic product (GDP) that is devoted to health care has increased steadily (although, of late, at a slower rate of increase). In 1996, it was 14%, and is anticipated to grow to 16% by the year 2000 and 18% by 2005. The per capita health care expenditure is anticipated to increase from $3759 in 1996 to $5198 in 2000, and to $7352 in 2005. Predicting health care costs, however, is notoriously unreliable. For instance, in 1965, when Medicare and Medicaid were implemented, it was anticipated that in 1990 total expenditures for Medicare would be $9 billion, and for Medicaid would be $1 billion. Actual 1990 expenditures were $106 billion and $76 billion, respectively.

This trend of constantly increasing health care expenditures, whether on a per capita basis or as a percentage of GDP, clearly cannot continue. As a consequence of the stabilization of total health care expenditures (as a percentage of GDP), as they almost certainly must by the year 2010, per capita expenditures will obligatorily decrease as the population of persons older than 65 begins to increase rapidly (per capita expenditure equals total health care costs divided by number of patients). Thus, despite more patients and more sophisticated technology, it is almost certain that fewer dollars will be available after the year 2010 for per capita health care.

Aging Population

World War II resulted in a low birth rate throughout the industrialized world during the conflict. In the succeeding prosperous years, starting in 1945, the birth rate in the United States accelerated dramatically with what is now known as the Baby Boom. The members of this cohort will begin to reach 65 in the year 2010 with unsettling consequences. It is instructive to reflect on the circumstances surrounding the beginning of Social Security in the United States in 1935. Life expectancy was 62 years and it was expected that 7% of adult life would be spent in retirement. In 1995 those figures were 76 years and 26%, respectively, a substantial difference with enormous actuarial consequence. Another way to view this issue is to look at the ratio of workers to retirees. As Table 1–1 indicates, in 1995 there were about 2 retirees for every 10 workers; in the year 2025, there will be about 3 retirees for every 10 workers, and this may rise (as predicted for France and Japan) to as much as 5 retirees for every 10 workers. In other words, people who retire after 2010 will have to rely on a diminishing base of workers to provide support.

Of note is the fact that the premiums Medicare recipients pay do not come close to meeting the cost of Medicare. Moreover it is estimated that the average married worker retiring in 1995 will receive $182,000 more in Social Security benefits than was paid into the system; that is, current Social Security payments are funded by current taxpayers, not by the invested income that the retired contributed.

The consequences of these statistics are that retirees will need to save more and will likely be provided with fewer benefits (later retirement age, means testing for Social Security and Medicare benefits, increased deductibles and premiums for Medicare) than are currently provided.

Enhanced Technology

In most industries enhanced technology increases convenience, expands utility, and usually reduces cost, especially over time. In health care it seems to enhance care, expand utility, and *increase* cost. At the beginning of the 20th century, it was estimated that going to a physician was more likely to result in harm than in good. Although that probably changed within the first decade, there were relatively few effective treatments for any diseases. There were no antibiotics, few drugs, and little understanding of the pathophysiology of disease. After the advent of total parenteral nutrition (one person's view of the transition point), wondrous improvements were made in the treatment of severe disease even when long-term prognosis remained grim. Indeed, medical technology has progressed so far and is so effective that it is impossible for any society (with the possible exception of small oil-exporting countries) to provide all the possible legitimate health care to its entire populace. Moreover, the expansion of technological capabilities within health care is expanding, not contracting. Consider the possibilities of the current ongoing investigations of cloning, fetal research, regeneration, artificial materials, small biosensors, and gene therapy.

The underlying conundrum, of course, is that when a child or active worker has life or health preserved, that person returns to work and pays taxes, which supports society. When the same happens to someone who is retired, that person lives to consume more Social Security benefits and will almost certainly consume more health care. This is not to imply that persons older than 65 have any obligation whatsoever to die or

TABLE 1–1. WORKERS PER RETIREE

Country	Year	
	1995	*2025*
United States	4.7	3.3
France	2.8	1.7
Japan	2.8	2.1
Canada	5.2	2.7
Germany	3.1	2.3
Italy	2.4	1.8

not receive care, but it is intended to point out the actuarial facts that policy makers must grapple with.

The consequences of enhanced technology within health care is that either people or technology must be rationed (the best technology can be provided to relatively few people, or all people will get the same access to technology but the availability of technology will be restricted). The probability is that there will be a combination of placing restrictions on the technology available and also on those who receive the available technology. What is certain is that health care will be rationed (as it already is). The basis for how this is done, other than the current capricious methods, awaits public debate. The underlying principle, however, is likely to be value as defined as quality divided by cost.

A factor in the debate concerning what to do about the technological expansion in health care now being experienced is the impact that overly severe restrictions might have in providing incentives for innovative companies to move their development efforts to other countries. This is an increasingly attractive option and carries few disadvantages in the developing global market. Stifling innovation rarely produces productive outcomes for companies or societies.

Health Care Workforce

In 1967, Senator Edward Kennedy and then Health, Education and Welfare Secretary (HEW) Joseph Califano proclaimed that there was a looming doctor shortage and proposed legislation that provided incentives for US medical schools to double the number of doctors they produced. The legislation was passed by Congress and President Johnson, and the number of yearly graduates increased from 8000 per year to 16,000 per year. Mr. Califano has subsequently confessed to knowing at the time that there was no doctor shortage. He has acknowledged his intent was to increase the number of doctors in order to increase competition and reduce prices. If ever there were a classic example of the public policy law of unintended consequences, this is it. Almost anyone with any substantive understanding of physician behavior would have pointed out that physician fees represent less than 20% of the health care expenditures in the United States and that more than 80% of expenditures are generated by doctor's decisions and orders. Thus, the more physicians, the more the costs, regardless of what the physicians are paid.

The adverse public policy consequences of ill-conceived legislation have now become apparent, as predictable (unfortunately, those responsible for such massive miscalculations are rarely held accountable as the effects take place long after they have left office). Every year in the United States, 16,000 allopathic medical students, 1700 osteopathic medical students, 1400 graduates of international medical schools, and 5600 foreign graduates of international medical schools are produced. Thus there are about 25,000 new graduates entering training programs in the United States each year. The need is probably 12,000.

Currently, there are 220 active MDs per 100,000 population. To run an effective fee-for-service system, it is estimated 180 MDs per 100,000 population are needed. A health maintenance organization (HMO) system requires 146 MDs per 100,000 population, and a tightly integrated network (Mayo Clinic, Cleveland Clinic, etc.) needs 124 MDs per 100,000 population.

Not only are there too many physicians, but there are also too many specialists in almost every surgical specialty, although the gastroenterologists (1073% growth since 1965) and cardiologists (740% growth since 1965) have done little to curtail their growth.

Current conventional wisdom promotes the concept that we need generalists as "gatekeepers" to restrict inappropriate use of specialty care. The inanity of this concept is demonstrated by the increasing use of nonphysician providers (NPPs), especially by managed care entities, to triage patients. Although the HMOs seem to have finally discovered that "gatekeepers" cost rather than save, this message has not yet reached those who continue to advocate the production of yet more primary care doctors.

In sum, there is a surplus of physicians, a surplus of specialists, and probably a surplus of primary care doctors. Whether there is a distorted ratio of specialists to generalists (in the United States the current ratio is 66:34; it is 47:53 in Canada and 55:45 in France) is not yet clear to policy makers (my guess is that the current ratio in the United States is probably close to the correct one). Given the increasing role of NPPs and the begrudging recognition that specialty care, if provided by ethical individuals who restrict the tests they order to those that are truly indicated, is the best and, often, the cheapest care. For instance, the 75-year-old male diabetic former smoker with classic three-block claudication for the prior 4 years that interferes minimally with his lifestyle and who, on physical examination, does not have palpable pedal pulses does not need an arteriogram or even arterial Doppler studies. The diagnosis is clear and treatment will be noninterventional in almost all instances. Similarly the orthopedist can often be highly accurate after a history and physical, supplemented by a special view x-ray, often performed in the office. Surely there is little advantage to having a primary care physician inject a painful joint or order sophisticated imaging studies without the patient having seen someone who is knowledgeable about orthopedic issues.

The consequence of a physician and specialty surplus is hard to ascertain, but is probably extremely damaging not only to physicians, but also to society. Physicians who do not have enough to do within their area of expertise will not retain their skills at the maximum level, and will have a strong incentive to create more business for themselves, even if the care they provide is unnecessary or inappropriate.

Other Issues

A number of other issues, although less important than those discussed previously, also have an impact on the cost of health care. The medicolegal system is inefficient and distorting. Many expensive tests are ordered to protect a physician or a hospital from a perceived threat of possible litigation rather than because the test is indicated. Moreover, few of those who suffer the consequences of malpractice are ever awarded payments; less than 25% of malpractice premiums are paid to patients or their families (the rest goes to insurance companies and lawyers). Ironically, fear of lawsuits seems to be one of the few factors that restrains HMOs from even more unconscionable behavior than they now exhibit.

Those that pay get to make the rules. This generally works, but in health care, problems frequently arise because those paying (Congress) do not have the expertise to know what to pay for. Parenthetically, this is not easy, and it probably would not be easy even if the information on which to make our choices were far better. Nonetheless, decisions about health care delivery are often based on political pressure rather than scientific data. An example of this phenomenon is Congress mandating expenditures for human immunodeficiency virus (AIDS) research to an extent far greater than the prevalence of the disease. Another example is the overwhelming vote of the Senate mandating payment for mammography for women aged 40 to 50 years when an expert National Institutes of Health (NIH) panel could not agree on whether the available data warranted such a policy. Scientific decisions made by political whim is rarely a prescription for sound policy.

No country has resolved the problem of how to align incentives for health care providers to supply the appropriate amount of care. A fee-for-service system provides incentives for an excess of care with few restraints; an HMO does the reverse. Physicians are, in a very real sense, pieceworkers. Thus, one of the many reasons to reduce the number of providers is to reduce the incentives for unnecessary care.

Finally, the pace of change in health care challenges our legal and ethical values. The public has become accustomed to the view that heroic life-saving measures are possible and fruitful. Although this is sometimes true, often these measures cause prolongation of the process of dying, resulting only in expensive bills and much family agony. Moreover, many families have financial or other incentives for prolongation of life when the measures necessary to do this are wholly inappropriate. A classic example is the moribund or completely disorientated patient on prolonged hemodialysis. No other health care system in the world tolerates such a misuse of limited resources.

SHORT-TERM INITIATIVES

As one reflects on the forces enumerated previously that are driving the changes in health care delivery, it is obvious that Congress will need to control the costs of health care. The broad initiative by President Clinton failed, so the next efforts to effect change are likely to be incremental. These have begun. As is typical with efforts to control or change mammoth bureaucracies, general concepts are established to guide regulation. Unfortunately, when these concepts turn out to be incorrect or inflexible, the regulators are often unable to change direction; they then tend to adhere much more to the process rather than to apply judgment or try to modify the objectives. This phenomenon of concentrating more on the process than the result allows regulators and lawyers to justify their pursuit of goals that are often inequitable or irrational, with the rationalization that the system required the result. Such seems to be occurring in the changes being implemented in health care.

Resource Based Relative Value System

In 1992, Congress passed a law requiring that Medicare reimbursement be based on a formula consisting of three components—work, practice expense, and malpractice costs multiplied by a conversion factor, known as Resource Based Relative Value System (RBRVS). This was intended to reimburse physicians more equitably while, at the same time, control costs.

Work Values
The first element to be studied was the work component. Unfortunately, vascular surgeons were not included in the original valuation process, so their values were determined almost entirely by surgeons, who only rarely performed the services they were assessing. To no one's surprise, the work values assigned for vascular procedures were distorted and bizarre when compared to other specialties. The only consistent component was that all vascular work values were substantially undervalued. This has been corrected to a slight extent, but vascular work values still lag behind other surgical specialties.

Practice Expense Values

Given the successful control of rising costs with the work value initiative, Congress mandated that the Health Care Financing Administration (HCFA) next adjust the practice expense component to transfer additional reimbursement from specialists to primary care physicians in the belief that primary care was a critical component in the health care delivery system and needed to be encouraged. Although the assumptions about how to measure the cost of maintaining a medical practice varied widely (the method of analyzing the actual expenses of running a group of medical practices was rejected, presumably because it would not meet the presumption that specialists had far fewer costs of maintaining a practice than did primary care physicians) and did not approximate any rational accounting principles, a system was finally decided on that seemed to meet the needed political goals and was imposed. Almost all specialties experienced a further decline in their incomes as a result.

Fraud and Abuse (Evaluation and Management Documentation Guidelines)

Although fraud and abuse accounts for little loss to Medicare in the aggregate, curtailing dishonest medical practice has acquired an attractive patina. Politicians have been quick to rail against many of these nefarious practices and have encouraged the HCFA, backed by funding, to seek out and punish offenders. It should be relatively easy, by examining the frequency of charges of some practitioners compared to others in the same field, to detect the more flagrant abusers and prosecute them for criminal behavior with resulting widely publicized incarceration. This would likely be a swift, cheap, and effective deterrent. Although the HCFA may well opt for this strategy, their current efforts are directed to codifying what must be included in the physician notes of their evaluation and management (E&M) of patients seen and billed for. The American Medical Association (AMA) and the HCFA reached an agreement and guidelines were issued in 1997. These guidelines were intended to make it easy for billing clerks with no medical background to confirm that requisite checkpoints were met to justify the level of charge. Unfortunately, these guidelines attempted to impose a one-form-fits-all approach. This obviously did not reflect the realities of specialty practice, and immense opposition arose to their implementation. In a belated response, the AMA acknowledged that it was important to consult with specialists before agreeing to guidelines that were likely to be cumbersome, ineffective, and would encourage physicians to spend time on paperwork rather than taking care of patients. New guidelines are now being devised for each specialty. It is too early to know whether the new guidelines will reflect that the evaluation of a patient with carotid disease is markedly different than that for a patient with distal lower extremity ischemia.

This is a wonderful example of how difficult it is to convert an entirely appropriate concern into a workable policy. There are no doubt physicians who bill for E&M services that are not provided. A clerk should be able to be provided with a checksheet that allows disallowance of a submitted bill if certain specified conditions are not met. Creating that checksheet, however, is difficult. If each disease has its own checksheet, the amount of time the clerks would have to spend looking them up and checking against the submitted bill would overwhelmingly negate any savings accrued from reducing fraudulent behavior. If the checksheet is a generic one, then a patient with a carotid stenosis may need a breast exam, a rectal exam, and a careful documentation of the status of their pedal pulses. This would, of course, leave less time making sure that the patient and the family understood the implications of the procedure they are being asked to agree to. Further complicating the process is the high likelihood that the unscrupulous physician would employ computer help in generating varying boilerplate detailed physical examination sheets to submit; whereas the physician who concentrates on addressing the patient's problem may inadvertently be fined many thousands of dollars for failure to comply completely with the terms specified on the checksheet, few of which may be at all pertinent to the disease being assessed and treated.

FUTURE

The political pressures to force physicians into large organizations, regardless of what they are called, that resemble integrated networks will be unending. Time and money are on the side of these forces. The public, as relatives of patients or as potential patients themselves, seem less than enthusiastic about this transformation. How the struggle to refine our health care system will turn out is not at all apparent. Several trends, however, are likely:

1. Per capita spending for health care will decrease shortly after 2010 as the percentage of GDP devoted to health care stabilizes and the elderly population grows.
2. Overt rationing of health care will be acknowledged.
3. Restrictions on the number of international medical graduates will occur.
4. Some means testing will be required in order to receive some benefits.
5. Medicare recipients will need to assume more financial responsibility for some of the cost of their health care.
6. An assessment of value as defined as a measure of quality per cost will gain favor among policy makers. Accordingly, methods of assessing quality will be important in determining the degree of value accorded various surgical procedures.
7. Physicians will be encouraged/required to adopt and follow practice protocols. This will tend to raise substantially the quality of care that many patients receive; at the same time, it will stifle innovative and customized care that now often occurs at the high end of the quality spectrum.
8. Coding of diseases and procedures will improve. International Classification of Diseases, Current Procedural Terminology, and Diagnosis Related Group (ICD, CPT, and DRG) will likely be combined so that data analysis will be much more reflective of reality.
9. The amount, quality, and accessibility of information will improve dramatically.
10. Specialty care, when the volume is controlled by protocol rather than whim, will be acknowledged as the best quality and also the cheapest health care.
11. The number of acute care hospital beds will decrease substantially (30% to 40% less than in 1998).

Change is usually painful and the enormously disruptive and frequent changes now occurring in health care are certainly no exception. It is not at all clear that physicians will have much of a role in determining the direction or extent of these changes. Furthermore, with the coming of even tighter cost constraints, it is not apparent whether being a physician will be sufficiently satisfying to justify the cost and years of training necessary.

What does become obvious, however, is that the physician who understands the forces that are driving these changes in health care delivery will be better prepared to adopt the measures that will best position him or her to compete for the more desirable positions. These measures include obtaining high quality training with full credentialing for the chosen specialty, developing a spirit of affability and collegiality, demonstrating a willingness to allow cost to be a factor in health care decisions, and participating in community and hospital activities as an advocate of community health rather than self-interest.

Change is interesting, disruptive, and difficult. Physicians over the next few decades face interesting, disruptive, and difficult times.

2

Impact of Critical Pathways on Surgical Outcome and Hospital Stay

Joseph R. Schneider, MD, PhD,
Julie S. Droste, BSN, RN, and John F. Golan, MD

Health care delivery is evolving rapidly in the United States. Results of health care organizations, groups, and, indeed, individual practitioners are increasingly scrutinized for evidence of quality and also for amount of resource utilization. Patients and doctors increasingly ask practitioners about the risks of interventions in the individual practitioner's hands. It is becoming more important to have a current tabulation of one's own results. It is no longer acceptable to quote published estimates of success, morbidity, and mortality of interventions (unless the published results are one's own). Physicians whose patients' outcomes are significantly inferior to established benchmarks of quality or whose resource utilization is significantly greater than their peers may find themselves "deselected" from various health plans.

Physicians cannot afford to follow this revolution. We must lead it, and this applies to virtually all aspects of clinical medicine, including vascular surgery and medicine. A key element of assessing and improving both quality and outcomes is collection of quality data and good information systems within the health care organization. Once such data has been gathered, it can be examined for quality and resource utilization and, hopefully, identify potential areas for improvement.

CONTINUOUS QUALITY IMPROVEMENT VERSUS REDUCING RESOURCE UTILIZATION

Surgeons are used to measuring quality in terms of perioperative complication rates and long-term durability of interventions, and may feel that current results are so good that they cannot be improved. However, continued improvements in quality as measured by surgical outcomes and patient satisfaction can probably be achieved in virtually all aspects of vascular surgery. As interest in outcomes and resource utilization has increased, the industrial concepts of continuous quality improvement of Deming[1] and Juran[2] have been found to be increasingly applicable to health care delivery. The phenomenal industrial success of Japan has been attributed in part to the recognition of Deming's genius decades before North America recognized the genius of one of its own.

The goals of individuals trying to improve any process, including patient care, may be diverse. Physicians may be interested in quality improvement. The conditions of the health care market may affect the hospital's or clinic's interest in decreasing costs. Under the old reimbursement conditions, hospitals could simply bill patients for every service and hospital day and were not anxious to shorten hospital stays. Under conditions of prospective fixed payment such as the Medicare diagnosis related group (DRG) system, hospitals are more interested in cost control. As markets move toward capitated reimbursement systems, hospitals inevitably become aggressive with respect to controlling costs. Health care professionals traditionally have argued that quality needs to be defended at any cost, but ultimately the financial issues must be at least considered if there is to be a place to work in the future. A critical point is that there is no reason why both of these goals cannot be satisfied simultaneously.

One must acknowledge that in health care, there are ill-defined limits of resource utilization below which quality may suffer,[3] but that just as in industry, variations from the plan or, more commonly in the medical setting, complications are what are most expensive. It is becoming more apparent that in patient care, just as in industry, quality and cost are inversely related, or "quality is cheap."[4] Industry has learned that quality problems do not usually reflect failure of the workers; rather, quality problems usually reflect inadequate engineering of the production process. Health care providers must recognize that traditional hospital stays and utilization of other resources for specific interventions may often be reduced with no decrease and, perhaps even with some improvement in quality.

CRITICAL (CLINICAL) PATHWAYS

One mechanism to try to formalize the process, improve quality, and reduce resource utilization in health care is the "clinical pathway" or "critical pathway" (CP).[5,6] CPs are guidelines for quality care. They include explicit routine orders, expectations for outcomes and length of each stage of treatment, thresholds for graduation to the next stage of treatment, and ultimately to discharge from the treatment setting. CP may be appropriate for treatment in the inpatient or outpatient setting. Collection of good quality data and continuous examination of this data during the process are a vital part of a successful CP implementation.

A search of the literature in preparation for this chapter revealed that CPs have been implemented for a large and diverse number of clinical problems including but not limited to anesthesia,[7,8] asthma,[9] AIDS,[10] colectomy,[11] trauma,[12] chest pain,[13] pneumonia,[14–16] pulmonary lobectomy,[17] cardiac transplantation,[18] coronary artery bypass,[19] stroke,[20,21] total joint replacement,[22] prostatectomy,[23] head and neck surgery,[24] and, apropos of this presentation and symposium, vascular surgery, including carotid endarterectomy.[25–28] A CP may be appropriate for any clinical problem that may be expected to be encountered more than a few times per year. This chapter discusses the rationale for CPs and their development and provides examples of the manner in which outcomes can be improved using a CP.

CAROTID ENDARTERECTOMY PATHWAY (THE SURE BET)

Our own experience with CPs began with carotid endarterectomy (CEA) in 1994. We chose CEA first because it is the most commonly performed arterial reconstructive operation in our own practice and in the United States.[29] Thus, we believed even small improvements in quality and resource utilization would have a large aggregate effect on overall system performance. This proposal was not financially driven nor was it a response to concerns with quality. Our outcomes were quite satisfactory compared to established quality benchmarks and our hospital did not ask us to implement a CP for CEA.

Previous investigators had examined the impact on quality and resource utilization in CEA with respect to type of anesthesia[30] and routine postoperative use of the intensive care unit.[31–34] Others had examined the impact of length of stay[35–41] and still others had examined the effect of multiple alterations in the process of CEA, in particular on costs.[42–45] Our view was that many patients were spending unnecessary postoperative days in the hospital. Many patients were undergoing too many postoperative tests and receiving too many pharmaceuticals, which we believed was due to suboptimal supervision and education of surgical residents and students. We believed CEA was the ideal procedure to try to standardize a pathway, and ultimately we were able to design and implement a successful pathway. Our initial goal was to eliminate unnecessary postoperative hospital days and laboratory studies. We have never had to transfuse a postoperative CEA patient in more than 600 cases and believed that blood counts, electrolytes, and coagulation studies, so often routinely ordered in postoperative patients, were superfluous after CEA.

Success of a CP depends on identification and involvement of all members of the health care team with significant contact with these patients. In the case of CEA, we believed it was necessary to involve the following departments: Anesthesia, Ambulatory Surgery Nursing, Recovery Room Nursing, Operating Room Nursing, Intensive Care Unit Nursing, Nursing from the Medical–Surgical floor where these patients would be postoperatively, Neurology, and Hospital Quality Improvement. However, we believe that a single individual must take charge of educating involved nursing and other personnel, surveillance to make sure that patients stay on the pathway, and data collection. In our case, this role was filled by the Vascular Surgery Nurse Coordinator, the second author of this chapter. Previous published experience with CPs has reinforced the concept that nursing staff are critical at every stage of the pathway.[46] Indeed, review of the references at the end of this chapter shows that much of the literature of CPs is written by nurses and published in nursing journals. Once the pathway was designed to the satisfaction of all members of the team, we received approval to implement the pathway from the hospital Steering Committee, a step in the process that is certain to be required in virtually any North American hospital. The corollary to this is that periodic reporting of results to the hospital board has been required in our hospital.

We believed that preoperative education of patients was critical to success of the pathway. CEA pathway patients, families, and, in some cases, referring physicians were reassured that CEA is not a severe metabolic injury to most patients.[47] Most patients are ready for discharge on the day after CEA and although discharge on postoperative day 1 was a goal, discharge would occur only when the patient was medically ready. We were concerned that some patients might think early discharge was a response to demands of insurance carriers or hospital administration, a problem in some others' experience.[25] We told patients explicitly that the pathway had been initiated by vascular surgeons and that the goal of day 1 discharge was medically, and not financially, driven.

We prospectively collected control data for an entire year prior to implementing our CEA pathway. Once we were satisfied that the appropriate hospital staff were fully educated about the rationale and conduct of the pathway, we instituted the CEA pathway on June 1, 1995, and have reviewed the data regularly throughout the following 3 years. A detailed analysis of results 1 year after initiation of the pathway showed that prepathway and pathway patients were indistinguishable with respect to patient characteristics, medical comorbidities, indications for surgery, and anatomic severity of disease. In addition, there was no evidence of a decline in quality of outcomes. However, we noted a decrease from 2.1 to 1.6 days in average postoperative hospital stay and a decrease of 22% in direct costs, both of which were statistically significant. Furthermore, despite the lack of shorter preoperative stay as a goal of the CP, there was a pronounced trend toward greater likelihood of CEA on the day of admission in CP patients. These results have been published previously.[29]

CAROTID ENDARTERECTOMY PATHWAY MODIFICATION IN PROGRESS—CHANGING "ON THE FLY"

Critical pathways are a far more effective tool if there is good data collection, frequent review of results, and pathway modification when appropriate to improve patient care. Although we were quite pleased with our initial results in terms of maintenance of quality and decreased resource utilization, ongoing review of our experience led to several modifications of the CEA pathway. More than 40% of our patients required (IV) intravenous vasoactive medication for postoperative hypertension or hypotension. We initially found this difficult to reconcile with others' minimal use of the intensive care unit following CEA.[31-34] Initially, we had designed the pathway to trigger administration of antihypertensive medications for systolic blood pressure exceeding 160 mm Hg in order to avoid the complications of perioperative hypertension after CEA,[48-50] but after examining our data, we thought this standard might be too strict. We relaxed the threshold for treatment of hypertension to 180 mm Hg systolic. We also decided that patients without severe uncompensated cardiac or pulmonary disease who were hemodynamically stable on no continuous IV vasoactive medications after 1 h in the recovery room would be candidates to be transferred to a nonintensive care medical–surgical nursing unit after 4 h of observation in the recovery room. We initiated this change in the pathway in May 1997. We have noted no apparent decrement in quality and there have been no strokes and no deaths in nearly 100 patients who have undergone CEA since that time. Fewer than 10% of patients have required continuous drip vasoactive medications since that time. Furthermore, 36% of patients undergoing CEA in 1997 spent their postoperative night in a nonintensive care nursing unit. In our most recent experience, this number approaches 50%, and no patient has required transfer from the nonintensive care to the intensive care unit.

Cerebral angiography is associated with significant stroke risk (1.2%–1.3% in the NASCET and ACAS studies[51,52]) and expense. Furthermore, carotid duplex has been shown to be very sensitive and specific for high grade stenosis of the carotid bulb and internal carotid artery when compared to conventional contrast angiography, and several investigators have found duplex scanning alone to be sufficient preoperative imaging prior to CEA.[53-55] Ongoing comparison of conventional angiography with duplex scanning from our vascular laboratory had shown excellent correlation and we proposed to eliminate conventional angiography in selected patients with high quality duplex scans beginning in mid-1997. We now reserve angiography for patients with suboptimal duplex scans, "redo" CEA, or suspicion of more proximal great vessel or aortic arch level lesions. In 1998, 75% of CEAs have been performed with duplex scanning only, and of the remaining 25%, more than two-thirds of CEAs have had magnetic resonance (MR) angiography and not conventional contrast angiography. Again, there has been no apparent decrement in quality, with no strokes and no deaths since that time.

In summary, we have made substantial changes in our practice of CEA. In 1993, nearly all patients were admitted with conventional angiography on the day of admission, stayed in the hospital overnight, underwent CEA the next day, spent the first postoperative night in the intensive care unit, and spent at least the next night in the hospital, for a total of at least 3 nights in the hospital. Since initiation of the CEA pathway, we have moved to reduce the use of angiography, selective use of the intensive care nursing unit, and nearly all patients are discharged home on the first postoperative day. Mean postoperative length of stay for CEA was 1.2 days for 1997. Despite these changes, quality has been maintained or even improved, with no deaths and only one stroke in more than 250 patients treated since initiation of the pathway. Our CEA volume continues to increase and patient satisfaction is high. In fact, patients who need to spend a second night in the hospital seem genuinely disappointed not to be able to go home on day 1.

These favorable results cannot be attributed to selection of lower risk patients. Patients in our most recent experience have similar presentation compared to earlier patients both with respect to symptomatology and anatomic disease severity, medical comorbidities if anything are slightly worse, and there is a trend toward increasing age (current average 73 years). In addition to these stable to improved measures of quality, direct costs have been reduced by 41% (unadjusted dollars). We continue to try to find ways to decrease variability, improve quality, and limit resource utilization. We view this experience as a great demonstration not only of the concepts of decreasing variability to both improve quality and reduce resource utilization, but also of the ability to improve quality continuously by ongoing review of data and modification of the process where it seems prudent.

AORTIC SURGERY PATHWAY (LESS THAN CERTAIN SUCCESS)

Enthusiastic after our success with a CEA critical pathway, we decided to try to design and implement a critical pathway for elective aortic surgery. Once again, our results with aortic aneurysm surgery[56] and aortic surgery for occlusive disease[57] compared favorably with published benchmarks in terms of morbidity and mortality and we proposed to standardize our approach to care of aortic surgery patients as much as was possible. We included essentially all of the participants in the CEA pathway except the neurology service, but solicited input from Occupational Therapy and Physical Therapy because we believed that early mobilization would both reduce complications of immobility and contribute to earlier hospital discharge. We planned for all patients to be extubated in the operating room, recovery room, or intensive care unit on the day of surgery, to spend only the first postoperative night in the intensive care unit, to begin physical and occupational therapy on the second postoperative day, to expect return of bowel function on the third postoperative day, and targeted discharge on postoperative day 6.

The aortic surgery pathway was initiated in June 1997. We found that our goals of early extubation, early transfer to nonintensive care nursing units, and day 6 discharge were difficult to achieve. Review of our experience in the first eight patients showed an average intensive care unit stay of 1.6 days and an average postoperative length of stay of 7 days. Examination of each case suggested this might just represent an atypical patient sample that did not represent our typical aortic surgery patient. Therefore, we made no modification in the pathway and continued enrolling patients. Our subsequent experience has been more satisfactory. The average time in intensive care was 1.3 days and the average total postoperative length of stay was 6.0 days for eight subsequent patients treated in 1997.

This elective aortic surgery pathway was certainly not the immediate success that we enjoyed with the CEA pathway. We were not so naive as to not recognize that patients would reach the thresholds for advancement along the aortic surgery pathway much less predictably than they did on the CEA pathway. Clearly, the course of aortic surgery patients is much more variable than that of CEA patients. However, to have reviewed the disappointing length of stay information from our initial aortic surgery pathway patients without having the appropriate comorbidity and other patient data, one might have simply abandoned the aortic pathway. Just as the availability of prospectively acquired quality patient data allowed us to alter the CEA pathway "on the fly," we believe our ability to persevere with the aortic pathway was due in large part to the availability of the same quality prospectively acquired data and our experience with subsequent patients and no change in the pathway has been more satisfactory.

FUTURE PROJECTS

Critical pathways have the most potential utility in high volume interventions. We have considered designing a pathway for infrainguinal arterial reconstruction. We also perform a significant number of primary and secondary procedures for hemodialysis access, which may also be appropriate for a CP. We have assisted our internal medicine colleagues in design of a pathway for acute lower extremity deep venous thrombosis and expect that our colleagues in other fields may wish to ask us to participate in the design of other new pathways. There are 43 active CPs in our hospital, and they are excellent tools to examine the manner in which care is provided for almost any diagnosis, and their application is limited only by one's level of interest in quality improvement.

EDUCATION—WILL IT SUFFER FROM CRITICAL PATHWAYS?

Critical pathways are often criticized as being a "cookbook" approach to patient care. These criticisms imply some decrement in quality of the education of medical students and residents. Both these groups have participated in the care of all our CP patients. In retrospect, the way we traditionally "reinvented the wheel" by writing new orders with a resident or student after each case was inefficient and clearly risked variation from the treatment plan.

We have approached the pathway as an educational opportunity, not a liability. The pathway and the preprinted orders are reviewed and the rationale explained where not immediately apparent to the student or resident. We do not suggest that our approach is the only method, but we rely on the data we have collected showing nearly uniformly favorable outcomes in the face of decreased costs as proof of concept. Furthermore, CPs are likely to be with us for some time. Residents have participated and will likely continue to participate in the development, implementation, and revision of CPs. Therefore, it is only reasonable that they should be introduced to CPs early in their clinical education.

SUMMARY

The design and modification of medical treatment may be compared to process engineering. Industrial techniques of continuous quality improvement can be applied to medicine and, within limits, quality can be maintained or even improved while lowering costs. Health care professionals must continually reexamine the manner in which we provide care in order for our practices to remain viable. CPs represent one proven tool to examine the manner in which care is provided and to facilitate both continuous quality improvement and decreased resource utilization.

REFERENCES

1. Deming WE. *Out of the Crisis.* Cambridge, MA: Massachusetts Institute of Technology Press, Center for Advanced Engineering Study, 1989.
2. Juran JM, Gryna FM Jr. *Quality in Planning and Analysis.* New York: McGraw-Hill, 1980.
3. Pearson SD, Goulart-Fisher D, Lee TH. Critical pathways as a strategy for improving care: problems and potential. *Ann Intern Med.* 1995;123:941–948.
4. Goldstone J. Sony, Porsche, and vascular surgery in the 21st century. *J Vasc Surg.* 1997;25: 201–210.
5. Gadacz TR, Adkins RB Jr, O'Leary JP. General surgical clinical pathways: an introduction. *American Surgeon.* 1997;63:107–110.
6. Campbell H, Hotchkiss R, Bradshaw N, Porteous M. Integrated care pathways. *BMJ.* 1998;316:133–137.
7. Butterworth J. Clinical pathways for the high-risk patient. *Journal of Cardiothoracic & Vascular Anesthesia.* 1997;11(2 Suppl 1):16–18; discussion 24–25.
8. Rietz C, Erickson S, Deshpande JK. Clinical pathways and case management in anesthesia practice: new tools and systems for the evolving healthcare environment. *AANA Journal.* 1997;65:460–467.
9. Bailey R, Weingarten S, Lewis M, Mohsenifar Z. Impact of clinical pathways and practice guidelines on the management of acute exacerbations of bronchial asthma. *Chest.* 1998;113: 28–33.
10. Jones SG. Implementing a multidisciplinary HIV diarrhea critical pathway in the acute care setting. *Journal of the Association of Nurses in AIDS Care.* 1997;8:59–68.
11. Archer SB, Burnett RJ, Flesch LV, Hobler SC, et al. Implementation of a clinical pathway decreases length of stay and hospital charges for patients undergoing total colectomy and ileal pouch/anal anastomosis. *Surgery.* 1997;122:699–705.
12. Danne P, Brazenor G, Cade R, Crossley P, et al. The major trauma management study: an analysis of the efficacy of current trauma care. *Australian & New Zealand Journal of Surgery.* 1998;68:50–57.
13. Nichol G, Walls R, Goldman L, Pearson S, et al. A critical pathway for management of patients with acute chest pain who are at low risk for myocardial ischemia: recommendations and potential impact. *Ann Internal Med.* 1997;127:996–1005.

14. Gottlieb LD, Roer D, Jega K, D'arc St Pierre J, et al. Clinical pathway for pneumonia: development, implementation, and initial experience. *Best Practices and Benchmarking in Healthcare.* 1996;1:262–265.
15. Borawski DB, Snow MD. Pneumonia pathway streamlines care. *Nursing Case Management.* 1996;1:180–182.
16. Phillips KF, Crain HC. Effectiveness of a pneumonia clinical pathway: quality and financial outcomes. *Outcomes Management for Nursing Practice.* 1998;2:16–22.
17. Wright CD, Wain JC, Grillo HC, Moncure AC, et al. Pulmonary lobectomy patient care pathway: a model to control cost and maintain quality. *Ann Thoracic Surg.* 1997;64:299–302.
18. Noedel NR, Osterloh JF, Brannan JA, Haselhorst MM, et al. Critical pathways as an effective tool to reduce cardiac transplantation hospitalization and charges. *Journal of Transplant Coordination.* 1996;6:14–19.
19. Velasco FT, Ko W, Rosengart T, Altorki N, et al. Cost containment in cardiac surgery: results with a critical pathway for coronary bypass surgery at the New York hospital–Cornell Medical Center. *Best Practices and Benchmarking in Healthcare.* 1996;1:21–28.
20. Wentworth DA, Atkinson RP. Implementation of an acute stroke program decreases hospitalization costs and length of stay. *Stroke.* 1996;27:1040–1043.
21. Ross G, Johnson D, Kobernick M. Evaluation of a critical pathway for stroke. *Journal of the American Osteopathic Association.* 1997;97:269–272, 275–276.
22. Meyer T. Clinical pathway for total knee replacement. *WMJ.* 1997;96:44–47.
23. Koch MO. Cost-efficient radical prostatectomy. *Seminars in Urologic Oncology.* 1995;13:197–203.
24. Cohen J, Stock M, Andersen P, Everts E. Critical pathways for head and neck surgery. *Archives of Otolaryngology—Head & Neck Surgery.* 1997;123:11–14.
25. Calligaro KD, Dougherty MJ, Raviola CA, Musser DJ, et al. Impact of clinical pathways on hospital costs and early outcome after major vascular surgery. *J Vasc Surg.* 1995;22:649–660.
26. Edwards WH Sr, Edwards WH Jr, Martin RS III, Mulherin JL Jr, et al. Resource utilization and pathways: meeting the challenge of cost containment. *Amer Surgeon.* 1996;62:830–834.
27. Back MR, Harward TR, Huber TS, Carlton LM, et al. Improving the cost-effectiveness of carotid endarterectomy. *J Vasc Surg.* 1997;26:456–464.
28. Schneider JR, Droste JS, Golan JF. Impact of carotid endarterectomy critical pathway on surgical outcome and hospital stay. *Vasc Surgery.* 1997;31:685–692.
29. Gillum RF. Epidemiology of carotid endarterectomy and cerebral arteriography in the United States. *Neurology.* 1995;26:1724–1728.
30. Godin MS, Bell WH III, Schwedler M, Kerstein MD. Cost effectiveness of regional anesthesia in carotid endarterectomy. *Amer Surgeon.* 1989;55:656–659.
31. O'Brien MS, Ricotta JJ. Conserving resources after carotid endarterectomy: selective use of the intensive care unit. *J Vasc Surg.* 1991;14:796–802.
32. Lipsett PA, Tierney S, Gordon TA, Perler BA. Carotid endarterectomy—is intensive care unit care necessary? *J Vasc Surg.* 1994;20:403–410.
33. Morasch MD, Hodgett D, Burke K, Baker WH. Selective use of the intensive care unit following carotid endarterectomy. *Ann Vasc Surg.* 1995;9:229–234.
34. Ammar AD. Is intensive care necessary following carotid endarterectomy? *Kansas Medicine.* 1995;96:125–126.
35. Kraiss LW, Kilberg L, Critch S, Johansen KH. Short-stay carotid endarterectomy is safe and cost-effective. *Amer J Surg.* 1995;169:512–515.
36. Harbaugh KS, Harbaugh RE. Early discharge after carotid endarterectomy. *Neurosurgery.* 1995;37:219–225.
37. Collier PE. Are one-day admissions for carotid endarterectomy feasible? *Amer J Surg.* 1995;170:140–143.
38. Katz SG, Kohl RD. Carotid endarterectomy with shortened hospital stay. *Arch Surg.* 1995;130:887–891.
39. Friedman SG, Tortolani AJ. Reduced length of stay following carotid endarterectomy under general anesthesia. *Am J Surg.* 1995;170:235–236.
40. Musser DJ, Calligaro KD, Dougherty MJ, Raviola CA, et al. Safety and cost-efficiency of 24-hour hospitalization for carotid endarterectomy. *Ann Vasc Surg.* 1996;10:143–146.

41. Kaufman JL, Frank D, Rhee SW, Berman JA, et al. Feasibility and safety of 1-day postoperative hospitalization for carotid endarterectomy. *Arch Surg.* 1996;131:751–755.
42. Collier PE. Carotid endarterectomy: a safe cost-efficient approach. *J Vasc Surg.* 1992;16: 926–933.
43. Gibbs BF, Guzzetta VJ, Furmanski D. Cost-effective carotid endarterectomy in community practice. *Ann Vasc Surg.* 1995;9:423–427.
44. Luna G, Adye B. Cost-effective carotid endarterectomy. *Amer J Surg.* 1995;169:516–518.
45. Hirko MK, Morasch MD, Burke K, Greisler HP, et al. The changing face of carotid endarterectomy. *J Vasc Surg.* 1996;23:622–627.
46. Calligaro KD, Miller P, Dougherty MJ, Raviola CA, et al. Role of nursing personnel in implementing clinical pathways and decreasing hospital costs for major vascular surgery. *Journal of Vascular Nursing.* 1996;14:57–61.
47. Hoyle RM, Jenkins JM, Edwards WH Sr, Edwards WH Jr, et al. Case management in cerebral revascularization. *J Vasc Surg.* 1994;20:396–402.
48. Bove EL, Fry WJ, Gross WS, Stanley JC. Hypotension and hypertension as consequences of baroreceptor dysfunction following carotid endarterectomy. *Surgery.* 1979;85:633–637.
49. Towne JB, Bernhard VM. The relationship of postoperative hypertension to complications following carotid endarterectomy. *Surgery.* 1980;88:575–580.
50. Corson JD, Chang BB, Leopold PW, et al. Perioperative hypertension in patients undergoing carotid endarterectomy: shorter duration under regional block anesthesia. *Circulation.* 1986;74S:1–4.
51. North American Symptomatic Carotid Endarterectomy Trial Collaborators. Beneficial effect of carotid endarterectomy in symptomatic patients with high grade carotid stenosis. *N Engl J Med.* 1991;325:445–453.
52. Executive Committee for the Asymptomatic Carotid Atherosclerosis Study. Endarterectomy for asymptomatic carotid artery stenosis. *JAMA.* 1995;273:1421–1428.
53. Gelabert HA, Moore WS. Carotid endarterectomy without angiography. *Surg Clin North Am.* 1990;70:213–223.
54. Dawson DL, Zierler RE, Strandness DE Jr, Clowes AW, et al. The role of duplex scanning and arteriography before carotid endarterectomy: a prospective study. *J Vasc Surg.* 1993;18:673–683.
55. Horn M, Michelini M, Greisler HP, Littooy FN, et al. Carotid endarterectomy without arteriography: the preeminent role of the vascular laboratory. *Ann Vasc Surg.* 1994;8:221–224.
56. Schneider JR, Gottner RJ, Golan JF. Supraceliac versus infrarenal aortic cross-clamp for repair of non-ruptured infrarenal and juxtarenal abdominal aortic aneurysm. *Cardiovasc Surg.* 1997;5:279–285.
57. Schneider JR, Zwolak RM, Walsh DB, McDaniel MD, et al. Lack of diameter effect on short-term patency of size-matched Dacron aortobifemoral grafts. *J Vasc Surg.* 1991;13:785–791.

3

The Vascular Laboratory

Quality Control and Accreditation

J. Dennis Baker, MD

TEST DEVELOPMENT

The first noninvasive laboratories were research facilities dedicated to the investigation of circulation. These were established and supervised by physicians with a special interest in developing objective methodologies for studying patients. Extensive efforts went into the correlation of the tests with the clinical status of the patient or with objective determinations. Often the results of physiologic tests were compared to anatomic information such as measurements made of disease demonstrated on contrast angiography.

A key to developing a diagnostic test is to establish the parameters or criteria that define an abnormal results or a range of abnormality. An important initial step is the determination of the variability of the results in normal subjects. The second step is to determine how much the findings in patients with known pathology differ from the normal subjects. Most screening tests simply aim at identifying an abnormal status without defining the severity of the abnormality. Ocular pneumoplethysmography (OPG) is an example of such a screening. The simplest situation is when a numeric value falls outside of a range defined as normal, but some tests have multiple criteria. The need for multiple criteria is found in the OPG, with abnormality defined both in terms of a difference in ophthalmic artery pressure and in the ratio of the ophthalmic artery to the brachial artery pressure. As the field of noninvasive testing expanded there was increasing interest in being able to determine the severity of an abnormality. A good example can be seen in the evolution of carotid studies. As routinely used, OPG simply screened for the presence or absence of a "hemodynamically significant" lesion in the carotid system. The great advantage offered by duplex scanning was the ability to detect various levels of stenosis, and an important evolution came with adoption of criteria to subdivide the 50% to 99% stenosis category into two subgroups. Strandness has provided a valuable summary of this evolution.[1]

An important part of development of diagnostic criteria is the comparison of test parameters with a reference standard. Most commonly, the contrast angiogram is used and severity of disease is measured as residual lumen diameter or as percentage reduction of lumen diameter. The best way to determine the cut-point separating normal from abnormal range of test values is to use receiver operating characteristic (ROC) curves to evaluate the relative sensitivity and specificity (Sumner[2] provides a good review of this technique). Once the criteria have been selected, a validation phase is required. A separate group of examinations must be carried out on normal subjects and patients with varying extents of disease. The results are then subjected to statistical analysis to determine the accuracy achieved using the criteria established on the first group. When the tests results are binary (normal vs. abnormal), the sensitivity and specificity can be used, but when more than two categories are used, the kappa analysis is used.[2]

Once a test is shown to have appropriate accuracy to make it a reasonable clinical tool, it is useful to carry out additional investigation. Reproducibility of test results by different examiners is an important factor, because a test will not be practical if it is difficult to obtain consistent results. Another issue is how much variability in tests results from exam to exam when repeated over a short period of time.

TRANSFER TO ROUTINE TESTING

As experience was gained with the early methods, increasing numbers of publications appeared in the medical literature. The potential benefit of routine clinical application of noninvasive techniques resulted in a transition from the research setting into everyday practice, and gradually there was an increasing demand for routine testing. Noninvasive laboratories were established in many hospitals and clinics. In most cases the new facilities simply reproduced techniques and applied the diagnostic criteria that appeared in literature. In some places the results were compared to objective standards to ensure that the published results could be reproduced; however, in many settings this validation phase was omitted. The simple assumption was made that the diagnostic accuracy would be similar to that published from the different research centers.

When validation studies are carried out by new laboratories a variety of findings result. In the best situation the published accuracy can be achieved, but, unfortunately, in other cases the correlation is not as good as expected or hoped for. Over the years there have been different reasons for failure to duplicate initial results that appeared in literature. The makeup of the original study population, often highly selected, may account for some of the problems. When the technique in question is later applied to a more heterogeneous patient group, the difference in incidence of disease state can result in considerable difference in sensitivity or specificity. The second type of error can arise from the fact that some of the tests are very operator dependent. The personnel performing the test in research labs usually have spent considerable time developing the testing techniques, giving great attention to detail. When personnel in the new laboratory learn the techniques, they often do so with less instruction and supervision, leading to more variability in technique and a lower accuracy. In a few cases there can be additional variability resulting from the purchase of different equipment from that used when the test was developed.

INCREASING NEED FOR QUALITY

In the early days of physiologic methods, high accuracy was desirable but not critical. Most of the tests were used to screen patients and the diagnosis was usually verified with additional examinations, usually arteriograms. With the introduction of duplex scanning and the substantial improvement in this technology, ultrasound studies have come to provide the definitive diagnosis in a number of areas. This phenomenon arose in the diagnosis of deep vein thrombosis and advanced to such a level that in most hospitals venograms are rarely performed. Since the early 1990s there has been a trend toward performing carotid endarterectomy based on the duplex scan review without obtaining a confirmatory angiogram, and more recently surgeons are investigating a similar approach to the decision regarding revascularization procedures in the leg. The fact that definitive diagnoses are being made and patient management planned based on noninvasive studies increases the pressure for greater attention to accuracy in the vascular laboratory.

PROBLEMS WITH REFERENCE STANDARDS

For many years the basic reference standard was the contrast angiogram. This practice certainly resulted from the fact that vascular surgeons were comfortable with interpretation of arteriography. Given standardized techniques, measurements made from the films could be corrected for magnification to yield actual vessel sizes. Use of views in two or more planes helped to offset the problem of plaque asymmetry. (In spite of the high confidence in diagnoses made from angiograms, there is considerable interobserver variation in the measurement of stenoses.[3]) In the 1980s there was a shift from conventional cut-film arteriograms to the smaller format usual with digital subtraction angiography. There is no simple mechanism for scaling the images to achieve actual measurements of the lumen diameters. All definition of stenosis had to be made based upon percent stenosis. Due to the small sizes involved, attention must be paid to careful measurement. This can be facilitated with a magnified comparator, which permits reading the scale in tenths of a millimeter. When this is done, one can achieve accuracy of measurement that approximates that usually obtained with cut-films.[4,5]

In more recent years the introduction of magnetic resonance angiography (MRA) added another possible "gold standard" to be considered. Although the early studies produced with the technique had low resolution, there have been substantial improvements in image quality. There are some inherent problems with signal dropout, which can produce failure to image the site of maximal disease or overestimation of the severity of stenosis. Further improvement in the MRA studies may be achieved through gated signal acquisition or with the use of contrast agents, but these are not yet the standard of practice. Another test in the category of a potential reference standard is the computerized tomographic angiogram. Further comparison with conventional contrast angiography is needed before either of these studies is accepted as a reference standard for noninvasive tests.

A growing problem is the loss of standards for some testing areas. As discussed previously, duplex scanning is becoming a primary diagnostic modality. This first occurred with evaluation of deep venous thrombosis, to the extent that except for a few academic centers carrying out research projects, it is nearly impossible to get validation of the results of venous scans. Consideration is being given to developing new approaches such as outcome analysis; however, to date there has been little experience in this area. Another problem area is the carotid scan, with which at least there is the possibility of using intraoperative findings to confirm diagnostic impressions.

ADDITIONAL IMPETUS TO QUALITY ASSURANCE—ACCREDITATION AND CREDENTIALING

Unlike most aspects of medicine, there has been no regulation of vascular laboratories. As a result there have been no standards by which to judge these facilities. In the

1980s there was rapid growth in the number of laboratories, resulting not only from increased clinical demand but also from the fact that the level of reimbursement made provision of these services profitable. By the end of the decade there was growing concern about the lack of standards and the increasing evidence of poor quality work being done. Some high visibility cases of extreme fraud raised questions about the whole field and some medical insurance carriers went so far as to suggest abolishing payment for noninvasive tests. Individual leaders within different specialties called for reforms but had little power initiate any action. In 1989 an ad hoc group started working on developing a multidisciplinary, voluntary accreditation for noninvasive laboratories. In 1991 these efforts resulted in the incorporation of the Intersocietal Commission for the Accreditation of Vascular Laboratories (ICAVL) as a not-for-profit organization. The broad base of support is demonstrated by the list of original sponsoring groups: the American Academy of Neurology, the American College of Radiology, the American Institute of Ultrasound in Medicine, the International Society for Cardiovascular Surgery (North American Chapter), the Society for Vascular Surgery, the Society for Vascular Medicine & Biology, the Society of Diagnostic Medical Sonographers, and the Society of Vascular Technology. The initial work of the ICAVL was to develop the standards for all the aspects of the vascular laboratory to be evaluated in the accreditation process. A critical principle was that the most important aspect of the evaluation process was to judge the quality of the work produced. Considerable effort went into developing the self-studies, which would provide the data for the primary review of each laboratory. In January 1992, the first 36 laboratories were granted accreditation for a 3-year period. Since then, there has been a continuing increase in the number of accredited facilities.

The application is divided into a review of the organization of the laboratory and separate sections for each testing area (extracranial cerebrovascular, intracranial cerebrovascular, peripheral arterial, peripheral venous, and visceral vascular). The organization section requires information about the training, experience, and continuing education for physicians and technical staff. There are numerous pathways to learning performance and interpretation of noninvasive techniques, so the education and training is not specified in the standards but the total background of the individual is reviewed. Because all personnel are expected to remain up to date with the field, there is a requirement for a minimum of 15 h of continuing education specifically related to vascular testing every 3 years. At present, credentialing of technical personnel is recommended but not required. The organization section also covers items of the specifics of report preparation, patient safety, and equipment maintenance. The testing sections require listing of the examination protocols, the specific diagnostic criteria, sample cases studied (including normals and a range of abnormals), and validation data reflecting the quality control carried out. The greatest emphasis of the review is focused on the cases submitted. For duplex scans both the quality of the images and the Doppler velocity tracings are important. Other factors include how closely the protocol was followed and whether the diagnostic criteria were applied consistently on all examples submitted.

From the beginning, the primary focus of the accreditation has been the evaluation of quality. The practices of the laboratory are compared to the standards. An important principle is that of inclusivity: the decision for accreditation is based on substantial compliance rather than requiring absolute compliance with every subsection. There are few absolute goals that must be reached. The ICAVL has always considered education as part of its role. The working hypothesis has been that by bringing labs with some weaknesses into the process, these facilities can be assisted in identifying and correcting these problems. Once accredited, each laboratory receives a critique letter specifying deficiencies that need to be addressed before application for reaccreditation, which is required at 3-year intervals.

Since 1992, sample cases have been found to contain a variety of errors or weaknesses including: (1) substantial variation from the written protocol (e.g., frequent failure to use appropriate setting of angle on the Doppler beam), (2) use of different diagnostic criteria for the same examination, (3) failure to apply or inconsistent application of diagnostic criteria, and (4) use of inadequate images or waveforms for diagnosis. Multiple occurrences of such problems in a single application point to serious quality deficiencies, for these reflect lack of consistency. Standardized testing procedures and diagnostic algorithms are critical for making a test reproducible, which is an important component of overall accuracy.

The question has been raised about the effectiveness of accreditation. From the beginning there has been feedback from the laboratories stating that in spite of the tedium of completing the application, the process forced a detailed review of all aspects of the operation, identifying weaknesses that needed correction. For laboratories with major deficiencies a site visit is required prior to making a final decision about accreditation or denial. In many cases the site visitors have found that some of the problems documented in the self-study are being addressed. Further validation was obtained once laboratories started applying for reaccreditation; many had corrected the deficiencies listed in the critique letters.

Another important component to improving the quality of the work of vascular laboratories is the credentialing of technologists. In the late 1970s the leaders of the precursor of the Society of Vascular Technology (SVT) became concerned about the competence of new workers entering the field of vascular testing and the desirability of defining an entry-level standard. They approached the American Registry of Diagnostic Medical Sonographers (ARDMS), which had been administering credentialing examinations in different areas of medical ultrasound since 1975. This cooperation led to the establishment of the Registered Vascular Technologist (RVT) certificate. An examination was developed specifically to cover topics related to the work of the noninvasive vascular laboratory. The first credentials were issued in 1983, and in 1998 there were 6740 active RVTs. An important requirement for RVT certificate holders is that they must report a minimum of 30 h of continuing medical education (CME) every 3 years in order to renew the credential. Critics of the RVT point out that the test evaluates only knowledge, not practical experience or skills; however, in its current form the process at least tests for an appropriate entry-level understanding of the technology and of the clinical considerations involved in the noninvasive laboratory. In the experience of people who have worked for a long time in the field, a person who cannot pass may be able to learn to perform tests by rote but usually does not master the subtleties required to do good work.

Both accreditation and technologist credentialing were developed as voluntary processes, but there is increasing pressure to mandate these. There has been growing concern about the quality of the testing performed by noninvasive laboratories. The medical insurance payers are looking for ways to improve the chances of getting good studies. In March 1998 the Medicare carrier in Virginia started requiring ICAVL accreditation as a condition for payment of vascular tests. Six other carriers have taken a different approach requiring either that the facility be accredited or that the testing be performed by RVTs. Four additional companies have served notice that they will implement this policy in 1999. Other insurance groups are following this lead and it is expected that the trend will continue to grow.

RECOMMENDATIONS

The goal of every vascular laboratory should be to produce consistent high quality testing. There are several components that need to be in place in order to achieve this end. Knowledgeable and experienced personnel are the first step. For the technologists, the RVT credential indicates a reasonable entry-level base of knowledge, but the examining skills need to be monitored by the medical director for proof of clinical experience. Until a high level of clinical competence is achieved, close supervision and assistance are necessary. It may be helpful to send the person to a course or workshop with a heavy dose of hands-on experience. It is equally important to make sure of the knowledge of the medical staff working with the laboratory. The majority of vascular surgery fellowships currently offer instruction and experience in noninvasive techniques, so that many recent graduates are well prepared. It is still important to verify the skills by having an established member of the medical staff verify the interpretations made by the new physician. A reasonable check should be possible by double reading 50 tests in each testing area performed by the laboratory. Physicians who have not received the laboratory experience during a fellowship should seek to obtain 40 to 50 h of formal learning through CME courses focused specifically on the principles of testing and result interpretation. In addition, they should spend some time observing testing. This phase is intended more for them to learn the practical aspects and limitations of the specific tests rather than to become skilled examiners. As is recommended for the new graduates, the initial interpretations should be monitored by the medical director.

Standardization is a second key to quality work. A specific examination protocol should be adopted and a detailed written description prepared. The written document is important for ensuring that all the tests are done the same way by all technologists. It is also an important training tool when new staff are added. Similarly, a single set of diagnostic criteria are needed for each test. The final reports must always use the diagnostic categories defined, for this is a critical element in the consistency in interpretation. In laboratories found to have variability in results, the problem is often a reflection of the fact that the physicians use differing criteria.

As it is in other areas, specific quality control is essential in the noninvasive laboratory. When a facility is first established, it is important to demonstrate that the techniques are yielding the expected accuracy in terms of low false-positives and false-negatives. The most common procedure is to compare the tests with contrast angiograms. As discussed previously, in some areas this is becoming more difficult and the use of intraoperative findings as a reference standard may be necessary. Some laboratories carry out a validation study when they first start out, then stop the process. It is necessary to carry out ongoing or at least periodic validations in order to detect new sources of error such as might result from introduction of new equipment or addition of new staff. Another way of detecting problems is to have blinded repeat studies performed by different technologists with subsequent comparison of the studies. Studies showing substantial variance point to the need for analysis and correction.

The best approach to these steps is to go through the formal process of preparing an application for accreditation. The documentation requested in the ICAVL self-studies sets out the paper trail covering the major items related to quality in vascular testing. Having the external review certainly forces us to be more critical of the work done.

APPENDIX

For information regarding accreditation, contact:
   Intersocietal Commission for the Accreditation of Vascular Laboratories
   8840 Stanford Blvd., Suite 4900
   Columbia, Maryland 21045
   Telephone: (410) 872-0100
   Fax: (410) 872-0030
   Home page: www.icavl-icael.org

REFERENCES

1. Strandness DE. Extracranial arterial disease. In: *Duplex Scanning in Vascular Disorders,* 2nd ed. New York: Raven Press; 1993:113–157.
2. Sumner DS. Evaluation of noninvasive testing procedures: data analysis and interpretation. In: Bernstein EF, ed. *Vascular Diagnosis* (4th ed.) St. Louis: Mosby; 1993:39–63.
3. Chikos PM, Fisher LD, Hirsch JH, et al. Observer variability in evaluating extracranial carotid stenosis. *Stroke.* 1983;14:885–892.
4. Moll FL, Baker JD. Observer variability with conventional and digital subtraction carotid angiograms. *Eur J Vasc Surg.* 1987;1:297–303.
5. Baker JD. Quality assurance in the vascular laboratory. *Semin Vasc Surg.* 1994;7:241–244.

4

The Vascular Center

The Concept of a Multidisciplinary Approach

Anthony D. Whittemore, MD

INTRODUCTION

Every clinician involved in the care of our aging population is only too well aware of the increasing complexity required for the management of systemic atherosclerosis and interrelated comorbidity, particularly in the larger teaching settings where the acuity index is rapidly rising. Treatment of atherosclerosis and its associated risk factors requires a facility with management algorithms made increasingly complex by expanding alternatives, both pharmacological and interventional. From the patient's perspective, medical management often requires a neverending schedule of appointments with not only primary care physicians, but also a multitude of subspecialists as well. Transportation difficulties often present insurmountable problems for patients with limited ambulatory ability and economic means. As such they depend on public transportation for the frequent office visits required and their medical care becomes an all-encompassing ordeal. Because these patients are seen by a plethora of medical specialists, communication among physicians often lags behind therapeutic decisions. As a result, patients may suffer from insufficient oversight, delays in initiation in therapy, and adverse drug interactions. Finally, risk factor management presents an extraordinary challenge for individuals who may suffer from disabling claudication in addition to symptomatic coronary artery disease, cerebrovascular disease, hypertension, diabetes mellitus, and dyslipidemia. Such risk factor reduction programs are not readily available and follow-up protocols often lack compliance.

Although the prime factor underlying the creation of the Vascular Center was a desire to provide expeditious clinical care for patients with atherosclerosis, other objectives included an effort to educate medical subspecialists and primary care physicians regarding appropriate guidelines for a variety of interventions, an important goal with the reemergence of the gatekeeper concept so critical to increasing managed care penetration. Although vascular surgeons have been conscientious with regard to self-education and have expended considerable energy in providing up-to-date education for residents and medical students, consistent efforts directed toward the education of primary care physicians regarding developments in peripheral vascular disease have been lacking. Vascular surgeons frequently see patients with high-grade internal carotid artery lesions that have been symptomatic for many months, and excessively large aneurysms that have been observed to grow at alarming rates under the watchful eye of their primary care physician. Many of our primary care colleagues, as diligent as they may be, are simply unaware of contemporary morbidity and mortality statistics associated with a variety of vascular reconstructions and are therefore imparting inappropriate advice based on outcome figures referenced to their period of training. In similar fashion, vascular surgeons in the past had been able to maintain a working knowledge of cardiac pharmacology, antihypertensive therapy, and diabetic management, but it is a rare individual who is able to master the impressive spectrum of cardiovascular pharmacological therapy with all its idiosyncrasies.

The evolution of two associated disciplines during the late 1970s and early 1980s contributed significantly to the need for the institution of the Vascular Center concept. Many clinical cardiologists understandably became focused on the management of myocardial dysfunction to the exclusion of comorbidity from peripheral vascular disease initially within their pervue. There arose a need for fully trained cardiologists, well versed in the medical management of systemic atherosclerosis and associated risk factors. Simultaneously, the proven efficacy of percutaneous transluminal approaches to vascular disease spawned interventional radiologists who rapidly established an important role in the management of these patients. As these individuals were not accustomed to assuming primary care with admitting privileges in most institutions and lack the associated infrastructure to ensure the longitudinal follow-up, appropriate integration with other disciplines seemed sensible.

Finally, an important factor that motivated a multidiciplinary effort in our academic setting stemmed from the increasing demands placed on clinical and basic science investigators. The current environment encourages most in our specialty to declare themselves primarily one or the other, but not both. The effort required for efficient patient care in the setting of volume-related outcome and managed care requires the full time attention of clinicians. Similarly, the maintenance of a well-disciplined laboratory infrastructure in compliance with a variety of regulatory agencies requires the efforts of a full-time investigative presence in the laboratory.

The Vascular Center at the Brigham and Women's Hospital was initiated in 1984 in an attempt to provide a multidiciplinary approach toward the solution of the aforementioned deficiencies. The divisions of Vascular Surgery, Interventional Cardiovascular Radiology, and a newly created Division of Vascular Medicine began to share resources and wrestle with the constraints imposed by conventional departmental boundaries under the administrative structure of the hospital (Fig. 4–1).

CLINICAL CARE

The mission of the Vascular Center as initially formulated was to provide expeditious comprehensive care for a patient referred for management of an acute manifestation of underlying systemic atherosclerosis. As the initial referral was usually prompted by a desire on the part of the referring physician for an interventional solution for a specific problem, considerable efforts were directed toward delivering focused in-hospital tertiary care, critical components that included vascular medical management, and appropriate utilization of evolving endovascular approaches. As the role of the interventional

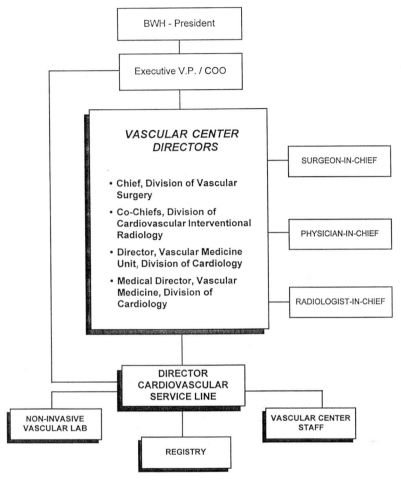

Figure 4–1. Brigham and Women's Hospital Vascular Center organization chart (as of January 1997).

radiologist continued to increase, the vascular internists provided appropriate primary clinical care for patients not necessarily under the direct supervision of the vascular surgeon. Whereas the vascular internist and surgeon maintain primary responsibility for the in-hospital care in our current setting, the interventional radiological service has been granted admitting privileges for patients hospitalized for brief periods following a procedure, often for a short course of parenteral anticoagulation. As the vast majority of referrals are directed toward the primary clinicians, decisions to intervene with conventional surgery or endovascular techniques are made jointly, yet those patients managed from a technical point of view by the interventionalist are no longer admitted to the surgical service, thereby relieving an overworked house staff of a significant burden of paperwork.

During the acute hospitalization, the medical team is charged with the additional responsibility of formulating a patient-specific longitudinal management plan, which encompasses comprehensive care directed at all manifestations of underlying atherosclerosis and at risk factor reduction. This plan is then transmitted to both primary care and referring physicians at the time of discharge in hopes of fulfilling two objectives. First, such a plan facilitates the transmission of current recommendations that may or may not be utilized by the primary care physician as they see fit. Second, there is a considerable educational benefit for primary practitioners that for the most part has been received with appreciation. Reservations that the vascular medical specialist, serving in the capacity of gatekeeper, might obstruct referral for appropriate intervention was rapidly put to rest as our surgical volume has increased steadily since the opening of the center and as the vascular internists became aware of accurate morbidity and mortality figures. Internists referring patients for vascular medical consultation were thereby reassured and educated with respect to anticipated outcome. As a result, new patient primary referral to the vascular medical team has increased dramatically in recent years (Fig. 4–2). Whereas the potential for diverting future patient flow certainly existed initially and the interposition of vascular internist might have been perceived as meddlesome, this has not been the case as judged by the growth of our referral base (Figs. 4–3 and 4–4). Since 1992, our volume of arterial reconstructions has increased by 40% and percutaneous interventions by 40%. A significant proportion of our surgical volume at present derives from our group of vascular internists, and our primary care physicians have, for the most part, been grateful for both the practical and educational aspects of the comprehensive longitudinal care plans transmitted to them following an acute hospitalization.

The vascular internists have also enhanced the care of patients with nonsurgical vascular problems, including both inflammatory and thrombotic disorders. Focused expertise in the management of these specific disorders has been developed along with clinical and basic science investigative efforts.

A major objective in providing optimal care for the atherosclerotic patient has been the "one-stop shopping" concept. A patient initially referred to one of the three disciplines ideally should be seen in consultation as needed by any other specialist on

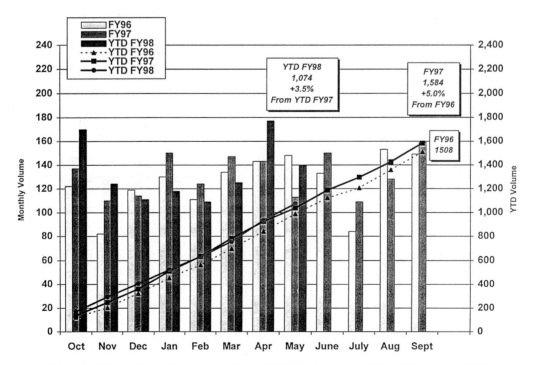

Figure 4–2. Total visits to the Vascular Medical Clinic for fiscal year 1998. FY, fiscal year; YTD, year-to-date.

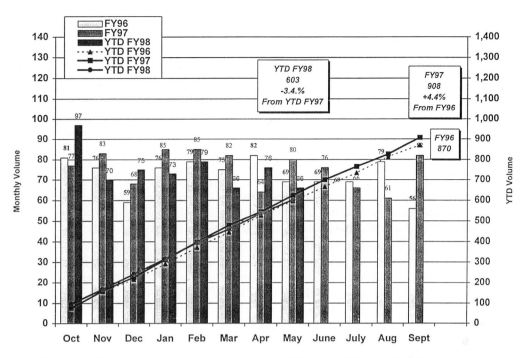

Figure 4–3. Vascular surgery procedure activity at Brigham and Women's Hospital as of June 1998. FY, fiscal year; YTD, year-to-date.

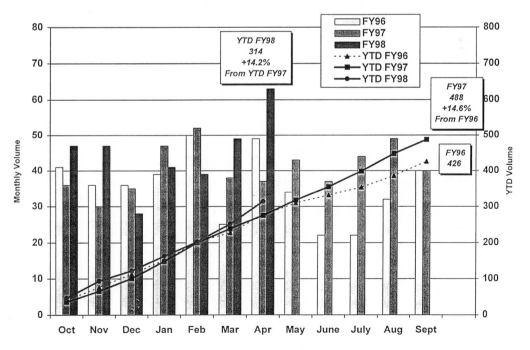

Figure 4–4. Vascular angiography—total vascular interventions at Brigham and Women's Hospital as of June 1998. FY, fiscal year; YTD, year-to-date.

the same day as the initial referral visit and a decision should be reached regarding management strategy. From the surgeon's standpoint, patients referred for a specific procedure are seen by a vascular medical specialist and/or interventional radiologist on the same day and the optimal course of action formulated. Often the patient is referred to our Pre-Admitting Test Center on the same day for appropriate laboratory studies and consultation with an anesthesiologist. The next visit to the hospital ideally occurs on the morning of the proposed intervention. Should further cardiopulmonary evaluation prove necessary, however, diagnostic studies to determine the presence and severity of coronary artery disease, left ventricular dysfunction, or significant comorbidity often require a second preoperative visit. An important component of this patient-flow scheme is the role of the scheduling coordinator, who remains in telephone contact with the patient and family throughout the entire perioperative experience. The second major component of our clinical team is provided by our Nurse Specialist, who is introduced to the patient on the first visit and whose responsibilities include ensuring that preoperative anxieties are minimized and appropriate evaluations are completed. The Nurse Specialist also makes daily rounds during hospitalization to facilitate discharge planning, postoperative office visits, and appropriate nursing services following discharge.

EDUCATION

We have been successful in instituting a multidisciplinary weekly teaching conference during which specific cases are presented and discussed and pertinent review topics are presented. Daily multidisciplinary work rounds, however, have proved nearly impossible due to the scheduling logistics characteristic of each team. Although the radiologists are most flexible with regard to timing, the intrinsic circadian rhythm of surgeons continues to differ so radically from that characteristic of internists that daily rounds present a challenge. At the resident or fellow level, however, measurable interdisciplinary interaction occurs several times daily, and the same proves true at the attending level on a one-to-one consulting basis.

The institution of an effective patient education and risk reduction program represents yet another challenge. We have instituted a lipid clinic as part of our vascular center for management of patients with complex dyslipidemia. The clinic is staffed by vascular physicians with expertise in lipid disorders and by nutritionists and a coordinator. A smoking cessation program offering counseling and pharmacological supervision is scheduled to begin soon after an initial disappointing attempt thwarted by poor patient compliance. Unfortunately, plans for exercise rehabilitation have been curtailed by the failure of the Health Care Finance Administration and insurers to provide reimbursement for this modality despite its proven efficacy.

RESEARCH

For the academic community at the Brigham and Women's Hospital, this multidisciplinary approach has provided unique opportunities for integrated research endeavors in both basic and applied sciences.

As the demands for clinical intervention become more time consuming for clinical specialists, and as responsibilities for senior investigators in the laboratory have expanded dramatically, a team approach to vascular research seems advantageous from several points of view, as funding agencies look most favorably on a laboratory supervised by a full-time investigator. Such an individual maintains the necessary technical infrastructure, on-site supervision of increasingly sensitive assays and procedures, and compliance with numerous regulatory agencies with routine inspections to enforce compliance criteria. A coordinated research team under the supervision of such an individual is far more likely to be productive and maintain funding than a clinician whose time is increasingly consumed by clinical obligations. Full-time principal investigators in vascular wall biology, atherogenesis, and the pathology of fibrous intimal hyperplasia have remained well supported and are provided an opportunity to interact with clinicians to mutual benefit. Within the framework of The Vascular Center, research space and redundant equipment and personnel have been combined into a more coordinated and well-funded core resource. Funding currently supports a score grant, a program project grant, a career development award, a clinician scientist award, a merit (R-37) award, five R-01 awards, and four sponsored research endeavors. These grants provide partial salary support for 5 of the 6 internists and full support for 19 fellows and 8 technical positions.

CONCLUSION

A potentially divergent course between specialists has thus far been avoided among the three primary components of The Vascular Center in a constructive collaborative effort to provide optimal multidisciplinary care. The mortality rate on the vascular surgery service remains below 2%, in spite of the fact that both age and acuity of our patients continue to increase. This statistic reflects favorably on a number of factors, including the focused attention provided by our vascular medical colleagues during the perioperative period. The transition between in-hospital and outpatient care has been facilitated significantly with vastly improved communication among the various members of an expanding health care team, yet the academic mission of all three disciplines moves forward.

II

Practical Application of the Noninvasive Vascular Laboratory

5

Increasing Use of Autogenous Fistulas

Selection of Dialysis Access Sites by Duplex Scanning and Transposition of Forearm Veins

*Michael B. Silva, Jr., MD, Peter J. Pappas, MD,
Frank T. Padberg, Jr., MD, and
Robert W. Hobson II, MD*

INTRODUCTION

The arena of dialysis access is one filled with contradictions and paradox for the vascular surgeon. Often relegated to a position of second-tier interest, frequently passed over as a topic of study and discussion at national forums for vascular research, one might suspect that this is an area of only marginal importance. A review of the facts would suggest otherwise.

Surgical procedures for hemodialysis access are the most common vascular surgical operations performed in the United States, and although a number of subspecialists (general surgeons, transplant surgeons, urologists, and interventional radiologists) participate in this field, vascular surgeons are the primary providers of service, with responsibility for 72% of the dialysis-access procedures performed in 1992.[1] By comparison, vascular surgeons were responsible for only 68% of aortic aneurysmorraphies and 64% of carotid endarterectomies (CEAs) performed during the same period. For general surgeons, hemodialysis access procedures remain their most commonly performed vascular surgical procedure.[2] Furthermore, performance rates for dialysis-access procedures are on the rise, whereas many other standard vascular surgical bypass procedures have been declining in frequency.

The importance and impact of these procedures is further highlighted by the magnitude of the numbers involved: more than 200,000 Americans are dependent on dialysis (growing at a rate in excess of 10% per year), and more than $9.5 billion are spent annually on the treatment of end-stage renal disease (ESRD).[3] The average yearly cost per patient with ESRD to the Medicare system is in excess of $50,000, with a substantial percentage spent on placement and maintenance of access sites. Poor patency rates for hemodialysis access procedures contribute to these costs by requiring revisions and new procedures.

Patency data for vascular access procedures are worse than those for almost all other types of vascular surgical therapeutics. In no other instance would we accept a vascular procedure as a viable alternative with primary patency results presented in categories of 30-, 60-, or 90-*day* cumulative patencies (as in the case of either surgical or lytic thrombectomy of thrombosed access grafts). This probably accounts for some of the unpopularity of reporting on, or researching topics associated with, dialysis-access surgery within the vascular surgical community.

Clearly, the most salient difference responsible for lower patency rates with access procedures compared to other bypass grafts is the nature of repetitive instrumentation. Six cannulation sites per week, with subsequent pressure for hemostasis, would be expected to trend patency rates for any graft downward. However, there are other less obvious factors that have contributed to the reduced expectations for dialysis-access grafts and fistulas that, when introduced in the 1960s, were greeted with promise and enthusiasm.

The patients are different. A review of data from the US Renal Data System's 1995 Annual Report demonstrates that patient characteristics have changed significantly since the initial description of successful hemodialysis by the autogenous radiocephalic fistula. The average age of the 17 patients described by Brescia, Cimino, and colleagues in their initial description of the autogenous fistula was 45 years.[4] Our average age for initial placement of access is now 63 years, and patients present for hemodialysis access in more debilitated states with additional comorbid conditions. Life expectancy on dialysis, however, is increasing. This latter fact combined with poor access patency rates means that each dialysis patient requires numerous access procedures and revisions during their dialysis lifetime. These factors underscore the need to develop a strategy to improve our performance data in the placement of dialysis access grafts and fistulas.

TYPES OF ACCESS PROCEDURES AND CHANGING PRACTICE PATTERNS

Three common procedures are performed for hemodialysis access: autogenous fistulas (AF), prosthetic bridging grafts (BG), and indwelling central venous catheters. Most vascular surgeons regard AF as king of dialysis access; however, the numbers suggest their loyalty is fading as utilization of AF steadily declines and placement of BG continues to increase. The most recently available data for the United States confirmed that prosthetic BG was utilized 1.7 times more commonly than AF [51.9% for BG vs. 30.5% for AF and 9.3% for permanent catheters (PC)].[3]

This trend is disconcerting because once established, mature AFs (those with arterialized venous segments that can be cannulated successfully and support flow rates adequate for effective dialysis) have improved patency rates and lower complication and infection rates compared with BGs. Several authors have reported higher early patency rates for BG than for AF when all attempted AFs are included in the evaluation.[5-10] This is because of the high failure to mature rates for AF (as high as 30% to 40%). These studies correctly count AFs that remain patent but fail to mature sufficiently to support dialysis as early failures. In many cases, these failures may be attributed to the difficulty in selecting adequate veins that reliably produce mature AFs.

Although BG may have a higher early patency rate than AF, they have poor 1- and 2-year patency rates and higher complication rates when compared to mature AF. The two common sites for BG are the forearm and the upper arm. Difficulty in predicting adequacy of venous outflow in the antecubital space has led some authors to recommend the routine placement of brachial–axillary bridging grafts where the inflow and outflow vessels are commonly satisfactory.

This type of policy has the advantage of achieving high early success rates in the greatest number of people but has the disadvantage of minimizing access possibilities, and may be at the expense of decreased long-term dialysis options. Failed brachial–axillary grafts may precipitate upper extremity venous outflow obstruction and limit subsequent options for ipsilateral forearm access. The optimal strategy for maximizing options preserves more proximal sources for future development.

There are other explanations for the shift in placement patterns away from autogenous fistulas. The radiocephalic fistula, as performed through a single incision, became the preferred method for hemodialysis access after its initial description in 1966. However, in the population of older, sicker patients with multiple prior hospitalizations who present for hemodialysis today, arteries and veins in close proximity that are suitable for radiocephalic fistulas are uncommon.

In addition, visual inspection and physical examination of upper extremities may be inadequate to assess the quality of arterial inflow and continuity of venous outflow. Segmental stenoses may not be appreciated, and deeper suitable veins may be overlooked. Furthermore, spared veins that are adequate for AF formation may be encountered in the forearm, but their anatomic position may lie in a deeper subcutaneous location. Needle cannulation for hemodialysis of AF formed with these deeper veins *in situ* is technically more difficult than for BG. The basilic vein in the forearm may also be spared and suitable for AF formation, but in its *in situ* position may necessitate awkward forearm positioning for needle cannulation and subsequent hemodialysis.

OUR STRATEGY

We are committed to a policy of maximizing our use of AF for dialysis access. We use routine preoperative noninvasive assessment of the upper extremity to enhance our ability to identify arteries and veins suitable for hemodialysis access.[11,12] Duplex ultrasound (DU) has been used effectively in mapping lower extremity arteries and veins for infrainguinal bypass procedures as well as for surveillance of infrainguinal vein grafts.[13,14] We have used DU in the upper extremity for selection of patients for AF hemoaccess and for clinical follow-up of patients undergoing hemodialysis access procedures. We hypothesized such a strategy would increase our options for AF by identifying veins not clinically evident and reduce AF early failure rate by improved selection. When anatomy not suitable for autogenous fistulas is identified, optimal locations for BG are investigated. This strategy was developed to increase our use of AF, enhance cumulative patency for all types of access procedures by improving selection, and maximize options for hemodialysis access in our dialysis population.

Noninvasive Assessment

All patients referred for hemodialysis-access procedures at our institution are entered into a dialysis-access registry. Demographic and medical history information is obtained and recorded in a prospective manner. All patients undergo preoperative evaluation by DU to assess the suitability of upper extremity arteries and veins and to facilitate planning of dialysis access. Table 5–1 summarizes criteria utilized to define satisfactory venous outflow and arterial inflow. In addition, suitability of upper extremity arteries and veins for AF is evaluated by clinical examination alone in all cases by the operating surgeon prior to noninvasive evaluation and recorded separately for later comparisons.

Ultrasound Technique

Ultrasound scans of the superficial venous system are initiated at the wrist of the nondominant arm with a tourniquet placed at midforearm. Superficial veins in the forearms are dilated by tapping and stroking maneuvers. Warm ultrasonic gel (Thermasonic, Parker Labs, Orange, NJ) is applied and the veins insonated using a 5 MHz or 7 MHz scanning probe (Accuson, 128 XP-10). Veins are assessed for compressibility and diameter. The tourniquet is then moved to the arm and forearm, and veins of acceptable diameter are followed proximally for continuity and size. At the antecubital space, continuity with arm veins is verified. The tourniquet is then removed and continuity of the deep system determined through the axillary and subclavian veins. The superficial forearm veins most suitable for use, as identified by DU, are mapped by skin markings for use in the operative procedure.

Once the venous anatomy is determined to be acceptable for AF, segmental arterial pressures are measured and the status of the radial artery is evaluated. Diameter of the radial artery at the wrist is measured and the radial artery scanned by DU. The patency of the palmar arch is verified. If the radial artery is not suitable, the ulnar and brachial arteries are examined for possible use as alternative sources of arterial inflow. Evaluation of the dominant arm is performed only if evaluation of the nondominant arm proves unsatisfactory. Skin overlying the most suitable segment of artery is marked.

Patients requiring immediate dialysis and yet noted to have suitable arteries and veins for AF formation are evaluated for concomitant placement of a contralateral internal jugular hemodialysis catheter for use during the period of maturation. A period of 4 to 6 weeks is allowed for AF maturation prior to attempts at cannulation. Prior to initial access, AF are evaluated by DU, and the areas of maximal diameter are marked on the skin to facilitate needle cannulation by dialysis nursing personnel.

Access procedures are performed on an outpatient basis utilizing the same-day surgery unit. Intraoperative measurements of arterial and venous diameters are per-

TABLE 5–1. NONINVASIVE CRITERIA FOR SELECTION OF UPPER EXTREMITY ARTERIES AND VEINS FOR DIALYSIS ACCESS PROCEDURES

Venous Examination
    Venous luminal diameter ≥2.5 mm for AF
    Venous luminal diameter ≥4.0 mm for BG
    Absence of segmental stenoses or occluded segments
    Continuity with the deep venous system in the upper arm
    Absence of ipsilateral central venous stenosis or occlusion

Arterial Examination
    Absence of pressure differential ≥20 mm Hg between arms
    Arterial lumen diameter ≥2.0 mm
    Patent palmar arch

AF, autogenous fistula; BG, bridging graft.
Reprinted with permission: Silva MB Jr, Hobson RW II, Pappas PJ, et al. A strategy for increasing use of autogenous hemodialysis access procedures: impact of preoperative noninvasive evaluation. *J Vasc Surg.* 1998;27(92):302–308.

formed using intravascular dilators to evaluate accuracy of preoperative DU measurements.

Bridging grafts are performed using 6-mm polytetrafluoroethylene (PTFE) grafts as either forearm antecubital loop grafts or upper arm brachial–axillary grafts. If both anatomical locations are acceptable, the forearm loop is used preferentially in all cases.

A successful AF or BG is defined as one that remains patent and sustains a velocity of blood flow (≥250 ml/sec) sufficient for successful hemodialysis. AF or BG that thromboses prior to initiation of dialysis are considered early failures. In addition, AF that remains patent but fails to mature sufficiently to allow successful needle cannulation and provide flow rates adequate for dialysis must be considered as failures for determination of life table cumulative patency rates. DU is performed at 3-month intervals or as indicated by reduced flow rates during dialysis.

Superficial Venous Transposition

Routine upper extremity evaluation of all prospective dialysis patients by DU has led to the identification of numerous patients with veins suitable for AF that are not easily identifiable by clinical examination alone, usually because of their depth or location. These qualities, which probably impart some protective status from previous venipuncture, nonetheless make standard Brescia–Cimino type fistula formation difficult or impossible.

In order to expand our options for formation of AF, we have utilized modifications of the single-incision radiocephalic fistula technique described by Brescia, Cimino and associates, which allows for the use of veins identified by DU as suitable for selection but remote from the arterial source of inflow. These modifications involve separate incisions for exposure of arteries and veins, extended venous dissection with dilation, and subsequent transposition of the vein to a more superficial and subcutaneous position on the volar aspect of the forearm. In addition to maximizing options for AF formation by identifying and utilizing veins remote from the arterial inflow source, these technical modifications facilitate needle cannulation by the dialysis nursing personnel once the fistula has matured, and allow for comfortable arm positioning during hemodialysis.

Surgical Technique

Most patients' arms are examined and marked in the vascular laboratory in the days prior to the planned surgical procedure and the patients are instructed on methods to preserve the markings at home.

In the operating suite, a local 1% lidocaine infusion is the usual anesthetic choice, supplemented by judicious use of intravenous sedatives. Because of its vasoconstrictor properties, the use of 1% lidocaine with epinephrine is avoided. The entire arm is prepared in a sterile fashion, the hand is excluded, and the procedure is performed by the surgeon and the surgical assistant from a seated position. The use of surgical magnifying lenses with 2.5× magnification is routine.

Once the skin and subcutaneous tissue overlying the vein has been properly anesthetized, a longitudinal incision is made directly over the vein beginning at its distalmost usable aspect and carried towards the antecubital fossa for a distance of at least 15 cm (Fig. 5–1). The vein is transected at the wrist, and a 3-0 silk suture ligature is used to ligate the portion of vein remaining in its distal bed. The vein is dissected free from its surrounding tissue so that it may be completely transposed to a superficial tunnel in the mid-portion of the volar aspect of the forearm. Venous branches that will not

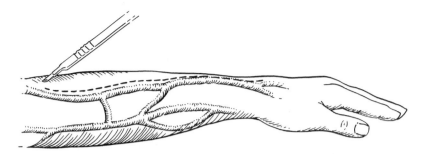

Figure 5–1. Incision along length of vein marked by Duplex ultrasonography. (*Reprinted with permission: Silva MB Jr, Hobson RW II, Jamil Z, et al. Vein transposition in the forearm for autogenous hemoaccess.* J Vasc Surg. *1997;26(6):981–988.*)

interfere with transposition are left intact to maximize outflow. Heparinized saline is injected through the open end of the vein with digital compression for occlusion of outflow at the antecubital fossa (Fig. 5–2). This results in substantial dilation of the freed segment of vein. The vein is wrapped in a heparinized saline–soaked sponge, and attention is then turned to the arterial dissection.

The portion of the artery that has been identified as suitable for inflow is then dissected. In most instances, the radial artery is identified between the brachial radialis and the flexor carpi radialis tendons. The superficial branch of the radial nerve lies lateral to this, and is separated from the radial artery by the brachial radialis muscle. The nerve is sensory at this level, and care must be taken not to injure it. There are concomitant veins running parallel to the artery on either side. These should be dissected free from the artery with care, which facilitates identification of the numerous small

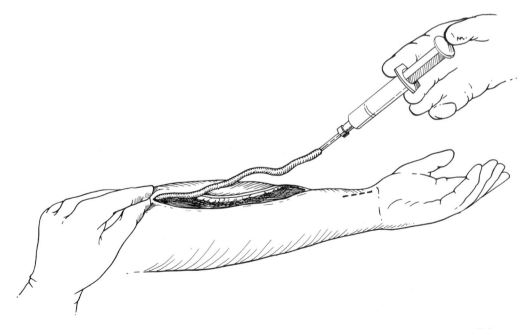

Figure 5–2. Complete dissection of the vein and dilation with heparinized saline; separate radial artery incision marked. (*Reprinted with permission: Silva MB Jr, Hobson RW II, Jamil Z, et al. Vein transposition in the forearm for autogenous hemoaccess.* J Vasc Surg. *1997;26(6):981–988.*)

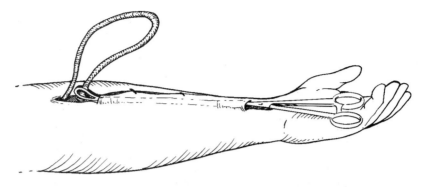

Figure 5–3. Construction of subcutaneous tunnel. (*Reprinted with permission: Silva MB Jr, Hobson RW II, Jamil Z, et al. Vein transposition in the forearm for autogenous hemoaccess. J Vasc Surg. 1997;26(6):981–988.*)

arterial branches. Although there typically are no arterial branches on the anterior aspect of the artery, there are usually several paired arterial branches leaving the radial artery on each side that must be addressed. We ligate these in continuity, with the ligature placed approximately 2 mm away from the radial artery to avoid impingement once dilation has occurred. Vessel loops are placed proximally and distally along the artery for vascular control.

A tunneling instrument is passed to develop the superficial subcutaneous tunnel (Fig. 5–3). The vein is marked along its length with a sterile marking pen to facilitate passage through the tunnel without twisting or kinking. Once the vein has been passed through the tunnel (Fig. 5–4) and hemostasis has been assured, the patient is typically given a bolus of 3000 units of intravenous heparin and a 1- to 2-mm arteriotomy is made with a number 11 blade on the volar surface of the artery. The arteriotomy is extended to approximately 15 mm to 20 mm using fine Potts' scissors. Using an 18-gauge angiocatheter, the artery is locally heparinized by injecting heparinized saline distally and then proximally while simultaneously opening the vessel loops.

An end-to-side anastomosis is performed using either 7-0 polypropylene with double-armed CV1 needles or, alternatively, Gortex CV6 on TT-9 needles can be used. Prior to completion of the anastomosis, vascular dilators are used to size both the vein and the radial artery. This has the benefit of allowing enlargement of blood vessels in spasm from vessel loops and manipulation. We use the dilators to verify the size of the arteries and veins predicted by the noninvasive evaluation. It should be noted that

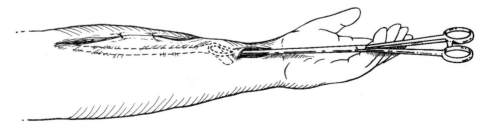

Figure 5–4. Vein transposed through mid-forearm volar subcutaneous tunnel. (*Reprinted with permission: Silva MB Jr, Hobson RW II, Jamil Z, et al. Vein transposition in the forearm for autogenous hemoaccess. J Vasc Surg. 1997;26(6):981–988.*)

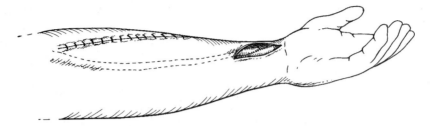

Figure 5–5. Completed fistula. Mid-forearm volar location facilitates cannulation and comfortable arm positioning during dialysis. (*Reprinted with permission: Silva MB Jr, Hobson RW II, Jamil Z, et al. Vein transposition in the forearm for autogenous hemoaccess.* J Vasc Surg. *1997;26(6):981–988.*)

self-retaining retractors are not used as the portion of the retractor above the skin level is cumbersome and the increased distance above the anastomotic line makes suturing more difficult.

Following the anastomosis, it is essential that a thrill be felt within the vein. Absence of a thrill indicates a probable technical or anatomic defect and requires further investigation with exploration of the anastomoses as indicated. Wounds are closed using a running subcuticular absorbable stitch (Fig. 5–5). Care is taken to maintain strict atraumatic technique when handling the skin edges in order to limit wound complications. Adhesive strips or tape applied directly to the skin are not used.

Adequate arterialization of the vein usually occurs within 4 to 6 weeks. Hand exercises are advocated to encourage fistula maturation. Prior to the initial use by our dialysis-access personnel, the patient is reevaluated in the noninvasive laboratory and the sites most suitable for needle insertion are marked on the skin to facilitate needle cannulation.

RESULTS AND IMPACT OF NONINVASIVE PROTOCOL

From September 1994 through January 1997, we evaluated 172 patients for dialysis-access procedures. The patients were 60% men and 40% women. The mean age of the patients was 63.3 years, with a range of 25 to 82 years. The causes of ESRD and the incidence rates were 36% for hypertension, 31% for diabetes mellitus, 12% for glomerulonephritis, 4% for human immunodeficiency virus (HIV)-related nephropathy, and 17% for other causes.

The records of 183 patients receiving access procedures performed at our institution from June 1, 1992, to August 31, 1994, before the initiation of this protocol, were reviewed to evaluate its impact on choice of dialysis-access procedures. The incidence of each procedure's use was recorded and compared between the two periods of observation.

Apparent differences in the frequency of various procedures performed for hemodialysis were analyzed for statistical significance. Cumulative patency for AF and BG performed on the 172 patients evaluated using our DU protocol were determined and compared using life-table analysis.

Of the 172 patients evaluated by DU protocol during the study period, 108 (63%) were identified as having arteries and veins suitable for AF, 52 (30%) were suitable for BG, and the remaining 12 patients (7%) had PCs placed.

It is interesting to note that of the 108 AF cases, 58 (53%) were performed in forearms that did not appear clinically suitable for AF when inspected visually by the surgeon prior to ultrasound mapping, confirming our prejudice that visual inspection and physical examination of upper extremities are commonly inadequate for the identification of suitable arteries and veins.

In addition, only 16 of the 108 AF procedures were radiocephalic fistulas, which could be performed through a single incision. The remaining 92 fistulas were performed using separate incisions for arteries and veins, with transposition of superficial veins to subcutaneous tunnels, demonstrating the utility of this technique as an adjunct to information obtained by upper extremity DU in expanding options for AF.

Successful cannulation and hemodialysis was accomplished with 99 of the 108 AF for a maturation rate of 91.6%. Of the 9 fistulas that did not initially support dialysis, 4 occluded postoperatively, 3 had stenoses detected at the initial DU exam and underwent successful revision, and 2 remained patent but with flows insufficient for adequate dialysis (<250 ml/sec). An additional 12 of the 99 functioning AF failed during the follow-up period.

In total, 21 AF failed. Five were successfully salvaged by revision, 4 were converted to contralateral forearm AF, 6 were converted to ipsilateral BG (3 forearm, 3 upper arm), 3 were converted to contralateral forearm BG, 2 received permanent central venous catheters, and the last patient, one of the early failures with a patent fistula not supporting adequate dialysis, died prior to revision.

The early failure rate for procedures performed under the direction of the protocol was 8.3% (9/108) for AF and 7.6% (4/52) for BG. Clinical follow-up by repeat DU was performed (mean: 15.2 months) and confirmed primary cumulative patency rates for AF of 83%, and 73% at 12 and 21 months, respectively (Table 5–2 and Fig. 5–6). Primary cumulative patency rates for BG were 74% and 62% at the same time intervals (Table 5–3 and Fig. 5–7). The number of PC was inadequate for life-table analysis, but during the follow-up period, 7 of the 12 PC failed for an absolute patency rate of 42%.

Table 5–4 compares relative frequencies of each access type performed during the two time periods. For the period prior to implementation of the protocol (6/1/92 to

TABLE 5–2. LIFE-TABLE ANALYSIS OF CUMULATIVE PRIMARY PATENCY RATES FOR AUTOGENOUS FISTULA

Interval (mo)	No. at Risk at Start of Interval	No. of Failures	No. Withdrawn Patent	Interval Patency Rate	Cumulative Patency	SE (%)
0–1	108	4	0	0.96	100	0.00
1–3	104	5	10	0.95	96	1.88
3–6	89	2	11	0.98	91	2.89
6–9	76	3	8	0.96	89	3.39
9–12	65	1	9	0.98	85	4.08
12–15	55	2	10	0.96	83	4.61
15–18	43	2	12	0.95	80	5.45
18–21	29	1	8	0.96	76	6.91
21–24	20	1	6	0.94	73	8.48
24–27	13	0	7	1.00	69	10.65
27–30	6	0	5	1.00	69	15.68
30–33	1	0	1	1.00	69	38.41

SE, standard error.
Reprinted with permission: Silva MB Jr, Hobson RW II, Pappas PJ, et al. A strategy for increasing use of autogenous hemodialysis access procedures: impact of preoperative noninvasive evaluation. *J Vasc Surg.* 1998;27(92):302–308.

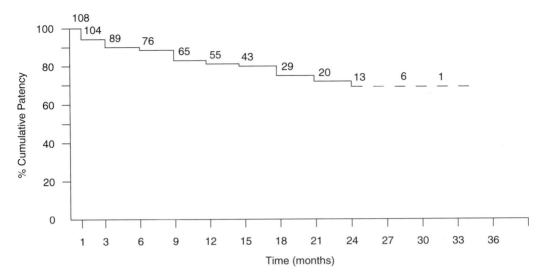

Figure 5–6. Life-table plot of cumulative patency rates for autogenous fistula performed during protocol period. (*Reprinted with permission: Silva MB Jr, Hobson RW II, Pappas PJ, et al. A strategy for increasing use of autogenous hemodialysis access procedures: Impact of preoperative noninvasive evaluation.* J Vasc Surg. *1998;27(92):302–308.*)

8/31/94), 183 procedures were performed with the following distribution: 25 AF (14%), 114 BG (62%), and 44 PC (24%). AF early failure rate during this period was 38% (10/25) and BG early failure rate was 11% (13/114). Patency rates of 48%, 63%, and 48% were obtained for AF, BG, and PC, respectively (mean follow-up: 13.8 months).

Comparisons between the two periods demonstrated significant differences in utilization rates of AF, BG, and PC ($p < 0.05$), with a marked increase in the placement of AF and a concomitant reduction in placement of BG and PC. Early failure rates were

TABLE 5–3. LIFE-TABLE ANALYSIS OF CUMULATIVE PRIMARY PATENCY RATES FOR BRIDGING GRAFTS

Interval (mo)	No. at Risk at Start of Interval	No. of Failures	No. Withdrawn Patent	Interval Patency Rate	Cumulative Patency	SE (%)
0–1	52	2	0	0.96	100	0.00
1–3	50	2	2	0.96	96	2.72
3–6	46	3	3	0.93	92	3.84
6–9	40	3	4	0.92	86	5.08
9–12	33	2	3	0.94	79	6.30
12–15	28	1	4	0.96	74	7.13
15–18	23	1	4	0.94	71	7.97
18–21	18	1	1	0.94	66	9.07
21–24	16	1	2	0.93	62	9.55
24–27	13	1	6	0.90	58	10.42
27–30	6	1	3	0.78	52	14.70
30–33	2	0	2	1.00	40	21.90

SE, standard error.
Reprinted with permission: Silva MB Jr, Hobson RW II, Pappas PJ, et al. A strategy for increasing use of autogenous hemodialysis access procedures: impact of preoperative noninvasive evaluation. *J Vasc Surg.* 1998;27(92):302–308.

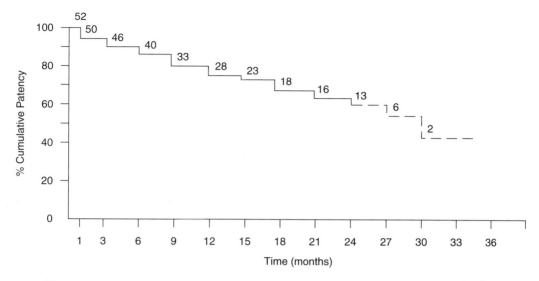

Figure 5–7. Life-table plot of cumulative patency rates for bridging grafts performed during protocol period. (*Reprinted with permission: Silva MB Jr, Hobson RW II, Pappas PJ, et al. A strategy for increasing use of autogenous hemodialysis access procedures: impact of preoperative noninvasive evaluation.* J Vasc Surg. *1998;27(92):302–308.*)

significantly lower for AF during the period utilizing the noninvasive protocol as compared to the previous period (p <0.05), suggesting the increased efficacy of DU in identifying arteries and veins as compared to visual inspection alone. In addition, comparisons of patency rates by access type also showed a significant increase in patency rates for AF and BG performed during the protocol period (p <0.05) confirming our bias for the preferential placement of AF. PC patency rates are comparable in the two periods.

As would be expected, the accuracy of DU measurements compared to intraoperative findings was 98%. In only three instances, veins measured as 2.5 mm by DU were found to have internal lumens of less than 2 mm at operation and were not used.

Table 5–5 compares dialysis unit census records for the two periods. Of the 60 patients undergoing chronic hemodialysis in June 1994, prior to initiation of our protocol, 5 (8%) were being dialyzed by AF, 39 (65%) by BG, and 16 (27%) by PC. In April 1997, at the end of our study period, of 64 patients undergoing chronic hemodialysis,

TABLE 5–4. RELATIVE FREQUENCIES OF EACH ACCESS TYPE PLACED DURING THE TWO PERIODS

	Before Institution of Protocol (%)	Noninvasive Protocol (%)
Autogenous fistula[a]	14	63
Bridging grafts	62	30
Permanent catheter	24	7

[a] Prevalence significantly different in each group (p <0.05). From June 1992 to August 1994, 183 procedures were performed before institution of protocol. From September 1994 to April 1996, 172 procedures were performed with noninvasive protocol.
Reprinted with permission: Silva MB Jr, Hobson RW II, Pappas PJ, et al. A strategy for increasing use of autogenous hemodialysis access procedures: impact of preoperative noninvasive evaluation. *J Vasc Surg.* 1998;27(92):302–308.

TABLE 5–5. IMPACT OF PROTOCOL ON PATIENT ACCESS PROFILE FROM IN-HOSPITAL DIALYSIS UNIT CENSUS RECORDS

	Before Protocol (%) (June 1994; $n = 60$)	After Protocol (%) (April 1997; $n = 64$)
Dialysis accomplished by:		
AF	8	64
BG	65	30
PC	27	6

Differences are significant for each access type ($p < 0.05$).
Reprinted with permission: Silva MB Jr, Hobson RW II, Pappas PJ, et al. A strategy for increasing use of autogenous hemodialysis access procedures: impact of preoperative noninvasive evaluation. *J Vasc Surg.* 1998;27(92):302–308.

41 were being dialyzed by AF (64%), 19 (30%) by BG, and 4 by PC (6%), which confirms a significant ($p < 0.01$) increase in the use of AF.

No postoperative infections were observed with AF, whereas 6 were seen with BG and 2 with PC insertion. Symptomatic steal was observed in 1 BG, whereas none were observed with AF. Pseudoaneurysm developed in 2 BG. One AF developed diffuse aneurysmal dilatation with maximal diameters of 2.0 cm, but continues to function successfully more than 2 years following placement.

SUMMARY

Higher early failure rates for AF as compared to BG may be attributed to the difficulty in selecting adequate veins and arteries that will mature reliably into functioning AF by clinical examination alone. Use of preoperative assessment by DU for vascular selection reduces early failures significantly and correlates with the improved patency rates and decreased rates of infection reported for mature AF as compared to BG. Because of their location in the forearm, AF performed in this manner fulfills the goal of preservation of more proximal vasculature for future hemodialysis-access procedures.

Duplex ultrasound has been used effectively in mapping lower extremity arteries and veins for infrainguinal bypass procedures as well as for surveillance of infrainguinal vein grafts. We have used DU in the upper extremity for selection of patients for AF hemoaccess and for clinical follow-up of patients undergoing hemodialysis access procedures. DU has enhanced our ability to identify arteries and veins suitable for AF. In addition to selection of patients for radiocephalic fistulas, a larger group of patients has been selected for superficial venous transposition in the forearm, described by our group.

In our series, utilization of AF has increased significantly as a result of preoperative noninvasive evaluation of the upper extremity. Early failure rates for AF were significantly reduced, from 36% prior to implementation of the protocol to 8.3% in our current experience. Patency rates for AF and BG also have improved significantly. In addition, reduced infection rates for AF also support our recommendation for the preferential use of AF.

Our strategy for management of dialysis-dependent patients has significantly altered our use of procedures for hemodialysis access. Since the introduction of a preoperative noninvasive protocol, we have significantly increased use of AF. Currently, 64% of our patients undergo successful hemodialysis using AF.

We recommend the use of noninvasive DU evaluation of the upper extremity in concert with application of the technique of superficial venous transposition in the forearm to increase opportunities for the placement of AF, thereby reducing dependency on BG and PC with their attendant shortcomings.

REFERENCES

1. Stanley JC, Barnes RW, Earnst CV, et al. Vascular surgery in the United States: workforce issues. *J Vasc Surg.* 1996;23:172–181.
2. Hobson, RW II. Presidential address: practice patterns in vascular surgery—implications for the certification and training of vascular surgeons. *J Vasc Surg.* 1997;26:905–912.
3. United States Renal Data System. USRDS 1995 Annual Data Report. The National Institutes of Health, National Institute of Diabetes and Digestive and Kidney Diseases, Bethesda, MD, 1995. *Am J Kidney Dis.* 1995;26:4.
4. Brescia MJ, Cimino JE, Appel K, Hurwich BJ. Chronic hemodialysis using venipuncture and a surgically created arteriovenous fistula. *N Engl J Med.* 1966;275(20):1089–1092.
5. Palder SB, Kirkman RL, Whittemore AD, et al. Vascular access for hemodialysis. *Ann Surg.* 1985;202(2):235–239.
6. Rivers SP, Scher LA, Sheehan E, et al. Basilic vein transposition: an underused autologous alternative to prosthetic dialysis angioaccess. *J Vasc Surg.* 1993;18:391–396.
7. Sands J, Miranda CL. Increasing numbers of AV fistulas for hemodialysis access. *Clin Nephrol.* 1997;48:114–117.
8. Rohr MS, Browder W, Frenz GD, McDonald JC. Arteriovenous fistulas for long-term dialysis. *Arch Surg.* 1978;113:153–155.
9. Lazarides MK, Iatrou CE, Karanikas ID, et al. Factors affecting the lifespan of autologous and synthetic arteriovenous access routes for haemodialysis. *Eur Surg.* 1996;162:297–301.
10. Limet RR, Lejeune GN. Evaluation of 110 subcutaneous arteriovenous fistulae in 100 chronically hemodialysed patients. *J Cardiovas Surg.* 1974;15:573–576.
11. Silva MB Jr, Hobson RW II, Jamil Z, et al. Vein transposition in the forearm for autogenous hemoaccess. *J Vasc Surg.* 1997;26(6):981–988.
12. Silva MB Jr, Hobson RW II, Pappas PJ, et al. A strategy for increasing use of autogenous hemodialysis access procedures: impact of preoperative noninvasive evaluation. *J Vasc Surg.* 1998;27(92):302–308.
13. Leopold PW, Shandall A, Kupinkski AM, et al. Role of B-mode venous mapping in infrainguinal *in situ* vein–arterial bypasses. *Br J Surg.* 1989;76:306–307.
14. Beidle TR, Brom-Ferral R, Letourneau JG. Surveillance of infrainguinal vein grafts with duplex sonography. *AJR* 1994;162:443–448.

6

Appropriateness of Noninvasive Follow-Up for Vascular Procedures

Dennis F. Bandyk, MD

The application of noninvasive vascular testing for surveillance of arterial reconstructive procedures and endovascular interventions has evolved to the point of becoming a recommended standard of vascular surgery. The vascular laboratory can assist in the evaluation of patients with suspected early technical failure and identify problems in clinically successful arterial repairs before failure develops (i.e., vein graft thrombosis caused by myointimal hyperplasia). For surveillance to be worthwhile, the arterial repair must be subject to modes of failure that are preventable, the incidence of late failure must be sufficient to warrant concern, and secondary procedures to correct identified abnormalities should be associated with a high success rate and low morbidity. Noninvasive testing following carotid surgery, infrainguinal bypass grafting, and peripheral arterial angioplasty have been recommended, but concerns remain regarding both the extent and frequency of testing.[1-3] Appropriateness of follow-up testing is based on the premise that serial patient follow-up will improve outcome, whether it be stroke prevention or limb salvage. The additional health care costs and demands on vascular laboratory personnel mandate that postoperative testing is limited to instances that affect clinical decision making or ensure continued patency. At present, intensive surveillance of aortic reconstructions, visceral arterial repairs, or procedures for portal hypertension is not recommended, but noninvasive testing is useful to confirm initial anatomic and hemodynamic success, and then to evaluate patients when recurrent symptoms or signs occur. If a vascular prosthesis has been implanted, assessment of anastomotic and graft integrity should be performed annually by physical examination and, if necessary, duplex ultrasonography.

In a number of prospective studies, duplex surveillance has demonstrated residual and acquired postimplantation lesions that developed in a significant number of patients after peripheral transluminal angioplasty (PTA), carotid endarterectomy (CEA), or infrainguinal bypass. Within a year, focal flow abnormalities (increase in peak systolic velocity, spectra broadening) have been detected in 10% to 20% of repairs.[2,4-8] The majority of these abnormalities are asymptomatic when first identified, but long-term follow-up has confirmed a higher failure rate in reconstructions with abnormal scans. Although the natural history of duplex-detected abnormalities has not been determined for each type of arterial reconstruction with respect to the likelihood of regression, persistence, or progression, in approximately one-half of cases progression to a high-grade stenosis occurs; thus caution is warranted regarding the repair of all early appearing lesions.[8,9] Many defects detected during the early postoperative period (<3 months) represent a *residual defect* caused by technical imperfection or residual disease rather than a *de novo* lesion.[9,10] These residual defects have the velocity spectra of a moderate (30% to 60% diameter reduction) stenosis and thus are not associated with impairment of blood flow or perfusion pressure. It does appear that such residual defects in an arterial reconstruction or a PTA site increase the likelihood of clinical failure, usually as a result of progressive myointimal hyperplasia. If the site develops velocity spectra of high-grade stenosis, the potential for thrombosis of the involved arterial segment is increased. Thus, an important strategy to reduce the need for postoperative surveillance is emphasis on using operative and endovascular procedures combined with monitoring techniques, such as intraoperative duplex ultrasound, to ensure technical precision and normal blood flow patterns.

A goal of postoperative surveillance is not only to detect lesions with a potential for precipitating failure, but also to assist the surgeon in deciding when to recommend a revision procedure. Clinician evaluation by patient interview and physical examination of the arterial system (pulse palpation, auscultation for bruit, hand-held continuous-wave Doppler survey) is not as accurate as duplex ultrasonography in the detection of postintervention stenosis or grading severity. When a lesion progresses to or presents as a high-grade stenosis, symptoms of ischemia may also be present. The subsequent time interval for these lesions to trigger thrombosis is unpredictable but may be quite brief when associated with a low flow state. Intervention should be instituted before an embolic or thrombotic complication occurs, with secondary procedures being performed electively on arterial segments while still patent.

Postoperative noninvasive testing requires the use of serial duplex scans for optimum diagnostic accuracy and to identify lesion progression. Scans should be performed using the same ultrasound system and transducer with duplex-derived velocities acquired using a Doppler angle of 60° or less. When serial studies are compared, the same Doppler correction angle should be used to minimize interpretation errors based on changes in systolic or diastolic velocity spectra. In general, a change in stenosis severity category [i.e., for <75% diameter reduction (DR) to a greater than >75% DR] is necessary to report disease progression. Critics of postoperative noninvasive testing feel duplex surveillance cannot be justified based on its costs and limitations in diagnosis, representing another tier of costs and testing because it does eliminate the need for other confirmatory vascular imaging studies (contrast or magnetic resonance angiography). Thus, in evaluating the risk–benefit aspects of postoperative surveillance, the morbidity and expense—which includes serial testing, on occasion confirmatory arteriography prior to revision, and the secondary revision procedures—must be balanced against the costs and morbidity of arterial repair failure. At present, a surveillance program, combined with corrective intervention after duplex-detected stenosis is identified can be recommended after CEA, infrainguinal vein bypass, and femoropopliteal PTA. A precise definition of "cost-effective" or appropriate noninvasive testing has not been agreed on, but following intervention for atherosclerotic arterial occlusive disease, "quality-of-life" outcome assessments and assurance of long-term patency are just as important as the medical expenses incurred.

SURVEILLANCE AFTER CAROTID ENDARTERECTOMY

Rationale

Occlusion or stenosis following CEA represents a procedure failure, even in the asymptomatic patient. The incidence of neurological symptoms following successful CEA is known to be low (1% to 4%), but when the reconstructions have been studied by duplex scanning, an alarming high incidence (7% to 22%) of restenosis has been reported.[5,10–18] The natural history of early recurrent stenosis is generally felt to be benign, and in some instances has been noted to regress.[17] Stroke after CEA is uncommon (0.3% to 1% per year) with a similar incidence of ipsilateral and contralateral hemispheric events.[14,15,18] Approximately one-half of ipsilateral strokes are related to high-grade stenosis or occlusion of the endarterectomized internal carotid artery (ICA).[5,15,18,19] Kinney et al.[15] reported the incidence of late stroke was increased ($p < .0001$) in patients with restenosis or occlusion (3 of 35) compared to patients with duplex scans showing normal operated ICAs or less than 50% restenosis (3 of 426). In some patients, "recurrent" carotid stenosis is actually a residual stenosis, and progression of these defects to a high-grade (>80% diameter reduction) occlusive lesion or ICA occlusion has been observed.[5,13,19] Thus, technical precision or carotid reconstruction can have an impact on both early and late stroke prevention.

Duplex surveillance following CEA has been recommended by an expert panel of vascular surgeons commenting on vascular laboratory utilization and payment.[1] Scans at 6 weeks, 1 year, and annually thereafter were recommended to establish a baseline and determine whether myointimal hyperplasia develops within the operative site and to what degree. No studies have verified the cost–benefit of duplex surveillance. The efficacy of this approach can be influenced by a number of factors, including the use and type of intraoperative assessment, the prevalence of contralateral (>50% DR) ICA stenosis, and the frequency of high-grade (>80% DR) postendarterectomy stenosis in an individual surgeon's practice. Bilateral extracranial carotid disease is common in patients identified as candidates for surgical intervention. Approximately one-third of patients will have severe (>50% DR) disease, of which one-quarter are high-grade (>70% to 80% DR) stenosis severe enough to warrant staged endarterectomy and one-quarter are total occlusions.[13,18] The remainder have a 50% to 74% DR asymptomatic stenosis, which should be followed using duplex ultrasound. The frequency of disease progression of the unoperated carotid bifurcation increases with time: 5% to 10% at 3 years; 10% to 18% by 5 years; and 30% by 7 to 10 years.[18] In a 1992 report, Mackey et al.[5] estimated the cost of duplex surveillance per stroke prevented was approximately $25,000. Although most vascular surgeons recommend duplex surveillance after CEA, the essential features (timing of postoperative studies, criteria for intervention) of the diagnostic and management algorithm varies. It is generally agreed that with careful patient selection, reoperation for high-grade ICA stenosis is appropriate, associated with a reduction in stroke risk, and can be performed with perioperative complication rates and long-term outcome similar to that of primary procedures. A conservative approach to asymptomatic carotid restenosis is recommended, as several studies have documented a similar stroke rate for patients with or without more than 50% DR stenosis.[13,14] Intervention is typically recommended for asymptomatic recurrent stenosis when progression to more than 75% DR based on duplex velocity criteria are demonstrated and the lesion is amenable to surgical or endovascular (stent angioplasty) intervention.

Noninvasive Testing Follow-up

Postoperative duplex scans (CPT 93880) are indicated to confirm normal healing of the operated carotid bifurcation, identify repair site abnormalities (stenosis, residual plaque, mural thrombus, aneurysm change), follow sites of restenosis for progression, and detect progression to a high-grade stenosis for patients with contralateral disease. After CEA, duplex testing is recommended during the early postoperative period and at intervals thereafter, the frequency determined by initial scan findings and the presence of contralateral disease. For lesions that are progressive and have narrow lumen diameter of more than 75% based on velocity spectra criteria (Table 6–1), operation is recommended in otherwise healthy, active patients without severe concomitant cardiopulmonary disease.

University of South Florida Experience and Surveillance Protocol

From 1992 to 1997, 190 patients who underwent 212 CEAs were enrolled in a postoperative stroke prevention program that included duplex scan surveillance at 6 month intervals. High-grade ICA stenosis [peak systolic velocity (PSV) > 250–300 cm/s; diastolic velocity >125 cm/s] prompted recommendation for repair. An average of five postoperative scans were performed during the mean follow-up of 27 months, including an intraoperative scan, one at 3 months, and every 6 months thereafter.

Intraoperative duplex scanning resulted in immediate revision of 9 (4%) of repairs. One perioperative (30-day) stroke occurred; a patient who developed ICA thrombosis in the recovery room following carotid repair with vein-patch angioplasty, and intraoperative revision, but the final scan showing residual stenosis (PSV = 200 cm/s). During follow-up, 1 occlusion occurred and 6 carotids developed more than 50% DR restenosis. One 1 patient progressed to more than 75% stenosis and underwent reoperation (<1% yield for duplex surveillance). The yield of duplex surveillance for the unoperated ICA was higher ($p = .003$); 12% of unoperated carotids experienced disease progression (stenosis, $n = 21$; occlusion, $n = 2$), leading to 7 CEAs for high-grade stenosis. Disease progression to more than 75% stenosis and carotid surgery was five times higher in patients with 50% to 74% DR stenosis versus less than 50% DR stenosis of the unoperated carotid. All but 1 patient requiring contralateral CEA had more than 50% ICA stenosis when first seen. No disabling strokes ipsilateral to the operated carotid artery occurred during follow-up, but 3 contralateral strokes occurred. Overall, only 8 (4%) patients developed disease severe enough to warrant additional intervention, and the incidence of disabling stroke was 1.6%.

TABLE 6–1. UNIVERSITY OF SOUTH FLORIDA DUPLEX SCAN CRITERIA
FOR GRADING PRIMARY AND RECURRENT INTERNAL CAROTID ARTERY
OCCLUSIVE DISEASE

| Disease Category (DR) (%) | Internal Carotid Artery | | | |
	PSV (cm/s)	ICA/CCA Ratio	End-Diastolic Velocity (cm/s)	Color Doppler Image
0–15	<100	<2	NA	Minimal or no lumen reduction
16–49	<125	<2.5	NA	Moderate lumen reduction
50–74	>125	>4.5	<125	Severe lumen reduction
75–99	>290	>4.5	>125	High-grade stenosis
Occlusion	NA		NA	No flow visualized

DR, diameter reduction; NA, not applicable

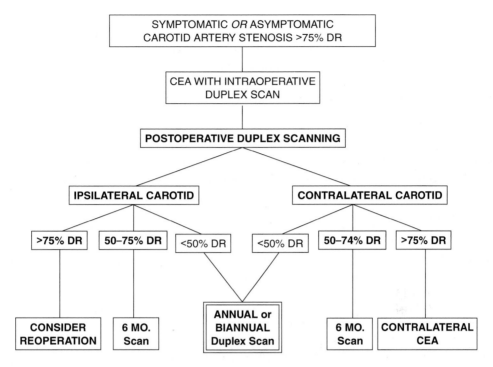

Figure 6–1. Algorithm used at the University of South Florida (USF) for frequency of duplex scan surveillance following carotid endarterectomy (CEA) based on intraoperative duplex findings and the severity of contralateral carotid artery stenosis.

Based on this experience, the duplex surveillance protocol at USF was modified to that outlined in Fig. 6–1. The need and frequency of duplex scans is based on the result of intraoperative scanning and the presence of contralateral disease (>50% DR stenosis). An annual or biannual duplex scan (cost $125) is adequate when a technically precise repair is achieved and minimal contralateral disease is present. For patients found to have residual ICA stenosis or contralateral 50% to 74% DR ICA stenosis, duplex scans at 6-month intervals are recommended. Using these guidelines, approximately one-quarter of patients required duplex surveillance at 6-month intervals (cost $250/year).

SURVEILLANCE AFTER INFRAINGUINAL BYPASS GRAFTING

Rationale

Autologous vein bypass grafts constructed by either the reversed or *in situ* grafting technique are prone to develop intrinsic lesions during the first months to years after implantation into the arterial circulation.[6-8,20-23] Despite careful operative technique and assessment of technical adequacy by completion arteriography, a spectrum of abnormalities can be present within the arterial repair or develop as a result of arterialization of the vein graft. Clinical examination detects only the most severe lesions and, in general, development of recurrent limb ischemia is most commonly associated with graft thrombosis. Prospective observational studies that utilized duplex scanning to monitor vein bypass grafts have confirmed that fibrous strictures develop in 20% to 30% of infrainguinal bypasses during the first postoperative year.[6-9,23] The development of these lesions, which are typically the result of myointimal hyperplasia, was associated with a threefold increase in graft occlusion and accounted for up to 80% of graft failures within 5 years of operation. Lesions with duplex-derived velocity spectra of a high-grade stenosis (peak systolic velocity >300 cm/s, end-diastolic velocity >20 cm/s, velocity ratio across the stenosis >3.5) and more than 70% DR by arteriography are associated with graft failure if not corrected promptly.[7] Multiple investigators have observed an approximate 25% incidence of graft thrombosis in stenotic bypasses when a policy of no intervention was followed. Idu et al.[7] reported all infrainguinal vein grafts with a 70% DR stenosis eventually occluded, compared to 10% of grafts with similar lesions that were revised. Mattos et al.[24] reported similar results when color-duplex scanning identified a stenosis (velocity ratio at the stenosis >2). Grafts with a duplex-detected stenosis had lower patency rate (57%) compared to grafts with a normal scan (83%). Surveillance programs based on duplex scanning have resulted in assisted-primary patency rates of 82% to 93% at 5 years, compared to 60% to 70% patency for bypasses followed clinically, and 30% to 50% patency rates after secondary procedures to salvage thrombosed vein grafts.[6,24-26] The enhanced patency associated with duplex surveillance has also been verified in a randomized, prospective clinical trial conducted in Malmo, Sweden.[26] A 25% improvement in infrainguinal vein bypass patency at 3 years (78% versus 53%) occurred with duplex surveillance, but no significant benefit was documented in polytetrafluoroethylene (PTFE) or PTFE-composite graft patency. These observations are important measures of efficacy because "redo" bypass procedures are difficult or may not be possible if no suitable outflow artery or other vein conduit is available.

Important issues regarding graft surveillance include when the duplex surveillance program should begin, how long it should continue, and at what frequency testing should be performed. The first duplex scan should be performed at operation, if feasible; if not, prior to discharge from the hospital. The "predischarge" duplex examination permits identification of bypasses with residual graft defects. Such duplex abnormalities are prone to progress in severity, which, if it occurs and is corrected in a timely fashion, dramatically reduces the incidence of graft thrombosis within first year after surgery. Graft surveillance should be indefinite, with the majority of patients requiring an annual evaluation after the first year. It has been suggested that if limb loss could be prevented in only 2% of patients, a duplex surveillance program would be cost-effective.

The decision to recommend graft revision has not been clearly defined, except when patients have recurrent symptoms of claudication or develop ischemic lesions. Studies at the University of South Florida have documented symptomatic limb ischemia in only one-third of patients, despite conclusive vascular laboratory evidence for a "hemodynamically failing" bypass graft. Our experience indicates graft revision should be recommended to asymptomatic patients whenever a correctable lesion has been identified by duplex scanning or arteriography and a low-flow state has developed in the graft (compared to prior studies). Typically, a decrease in ankle–brachial index (ABI) (>0.15) has been measured. Essentially, all revised graft lesions repaired have had velocity spectra of greater than 75% DR stenosis (Table 6–2).

Noninvasive Testing Follow-up

Infrainguinal graft surveillance should consist of measurement of ABI and color-duplex imaging of the entire bypass, including anastomosis and adjacent inflow and outflow

TABLE 6–2. DUPLEX CLASSIFICATION OF RESIDUAL OR ACQUIRED GRAFT STENOSIS

DR (% stenosis)	Vr and Velocity Spectra
<20	Vr < 1.5; mild spectral broadening in systole; PSV < 150 cm/s
20–50	Vr 1.5–2; spectral broadening throughout systole; no change in waveform configuration across stenosis; PSV < 180 cm/s
50–75	Vr > 2; severe spectral broadening in systole with reversed flow components; PSV > 180 cm/s
>75	Vr > 3.5; severe lumen reduction and "flow jet" present by color Doppler imaging; PSV >300 cm/s; end-diastolic flow velocity in flow jet >40 cm/s

DR, diameter reduction; Vr, velocity ratio; PSV, peak systolic velocity.

arteries. The hemodynamics of graft flow is characterized by duplex-derived PSV measurements along the length of the bypass, recorded at a Doppler angle of 60°, and configuration of the velocity spectra waveform. The frequency of surveillance can be based on the type of bypass and the results of the intraoperative/predischarge duplex scan (Table 6–3). Grafts modified at operation, grafts requiring early thrombectomy, grafts with residual flow abnormalities, and low-flow grafts require more intensive surveillance than vein bypasses with a normal intraoperative duplex scan.[6,22,23,27] The incidence of graft revision is two to three times more frequent, typically within the first 6 months postoperatively. A baseline duplex scan and ABI is obtained prior to hospital discharge (scan 1). Graft assessment is repeated approximately 4 to 6 weeks postoperatively (scan 2), once all surgical wounds have healed. If no graft abnormality is detected, scan 3 is obtained 3 months later (4–6 months postoperatively). Subsequent intervals of surveillance depend on graft type and risk of graft stenosis, the time intervals being either 3 or 6 months. Despite a normal intraoperative duplex scan, reversed vein bypasses have higher incidence of "acquired" stenosis (28%) than an *in situ* saphenous vein bypass (10%), accounting for the 3-month surveillance schedule during the first 18 months after implantation.[23] Beyond 2 years if the graft duplex scan is normal and atherosclerotic disease risk factors are controlled, annual graft

TABLE 6–3. SURVEILLANCE SCHEDULE FOR GRAFTS WITH NORMAL DUPLEX SCANS

Bypass Type	Surveillance Interval	
	3 Months	*6 Months*
Alternative vein bypass	X	
Vein bypass modified at operation	X	
Reversed saphenous vein bypass	X	
Nonreversed saphenous vein bypass		X
In situ saphenous vein bypass		X
Second postoperative year: two scans at 18 and 24 months		
Third year and annually thereafter: duplex scan and ABI measurement		

Time 0: vein bypass with normal intraoperative or predischarge duplex scan.
Scan 1: 4–6 weeks postoperatively [grafts with residual or *de novo* stenosis detected required surveillance every 6-weeks to evaluate for lesion resolution or progression (see Fig. 6–2)].
Scan 2: 3 months postoperatively.
Scans 3 and 4: 3- or 6-month interval, depending on graft type.

surveillance can be recommended to the patient. Although the value of surveillance after prosthetic grafting has not been proved, Calligaro et al.[28] found duplex scanning was more sensitive (81%) than ABI and clinical evaluation (24%) in predicting failure or the need for revision. Duplex surveillance of failing prosthetic grafts found 48% of stenoses were located at anastomotic site, 38% at inflow or outflow arteries, and 14% within the graft. It should be noted that, in general, thrombosis of a prosthetic graft is not as detrimental as vein graft occlusion because both thrombolysis and surgical thrombectomy are more effective in restoring patency. Some vascular groups have recommended vein graft replacement, if feasible, when repetitive prosthetic graft thrombosis is encountered.

Grafts with low flow and high outflow resistance are at increased risk for thrombosis.[13,20] The measurement of low blood flow velocity ($Vp < 40$ cm/s) in the normal (no stenosis, diameter 5 mm or less) vein bypass indicates low volume flow, particularly if no flow during diastole is present. In these patients, I have prescribed oral sodium warfarin anticoagulation (INR 1.6–1.8) plus aspirin (325 mg/day), and made a diligent search for any inflow or outflow occlusive lesion. This regimen is also prescribed following femorodistal PTFE bypass grafting when $Vp < 60$ cm/s is measured in the graft by duplex scanning prior to discharge. The rationale for this practice is based on the concept of "thrombotic threshold velocity," which is different between autologous vein and prosthetic bypasses.

Our recommendations for infrainguinal vein graft surveillance, including duplex criteria for intervention, are outlined in the algorithm shown in Fig. 6–2. When a focal color-flow disturbance is detected in the bypass, careful interrogation of the stenosis

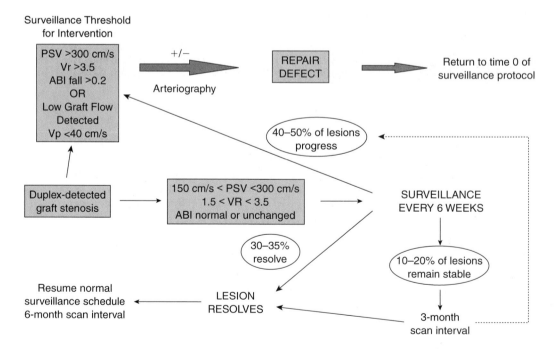

Figure 6–2. Algorithm of infrainguinal vein graft surveillance based on duplex scanning and measurement of ankle–brachial indices (ABI). Intervention is based on velocity spectra criteria. Vp, peak systolic velocity in normal caliber (4 mm) mid- or distal graft segment; PSV, peak systolic velocity at lesion; Vr, velocity ratio across a stenosis (PSV proximal to stenosis/maximum PSV at or immediately distal to stenosis).

with measurement of maximum peak systolic velocity (PSV) and the velocity ratio (Vr) should be performed. A PSV that exceeds 150 cm/s accompanied by a Vr ≥ 1.5 indicates a graft abnormality, and when detected within 6 months of the primary procedure should be monitored for progression to a high-grade stenosis. Pressure- and flow-reducing stenoses have the color Doppler features of "flow jet" in systole, an apparent reduction in lumen caliber, and increased flow velocity both systole (>300 cm/s) and diastole (40–100 cm/s). The peak systolic Vr across the stenosis is greater than 3.5. Stenoses with these velocity spectra are flow-limiting in systole with compensatory flow in diastole, accounting for loss of the normal triphasic velocity waveform and decrease in ABI. Intermediate graft stenoses (Vp of 150–300 cm/s, Vr < 3.5) are not pressure- or flow-reducing at basal flow, and when detected within the first 3 months of surgery may regress (30% to 35% likelihood), remain stable, or progress (40% to 50% likelihood) to a high-grade stenosis. Serial scans at 4- to 6-week intervals are recommended to follow the hemodynamic course of these lesions for progression. In general, the lesion will stabilize or progress within 4 to 6 months of identification.[8,9,29,30] An important feature of a "graft-threatening" stenosis is its propensity to progress in severity or form surface thrombus, events that precipitate thrombosis. Duplex scanning is unable to predict which lesion will progress, accounting for the observation that some lesions with spectra of a severe stenosis are "benign" and do not progress with time.

Threshold Velocity Criteria for Graft Revision

Repair of all graft stenoses identified by duplex scanning with a Vp > 300 cm/s and Vr > 3.5 is recommended, especially if the lesion has progressed on serial scans or is associated with low graft flow velocity (<45 cm/s).[31] The combination of high- and low-velocity criteria identifies bypasses with low flow and a pressure-reducing stenosis. In a prospective study, the application of these threshold criteria identified all grafts at risk for thrombosis, and only one lesion with high-velocity criteria regressed.[29]

USF Experience

Over a 6-year time period (1991–1997), during which approximately 525 infrainguinal vein bypasses have been monitored using duplex scanning, 118 (22%) grafts underwent revision for a duplex-identified stenosis. Sixty-two lesions had open surgical revision, and 56 (47%) had PTA of an angiography confirmed greater than 70% DR vein graft stenosis. Stenosis-free patency at 2 years was identical for surgical (63%) and endovascular intervention (63%). Overall assisted graft patency (life-table analysis) was 91% at 1 year and 80% at 3 years. No patient died as a result of intervention for primary or recurrent graft stenosis. We have observed that early appearing (<3 month) or residual graft stenoses are not suited for PTA, as are diffuse vein graft stenosis or focal lesions in small diameter (<3.5 mm) vein grafts. Failure rate after PTA has been reported to be high (>50% within 3 months), and surgical repair by either interposition graft replacement or balloon angioplasty is recommended. Following balloon angioplasty or open surgical repair, the frequency of graft surveillance is based on beginning of the surveillance protocol again.

Lesions amenable to revision continue to develop years after infrainguinal bypass grafting. Erickson et al.[32] emphasized the need for indefinite bypass surveillance in a study of 556 bypasses followed for up to 13 years. Approximately one-fifth (18%) of initial interventions for a duplex-detected graft abnormality occurred 2 years after bypass grafting. The majority (63%) of the defects involved the conduit or its anastomoses, 17% were inflow procedures, 17% were outflow procedures, and 3% (one graft) required replacement. Our experience has been similar; approximately 20% of all graft revisions were performed 2 years after bypass grafting. These data support annual duplex evaluation of infrainguinal bypasses to detect atherosclerotic disease progression or aneurysmal changes in the venous conduit. In general, graft surveillance can be implemented by well-trained vascular technologists, and only when graft abnormalities are identified is a physician-directed evaluation required.

Cost-Effectiveness

The efficacy of vein graft surveillance requires comparison of the incidence of "graft-threatening" lesions, the cost of screening, the risk of untreated graft stenosis, and the benefit of surgical revision. The risk–benefit of surveillance should ultimately be expressed in limbs saved, graft failures avoided, and outcomes measures of patient function and well-being.

The vascular laboratory represents a significant cost of graft surveillance. In USF vascular laboratory, a duplex scanner and a vascular technologist are utilized for approximately one-third of the weekly hours for postoperative graft examinations, with an annual cost of approximately $38,000 for 1-year's surveillance (equipment lease, maintenance agreement, salary/benefits, overhead). Assuming 100 infrainguinal vein bypasses are performed each year, and each is scanned five times in the first postoperative year (predischarge; 6 weeks; 3, 6, and 12 months), the cost of each scan is $76. In Florida, the Medicare carrier reimburses for three postoperative studies during the first year, with any additional testing requiring justification (i.e., abnormal graft scan or recent graft revision). The graft duplex study that includes measurement of bilateral ankle–brachial indices is coded and charges as a limited duplex study (CPT 93926) with global fee of $200 (Medicare reimbursement of $147). Thus, reimbursement for graft surveillance is comparable to the cost of testing in an outpatient clinic vascular laboratory.

With an incidence of graft stenosis during the first year of approximately 25%, the cost of detecting each stenosis is $38,000/25 = $1520. Approximately 80% of detected stenoses progress to high-grade lesion and require revision. The estimated cost of stenosis revision is $5500 for percutaneous balloon angioplasty (used in 20% of lesions) and $9000 for direct surgical repair (vein-patch angioplasty, interposition grafting). The total cost of graft revision would be ($5500 × 4 PTAs) plus ($8000 × 16 surgical procedures) for a total of $150,000. Thus, the cost of 1-year's surveillance of 100 grafts, including revision of 20 grafts, is approximately $188,000. In the United States, the cost of amputation and rehabilitation has been estimated at approximately $22,000, and that of a re-do bypass procedure at approximately $21,000. A duplex surveillance program would need to save between seven and eight limbs or avoid a similar number of repeat bypasses to be cost-effective. The use of catheter-directed thrombolysis to salvage acutely thrombosed vein grafts followed by PTA or direct surgical revision would result in costs similar or higher than a re-do bypass procedure because of the expense of the thrombolytic agent and a late failure rate of approximately 40% to 50%.

Based on the costs of graft surveillance, the salvage of 7% to 8% of bypasses would indicate a beneficial effect. The 15% improvement in limb salvage reported by Moody et al.[25] and the 25% increase in graft patency shown in a randomized, prospective clinical trial suggest graft surveillance[26] should be "part of the service" vascular surgeons provide after infrainguinal vein bypass grafting. It should be emphasized that the benefit of surveillance is highly dependent on the durability and morbidity of procedures used to correct "graft stenoses." Most series have reported a mortality of less than 0.5%, early failure rate of less than 1%, and late failure rate of less than 15% with graft revision procedures.[6]

SURVEILLANCE OF PERIPHERAL TRANSLUMINAL ANGIOPLASTY

Rationale

The early failure rate of PTA, defined as technical failures plus technical success without clinical improvement 1 month after treatment, correlates with type (stenosis vs occlusion) and location (aortoiliac vs femoropopliteal–tibial) of lesion treated, the status of the distal runoff (focal vs diffuse atherosclerotic disease), and the severity of ischemia. Early failure rates of 9% to 47% have been reported, with factors such as restenosis at the PTA site due to elastic recoil, dissection, *in situ* thrombosis, or spasm being implicated.[2,33,34] Even in limbs with improved ABIs, flow hemodynamics in the treated arterial site affects PTA durability. Using duplex scanning, Mewissen et al.[2] found a PTA site with velocity spectra of a greater than 50% diameter residual stenosis can be masked by completion angiography but was predictive of clinical deterioration and PTA failure. Using life-table analysis, a diameter-reducing stenosis of more than 50% was associated with only a 15% 1-year clinical success rate, versus 84% rate when a functional residual stenosis of less than 50% was confirmed. Spikjkerboek et al.[35] also reported a residual duplex stenosis 1 day after PTA predicted failure within a year. These observations support duplex surveillance after PTA to assess technical adequacy of the procedure. A persistent stenosis appears likely to progress to a lesion with similar hemodynamics of the primary lesion or to lead to occlusion. One application has been the use of duplex scanning to evaluate carotid stent procedures.

Late failure of PTA can result from restenosis at the treated arterial site (typically the result of myointimal hyperplasia), progression of atherosclerosis remote from the PTA site, or a combination of both disease processes. Identification of a failing PTA does not preclude redilation or stent placement. In general, repeat PTA has been associated with a patency identical to a first-time procedure.

Noninvasive Testing Follow-up

Lower limb and carotid angioplasty sites should be evaluated by duplex scanning (CPT 93926 or 93882) and measurment of limb pressures if appropriate and incompressible arteries are not present. Examinations should be recorded on videotape and velocity spectra recorded at 60° Doppler-corrected angle. Arterial stents should be imaged in sagittal and transverse planes, and stent diameters measured to identify interval stent compression. Special attention should be directed at stent endpoints, where restenosis and disease progression typically occurs. Criteria for an abnormal PTA sites is a Vp of more than 150 cm/s and Vr at the site of duplex-detected stenosis of more than 2. A high-grade stenosis is associated with Vp of more than 300 cm/s, Vr greater than 3.5, and end-diastolic velocity greater than 80 cm/s. If the initial duplex scan demonstrates a residual stenosis of less than 50% and the ABI is greater than 0.2 compared to pre-PTA level, follow-up surveillance at 3 months and every 6 months thereafter is recommended. If the initial duplex scan detects a stenosis of more than 50% but less than 75% diameter, a repeat study in 1 to 2 weeks is recommended to assess for improvement or deterioration in functional patency. A progression PTA-site stenosis should be subjected to repeat dilatation, atherectomy, or stent placement depending on the anatomic characteristics of the lesion/arterial segment.

Cost-Effectiveness

No study has verified the cost–benefit aspects of routine duplex surveillance after PTA. Assumptions that PTA is less expensive therapy relative to surgical bypass grafting have proved to be correct, particularly when the efficacy of PTA is based on strict outcome criteria and reporting standards. One report has indicated the ratio of hospital costs of PTA to bypass surgery were 53% for patients with claudication but rose to 75% for patients with critical ischemia.[36] Angioplasty failure is expensive and efforts to improve the durability of these procedures must be encouraged. The predictive value of duplex-monitored angioplasty needs to be further evaluated. In approximately 20% of peripheral PTA procedures when duplex-monitored angioplasty has been performed, the duplex scan indicated a residual stenosis and led to additional dilation with a larger balloon, prolonged balloon inflation time, or placement. The goal of duplex-monitored PTA is to normalize the velocity spectra in the treated artery/graft segment. In general, the procedure is not terminated until the maximum systolic velocity is less than 150 cm/s and/or Vr is less than 2. A persistent duplex-detected stenosis at the PTA sites has correlated with early failure, with progression to a stenosis with similar hemodynamics as the primary lesion. Katzenschlager et al.[36] at the University of Vienna confirmed that the results of PTA of short stenosis or occlusion in the femoropopliteal arterial segment with duplex-scan guidance were similar to results of PTA performed under fluoroscopic control. In 3 of 25 successful duplex-guided PTAs, the scan detected residual stenosis and the PTA was repeated with a larger balloon. Duplex monitoring has also been used with an ultrasound-guided catheter system that permits PTA without ionizing radiation or use of pressure measurements to verify successful PTA. The criteria for success was a Vr less than 2 across the treated arterial segment. Using this system, Cluley et al.[37] found supplemental use of a high-pressure balloon redilation or an athrectomy device was necessary in 5 (29%) of 17 patients because of a residual duplex-detected stenosis. Because PTA has a failure mode similar to vein bypass, the cost-effectiveness of surveillance should be comparable.

OUTCOME OF SURVEILLANCE

The ability of duplex ultrasonography to identify postoperative arterial lesions during their preocclusive phase, coupled with a low potential for complication and high frequency of interpretable studies, make it the preferred technique for monitoring arterial procedures and endovascular interventions. The development of color Doppler and availability of suitable probes/standoffs minimize many of the cumbersome aspects of intraoperative imaging. Such initial surveillance offers the possibility of minimizing subsequent surveillance (i.e., if a normal repair site void of focal flow abnormalities can be documented). Ideally, a cost-effective surveillance program should identify arterial reconstructions at risk for thrombosis; help clarify the mechanism of failure should unexpected thrombosis occur (embolism, hypercoagulable state); be applicable to all patients; and be practical in terms of time, effort, and cost. After infrainguinal vein bypass, the unexpected failure rate with normal surveillance studies should be less than 2% per year. Institution of a vein graft surveillance program in our Division of Vascular Surgery helped achieve an assisted primary graft patency of 96% at 1 year and 88% at 3 years in patients undergoing *in situ* or reversed saphenous vein femoro-distal bypass grafting.[6,23,38] The ultimate fate of an arterial reconstruction depends on patient factors and mechanisms of arterial healing and disease, but the philosophy and commitment of the surgeon/interventionist to value of postoperative surveillance are also important. Certainly for vein bypasses, a premium must be placed on detection of the failing graft before thrombosis occurs. For other arterial interventions, the failure modes and accompanying patient outcomes may not warrant intensive surveillance, particularly if recurrent disease is not associated with adverse events. At present, a surveillance program combined with corrective intervention following stenosis detection can be recommended after CEA, infrainguinal vein bypass, and femoropopliteal PTA.

REFERENCES

1. Strandness DE Jr, Andros G, Baker JD, et al. Vascular laboratory utilization and payment: report of the Ad Hoc Committee of the Western Vascular Society. *J Vasc Surg*. 1992;16:163–170.
2. Mewissen MW, Kinney EV, Bandyk DF, et al. The role of duplex scanning versus angiography in predicting outcome after balloon angioplasty in the femoropopliteal artery. *J Vasc Surg*. 1992;15:860–864.
3. Strandness DE Jr. Indications for and frequency of noninvasive testing. *Semin Vasc Surg*. 1994;7:245–260.
4. Kinney EV, Seabrook GR, Kinney LY, et al. The importance of intraoperative detection of residual flow abnormalities after carotid artery endarterectomy. *J Vasc Surg*. 1993;17:912–923.
5. Mackey WC, Belkin M, Sindhi R, et al. Routine postendarterectomy duplex surveillance: does it prevent late stroke? *J Vasc Surg*. 1992;6:934–940.
6. Bandyk DF, Kinney EV, Bandyk DI, Mewissen MW, et al. Monitoring functional patency of *in situ* saphenous vein bypasses: the impact of a surveillance protocol and elective revision. *J Vasc Surg*. 1989;9:284–296.
7. Idu MM, Blankensteijn JD, de Gier P, et al. Impact of a color-flow duplex surveillance program infrainguinal graft patency: a five-year experience. *J Vasc Surg*. 1993;17:42–53.
8. Mills JL, Bandyk DF, Gahtan V, et al. The origin of infrainguinal vein graft stenosis: a prospective study based duplex surveillance. *J Vasc Surg*. 1995;21:16–25.
9. Caps T, Cantwell-Gab K, Bergelin RO, et al. Vein graft lesions: time of onset and rate of progression. *J Vasc Surg*. 1995;22:466–475.
10. Barnes RW et al. Reucrrent versus residual carotid stenosis: incidence detected by Doppler ultrasound. *Ann Surg*. 1986;203:652–660.
11. Cato R, Bandyk DR, Karp D, et al. Duplex scanning after carotid reconstruction: a comparison of intraoperative and postoperative results. *J Vasc Tech*. 1991;15:61–65.
12. Healey DA, Zierler RE, Nicholls SC, et al. Long-term follow-up and clinical outcome of carotid restenosis. *J Vasc Surg*. 1989;10:662–669.
13. Cook JM, Thompson BW, Barnes RW. Is routine duplex examination after carotid endarterectomy justified? *J Vasc Surg*. 1990;12:334–340.
14. Bernstein EF, Torem S, Dilley RB. Does carotid restenosis predict an increased risk of late symptoms, stroke, or death? *Ann Surg*. 1990;212:629–636.
15. Kinney EV, Seabrook GR, Kinney LY, et al. The importance of intraoperative detection of residual flow abnormalities after carotid endarterectomy. *J Vasc Surg*. 1993;17:912–913.
16. Carbello RE, Towne JB, Seabrook GR, et al. An outcome analysis of carotid endarterectomy: the incidence and natural history of recurrent stenosis. *J Vasc Surg*. 1996;23:749–754.
17. Nichols SC, Phillips DJ, Bergelin RO, et al. Carotid endarterectomy: relationship of outcome to early restenosis. *J Vasc Surg*. 1985;2:375–381.
18. Ricotta JJ, O'Brien MS, Deweese JA. Natural history of recurrent and residual stenosis after carotid endarterectomy: implications for post-operative surveillance and surgical management. *Surgery*. 1992;112:656–663.
19. Washburn WK, Mackey WC, Belkin M, et al. Late stroke after carotid endarterectomy: the role or recurrent stenosis. *J Vasc Surg*. 1992;15:1032–1037.
20. Sladen JG, Reid JDS, Cooperberg PL. Color flow duplex screening of infrainguinal grafts combining low- and high-velocity criteria. *Am J Surg*. 1989;158:107–112.

21. Mills JL, Harris EJ, Taylor LM, et al. The importance of routine surveillance of distal bypass grafts with duplex scanning: a study of 379 reversed vein grafts. *J Vasc Surg.* 1990;12:379–389.

22. Bandyk DF, Mills JL, Gahtan V, et al. Intraoperative duplex scanning of arterial reconstructions: fate of repaired and unrepaired defects. *J Vasc Surg.* 1994;20:426–433.

23. Gupta AK, Bandyk DF, Chenavechai D, et al. Natural history of infrainguinal vein graft stenosis relative to bypass grafting technique. *J Vasc Surg.* 1997;25:211–225.

24. Mattos MA, van Bemmelen PS, Hodgson KJ, et al. Does correction of stenoses identified with color duplex scanning improve infrainguinal graft patency? *J Vasc Surg.* 1993;17:54–66.

25. Moody AP, Gould DA, Harris PL. Vein graft surveillance improves patency in femoropopliteal bypass. *Eur J Vasc Surg.* 1990;4:117–120.

26. Kundell A, Linblad B, Bergqvist D, et al. Femoropopliteal graft patency is improved by an intensive surveillance program: a prospective-randomized study. *J Vasc Surg.* 1995;21:26–34.

27. Nielsen TG, Jensen LP, Schroeder TV. Early vein bypass thrombectomy is associated with an increased risk of graft related stenosis. *Eur J Endovasc Surg.* 1997;13:134–138.

28. Calligaro KD, Musser DJ, Chen AY, et al. Duplex ultrasonography to diagnose failing arterial prosthetic grafts. *Surgery.* 1996;120:455–459.

29. Westerband A, Mills JL, Kistler S, et al. Prospective validation of threshold criteria for intervention in infrainguinal vein grafts undergoing duplex surveillance. *Ann Vasc Surg.* 1997;11:44–48.

30. Gahtan V, Payne LP, Roper LD, et al. Duplex criteria for predicting progression of vein graft lesions. *J Vasc Tech.* 1995;19:211–215.

31. Erickson CA, Towne JB, Seabrook GR, et al. Ongoing vascular laboratory surveillance is essential to maximize long-term *in situ* saphenous vein bypass patency. *J Vasc Surg.* 1996;23:18–27.

32. Hewes RC, White RI Jr, Murray RR, et al. Long-term results of superficial artery angioplasty. *AJR.* 1986;146:1025–1028.

33. Milford MA, Weaver FA, Lundell CJ, Yellin AE. Femoropopliteal percutaneous transluminal angioplasty for limb salvage. *J Vasc Surg.* 1988;8:292–295.

34. Spikjerrboer AM, Nass PC, de Valois JC, et al. Evaluation of femoropopliteal arteries with duplex ultrasound after angioplasty. Can we predict results at one year? *Eur J Endovasc Surg.* 1996;12:418–423.

35. Hunink MGM, Cullen KA, Donaldson MC. Hospital costs of revascularization procedures for femoropopliteal arterial disease. *J Vasc Surg.* 1994;19:632–641.

36. Katzenschlager R, et al. Femoropopliteal artery: initial and 6-month results of color duplex US-guided percutaneous transluminal angioplasty. *Radiology.* 1996;199:331–334.

37. Cluley SR, Brener BJ, Hollier L, et al. Transcutaneous ultrasonography can be used to guide and monitor balloon angioplasty. *J Vasc Surg.* 1993;17:23–31.

38. Bergamini TM, Towne JB, Bandyk DF, et al. Experience with *in situ* saphenous vein bypasses during 1981 to 1989: determinant factors of long-term patency. *J Vasc Surg.* 1991;13:137–149.

7

Duplex Imaging for Chronic Venous Insufficiency

D. E. Strandness, Jr., MD

INTRODUCTION

For the practicing physician, chronic venous disease presents as a "black box."[1] He or she is aware that the disease is most likely on the venous side of the circulation, but understands little else. In general, we are taught that there are two common types of venous disease, and it is from this classification that we proceed. The first and most obvious diagnosis that all are aware of (including our patients) is varicose veins. These are evident to even the casual observer and it is often said that if you have seen one case, you have seen them all. However, the problem is not that simple and in order to plan therapy intelligently, more information is needed. There are really two scenarios that are often brought to our attention. The first and most simple scenario is the patient who appears with visible varicosities and wishes an opinion as to their natural history and the forms of therapy that might be available. The second and more difficult presentation is the problem of edema, pain, skin changes, and ulceration. When this is seen, the assumption is usually made that the underlying problem is secondary to a venous system that has been damaged by a previous episode of venous thrombosis. This entity is often referred to as the *postphlebitic syndrome.* However, this terminology is probably incorrect and should more appropriately be called the *postthrombotic syndrome.*[2] Its recognition is obviously important, but simply making the diagnosis is not enough if one is to treat the patient intelligently.[3]

It is well known that patients with primary varicose veins often have a strong family history of the problem.[4] Furthermore, these patients in general have a benign course and infrequently present with advanced skin changes and ulceration. The varices are often a cosmetic problem alone. However, patients can complain of pain, burning, and some edema, although it is rarely of the magnitude observed with the postthrombotic syndrome. Both primary varicose veins and the postthrombotic syndrome present different and challenging problems that are being addressed in more detail. In order to be more specific, it is necessary to review in some detail the information obtained by duplex scanning and how the problems can be sorted out.

VENOUS ANATOMY

The venous system is extremely complex for a host of reasons that are important to understand. From a physiologic standpoint, it has both a very important capacitance and thermoregulatory function.[1] The volume of blood found in the veins of the lower extremity depend on gravitational factors as well as systemic needs for an adequate cardiac output and organ perfusion. The superficial veins participate actively in the control of body temperature.

One of the unique aspects of the venous system is the very extensive system of valves that exist at nearly all levels of the venous system. These structures are subject to dramatic changes in venous pressure and volume either from gravitational effects or from the action of the muscle pump(s). The location of these valves tells us a great deal about their importance in the maintenance of normal pressure–flow relationships. In the abdomen, there are no valves in the inferior vena cava and very few persons (<10%) are found to have one valve in the common iliac vein. About 24% of subjects have a valve found in the external iliac, with 67% having a valve in the common femoral vein. Once we pass beneath the inguinal ligament, the situation changes drastically. There is a very common valve found at the termination of the greater saphenous vein at the level of the fossa ovalis. Varying numbers of valves are seen in the superficial femoral vein (usually less than five). A valve is often found in the popliteal vein that is considered by some practitioners to be critical in terms of its role in the prevention of the complications of the postthrombotic syndrome.[5] Below the knee there are hundreds of valves found at all levels, which says a great deal about this critically important region of the venous system. Why so many valves here as compared to other areas? This is no doubt related to the activity of the calf muscle pump and the amount of pressure generated with calf contraction. Because there are several points of entry for the draining veins in the calf, loss of valve function would result in serious derangement of the pressure–flow relationships in this area.

Normally the valves permit antegrade flow only. With each calf muscle contraction, the veins are emptied, with a resultant fall in pressure. With successive contractions, the distal venous pressure falls to very low levels and only very slowly return to the preexercise levels when the exercise is terminated. In fact, it is this fall and slow return in venous pressure that remains the "gold standard" for defining the status of the deep and superficial systems in this location.

One important anatomic landmark that must be recognized is the compression of the left common iliac vein by the overlying right common iliac artery. It is well known that compression at this level can lead to the iliac compression syndrome, with leg swelling and pain, which may in some circumstances lead to total occlusion with the development of iliofemoral thrombosis. The compression itself, if clinically significant, can be detected by ultrasonic duplex scanning. With the advent of thrombolysis in the treatment of iliofemoral thrombosis, investigation of this area should become routine for the vascular diagnostic laboratory.

Flow is normally phasic with respiration and variations in intraabdominal pressure.[6] Venous flow can become pulsatile if there is right heart failure, with distention of the inferior vena cava allowing retrograde pulsations from the right ventricle. With the patient in the supine position or −10° Trendelenberg, the flows detected at the level of the external iliac to the popliteal vein should be spontaneous and phasic with respiration. In the veins below the knee this may not be the case, due to the fact that vasoconstriction secondary to environmental factors may be present there. However, patency of the deep veins can be documented by carrying out augmentation maneuvers with compression of the foot. The venous valves are remarkable structures that appear flimsy but are extremely tough and able to withstand large swings and changes in venous pressure without becoming incompetent. The other remarkable feature in their design is the fact that the vein can undergo extensive changes in diameter and still remain competent. In other words, there is considerable redundancy built into the system.

Historically, it has been thought that most diseases of the venous system can be explained as a failure of the perforating veins that connect the superficial to the deep system. It is not often appreciated, but the two largest perforating veins are the greater and lesser saphenous veins. As is well known they are the most commonly involved veins in patients who present with varicose veins. An interesting observation was made by van Bemmelen and associates,[7] who noted that patients with a previous history of deep vein thrombosis (DVT) and who developed ulceration nearly always had associated incompetence of the greater and lesser saphenous veins. In a similar number of patients who did not develop ulceration, there was no incompetence of these major perforating veins. This raises several questions as to why and how these veins become incompetent because the greater and lesser saphenous veins are not commonly involved with the thrombotic process in the first instance. This is a very interesting problem to be investigated because it might well tell us more about the pathophysiology of the postthrombotic syndrome.

What about the perforating veins? The anatomy of the greater saphenous vein is remarkably constant, particularly in its point of entry into the deep venous system. For the surgeon there are very few surprises, except with perhaps the number of veins that join it just prior to the fossa ovalis. This is not true for the lesser saphenous vein, which has an extremely variable point of entry into the deep venous system. This fact has become very evident as duplex scanning has become more widely applied. The location of the perforating veins along the medial side of the lower leg and in proximity to the gaitre area have occupied a considerable amount of attention and conjecture. In fact, the "ankle blow-out" syndrome is a term that was often applied, implicating that communicating veins play an important role in the pathogenesis of pigmentation and ulceration.[8] Although many physicians believe that the perforating veins, which lie on a line starting just posterior to the medial malleolus, connect the deep system to the greater saphenous vein, this is not true. The perforating veins connect with the posterior arch vein, which then joins with the greater saphenous vein near the knee.[9]

Although it is commonly believed that the major perforating veins (so-called Cockett's perforators) have a fairly constant location, this would not appear to be the case.[10–12] In the study by Staubesand and associates,[11] only 7.3% of the veins belonging to this category of communicating veins are to be found where they are reported. Fischer and coworkers[10] noted similar findings. Thus one cannot rely on the reported locations as being accurate in planning therapy. It is also well known that not all communicating veins are along the medial side of the leg. For practitioners who have performed subfascial ligations by the method of Linton,[13] communicating veins can be found as far lateral as the fibula on the lateral side of the leg. A fact that has also become apparent is that, even in patients with postthrombotic syndrome, not all perforating veins are incompetent. Phillips and Cheng[14] studied the relationship between perforator size and incompetence. By using ultrasound, they found that reflux could be demonstrated in 60% of veins with a diameter greater than 4 mm. For veins with a diameter in the 3 to 4 mm range, reflux was demonstrated in 45%; this rate dropped to 25% for veins that were less than 3 mm in diameter.

A very important yet disputed factor relates to the importance of damage to each of the venous components and their contribution to the postthrombotic syndrome. It is necessary to review the relationship between physiology and function. It is accepted that adequate function of the calf muscle pump is critical for protection of the lower limb, not only in terms of the prevention of edema, but also in protecting the skin in the gaitre area, where most postthrombotic ulcers are found. In order for hyperpigmentation and ulceration to occur, there must be some derangement in the pressure–flow relationships of the deep, perforating, and superficial veins in this location. It is these facts that led Cockett and others[8] to propose the theory of the "ankle blow-out" syndrome. This theory ties together the problems of the deep system, the connecting perforators, and the superficial system as well. As noted previously, the greatest interest has been in the size and location of what are commonly referred to as the Cockett perforators, which traditionally were thought to play a critical role in the development of pigmentation and ulceration. The theory, which is quite simple, can be expressed as follows:

1. The deep system is damaged by a previous episode of DVT, which can lead to obstruction, valvular incompetence, or both.[3]
2. Flow that is normally from the superficial to the deep system is now directed outward through the incompetent perforators to the gaitre area.
3. The blood exits, producing what is referred to as a high-pressure leak.
4. Over time there is rupture of the capillaries, with leakage of red blood cells into the subcutaneous tissue.
5. The red cells break down with the hemoglobin further degraded to hemosiderin, which, over time, leads to atrophy, thinning of the skin, and what is commonly referred to as *lipodermatosclerosis,* which is an end stage of this process.
6. When lipodermatosclerosis develops, minor trauma to the area leads to the development of an ulcer.

Although this procession of events would appear to be a logical sequence, it is difficult to unify each of the elements of this scenario. Why, for example, should the perforating veins become incompetent? Is it due to the progressive enlargement that accompanies the reverse flow leading to valve incompetence? Does it occur because there are some perforating veins that do not have valves, so egress to the superficial system is unimpeded? Why is it as noted by Van Bemmelen and associates[7] that patients who develop ulceration nearly always show evidence of incompetence of the greater and lesser saphenous system, whereas patients without ulceration have competent greater and lesser saphenous systems? Why do the greater and lesser saphenous systems become incompetent when they were not involved in the thrombotic process in the first instance?

To further complicate the situation, we have to deal with the problem of the "floppy" valve syndrome. What is it, and how does it enter the picture? It is thought to be a congenital abnormality leading to valvular incompetence. This was brought to our attention by Kistner, who pioneered the use of valvuloplasty for the correction of incompetent valves in the superficial femoral vein. These patients were identified by descending venography, which identified the location and extent of the valvular reflux.[15] With the availability of duplex scanning, this can now be used to document findings and it is not necessary to use venography to detect the valvular incompetence, its location, and its long-term outcome.

Interruption of the perforating veins, with or without stripping, was a popular method for treatment of postthrombotic ulceration. A variety of surgical approaches were used to identify and interrupt these perforators. These involved the use of long incisions that were the frequent site of infection and wound breakdown. Because of this problem the operation was largely abandoned, but the concept and the approach has been reborn by the introduction of subfascial endoscopic perforator surgery (SEPs).[16] By virtue of the fact that the incisions are limited in both size and scope, it could become possible to prevent the high-pressure leaks by interrupting the key perforators along the medial side of the calf. The procedure is combined with ligation and stripping of the greater and lesser saphenous systems. The indications and results of this new approach are currently under evaluation.

PERFORMING THE EXAMINATION

It is clear to this author that the examination should be tailored to the specific clinical situation. A minimal examination should encompass the following items:

1. Document patency of the deep system.[3]
2. Assess the presence or absence of reflux.[17–19]
3. Identify the site(s) of reflux precisely.[20]
4. Provide a "road map" for the surgeon if operation is to be undertaken.

PROCEDURES

The proper use of duplex scanning involves the use of imaging (B-mode), color, and spectral Doppler display of the velocity patterns.[21] The studies are best done with the patient in −10° Trendelenberg position to ensure near maximal filling of the superficial and deep venous system. Although the testing for valvular incompetence is best done with the patient standing, this is not easy to learn and we have found that the −10° position is nearly as good for the detection of valvular incompetence. The examination procedure is as follows:

1. The procedure starts at the level of the common femoral–external iliac vein level.
   a. Imaging with compression is carried out. If the problem is chronic venous disease, one not need to go as high as the common iliac vein, which we do in cases of suspected acute DVT.
   b. The flow patterns should be examined both with the color flow and spectral Doppler to note its phasicity and spontaneity.
   c. Valvular reflux can be tested by performance of a Valsalva maneuver. With this test, the valves should close in less than 2 seconds.[22]
2. The same procedure should be done for the superficial femoral vein and the greater saphenous system at its termination and down to the level of the knee.
3. The popliteal vein is best studied with the patient prone. Valvular reflux can be tested by both Valsalva and limb compression. Flow patterns are assessed at this level as well.
4. For the below-the-knee segments, color flow is essential because it permits identification of the paired veins down to the level of the foot. Here, limb compression is used to document valve incompetence.
5. In examining for perforating veins, the examination is carried along the course of the posterior arch vein, using color to identify the veins themselves and to document both their size and the direction of flow.
6. In the case of primary varicose veins it is necessary to document the actual sites of incompetence and the identification of any perforators, such as midthigh, to

permit proper eradication of these channels at the time of operation, whether by a direct approach or by using the SEPs procedure.

7. If reflux testing is done with the patient upright, valve closure time should be less than 0.05 seconds.

DISCUSSION

The years since the late 1970s have seen an explosion in our knowledge of an area that had been relegated for much too long to the backseat of clinical problems. It was not long ago that the patient with the postthrombotic syndrome was simply given a diagnosis, with very little consideration given to the actual basis for the problem. For reasons that are difficult to understand, chronic venous disease has not excited much interest in medical circles, except perhaps with the general and vascular surgical groups. The reason for this probably lies in the limited number of therapeutic options that are available to the physician. In general terms, therapy, when considered, fell into the following categories:

1. For varicose veins, treatment was largely confined to three types:
   a. Vein ligation and stripping.
   b. Compression hose.
   c. Sclerotherapy.
2. For postthrombotic syndrome, compression therapy became the standby for nearly all physicians, who came to believe that this alone could result in healing of nearly all ulcers while minimizing the amount of edema and pain the patient suffered.
3. With the recognition that incompetence of the venous valves were implicated in nearly all cases of postthrombotic pain, swelling, and ulceration, attempts were made to correct this problem by surgical means. The initial attempts at valve repair were confined to the superficial femoral vein, in which it had been demonstrated by descending venography that the more proximal valves were indeed incompetent. It also turned out that it was possible to identify a group of patients with the "floppy" valve syndrome. The etiology of this problem remains a bit mysterious, but it appears that most practitioners feel this is not due to damage from venous thrombosis. This proves to be important because the remainder of the valves in the distal limb are often normal.
4. As noted earlier, the resurrection of the perforator concept and the new attempts to interrupt these by the SEPs procedure has brought new life to this procedure and concept as well. It is interesting that patients do well if the problem is not postthrombotic and there is no associated obstruction of the deep venous system. This procedure is under investigation at present, and in a few years we should have more definitive answers to this problem.

This resurgence of interest in the superficial and deep system has been possible because of the emergence of techniques such as ultrasonic duplex scanning. The major advantages of this approach are as follows:

1. All segments of the superficial, deep, and perforating veins can be examined.[17,18]
2. Patency can be established by simple compression maneuvers and the use of flow patterns.[23]
3. The sites of valvular incompetence can be assessed in a quantitative manner.[23]

The amount of information that can be obtained from a single complete examination can be overwhelming. However, this approach is the first and only one to date that has provided the kind of information that is needed to understand the pathophysiology of both acute and chronic venous disease. To what extent should the entire venous system be examined in the patient with chronic venous disease? The following suggestions are offered:

1. For primary varicose veins, the sites of incompetence must be determined if an intelligent surgical procedure is to be carried out.
2. Examination for perforating veins should be along the course of the posterior arch vein and at the knee and midthigh levels as well.
3. For patients with postthrombotic changes, the entire deep and superficial venous system must be studied to assess sites of occlusion and valvular incompetence.

ASSESSMENT OF DATA

Our group in Seattle has been most interested in using this method to follow patients over time after an episode of acute DVT to assess the effects of the disease on venous patency and valve function. This experience produced some interesting findings, the most important of which are as follows:

1. Spontaneous lysis of the thrombus is common.[24]
2. Recanalization occurs rapidly as the thrombus lyses.[18,23,24]
3. The more rapid the lysis of the thrombus, the more likely it is that valve function will be preserved.[23]
4. The combination of valvular incompetence and residual obstruction are the most common findings in patients who develop the postthrombotic syndrome.[3]
5. Rethrombosis, extension, or development of new thrombi during the acute and chronic phase of therapy is common.[23]

Other practitioners have also used this technology to document the relationship between reflux and outcome. Welch and associates[25] studied a total of 500 limbs using the cuff deflation technique in the upright position. They noted a relationship between reflux in the deep system and the severity of the limb involvement. Of interest was the finding that the incidence of isolated reflux in the superficial femoral vein and the popliteal vein did not differ by functional class, and that combined reflux in the popliteal vein and the superficial venous system was found in 53% of the class 3 limbs, as compared to 18.5% of the class 2 limbs. They concluded that as the amount of reflux in the deep system increases, the severity of the venous disease also increases.

A very important question relates to the extent of the valvular insufficiency in patients who are labeled as having primary varicose veins. This author has long maintained that the disease should be confined to the superficial venous system. Sakurai and coworkers[26] examined the legs of 240 patients with primary varicose veins using both color-flow ultrasound and photopethysmography with below-the-knee tourniquets. They concluded that femoropopliteal reflux contributed to the pathophysiology of venous stasis and was important in the symptoms related to involvement of the perforating and short saphenous vein.

In an exhaustive study of 776 limbs with primary varicose veins and 166 with lipodermatosclerosis, Myers and associates[27] documented the sites of involvement with duplex scanning. Most of the limbs with complications had either superficial reflux alone or in combination with reflux in the deep system. Reflux in the posterior tibial veins was more common with complications when compared to the patients with uncomplicated primary varicose veins. These authors concluded that attention to the superficial system alone may sufficient for most patients with complications. Abu and coworkers[28] found that patients with long saphenous reflux could possess it without having reflux at the level of the saphenofemoral junction. Although incompetent thigh perforators could be found in a minority of these cases, it was not inevitable. This study clearly showed that in some cases, ligation of the saphenofemoral junction alone will not suffice to treat the patient adequately.[28]

Duplex scanning is also of great value after operation in determining if the planned procedure was successful. McMullin and associates[29] investigated the findings after high ligation and multiple avulsions for the treatment of varicose veins. They found that in 54 limbs that underwent the procedure, there were 2 in which there was persistent reflux at the junction. In 24 limbs, there was persistent reflux down the greater saphenous vein, pointing out that high ligation alone was not a good method of treating this problem. Similarly, Nash[5] looked at the outcome following procedures to treat ulceration in 90 patients. When the popliteal vein was incompetent, the failure rate was unacceptably high. There were 12 patients with this finding who failed to heal. When 11 of these patients had a valve transplant, their venous pressures postexercise fell and the ulcers went on to heal.

Acknowledgment
Supported in part by NIH Grant 5RO1HL36095-12.

REFERENCES

1. Strandness DE Jr. Hemodynamics of the normal arterial and venous system. In: Strandness DE, Jr., ed. *Duplex Scanning in Vascular Disorders,* 2nd ed. New York: Raven Press, 1993:45–79.
2. Strandness DE Jr, Langlois YE, Cramer MM, et al. Long-term sequelae of acute venous thrombosis. *JAMA.* 1983;250:1289–1292.
3. Johnson BF, Manzo RA, Bergelin RO, et al. Relationship between changes in the deep venous system and the development of the postthrombotic syndrome after an acute episode of lower limb deep vein thrombosis: a one- to six-year follow-up. *J Vasc Surg.* 1995;21:307–313.
4. Strandness DE Jr, Thiele BL (eds). *Selected Topics in Venous Disorders: Pathophysiology, Diagnosis and Treatment.* New York: Futura Publ Co., 1981.
5. Nash TP. Venous ulceration: factors influencing recurrence after standard surgical procedures. *Med J Aust.* 1991;154:48–50.
6. Moneta GL, Bedford G, Beach K, et al. Duplex ultrasound assessment of venous diameters, peak velocities and flow patterns. *J Vasc Surg.* 1988;8:286–291.
7. Van Bemmelen PS, Bedford G, Beach KW, et al. Status of the valves in superficial and deep venous system in chronic venous disease. *Surgery.* 1991;109:730–734.
8. Cockett FB, Jones, DFE. The ankle blow-out syndrome: a new approach to the varicose ulcer problem. *Lancet.* 1953;1:17–23.
9. Hobbs JT. *The Treatment of Venous Disorders.* Philadelphia: J.P. Lippincott Co.; 1977.
10. Hanrahan LM, Araki CT, Fisher JB, et al. Evaluation of the perforating veins of the lower extremity using high resolution duplex imaging. *J Cardiovasc Surg Torino.* 1991;32:87–97.
11. Staubesand J, Hacklander A. Topography of the perforating veins on the medial side of the leg (Cockett's veins). *Clin Anat.* 1995;8:399–402.
12. Cockett FB. *The Pathology and Surgery of the Veins of the Lower Limb.* Dodd, H. (ed.). Edinburgh, Scotland: Churchill Livingstone; 1976.
13. Linton RR. Postthrombotic ulceration of the lower extremity: its etiology and surgical treatment. *Ann Surg.* 1953;138:415–432.

14. Phillips GW, Cheng LS. The value of ultrasound in the assessment of incompetent perforating veins. *Australas Radiol.* 1996;40:15–18.
15. Masuda EM, Kistner RL, Eklof B. Prospective study of duplex scanning for venous reflux: comparison of Valsalva and pneumatic cuff techniques in the reverse Trendelenburg and standing positions. *J Vasc Surg.* 1994;20:711–720.
16. Gloviczki P, Bergan JJ, Menawat SS, et al. Safety, feasibility, and early efficacy of subfascial endoscopic perforator surgery: a preliminary report from the North American registry. *J Vasc Surg.* 1997;25:94–105.
17. Johnson BF, Strandness DE Jr. Ultrasound and venous valvular reflux. *J Vasc Inv.* 1997;3(2):108–113.
18. Markel A, Manzo RA, Bergelin RO, Strandness DE Jr. Valvular reflux after deep vein thrombosis: incidence and time of occurrence. *J Vasc Surg.* 1992;15:377–384.
19. Tullis MJ, Meissner MH, Bergelin RO, et al. The relationship of venous diameter to reflux, cephalad thrombus and cephalad reflux following deep venous thrombosis. *Thromb Haemost.* 1997;77:462–465.
20. Meissner MH, Manzo RA, Bergelin RO, et al. Deep venous insufficiency: the relationship between lysis and subsequent reflux. *J Vasc Surg.* 1993;22:358–367.
21. Strandness DE Jr. *Duplex Scanning in Vascular Disorders,* 2nd ed. New York: Raven Press; 1993.
22. Markel A, Meissner MH, Manzo RA, et al. A comparison of the cuff deflation method with Valsalva's maneuver and limb compression in detecting venous valvular reflux. *Arch Surg.* 1994;129:701–705.
23. Meissner MH, Manzo RA, Bergelin RO, et al. Deep venous insufficiency: the relationship between lysis and subsequent reflux. *J Vasc Surg.* 1993;18:596–608.
24. Killewich LA, Bedford GR, Beach KW, et al. Spontaneous lysis of deep venous thrombosis: rate and outcome. *J Vasc Surg.* 1989;9:89–97.
25. Welch HJ, Young CM, Semegran AB, et al. Duplex assessment of venous reflux and chronic venous insufficiency: the significance of deep venous reflux. *J Vasc Surg.* 1996;24:755–762.
26. Sakurai T, Matsushita M, Nishikimi N, et al. Hemodynamic assessment of femoropopliteal venous reflux in patients with primary varicose veins. *J Vasc Surg.* 1997;26:260–264.
27. Myers KA, Ziegenbein RW, Zeng GH, et al. Duplex ultrasonography scanning for chronic venous disease: patterns of venous reflux. *J Vasc Surg.* 1995;21:605–612.
28. Abu OA, Scurr JH, Coleridge-Smith PD. Saphenous vein reflux with incompetence at the saphenofemoral junction. *Br J Surg.* 1994;81:1452–1454.
29. McMullin GM, Coleridge-Smith PD, Scurr JH. Objective assessment of high ligation without stripping the long saphenous vein. *Br J Surg.* 1991;78:1139–1142.

8

Vein Mapping for Infrainguinal Bypasses

Mark A. Mattos, MD and David S. Sumner, MD

The preferred conduit for infrainguinal bypass grafting is autogenous vein, especially for those grafts extending below the knee or to the ankle or foot.[1] Accurate knowledge of greater saphenous, lesser saphenous, cephalic, and basilic venous anatomy is important for optimal utilization of venous conduits for lower extremity revascularization. Unfortunately, seldom is the course and pattern of these venous systems as simple and straightforward as that described in the anatomy books. In a review of more than 1500 saphenous venous systems evaluated by duplex scanning, a standard greater saphenous vein (GSV) system, defined by a single dominant venous trunk in the thigh continuous with a single dominant vein in the calf, occurred in only 67% of patients. Double venous systems with or without branching were found in 8% and 25% of patients, respectively. The number of branching cutaneous tributaries were noted to be quite variable, whereas the number and location of deep perforating veins remained fairly constant.[2] Not infrequently, suitable veins are difficult to locate because of obesity, vein stripping or removal for previous vascular reconstruction, superficial phlebitis, trauma due to repeated venipuncture, or anatomic variations. In one series, rates of unavailable or inadequate GSV were found in 45% of patients who were candidates for lower extremity arterial revascularization.[3] Searching for veins at the time of operation is not only time-consuming, but is also traumatic; and despite extensive surgical dissection, no acceptable conduit may be found. Clearly, it is advantageous to the surgeon to know the location of veins that can be used and to know which sites need not be explored.

METHODS OF INFRAINGUINAL VEIN MAPPING

Preoperative evaluation of the saphenous vein and other potential venous conduits can be obtained by clinical examination, Doppler assessment, venography, and duplex scanning. Clinical examination by palpation or auscultation can identify the general course of the saphenous vein below the knee, but is inadequate in the thigh and in obese patients with excessive amount of subcutaneous fat. Continuous-wave venous Doppler assessment can be used to help determine patency of the venous segment, but is unable to identify the presence of varicosities, double segments, location of tributaries, or to determine the diameter of the vein.

Prior to the advent of duplex scanning, phlebography was the only method available for preoperative evaluation of potential autogenous grafts. Previous reports have described the usefulness of saphenous venography in delineating the anatomic variability of the GSV.[4-6] Anatomic variations and intrinsic venous abnormalities such as double segments, small diameter, and varicosities were found in approximately 30% of the veins studied, and were noted to influence decisions regarding patient management. Unfortunately, phlebography is invasive, carries a small risk of causing phlebitis in the veins being studied,[7] may fail to disclose anatomic variants,[4] does not predict vein diameters well,[5,8] cannot evaluate vein wall thickness,[9] and is impractical for examining multiple extremities. Furthermore, mapping of the vein and its tributaries on the skin surface is difficult and time-consuming, and because the venogram is typically viewed in only two planes, it fails to provide a true third dimension of tissue depth.

Duplex scanning, however, is noninvasive, subjects the patient to no risk or discomfort, can be used to examine all extremities as potential sources for vein, and has become the method of choice for preoperative vein mapping.[8,10-20] This chapter reviews the clinical goals and indications for preoperative venous mapping, relevant venous anatomy, and the duplex scanning techniques utilized to image potential venous conduits for use as infrainguinal arterial bypasses. Furthermore, the literature is reviewed and the results of duplex venous mapping for determining the location of the venous conduit, identifying anatomic and morphological abnormalities, measuring venous diameter, and predicting suitability of the vein as a conduit for infrainguinal arterial bypass are analyzed.

GOALS OF PREOPERATIVE VEIN MAPPING

The goals of preoperative venous mapping are designed to determine the suitability of venous conduits for use as infrainguinal arterial bypass grafts, and include the following:

1. To identify normal anatomic variations, such as double or bifid systems, that are frequent and may require modification of the surgical approach.
2. To identify areas of scarring or occlusion, that may render the vein unusable or necessitate splicing of two or more segments.
3. To determine whether the venous diameter is sufficiently large to allow it to function adequately as a bypass graft.
4. To identify residual patent segments suitable for bypass grafting in patients who have undergone previous vein harvest or ligation or stripping of varicose veins.
5. To search for alternate sources of vein when the ipsilateral GSV has been used (including the contralateral greater saphenous, the ipsilateral and contralateral lesser saphenous, and the cephalic and basilic veins).
6. To mark the course of all suitable veins on the skin. (This facilitates vein harvest, decreases the duration of the operation, and avoids cutaneous flaps by ensuring that incisions are placed directly over the vein.)

VENOUS ANATOMY

The GSV is the longest vein in the body. The origin of the vein arises from the medial side of the dorsal venous arch of the foot and ascends in front of the medial malleolus, along the medial side of the leg, behind the medial condyles of the tibia and femur, along the medial side of the thigh to the saphenous hiatus, where it terminates at the saphenofemoral junction approximately 4 cm below the inguinal ligament. The origin of lesser saphenous vein (LSV) is from the lateral side of the dorsal venous arch of the foot as it arises from the lateral plantar vein. The vein ascends from behind the lateral malleolus along the lateral side of the tendo calcaneus (Achilles tendon), crosses the tendon to the middle of the back of the leg, and runs straight upward to pierce the deep fascia in the lower popliteal space, where it ends in the popliteal vein between the heads of the gastrocnemius muscle.

The cephalic vein originates from the lateral side of the dorsal venous rete of the hand. The vein curves from the dorsum around to the lateral anterior side of the forearm, ascends in front of the elbow in the groove between the biceps and brachialis, continuing along the lateral side of the biceps to lie in the deltopectoral triangle (groove), where it pierces the clavipectoral fascia to terminate in the axillary vein below the clavicle. In contrast, the basilic vein origin is from the medial side of the dorsal venous rete of the hand. The vein ascends cephalad along the posterior side of the medial forearm, where it crosses to the volar side below the elbow; runs in the groove between the biceps and pronator teres muscles, continuing along the medial border of the biceps; pierces the deep fascia just below the midarm; and runs along the medial side of the brachial artery to the lower border of the teres major, where it joins the brachial vein and forms the axillary vein.

DUPLEX VEIN MAPPING TECHNIQUE

Studies are performed in a warm room with the patient resting comfortably on a bed in the supine position with a 10° to 20° tilt in the reversed Trendelenberg position. The lower extremity to be examined is exposed and externally rotated at the hip with the knee slightly flexed for GSV evaluation. Examination of the LSV requires that the patient be prone, with the bed flat and the leg elevated slightly with a pillow beneath the foot (Fig. 8–1).

A high-resolution duplex scanner with a 7.5 to 10 MHz linear array transducer is preferred. Color-flow facilitates longitudinal scanning and has been shown to expedite the process of venous examination.[21] The GSV is identified at or just distal to the saphenofemoral junction in the longitudinal axis. Scanning of the vein is performed proximally to locate and assess the saphenofemoral junction (Fig. 8–2), and then followed distally along it entire length to the level of the medial malleolus. During this initial longitudinal survey, the vein is inspected for patency and compressibility with light pressure from the transducer, acute and chronic thrombosis, narrow and occluded segments, intraluminal webs, and varicosities. Care must be taken to avoid excessive downward pressure with the transducer, which results in inadvertent compression and subsequent inaccurate assessment of the vein. Transverse imaging is then performed from the saphenofemoral junction to the medial malleolus to estimate venous diameter or compressibility and to identify double segments and tributaries. Special focus is paid to tributaries in the thigh. They must be followed to their termination to rule out the possibility of a double venous system. If a double system is identified, the diameters of each system are measured to determine the dominant system. Diameter measurements of the vein are obtained at the proximal, mid-, and distal thigh, and proximal, mid-, and distal leg. If the vein tapers, measurements should be obtained more frequently. Measurement of venous diameters can also be performed following venous

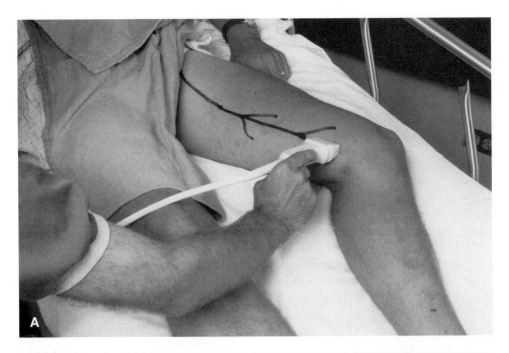

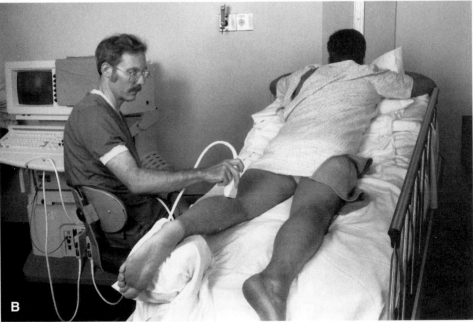

Figure 8–1. Photographs showing patient positions for preoperative vein mapping. (**A**) Greater saphenous vein (GSV). Note patient is in supine position with limb placed in slight flexion and externally rotated. (**B**) Lesser saphenous vein (LSV). Note patient is in the prone position with foot slightly elevated on a pillow.

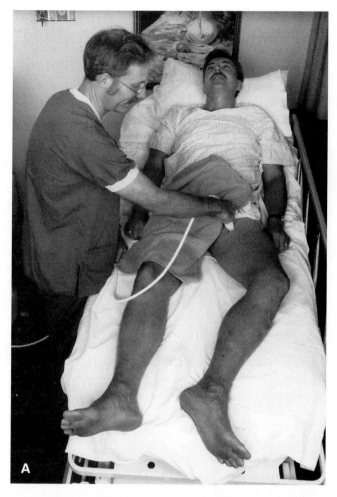

Figure 8–2. (A) Longitudinal scanning technique at the proximal thigh in the area of the sapheno-femoral junction. **(B)** Corresponding color-flow duplex scan showing location of saphenofemoral junction. Note that proximal GSV is dilated and is considered unusable because thrombus is visualized within the lumen.

occlusion for 3 min using a tourniquet or sphygmomanometer cuff (width 12 cm) inflated to 100 mm Hg around the proximal thigh, because the distended venous diameter may more closely approximate the diameter of the vein once it is arterialized.[15,16] As in other venous studies, proximal and distal compression may be used to increase venous flow, access obstructions, and identify sites of valvular incompetence. Unless there are varicosities, incompetence does not preclude using the vein for bypass grafting. As the veins are scanned, the technologist uses an indelible pen to mark the precise course of the vein on the overlying skin, indicating sites of stenosis, occlusion, tributaries, varicosities, bifurcations, or duplications (Fig. 8–3). Depending on the characteristics of the veins and number of sites surveyed, the process may require 20 min to 2 h.

The same technique is used to evaluate the LSV, which is examined with the patient in the prone position. Longitudinal and transverse views, with or without venous occlusion, are performed to locate the course of the vein, identify anatomic

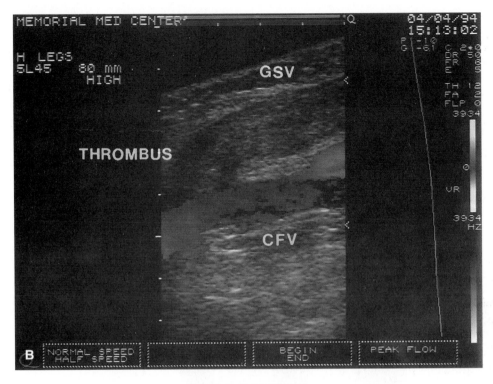

Figure 8–2. (*Continued*)

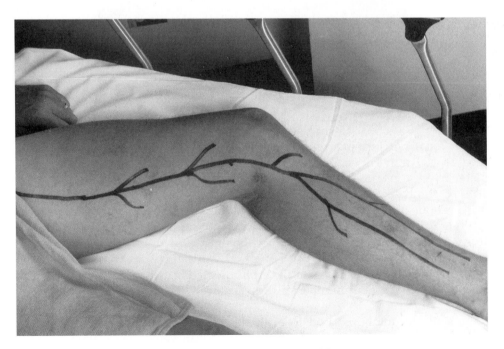

Figure 8–3. Venous map of the GSV.

characteristics, and determine the presence or absence of morphological abnormalities. Duplex mapping of the LSV begins immediately posterior to the lateral malleolus, where the vein arises from the lateral plantar vein, continues across the Achilles tendon at or just above level of malleoli, and proceeds in a cephalad direction along the posterior aspect of the leg until the knee crease is reached, where the lesser saphenous vein ends as it empties into the popliteal vein. Permanent ink is used to mark the course of the vein, internal venous diameters, and all relevant anatomic landmarks (Fig. 8–4).

Duplex mapping of the cephalic and basilic veins is performed with the patient in a supine position, the upper extremity externally rotated, and the palm facing upward in the traditional anatomic position. Similar to lower extremity venous evaluation, longitudinal and transverse views of the veins were obtained from the wrist to the shoulder and were marked and mapped with permanent ink (Fig. 8–5). Particular attention to imaging detail is paid to the veins at the level of the wrist and anticubital fossa. Great care is made to determine patency of the veins because repeated venipuncture trauma in these specific areas is likely to increase the risk of luminal stenosis secondary to intraluminal webs and venous sclerosis.

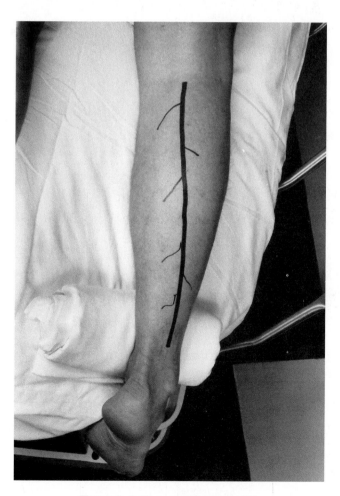

Figure 8–4. Venous map of the LSV.

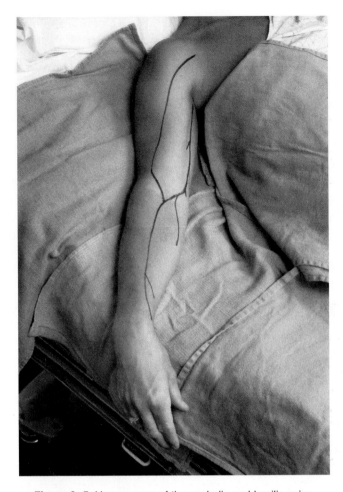

Figure 8–5. Venous map of the cephalic and basilic veins.

RESULTS OF VEIN MAPPING

The predictive value of duplex scanning for finding veins usable as infrainguinal bypass grafts has been reported to be 93% to 98%; but the predictive value for identifying inadequate veins is considerably less, ranging from 50% to 65%, suggesting that at least some veins thought to be unsuitable deserve further investigation (Table 8–1).

TABLE 8–1. PREDICTIVE VALUE OF PREOPERATIVE VENOUS DUPLEX MAPPING COMPARED WITH OPERATIVE FINDINGS

Author	Usable Vein	Inadequate Vein
Buchbinder et al.[19]	93% (14/15)	
Ruoff et al.[9]	96% (82/85)	65% (11/17)
Seeger et al.[7]	98% (50/51)	
McShane et al.[10]	95% (18/19)	
Leopold et al.[12]	98% (224/229)	
Bagi et al.[11]	96% (25/26)	50% (2/4)

Table 8–2 lists probable sources of error for false-positive and false-negative studies. Errors occurred primarily due to variant anatomy or errors in duplex scanning techniques. Failure to identify the presence of a double or triple venous system was the most frequently reported source of venous mapping errors.[10–12,22] The diagnosis of multiple venous segments requires the necessary demonstration of continuous parallel venous trunks to their endpoint in order to document the presence of an additional segment and to avoid one segment being misdiagnosed as a tributary.[10] Also, if one of the segments is considerably smaller than the other this may produce imaging problems, making it difficult to visualize the entire continuous course of the segment. Technical errors can occur as a result of technician inexperience, limitations of the duplex machine, improper patient positioning, or simply as a result of the superficial location of venous segments. It is imperative that the technician perform duplex imaging of the venous system in a continuous fashion over its entire length, otherwise areas of narrowing[22] or the presence or absence of acute or chronic thrombus will be missed.[10] Also, if the technician is not familiar with scanning superficially located vascular structures, the veins are likely to collapse beneath the force of the transducer during imaging, resulting in the inaccurate assessment of the vein segment. Furthermore, the superficial position of the saphenous and upper extremity venous systems places them at a distance where resolution of the vein with duplex scanning is suboptimal, resulting in an inadequate evaluation of the vein.[13] It is important to place the patient in the supine position with the limb dependent in order to optimize visualization and maximize venous distention. One false-negative result was reported when a patient underwent evaluation of the GSV in the recumbent position shortly after an episode of hypotension. The vein was initially believed to be unusable, but following restoration of the blood pressure to a normal range the patient was reexamined with the limb in a dependent position, and the vein was identified as being adequate for bypass.[8]

The use of an acceptable minimal internal venous diameter to determine adequacy of vein utilization for infrainguinal bypass has not yet been defined. Minimal resting internal vein diameters suitable for use as infrainguinal arterial bypass have been reported for diameters of 2.0 mm,[13] 2.5 mm,[14] and 3.0 mm,[15,16] respectively. Leopold and coworkers[14] reported a 98% vein utilization rate using a minimal vein diameter of greater than 2.5 mm in determining feasibility for performance of a successful bypass. Many surgeons consider a vein diameter of 3.0 mm as the lowest acceptable diameter necessary to ensure a successful infrainguinal bypass and abandon veins with resting diameters less than 3.0 mm as inadequate. However, diameters of undistended veins measured with duplex scanning average about 1.0 to 1.5 mm less than they do when they are subjected to arterial pressure or venous occlusion.[11,15–18] Using the technique

---

TABLE 8–2. SOURCES FOR ERROR IN PREOPERATIVE DUPLEX VENOUS MAPPING

False Positive

Failure to image stenotic area of GSV in proximal thigh; vein interpreted as adequate
Venous tributary misinterpreted as GSV; vein interpreted as inadequate.

False Negative

Double and triple venous segments not imaged
GSV collapsed in hypotensive patient; vein interpreted as inadequate
GSV collapsed secondary to increased flow to large perforator vein; vein interpreted as inadequate
GSV not identified due to superficial subcutaneous location; vein interpreted as unusable
GSV with internal diameter less than 2 mm; vein interpreted as unusable

---

GSV, greater saphenous vein.

of venous occlusion, Davies et al[15,16] were able to increase resting internal vein diameters of less than 3.0 mm to a diameter greater than 3.0 mm. Using a vein diameter of 3.0 mm as their lower limit for suitability for distal bypass, the authors concluded that the use of this technique would have theoretically increased their vein utilization rate by 14% to 22%. Furthermore, the authors demonstrated that the functional diameter and adaptive capability of the vein distended by venous tourniquet occlusion could be predicted, and that it coincided closely with the diameters of veins measured at 7 days and at 12 months after insertion in the arterial system.

Accurate preoperative determination of the presence or absence of adequate venous conduits by venous mapping has been shown to lower the incidence of vein graft stenosis,[16] improve the short- and long-term success of lower extremity arterial revascularization,[8,20,23] and decrease the incidence of wound complications following these extensive procedures.[8] Davies and associates[16] noted that vein graft stenoses were more likely to develop in bypasses with resting vein diameters, measured at midthigh and knee level, which did not increase by 10 mm or more with preoperative venous occlusion. Seeger and coworkers[8] prospectively evaluated 51 patients undergoing arterial reconstruction. The presence of an adequate venous conduit for arterial bypass was found to be predictive of significantly higher 30-day limb salvage, 12-month graft patency, and overall limb salvage. Very few patients without usable vein who required distal tibial–peroneal bypass achieved long-term limb salvage with a prosthetic bypass. Panetta and associates[23] observed that long-term graft patency out to 30 months was significantly greater for bypasses with veins without detectable disease compared to bypasses performed with diseased veins (73% vs. 32%). An additional benefit of preoperative vein mapping lies in its ability to avoid or at least minimize major wound complications. A comparison of patients who underwent preoperative vein mapping versus a historical control group of patients who did not receive vein mapping indicated that the performance of preoperative venous mapping was responsible for a significant decrease in venous wound complications following arterial reconstruction (17% vs. 2%).[8]

SUMMARY OF AND CLINICAL INDICATIONS FOR VEIN MAPPING

Duplex vein mapping is an accurate and reliable noninvasive method of evaluating and selecting multiple favorable veins of the lower and upper extremities to serve as suitable venous conduits for infrainguinal arterial bypasses. However, its predictive ability for identifying and excluding veins considered inadequate for use as bypass grafts, particularly veins with resting internal diameters of less than 2.0 mm, is relatively poor. Tourniquet venous occlusion to evaluate the adaptive response of the vein or local exploration of the vein should be undertaken prior to any decision to abandon a vein with resting internal diameter of less than 2.0 mm. The ability of duplex venous mapping to precisely map and simultaneously outline the actual course of the vein, location of tributaries, presence or absence of varicosities, and identification of double systems is a distinct advantage over other vein-mapping techniques. An accurate skin map decreases surgical complications as undermining and dissection of skin flaps are avoided and operating room time is shortened. Duplex scanning is the method of choice for preoperative vein mapping in patients scheduled to receive an infrainguinal arterial bypass.

Vein mapping is indicated in patients who have undergone peripheral arterial or coronary bypasses in which a portion of the ipsilateral GSV has been used, patients who have had venous ligation or limited stripping, patients who had a documented or historical episode of superficial phlebitis, patients who have been or are intravenous drug users, patients who have had trauma to their extremities or have been subjected to many previous vein punctures, and patients with obese extremities. In fact, a strong argument can be made for vein mapping in all patients prior to infrainguinal bypasses to minimize wound complications and to facilitate vein harvest, particularly when the lesser saphenous or the arm veins are to be used.

REFERENCES

1. Londrey GL, Ramsey DR, Hodgson KJ, et al. Infrapopliteal bypass for severe ischemia: comparison of autogenous vein, composite, and prosthetic grafts. *J Vasc Surg.* 1991;13:631–636.
2. Kupinski AM, Leather RP, Chang BB, et al. Preoperative mapping of the saphenous vein. In: Berstein EF, ed. *Vascular Diagnosis.* 4th ed. St. Louis, Missouri: Mosby-Year Book; 1993:897–901.
3. Taylor LM, Edwards JM, Porter JM. Present status of reversed vein bypass: five-year results of a modern series. *J Vasc Surg.* 1990;11:193–205.
4. Veith F, Moss C, Sprayregen S, et al. Pre-operative saphenous venography in arterial reconstructive surgery of the lower limb. *Surgery.* 1979;83:253–256.
5. Shah DM, Chang BB, Leopold PW, et al. The anatomy of the greater saphenous venous system. *J Vasc Surg.* 1986;3:273–283.
6. Mosely JG, Manhire AR, Raphael M, et al. An assessment of long saphenous venography to evaluate the saphenous vein for femoropopliteal bypass. *Br J Surg.* 1983;70:673–674.
7. Bettmann MA, Paulin S. Leg phlebography: the incidence, nature, and modifications of undesirable side effects. *Diagn Radiol.* 1977;122:101–104.
8. Seeger JM, Schmidt JH, Flynn TC. Preoperative saphenous and cephalic vein mapping as an adjunct to reconstructive arterial surgery. *Ann Surg.* 1987:205(6):733–739.
9. Buxton B, Lambert RP, Pitt TE. The significance of vein wall thickness and diameter in relation to the patency of femoropopliteal saphenous vein bypasses. *Surgery.* 1980;87:425–431.
10. Ruoff BA, Cranley JJ, Hannan LA, et al. Real-time duplex ultrasound mapping of the greater saphenous vein before *in situ* infrainguinal revascularization. *J Vasc Surg.* 1987;6:107–113.
11. Buchbinder D, Semrow C, Friedell ML, et al. B-mode ultrasound imaging in the preoperative evaluation of saphenous vein. *Am Surg.* 1987;53(7)368–372.
12. McShane MD, Field J, Smallwood J, Chant ADB. Early experience with B mode ultrasound mapping of the long saphenous vein prior to femorodistal bypass. *Ann R Coll Surg Engl.* 1988;70:147–149.
13. Bagi P, Schroeder T, Sillesen H, Lorentzen JE. Real time B-mode mapping of the greater saphenous vein. *Eur J Vasc Surg.* 1989;3:103–105.
14. Leopold PW, Shandall A, Kupinski AM, et al. Role of B-mode venous mapping in infrainguinal *in situ* vein–arterial bypasses. *Br J Surg.* 1989;76:305–307.
15. Davies AH, Magee TR, Jones DR, et al. The value of duplex scanning with venous occlusion in the preoperative prediction of femoro-distal vein bypass graft diameter. *Eur J Vasc Surg.* 1991;5:633–636.
16. Davies AH, Magee TR, Hayward JK, et al. Prediction of long saphenous vein graft adaptation. *Eur J Vasc Surg.* 1994;8:478–481.
17. Blebea J, Schomaker WR, Hod G, et al. Preoperative duplex venous mapping: a comparison of positional techniques in patients with and without atherosclerosis. *J Vasc Surg.* 1994;20(2):226–233.
18. Head HD, Brown MF. Preoperative vein mapping for coronary artery bypass operations. *Ann Thorac Surg.* 1995;59(1):144–148.
19. Salles-Cunha SX, Beebe HG, Andros G. Preoperative assessment of alternative veins. *Semin Vasc Surg.* 1995;8(3):172–178.
20. Levi N, Schroeder T. Preoperative ultrasound mapping of the saphenous vein: prognostic value on early post operative results, a prospective study. *Osaka City Med J.* 1997;43(1):77–80.

21. Mattos MA, Londrey GL, Leutz DW, et al. Color-flow duplex scanning for the surveillance and diagnosis of acute deep venous thrombosis. *J Vasc Surg.* 1992;15:366–376.
22. Leopold PW, Shandall AA, Corson JD, et al. Initial experience comparing B-mode imaging and venography and venography of the saphenous vein before *in situ* bypass. *Am J Surg.* 1986;152:206–210.
23. Panetta TF, Marin ML, Veith FJ, et al. Unsuspected preexisting saphenous vein disease: an unrecognized cause of vein bypass failure. *J Vasc Surg.* 1992;15:102–112.

III

Preoperative
Evaluation

9

Hypercoagulable Disorders

Donald Silver, MD

The vascular surgeon must have sufficient skills and "tools" to restore or preserve blood flow in the arterial and venous circulations. Most often, the vascular surgeon's armamentarium is quite adequate for the task—blood flow is restored or maintained, and limb, organ, or life are preserved. However, we occasionally encounter patients who develop venous thromboses yet have no obvious risk factors, or develop recurrent venous thrombosis in spite of the usual methods for preventing the recurrence. The vascular surgeon also occasionally encounters a patient with a technically satisfactory arterial reconstruction only to have the reconstruction fail immediately in the operating room or during the early postoperative period from unexplained thrombosis. Some of these patients have acquired or congenital disorders of the coagulation or fibrinolytic system that makes their blood likely to coagulate during conditions that are tolerated by most patients. These patients are said to be *hypercoagulable.* This chapter reviews the evaluation and management of the hypercoagulable syndromes with special emphasis placed on those syndromes likely to be encountered by vascular surgeons.

ACQUIRED HYPERCOAGULABLE DISORDERS

Most of the operative procedures performed by vascular surgeons predispose the patient, at least at the site of the operative procedure, to thrombosis. If there is inadequate anticoagulation during the time blood flow is diverted from the operative area, thromboses will form proximal and distal to the clamps and subsequently in the operative area. Endarterectomy, angioplasty, thrombectomy catheters, and so on remove or damage the intima and expose deep layers of the arterial wall, which activates platelets and the coagulation mechanism. Synthetic grafts are not protected by endothelial cells and thus are at risk for thrombosis. If adequate blood flow is restored to an operative site and the patient's blood is rendered hypocoagulable during the time of cessation of flow, the vascular surgical procedure is almost always successful. Small diameter prosthetic grafts or vascular reconstructions associated with low flow conditions are prone to thrombosis. Some of the causes of acquired hypocoagulability are discussed in the following sections and in Table 9–1.

TABLE 9–1. CAUSES OF ACQUIRED HYPERCOAGULABILITY

Smoking	Pregnancy
Heparin-induced thrombocytopenia	Oral contraceptives
Warfarin	Nephrotic syndrome
Antiphospholipid syndrome	Vasculitis
Diabetes mellitus	Malignancy
Hyperlipidemia	Surgery
Polycythemia vera	Thrombocythemia

Smoking

Smoking contributes to intervascular thrombosis and atherogenesis through a variety of mechanisms. Nicotine results in endothelial damage and desquamation, leading to platelet deposition, the release of platelet-derived growth factor, and platelet-mediated intimal and medial hyperplasia. The increased permeability of the endothelium results in the passage of low-density lipoprotein (LDL) cholesterol into the media, leading to the production of atheromas. Smoking increases the oxygenated modification of LDL cholesterol and has adverse effects on blood viscosity (increased), coagulation (increased), and platelet activation (increased).[1,2] Patients who continue to smoke after vascular reconstruction have a high risk of recurring ischemia and subsequent loss of limb or organ.[3] Management is, of course, to discontinue smoking.

Heparin-Induced Thrombocytopenia

Heparin-induced thrombocytopenia occurs in 2% to 3% of patients who receive heparin. Twenty-one percent of patients undergoing vascular reconstruction develop heparin-associated antiplatelet antibodies (Calaitges et al., unpublished data, 1998). When patients who have heparin-associated antiplatelet antibodies receive heparin, their platelets are activated to produce platelet aggregation and thrombosis, rarely hemorrhage. The development of the antibodies is independent of patient age or sex, of the route of the administration of heparin, or of the amount of heparin received. All forms of heparin, including low molecular weight heparin, can lead to the development of these antibodies. The antibodies usually occur in patients on the fifth to the eighth day during their first exposure to heparin and may (re)occur during the first day of a patient's reexposure to heparin. The clinical manifestations include: a falling platelet count; an increasing resistance to anticoagulation with heparin; or new thrombotic, rarely hemorrhagic, events. The paradox is that the exposure to heparin anticoagulation places these patients at risk for a heparin-induced thrombosis.

When the vascular surgeon completes a technically successful procedure, with normal postoperative angiograms or ultrasound studies, only to have a thrombosis occur in the operating room or in the recovery room, heparin-induced thrombocytopenia with thrombosis should be suspected. When this occurs, one must inhibit platelet function, usually with aspirin and/or dextran, and discontinue all forms of heparin administration. The patient's plasma should be tested for the presence of the heparin-associated antiplatelet antibodies. If the antibodies are found to be present, the patient should be warned not to accept any form of heparin in the future without retesting of the specific type of heparin to which that patient is to be exposed. Unlike most drug-induced antibodies, which tend to remit in a few weeks to months, we have found heparin-associated antiplatelet antibodies have persisted as long as 13 years. The heparin thrombocytopenia syndrome is one of the more common and potentially devastating disorders encountered in vascular surgery patients.

Management of the heparin-induced thrombocytopenia syndrome includes avoiding all forms of heparin to which the patient is sensitized. We routinely test the patient's antibodies against beef heparin, pork heparin, enoxaparin, and fragmin. Rarely, a patient may react with all four heparins; however, most patients do not. If a heparin is found to which a patient does not cross react, we offer a brief exposure to that type of heparin with retesting in a few days to determine whether the patient has now developed antibodies to the "new" type of heparin. We have found positive reactions by enoxaparin in 34% of our patients and a positive reaction by fragmin in 25.5% of our patients.[4,5]

Warfarin-Induced Thrombosis

The most serious nonhemorrhagic complication of oral anticoagulation is warfarin-induced skin necrosis, which is manifested by thrombosis and hemorrhage of venules and capillaries within the subcutaneous fat and the overlying skin. The skin necrosis occurs most typically in areas of increased subcutaneous fat as occurs in the breasts, thighs, buttocks, and legs. Warfarin inhibits the action of vitamin K in the liver, leading to reductions of functional factors II, VII, IX, and X, and proteins C and S. Protein C and factor VII have short half-lives of approximately 6 hr and are reduced early during warfarin therapy. The other vitamin K–dependent factors have significantly longer half-lives and therefore systemic therapeutic anticoagulation with warfarin requires 3 to 4 days. However, the induced deficiency of protein C (an anticoagulant that inactivates factors Va and VIIIa) induces a hypercoagulable state during the first 2 to 3 days of warfarin therapy. It is recommended that patients with risk factors for intervascular thrombosis, especially patients with protein C and S deficiencies or patients who have had previous episodes of warfarin-induced skin necrosis, be protected with heparin for the first 2 to 4 days of anticoagulation with warfarin. The low molecular weight heparins allow one to "protect" the patients more easily than has been possible in the past.

Antiphospholipid Syndrome

The antiphospholipid syndrome (APS) is another of the commonly acquired causes of hypercoagulability. It occurs in 1% to 5% of the population and increases with age so that 50% of patients older than 80 years have antiphospholipid antibodies.[6] APS occurs in patients with lupus anticoagulants or anticardiolipin antibodies. Patients with these disorders develop antibodies to protein–phospholipid complexes. The antibodies are directed against neoepitopes of the plasma proteins, especially those of $\beta 2$ glycoprotein I and prothrombin, which are formed when the substances bind to anti-anionic–phospholipids. Antibodies have also been identified that react to other phospholipid complexes with protein C or protein S, factors XI and XII, and high molecular weight kininogen. The antibodies also react with phospholipids on platelets and endothelial cells. The endothelial reactions block the antithrombin inactivation of thrombin and the thrombomodulin activation of protein C.

Recurrent venous thrombosis is a manifestation of APS.[7] The incidence of thrombotic complications in patients with lupus anticoagulant have been reported to be as high as 50%.[8] Patients with systemic lupus erythematosus, malignancies, and peripheral vascular occlusive disease who have circulating lupus anticoagulants or anticardiolipin antibodies have a high incidence of pulmonary embolism, vena cava thrombosis, myocardial infarction, acute arterial occlusion, and abortion.[7] Arterial thromboses are known to occur in the brain, eye, heart, as well as in the periphery. Another clinical manifestation of APS is that of mid- to late-pregnancy abortion. Thrombocytopenia is a common occurrence.

The diagnosis of APS includes testing for the lupus anticoagulant that is manifested by prolongation of clotting assays activated partial thromboplastin time, prothrombin time, and Russell's viper venom time (aPPT, PT, RVVT). These tests do not correct with a 1:1 mixture of normal plasma with the patient's plasma. Anticardiolipin antibodies are detected by enzyme-linked immunosorbent assay (ELISA). Patients should have both tests.

The management of APS includes eliminating risk factors in patients with known antibodies—for example, warn against pregnancies, avoid oral contraceptives, avoid major trauma, and so on. Patients with recurrent venous thromboses should be treated acutely with heparin and/or urokinase, and then later with lifelong administration of warfarin [international normalized ratio (INR) of 2.0–2.5]. Patients with an anticardiolipin antibodies who become pregnant should be treated during the pregnancy with heparin and after the pregnancy with warfarin. Warfarin should be continued as long as the antibodies and/or anticoagulants persist.

Clinical Disorders

Many clinical disorders predispose patients to thrombosis by activating the coagulation system or by causing platelet aggregation. Soft-tissue trauma, thermal injuries, and operative dissection predispose one to thrombosis through activation of the extrinsic pathway of coagulation by releasing tissue thromboplastin. Sepsis may predispose a patient to thrombosis by platelet activation/aggregation, alteration of endothelial cells, and/or tissue factor activation.

Malignancies are associated with increased incidences of venous thromboses. Many malignancies secrete tissue thromboplastin, whereas others are known to release proteases capable of activating factor X. Some patients with malignancies have increased concentrations of factors V, VIII, IX, and X.

Pregnant women and women taking exogenous estrogen have an increased tendency to develop venous thrombosis. The exact mechanism is unclear; however, these women frequently have increased levels of factors II,VII,VIII, IX, and X, and low levels of antithrombin.

Hyperlipidemia, myeloproliferative diseases, diabetes mellitus, and thrombotic thrombocytopenia all predispose the patient to thrombosis through their effects on platelets. Hyperlipidemia activates platelets by increasing thromboxane A_2, whereas it decreases platelet response to PGI_2.[9,10]

CONGENTIAL HYPERCOAGULABLE SYNDROMES

Hemostasis is usually maintained by the balance between the coagulation and the fibrinolytic systems. However, the presence of congenital defects of coagulation/anticoagulation proteins may result in an imbalance that leads to an increased thrombotic risk for the patient. Most of the congenital hypercoagulable disorders have resulted in increased venous thrombosis, but several of them also contribute to increased arterial thromboses. Table 9–2 lists congential hypercoagulable disorders and the more prevalent ones are discussed in the following sections.

TABLE 9–2. CONGENITAL COAGULATION DISORDERS

Antithrombin deficiency	Homocysteinemia
Protein C deficiency	Dysfibrinogenemia
Protein S deficiency	Increased factor VIII
Activated protein C resistance	Abnormal plasminogen
Prothrombin 20210A	Decreased plasminogen activator
Heparin cofactor II deficiency	Increased plasminogen activator inhibitor

Antithrombin (Antithrombin III) Deficiency

Antithrombin (AT) is the major plasma inhibitor of thrombin and also inhibits factors IXa, Xa, XIa, and XIIa. AT deficiency, described in 1965 by Egeberg[11] in a Norwegian family with repeated thrombotic episodes, has a prevalence of 1:5,000 in the population. Patients with low levels of AT are at risk for venous thromboses, especially lower extremity and mesenteric, but are also at increased risk for arterial thromboses. The risk of thrombosis increases as the functional AT activity decreases below 80% of normal, with the highest risk occurring when AT levels are below 60%.[12] The level of AT in heterozygotes is usually 40% to 70% of normal. AT levels are decreased in several disease states, including hepatic insufficiency, disseminated intravascular coagulation (DIC), venous thrombosis, sepsis, and in women on oral contraceptives. Thromboembolism is rare before the second decade of life. Whereas thromboembolism may occur spontaneously, it is usually associated with precipitating events such as surgery, trauma, or pregnancy. Although the optimal level of AT for treating thrombosis is unknown, it is recommended that the AT concentration be adjusted to more than 80% of normal activity prior to surgery in a patient with acquired or congenital AT deficiency. Management of a patient with AT deficiency includes infusions of fresh-frozen plasma or cryoprecipitate. AT concentrates are available. Long-term warfarin therapy is recommended for patients with AT deficiencies who have experienced thrombotic events. Patients from families with AT deficiencies should be studied, and if they have AT deficiencies, they should be protected with heparin or warfarin during times of increased risk (i.e., surgery, trauma, pregnancy, sepsis, etc.).

Protein C and Protein S Deficiencies

Protein C and protein S are vitamin K–dependent proteins that are synthesized in the liver. Consequently, their plasma levels may be decreased in patients with hepatic insufficiency, chronic renal failure, vitamin K deficiency, DIC, and in patients undergoing major operative procedures. The levels are also reduced during times of active thrombosis.

Congenital protein C deficiency is transmitted as an autosomal dominant trait, with a prevalence of 1:200 to 1:300. Incidences of thrombotic events in heterozygous patients range from 0% to 50%.[13,14] Homozygotes often die in early life from thrombotic complications. Congenital protein C deficiencies are responsible for 2% to 5% of venous thrombosis. Protein C may be reduced to 70% of normal in heterozygotes and 5% or less in homozygotes. Patients with protein C deficiencies have venous thromboses at an early age, especially in the lower extremity, cerebral, mesenteric, and renal veins. Arterial thrombosis is rare. Protein C and protein S deficiencies have been found in 15% to 20% of patients younger than 50 years of age with peripheral vascular disease.[7]

Management of the patient with protein C deficiency includes prophylaxis with heparin or warfarin during times of risk—for example, surgery, trauma, pregnancy, and so on. Fresh-frozen plasma infusions can restore functional levels of protein C. Lifelong anticoagulation with warfarin is recommended for patients with protein C deficiencies who have had idiopathic, recurrent, or life-threatening thromboses. The plasma concentration of protein C necessary to avoid life-threatening thrombotic events appears to be lower than 5%.

Cutaneous necrosis is more likely to occur when warfarin anticoagulation is offered to protein C–deficient patients. Consequently, all patients, especially those with protein C deficiency, should receive heparin during their first 3 to 4 days of warfarin therapy because protein C decreases more rapidly than coagulation factors II, IX, and X.

Histories of patients with congenital protein S deficiencies are very similar to those with deficiencies of protein C. Protein S has been identified as responsible for venous thrombosis and, rarely, arterial thrombosis. However, data suggest that many of the patients with protein S deficiency also have activated protein C resistance, which may have been the major factor leading to the thromboses.

Protein S circulates either as a free protein (30% to 40%) or bound to the complement pathway protein, C4b-binding protein. C4b is an acute phase reactant and is increased during times of acute inflamation, leading to a decrease in free protein S, and thus contributes to the increased tendency toward thrombosis during inflammatory conditions.[15] The management of protein S deficiency is similar to that of protein C deficiency.

Activated Protein C Resistance

Activated protein C resistance (APC-R), initially described by Dahlbäck and associates in 1993,[16] accounts for 52% to 64% of inherited thromboses.[17] The prevalence of APC-R in the general population ranges from 3% to 7%.[18,19] Many patients previously diagnosed with functional protein S deficiency have been found to have APC-R.

Activated protein C resistance is characterized by a poor anticoagulant response to APC. When protein C is activated, it degrades activated clotting factors V and VIII. The molecular defect in factor V occurs when arginine 506 is replaced with glutamine, rendering Va resistant to degradation by APC. The altered factor V (factor V Leiden) retains its procoagulant activity, thus favoring thrombosis.

Patients with the heterozygous form of APC-R have an increased risk of thrombosis by up to sevenfold; patients who are homozygous have an increased risk of approximately 80-fold and most will suffer at least one episode of thrombosis during their lifetime.[18,20] The risk for thrombosis is increased during pregnancy, surgery, trauma, by use of oral contraceptives, or other situations that increases one's risk for thrombosis. The optimal management of a patient with APC-R remains to be defined. However, APC-R patients in high-risk situations should receive thrombosis prophylaxis, and patients with recurrent or life-threatening thrombotic events should receive lifelong anticoagulation with warfarin.

Homocysteinemia

Homocysteine is a sulphur-containing amino acid formed during the metabolism of methionine. It is metabolized by remethylation to methionine or by transsulfuration to cysteine. Elevated homocysteine levels may result from inherited disorders that alter enzyme activity in the transsulfuration and methylation pathways. In addition, acquired hyperhomocysteinemia may occur in patients with deficiencies of vitamins B_{12}, B_6, and/ or folate. It was first suggested in 1969 that hyperhomocysteinemia was associated with arterial thrombosis and atherosclerosis.[21] It is now well established that hyperhomocysteinemia is a definite risk factor for atherosclerosis and atherothrombosis, as well as recurrent venous thrombosis.

Although severe hyperhomocysteinemia is rare, mild homocysteinemia occurs in approximately 5% to 7% of the population.[22] Homocysteinemia may be detected by measurement of fasting plasma homocysteine, or after a standardized methionine-loading test (100 mg/kg). Hyperhomocysteinemia is present if the homocysteine concentration after methionine loading is increased to more than 2 standard deviations above the mean. In addition to the patient with vitamin deficiencies, hyperhomocysteinemia has been found in patients with hypothyroidism, pernicious anemia, breast and pancreas carcinoma, and in patients who smoke cigarettes.

Hyperhomocysteinemia has been demonstrated to cause endothelial disruption and dysfunction, platelet activation, and thrombus formation. When homocysteine is oxidized, potent oxygen radicals, especially hydrogen peroxide, hydroxyl radical, and superoxide radical, are formed. These superoxide radicals induce endothelial damage, smooth muscle proliferation, and activation of platelets and leukocytes. Hyperhomocysteinemia alters the normal antithrombotic activity of the endothelium by enhancing the activity of factors VII and V and decreasing the activation of protein C by altering the expression of thrombomodulin. Hyperhomocysteinemia damaged endothelium has reduced nitric oxide production. Homocysteine inhibits the antithrombin binding activity of the endothelial heparan sulfate and indirectly stimulates platelet aggregation. Homocysteine interferes with the binding of tissue plasminogen activator. These toxic effects of hyperhomocysteinemia contribute to the development of atherosclerotic plaques, arterial atherothromboses (especially cerebral, coronary, and peripheral) events, and idiopathic venous thromboses.[23,24]

It is clear that elevated plasma homocysteine concentration is a risk factor for atherosclerosis and for arterial and venous thrombosis. Patients with premature atherosclerosis or unexplained atherothrombosis and/or venous thrombosis should be tested for hyperhomocysteinemia. Patients with high homocysteine levels should be treated with folate (1–5 mg/day) and/or with B_{12} and/or B_6. Normalization of the homocysteine level usually occurs within 4 to 6 weeks[23] and has been demonstrated to be protective.

Prothrombin Gene Variant (20210A)

In 1966, Poort and associates[25] examined the prothrombin gene in patients with a documented family history of venous thrombophilia. A nucleotide change (a G-to-A transition) was detected at position 20210 in 18% of the patients. In "a population based control study, the 20201A allele was identified as a common allele" (ref. 25, p. 3698), in 1.2% of patients which the authors suggested increased the risk of venous thrombosis threefold. Although patients with the 20201A allele are at risk for venous thrombosis, the mechanism for the increased risk is unclear, except that the patients have elevated levels of prothrombin (an identified risk factor for thrombosis). There are no reports of a patient with the homologous 20210AA genotype.

Initial reports suggested that the prothrombin 20210G/A genotype was not increased in patients with arterial disease.[26] Subsequent reports have indicated that the allele has a high prevalence (5.7%) in selected patients with arterial thromboses.[27,28] Patients with the 20210 allele have had increased frequency of cerebral and coronary thromboses. It has been suggested that the prothrombin 20210A allele and the factor V Leiden mutation will be found in 63% of families with thrombophilia.[29]

The management of patients with the thrombin gene variation has not been clearly defined, but is likely to require long-term anticoagulation with warfarin for those patients with early and/or recurrent thromboses.

Heparin Cofactor II Deficiency

Heparin cofactor II is produced by the liver and is a specific inhibitor of thrombin. Heparin cofactor II deficiency is a rare condition that is transmitted as an autosomal dominant. It inactivates thrombin by binding to it in a 1:1 relationship. Heparin enhances the rate of thrombin inactivation by heparin cofactor II. Patients with heparin cofactor II deficiencies are at risk for thrombosis when their cofactor level becomes 50% or less than normal.[30] Heparin cofactor II deficiencies have been reported in a few patients as a risk factor for venous, and fewer arterial, thromboses.

Deficient Plasminogen and Plasminogen Activator Activity

Increased thrombotic tendencies have been reported in patients with structural defects in plasminogen or defects in the plasminogen activator system. Twelve variant forms of the plasminogen molecule have been described.[31] These variants have functional abnormalities including altered active sites and the inability to form activator complexes. A few patients with recurrent thromboembolism have been identified as having decreased production of plasminogen activator by the endothelial cells. Patients with these deficiencies of fibrinolysis may suffer arterial and venous thromboses and are treated with long-term warfarin therapy.

SUMMARY

It is clear that most of the disorders of hypercoagulability can contribute to (cause) venous thrombosis. All patients with juvenile and/or idiopathic recurrent venous thrombosis should be tested for hypercoagulability. The initial screen should test for lupus anticoagulant and anticardiolipin antibodies, activated protein C resistance, proteins C and S, antithrombin, and prothrombin 20210A. If the patient is receiving heparin, the clinician should test for heparin antibodies. Patients with unexplained arterial thromboses should be tested for lupus anticoagulant, homocysteine, protein S, antithrombin, prothrombin 20210A, and, if the patient is receiving heparin, heparin-associated antiplatelet antibodies.

   If the initial screen does not reveal a hypercoagulable syndrome and the patient fits the pattern of juvenile and/or idiopathic recurrent thrombosis, then the patient should be screened for the remaining hypercoagulable conditions. The management of the hypercoagulable disorder is to remove the offending agents, such as smoking, warfarin, heparin, and so forth, and/or correcting homocysteine with folate B_{12} and/or B_6. Long-term anticoagulation with warfarin is recommended for most of the disorders. However, vascular surgeons must remember that despite the description of an increasing number of acquired and congenital hypercoagulable syndromes, most failures of vascular reconstruction are technical failures. Long-term anticoagulation cannot be a substitute for technical excellence.

REFERENCES

  1. Roald HE, Lyberg T, Dedichen H, et al. Collagen-induced thrombosis formation in flowing nonanticoagulate human blood from habitual smokers and nonsmoking patients with severe peripheral atherosclerotic disease. *Arteriolscler Thromb Vasc Biol.* 1995;15:128–132.

2. Blann AD, Steel C, McCollum CN. Influence of smoking and of oral and transdermal nicotine on blood pressure, and haematology and coagulation indices. *Thromb Haemost.* 1997;78:1093–1096.

3. Greenhalgh RM, Laing SP, Cole PV, et al. Smoking and arterial reconstruction. *Br J Surg* 1981;68:605–607.

4. Kikta MJ, Keller MP, Humphrey PW, et al. Can low molecular weight heparins and heparinoids be safely given to patients with heparin-induced thrombocytopenia syndrome? *Surgery* 1993;114:705–710.

5. Slocum MM, Adams JG Jr, Teel R, et al. Use of enoxaparin in patients with heparin-induced thrombocytopenia syndrome. *J Vasc Surg.* 1996;23:839–843.

6. Manoussakis MN, Tzioufas AG, Silis MP, et al. High prevalence of anti-cardiolipin and other autoantibodies in a healthy elderly population. *Clin Exp Immunol.* 1987;69:557–565.

7. Eldrup-Jorgensen J, Flanigan DP, Brace L, et al. Hypercoagulable states and lower limb ischemia in young adults. *J Vasc Surg.* 1989;9:334–341.

8. Ahn S, Kalunian K, Rosove M, et al. Postoperative thrombotic complications in patients with the lupus anticoagulant: increased risk after vascular procedures. *J Vasc Surg.* 1988;7:749–756.

9. Betteridge DJ, El Tahir KE, Reckless JP, et al. Platelets from diabetic subjects show diminished sensitivity to prostacyclin. *Eur J Clin Invest.* 1982;12:395–398.

10. Colwell JA, Winocour PD, Lopes-Virella M, et al. New concepts about the pathogenesis of atherosclerosis in diabetes mellitus. *Am J Med.* 1983;75:67–80.

11. Egeberg O. Inherited antithrombin deficiency causing thrombophilia. *Throm Diathes Haemorrh.* 1965;13:516–530.

12. Sagar S, Nairn D, Stamatakis JD, et al. Efficacy of low-dose heparin in prevention of extensive deep-vein thrombosis in patients undergoing total-hip replacement. *Lancet.* 1976;1:1151–1154.

13. Allaart CF, Poort SR, Rosendaal FR, et al. Increased risk of venous thrombosis in carriers of hereditary protein C deficiency defect. *Lancet.* 1993;341:134–138.

14. Broekmans AW, Veltkamp JJ, Bertina RM. Congenital protein C deficiency and venous thromboembolism: a study of three Dutch families. *N Engl J Med.* 1983;309:340–344.

15. D'Angelo A, Vigano-D'Angelo S, Esmon CT, et al. Acquired deficiencies of protein S: protein S activity during oral anticoagulation, in liver disease, and in disseminated intravascular coagulation. *J Clin Invest.* 1988;81:1445–1454.

16. Dahlback B, Carlsson M, Svensson PJ. Familial thrombophilia due to a previously unrecognized mechanism characterized by poor anticoagulant response to activated protein C: prediction of a cofactor to activated protein C. *Proc Natl Acad Sci USA.* 1993;90:1004–1008.

17. Griffin JH, Evatt B, Wideman C, et al. Anticoagulant protein C pathway defective in majority of thrombophilic patients. *Blood* 1993;82:1989–1993.

18. Rosendaal FR, Koster T, Vandenbroucke JP, Reitsma PH. High risk of thrombosis in patients homozygous for factor V Leiden (activated protein C resistance). *Blood.* 1995;85:1504–1508.

19. Svensson PJ, Dahlback B. Resistance to activated protein C as a basis for venous thrombosis. *N Engl J Med.* 1994;330:517–522.

20. Koster T, Rosendaal FR, deRonde H, et al. Venous thrombosis due to poor anticoagulant response to activated protein C: Leiden thrombophilia study. *Lancet.* 1993;342:1503–1506.

21. McCully KS. Vascular pathology of homocysteinemia: implications for the pathogenesis of arteriosclerosis. *Am J Pathol.* 1969;56:111–128.

22. Kang SS, Wong PW, Malinow MR. Hyperhomocyst(e)inemia as a risk factor for occlusive vascular disease. *Annu Rev Nutr.* 1992;12:279–298.

23. Welch GN, Loscalzo J. Homocysteine and atherothrombosis. *N Engl J Med.* 1998;338:1042–1050.

24. Guba SC, Fink LM, Fonseca V. Hyperhomocysteinemia: an emerging and important risk factor for thromboembolic and cardiovascular disease. *Am J Clin Pathol.* 1996;106:709–722.

25. Poort SR, Rosendaal FR, Reitsma PH, Bertina RM. A common genetic variation in the 3'-untranslated region of the prothrombin gene is associated with elevated plasma prothrombin levels and an increase in venous thrombosis. *Blood.* 1996;88:3698–3703.

26. Ferraresi P, Marchetti G, Legnani C, et al. The heterozygous 20210 G/A prothrombin genotype is associated with early venous thrombosis in inherited thrombophilias and is not increased in frequency in artery disease. *Arterioscler Thromb Vasc Biol.* 1997;17:2418–2422.

27. Arruda VR, Annichino-Bizzacchi JM, Goncalves MS, Costa FF. Prevalence of the prothrombin gene variant (nt20210A) in venous thrombosis and arterial disease. *Thromb Haemost.* 1997;78:1430–1433.

28. Rosendaal FR, Siscovick DS, Schwartz SM, et al. A common prothrombin variant (20210 G to A) increases the risk of myocardial infarction in young women. *Blood.* 1997;90:1747–1750.

29. Bertina RM. Factor V Leiden and other coagulation factor mutations affecting thrombotic risk. *Clin Chem.* 1997;43:1678–1683.

30. Tollefsen DM. Laboratory diagnosis of antithrombin and heparin cofactor II deficiency. *Semin Thromb Hemost.* 1990;16:162–168.

31. Robbins KC. Classification of abnormal plasminogens: dysplasminogenemias. *Semin Thromb Hemost.* 1990;16:217–220.

10

Guidelines for Preoperative
Cardiac Evaluation

John W. Hallett, Jr., MD

Few topics have engendered so much debate as preoperative cardiac evaluation and care in patients undergoing vascular operations. However, the controversy has begun to settle. The American College of Cardiology and the American Heart Association have approved "Guidelines for Preoperative Cardiovascular Evaluation for Noncardiac Surgery." This chapter summarizes those recommendations, placing them in the context of the wide variety of arterial reconstructions performed by vascular surgeons. In addition, the value of specific measures to decrease perioperative cardiac risk are discussed. Finally, new data on emergent revascularization for postoperative myocardial ischemia is presented.

BACKGROUND

From the earliest days of peripheral arterial reconstruction, surgeons recognized myocardial ischemia as the major danger in both the early and late postoperative periods. In 1984, Hertzer and associates[1] of the Cleveland Clinic reemphasized this key concept in a classic study of 1000 patients undergoing coronary angiography prior to peripheral vascular operations. They documented severe but correctable coronary artery disease (CAD) in 25% of patients presenting for surgical management of peripheral vascular disease. The prevalence was 31% in patients with abdominal aortic aneurysms (AAA), 26% in patients with cerebrovascular disease, and 21% in a third group presenting with arteriosclerosis obliterans of the lower limbs. Severe correctable CAD was present in approximately 50% of all patients with angina pectoris, as well as in one-third of patients with a previous myocardial infarction (MI) or with ischemia on routine electrocardiogram. These data stirred controversy concerning whether patients with severe correctable CAD should undergo myocardial revascularization before elective peripheral vascular operations, especially before aortic reconstructions. Subsequently, several large series documented reduced risk for cardiac death in patients who had coronary artery bypass grafting (CABG) or percutaneous transluminal coronary angioplasty (PCTA) before vascular operations.

In 1985, Boucher and associates[2] at the Massachusetts General Hospital (MGH) ushered in the era of preoperative noninvasive cardiac testing. They reported the determination of cardiac risk by dipyridamole–thallium imaging. Their work demonstrated that patients with clinically evident CAD and significant redistribution on thallium imaging were at heightened risk of perioperative cardiac events. A deluge of literature on noninvasive preoperative cardiac testing followed this report. Without correlation to clinical symptoms, some physicians and surgeons began to use these tests routinely before arterial reconstructive surgery. Since the mid- to late 1980s, the exorbitant costs of such routine testing became self-evident. Among an exponential proliferation of cardiologists, such noninvasive cardiac testing became an industry unto itself.

In 1989, Eagle and associates[3] at the MGH attempted to bring common sense back into the preoperative cardiac evaluation of vascular surgery patients. They began combining clinical and thallium data to optimize the preoperative assessment of cardiac risks before major vascular operations. Eagle identified five key clinical markers of increased cardiac risk: angina pectoris, prior MI, congestive heart failure, diabetes mellitus, and age greater than 70 years. They noted that the risk of perioperative cardiac events was remarkably low (2%) when the patient had none of these clinical characteristics. When one or two risk factors were present, the perioperative risk was 10%. With three or more risk factors, the perioperative cardiac risk rose significantly, to 30%. Their work documented that severe CAD was present on coronary angiography in 17% of patients with zero to one clinical risk factors, 44% in those with two to three risk factors, and 77% in those with three or more risk factors. They also established that the degree of ischemia seen on thallium scan correlated with perioperative cardiac events. Risk was highest when four or more segments appeared ischemic on redistribution. In an analysis of 606 peripheral vascular operations, they also emphasized that the cardiac event rate was highest (13%) for patients undergoing lower extremity bypass procedures, and actually lower for patients undergoing aortic (6%) or carotid (6%) operations.

Between 1990 and 1995, the American College of Cardiology and the American Heart Association recognized the need to develop guidelines for perioperative cardiovascular evaluation for noncardiac surgery. In 1996, they published their recommendations.[4,5] That same year, Mangano and colleagues[6] from the Multicenter Study of Perioperative Ischemia Research Group reported the beneficial effect of perioperative beta blockade on mortality and cardiovascular morbidity after noncardiac surgery.

Consequently, many of the controversies surrounding perioperative cardiovascular evaluation and treatment have been resolved—at least for now. Currently, the risk of perioperative cardiac evaluation and treatment can be minimized by familiarity with these guidelines. This chapter emphasizes a prudent approach to several general considerations, to coronary heart disease, to noncoronary heart disease, and to the value of specific perioperative measures.

GENERAL CONSIDERATIONS

Since the mid- to late 1980s, the following general concepts have evolved.[5–8]

1. Patients who suffer perioperative MI generally have severe coronary disease (left main or three vessel) and/or severe left ventricular dysfunction.
2. The predictive value of any noninvasive tests for myocardial ischemia is related not only to the sensitivity and specificity of the tests, but also to the probably of disease in the population being tested. For example, preoperative testing is

of least value in low- and high-risk situations, and is of greatest value for patients with intermediate risk.

3. Several reliable provocative tests for CAD are currently available, and one's choice must depend on local expertise.

4. The results of provocative testing for CAD should not be thought of as either positive or negative. Most tests can demonstrate a spectrum of ischemia, from relatively mild to diffusely profound.

5. Routine preoperative cardiac testing for all vascular surgery patients is neither beneficial nor cost-effective.

6. Currently, a selective approach to preoperative cardiac testing should be based on clinical markers (Table 10–1).

7. Although perioperative cardiac risk has received intense attention since the mid-1980s, long-term cardiac mortality and morbidity are, frankly, more important. Without modification of risk factors and lifestyle, many peripheral vascular surgery patients are doomed to a premature cardiac death (Figs. 10–1 and 10–2). Sometimes the long-term threat of cardiac death is forgotten after a successful reconstructive vascular procedure has been achieved. Many patients are lost to follow-up and do not receive adequate long-term health care maintenance.

8. For the patient's benefit, it is extraordinarily important for the vascular surgeon and the cardiologist to work together in the preoperative evaluation and perioperative management of patients undergoing major vascular reconstructions.

TABLE 10–1. CLINICAL PREDICTORS OF INCREASED PERIOPERATIVE CARDIOVASCULAR RISK[a]

Major
  Unstable coronary syndromes
    Recent myocardial infarction (MI)[b] with evidence of important ischemic risk based on clinical symptoms or noninvasive study
    Unstable or severe[c] angina (Canadian class III or IV)[d]
  Decompensated congestive heart failure
  Significant arrhythmias
    High-grade atrioventricular block
    Symptomatic ventricular arrhythmias in the presence of underlying heart disease
    Supraventricular arrhythmias with uncontrolled ventricular rate
  Severe valvular disease

Intermediate
  Mild angina pectoris (Canadian class I or II)[d]
  Prior MI based on history or pathological waves
  Compensated or prior congestive heart failure
  Diabetes mellitus

Minor
  Advanced age
  Abnormal electrocardiographic findings (left ventricular hypertrophy, left bundle branch block, ST-T abnormalities)
  Rhythm other than sinus (for example, atrial fibrillation)
  Low functional capacity (for example, unable to climb one flight of stairs while carrying a bag of groceries)
  History of stroke
  Uncontrolled systemic hypertension

[a] MI, congestive heart failure, or death.
[b] The American College of Cardiology National Database Library defines recent MI as greater than 7 days but less than or equal to 1 month (30 days).
[c] May include "stable" angina in patients who are unusually sedentary.
[d] Campeau L. Grading of angina pectoris. *Circulation.* 1976;54:522–523.

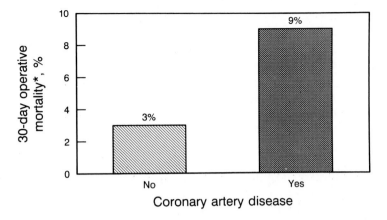

Figure 10–1. Risk of 30-day mortality following elective repair of an abdominal aortic aneurysm (AAA) based on whether the patient has no clinically evident or uncorrected coronary artery disease (CAD). (*Reprinted with permission from Roger VL, Ballard DJ, Hallett JW Jr, et al. Influence of coronary artery disease on morbidity and mortality after abdominal aortic aneurysmectomy: a population-based study, 1971–1987.* J Am Coll Cardiol. *1989;14:1245–1252.*)

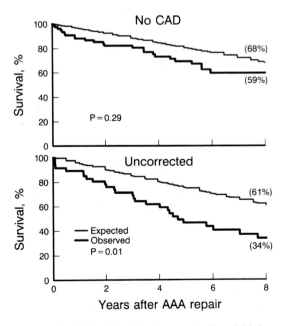

Figure 10–2. Long-term survival following elective repair of an AAA based on whether the patient has no clinically evident or uncorrected CAD. (*Reprinted with permission from Roger VL, Ballard DJ, Hallett JW Jr, et al. Influence of coronary artery disease on morbidity and mortality after abdominal aortic aneurysmectomy: a population-based study, 1971–1987.* J Am Coll Cardiol. *1989;14:1245–1252.*)

CORONARY HEART DISEASE

Numerous surgical series emphasize the dominance of CAD as the primary killer after major vascular surgery. Performed by different methods, three important studies document this critical point. In 1989, the Canadian Multicenter Aneurysm Study of more than 600 elective operations for AAA revealed a 4.8% hospital mortality.[9] Cardiac complications caused two-thirds of these deaths. In another referral-based study of 2452 elective operations performed for AAAs at the Mayo Clinic between 1980–1990, hospital mortality was 2.9%.[10] Cardiac complications accounted for 60% of these postoperative deaths. In a separate population-based study of elective AAA repair in Olmsted County, Minnesota, patients with clinically evident coronary heart disease (without revascularization) had a 30-day mortality of 9% compared to only 3% for patients without clinically evident coronary heart disease (Fig. 10–1).[11] This study also emphasized the discouraging 5-year survival of only 40% in patients with evident CAD (Fig. 10–2).

With this background, the American College of Cardiology and the American Heart Association developed consensus guidelines emphasizing the following concepts.[4,5,8,12,13] In brief, patients with any of the major clinical predictors of increased perioperative cardiovascular risk (eg, a recent unstable coronary syndrome; see Table 10–1) should be seen and evaluated by a cardiologist before the operation. Even in the setting of an emergent operation, a cardiology consultation should be made. At the other end of the clinical spectrum, patients at low clinical risk seldom require any further cardiac testing. The only exception would be patients who have poor functional capacity and are headed to a high-risk operation (major aneurysm or renovascular surgery).

Estimation of functional capacity is extraordinarily important in determining whether a patient needs any preoperative cardiac testing. Functional capacity can be expressed in metabolic equivalent levels (METs). The oxygen consumption of a 40-year-old man (weight, 70 kg) in a resting state is 3.5 mL/kg per minute, or 1 MET. In other words, 1 MET is the oxygen consumption of a middle-aged Minnesotan sitting on a couch, drinking a beer, and watching a Minnesota Vikings football game. Both perioperative cardiac and long-term risk are increased in patients who are unable to meet a 4-MET demand during most normal daily activities. Table 10–2 lists simple questions that can be used quickly in the office to ascertain whether a patient can normally do 4 METs of activity.

The patients who are most likely to benefit from preoperative cardiac testing are patients at intermediate risk for a perioperative cardiac event. For such patients of intermediate clinical risk (Table 10–1), provocative cardiac testing is advised for all except patients in good functional capacity about to have a low- or, at most, middle-risk surgical procedure. In an analysis of 1081 patients having a variety of vascular procedures, L'Italien and colleagues[14] at MGH correlated preoperative clinical risk stratification with postoperative cardiac event rates. Event rates for low-, intermediate-, and high-risk groups were 3%, 8%, and 18%, respectively.

Following stratification of patients by clinical risk factors, the next most important element in predicting cardiac events is the type of surgical procedure (Table 10–3). Highest risk (reported cardiac risk often >5%) is expected with emergent major operations, particularly in elderly patients, aortic and other major intra-abdominal vascular procedures, lower extremity bypasses, and anticipated prolonged procedures associated with large fluid shifts or blood loss. Intermediate cardiac risk (generally <5%) is associated with carotid endarterectomy.

Finally, a few caveats about preoperative cardiac evaluation deserve emphasis. Patients who have had definitive coronary revascularization within the preceeding 5

TABLE 10–2. ESTIMATED ENERGY REQUIREMENTS FOR VARIOUS ACTIVITIES

1 MET	4 METs
Can you take care of yourself?	Climb a flight of stairs or walk up a hill?
Eat, dress, or use the toilet?	Walk on level ground at 4 mph (or 6.4 km/h)?
Walk indoors around the house?	Run a short distance?
Walk a block or two on level ground at 2–3 mph (or 3.2–4.8 km/h)?	Do heavy work around the house like scrubbing floors or lifting or moving heavy furniture?
Do light work around the house like dusting or washing dishes?	Participate in moderate recreational activities like golf, bowling, dancing, doubles tennis, or throwing a baseball or football?
	Participate in strenuous sports like swimming, singles tennis, football, basketball, or skiing?
4 METs	**10 METs**

MET = metabolic equivalent; mph = miles per hour.
Adapted from the Duke Activity Status Index (Hlatky MA, Boineau RE, Higginbotham MB, et al. A brief self-administered questionnaire to determine functional capacity [the Duke Activity Status Index]. *Am J Cardiol.* 1989;64:651–654) and AHA Exercise Standards (Fletcher GF, Balady G, Froelicher VF, et al. Exercise standards: a statement for healthcare professionals from the American Heart Association. *Circulation.* 1995;91:580–615).

years and have no recurrent symptoms are at low risk for noncardiac surgery in general. Similarly, patients who are clinically stable within 2 years of a negative coronary risk assessment are also at low risk. In general, these two groups of patients do not need further cardiac evaluation prior to peripheral vascular surgery. Finally, it is essential to emphasize that many patients, especially patients undergoing urgent infrainguinal

TABLE 10–3. CARDIAC RISK STRATIFICATION FOR NONCARDIAC SURGICAL PROCEDURES[a]

High (reported cardiac risk often >5%)
  Emergent major operations, particularly in elderly patients
  Aortic and other major vascular operation
  Peripheral vascular operation
  Anticipated prolonged surgical procedures associated with large fluid shifts or blood loss (or both)

Intermediate (reported cardiac risk generally <5%)
  Carotid endarterectomy
  Head and neck operation
  Intraperitoneal and intrathoracic operation
  Orthopedic operation
  Prostate operation

Low (reported cardiac risk generally <1%)[b]
  Endoscopic procedures
  Superficial procedure
  Cataract operation
  Breast operation

[a] Combined incidence of cardiac death and nonfatal myocardial infarction.
[b] Further preoperative cardiac testing is generally unnecessary.

bypass for limb salvage, do not have time for extensive preoperative cardiac evaluation or revascularization. Their heightened perioperative risk must be recognized and managed with best medical management prior to operation, during anesthesia, and in the perioperative recovery.

Following these guidelines, eventually approximately 5% of patients with peripheral vascular disease who need preoperative coronary angiography and some type of revascularization will be identified. In our Mayo Clinic series of 2452 elective AAA repairs, 100 patients (4.1%) underwent preoperative coronary revascularization.[9] In most cases, the revascularization required CABG. In 15% of patients, PTCA was sufficient. This entire group of patients (CABG or PTCA) subsequently underwent AAA repair without any major cardiac events. The average time between coronary revascularization was 10 weeks for those undergoing CABG and 10 days for those undergoing PTCA. Other similar surgical series have also found that only 5% to 8% of patients undergoing elective peripheral vascular surgery need any type of preoperative coronary revascularization.

NONCORONARY HEART DISEASE

Valvular heart disease is relatively common in the aging population. In general, mitral and aortic regurgitation are well tolerated during peripheral vascular operations. Because these patients are at risk for perioperative heart failure, diuretics and other load-reducing agents are often beneficial. Patients with aortic insufficiency tend to do better with faster heart rates (eg, 100/min), and generally should be allowed to have such heart rates.

In contrast, patients with mild to moderate mitral stenosis do well as long as tachycardia is avoided. Patients with severe mitral stenosis should be considered for preoperative repair. Patients with significant but asymptomatic aortic stenosis (valve area <1 cm²) are especially vulnerable to labile perioperative hemodynamics. If they develop perioperative hypotension, acute coronary insufficiency can ensue. Such patients may deteriorate rapidly, and because of their fixed aortic valve, they are seldom resuscitated if they arrest. Patients with symptomatic aortic stenosis carry an even higher risk. They should be considered for preoperative aortic valve replacement or perhaps percutaneous aortic valvuloplasty in selected patients.

Recent congestive heart failure is an extraordinarily worrisome predictor of a bad outcome with noncardiac surgery. Several questions must be answered. Is the congestive failure systolic or diastolic in nature? Is it due to valvular or coronary disease? In general, perioperative heart failure can be expected if the ejection fraction is low (<35%) and the heart is already dilated. In such patients, a pulmonary artery catheter is essential. Arrhythmia is also fairly common in this group, and postoperative cardiac monitoring is mandatory.

Few physicians or surgeons would argue that hypertension should be controlled before operation. One must be cognizant that withdrawal of beta-blockers or clonidine may precipitate perioperative rebound hypertension and myocardial ischemia. In addition, hypertrophic cardiomyopathies also predispose to perioperative hemodynamic instability. These patients may move precariously between hypotension and oliguria, and subsequently hypertension and congestive failure. These hemodynamic swings can occur with little change in intravascular volume separating these two dangerous zones.

THE VALUE OF SPECIFIC PERIOPERATIVE MEASURES

With the previously described risk stratification, one must attempt to minimize perioperative cardiac events. A number of guiding principles must be considered.

In general, there is little difference in cardiac risk between regional and general anesthesia, except perhaps in patients with severely depressed left ventricular function and congestive failure. In such cases, a regional anesthesia may be better. Although commonly used, the data supporting perioperative use of nitrates and calcium channel blockers remain equivocal. Data are also equivocal for the routine use of pulmonary artery catheters, intra-aortic balloon pumps for acute coronary insufficiency, routine postoperative rule out MI protocols, and intraoperative transesophageal echocardiography.

However, data support perioperative beta-blockade as one method to reduce both early and late coronary morbidity and mortality. In a multicenter trial, treatment with Atenolol during hospitalization not only reduced perioperative mortality, but also the incidence of cardiovascular complications for as long as 2 years after surgery. This study emphasized the importance of starting the Atenolol approximately 1 hour before surgery. Event-free survival was 83% in patients receiving Atenolol, compared to only 68% at 2 years for patients receiving the placebo. Certainly, patients who have been taking beta-blockers preoperatively should continue to take them perioperatively and subsequently. Furthermore, if the preoperative evaluation shows clear or likely evidence of underlying coronary heart disease, it is probably appropriate to use beta-blockers perioperatively. Whether one should give beta-blockers routinely to patients who have cardiac risk factors but who have no clinical signs of coronary disease remains unclear.

Perioperative cardiac monitoring should be used in high-risk coronary patients and in patients with either risk for or a history of arrhythmia. In the patient with known silent myocardial ischemia, cardiac enzymes and serial electrocardiograms should be followed closely after operation for at least 24 hours. In general, pulmonary artery catheter monitoring is reasonable in any patient undergoing major vascular surgery (eg, aneurysm repair), especially if there is any clinical evidence of coronary heart disease.

Finally, the importance of perioperative pain control cannot be overemphasized. Several studies have documented transient but significant rises in serum catecholamines following operation. Catecholamine levels appear to correlate with the amount of perioperative pain. Such pain can usually be minimized or nearly eliminated by epidural analgesia or other continual methods of pain control, such as patient-controlled analgesia.

MANAGEMENT OF ACUTE PERIOPERATIVE MYOCARDIAL INFARCTION

Traditional wisdom, based on numerous clinical reports, emphasizes the high mortality of any postoperative MI. In most series, approximately 50% of these patients die in the early postoperative period.

At the Mayo Clinic, an unpublished clinical audit recently reviewed an aggressive approach to the management of early perioperative acute MI in 17 patients, all of whom had unstable ischemic events. Mean age was 72 years. Shock was present in 65%, and cardiac arrest had occurred in 35%. The most common sign of a perioperative MI, recognized at approximately 36 hours following operation, was congestive heart failure. These patients were taken to urgent cardiac catheterization at a mean of 7.3 hours following recognition of their acute MI.

In contrast to the usual perioperative death rate of 50% following acute MI, 71% of the patients in this aggressive revascularization protocol survived. Only one death (7%) was actually due to myocardial ischemia. In 77% of these patients, PTCA was successful. CABG was undertaken in 12%, whereas the remaining 12% had other intense medical therapy. Although these results are relatively preliminary, they are encouraging and indicate that urgent perioperative cardiac catheterization and revascularization should be considered in all patients who suffer a postoperative MI and are relatively unstable.

SUMMARY

Currently, clinical risk factors can be used to stratify patients into low-, intermediate-, and high-risk groups for perioperative cardiac events. Preoperative noninvasive cardiac testing should be guided by this risk stratification. Approximately 5% of patients undergoing elective peripheral vascular operations will have significant coronary heart disease that requires some type of intervention prior to elective surgery. Perioperative beta-blockade is the latest recommendation in minimizing both early postoperative cardiac events and in enhancing longer term survival. Improving late survival has probably not received as much attention as perioperative evaluation and treatment. Nonetheless, aggressive risk-factor modification is receiving more attention and must be the focus if late survival is to be improved following peripheral vascular surgery. Now that we have learned so much about perioperative cardiac evaluation and management, focus in the near future must be on a better long-term management of the heart.

Acknowledgments
The author acknowledges the special input to this chapter based on unpublished lectures by Drs. Kim A. Eagle and John R. Levinson.

REFERENCES

1. Hertzer N, Beven E, Young J, et al. Coronary artery disease in peripheral vascular patients: a classification of 1,000 coronary angiograms and results of surgical management. *Ann Surg.* 1984;199:223.
2. Boucher CA, Brewster DC, Darling RC, et al. Determination of cardiac risk by dipyridamole–thallium imaging before peripheral vascular surgery. *N Engl J Med.* 1985;312:389–394.
3. Eagle KA, Coley CM, Newell JB, et al. Combining clinical and thallium data optimizes preoperative assessment of cardiac risk before major vascular surgery. *Ann Intern Med.* 1989;110:859–866.
4. The American College of Cardiography and The American Heart Association. Guidelines for perioperative cardiovascular evaluation for noncardiac surgery. *Circulation.* 1996;93:1278–1317.
5. Guidelines for Perioperative Cardiovascular Evaluation for Noncardiac Surgery: An Abridged Version of the Report of the American College of Cardiology/American Heart Association Task Force and Practice Guidelines. *Mayo Clin Proc.* 1997;72:524–531.
6. Mangano DT, Layug EL, Wallace A, et al. Affect of Atenolol on mortality and cardiovascular morbidity after noncardiac surgery. *N Engl J Med.* 1996;335:1713–1720.
7. Mangano DT, Goldman L. Preoperative assessment of patients with known or suspected coronary disease. *N Engl J Med.* 1995;333:1750–1756.
8. Levinson JR, Guiney TE, Boucher CA. Functional tests for myocardial ischemia. *Ann Rev Med.* 1991;42:119.

9. Johnson DW. Multicenter prospective study of nonruptured abdominal aortic aneurysms. Part II. Variables predicting morbidity and mortality. *J Vasc Surg.* 1989;9:437.

10. Elmore JR, Hallett JW, Gibbons RJ, et al. Myocardial revascularization prior to abdominal aortic aneurysmorrhaphy: the impact of coronary angioplasty. *Mayo Clin Proc.* 1993; 68:637–641.

11. Roger VL, Ballard DJ, Hallett JW Jr, et al. Influence of coronary artery disease on morbidity and mortality after abdominal aortic aneurysmectomy: a population-based study, 1971–1987. *J Am Coll Cardiol.* 1989;14:1245–1252.

12. Hoeg JM. Evaluating coronary heart disease risk: tiles in the mosaic. *JAMA.* 1997;227:1387–1390.

13. Mason JJ, Owens DK, Harris RA, et al. The role of coronary angiography and coronary revascularization before known cardiac vascular surgery. *JAMA.* 1995;275:1919–1925.

14. L'Italien GJ, Paul SD, Hendel RC, et al. Development and validation of Beyesin model for perioperative cardiac risk assessment in a cohort of 1,081 vascular surgical candidates. *J Am Coll Cardiol.* 1996;27:779.

11

Choice of Diagnostic Tests in Patients Suspected of Having Extracranial Carotid Disease

William D. Turnipseed, MD

Our current knowledge about the risk factors for carotid disease and its association with stroke injury has emerged from a clinical database derived from surveillance and screening studies performed since the late 1970s. These risk factors include the presence of systolic hypertension, diabetes, hyperlipidemia, the presence of cervical bruits, and a previous history of transient cerebral ischemia. High-risk individuals exhibiting these risk factors within given sectors of the population must be detected, and preventive medical or surgical care must be provided whenever possible if the adverse consequences of stroke injury are to be averted. The need to more precisely evaluate patients at risk for stroke has been the stimulus for development of vascular imaging techniques. Information obtained from such tests has contributed to a better understanding of this disease's natural history.

X-RAY ARTERIOGRAPHY

The development of the contrast x-ray arteriography made it possible to evaluate directly the cervical carotid and intracranial circulation and to correlate distribution, configuration, and severity of atherosclerotic lesions with the development of focal hemispheric ischemic symptoms. Interventional arteriography was the first method for defining the presence of cerebral vascular disease objectively in stroke-risk patients identified by clinical screening and surveillance. Arteriography allowed us to better understand the anatomy of the cerebral circulation and pathologic changes that can cause ischemic brain injury. Arterial plaque disruption and ulceration, stricture formation, and occlusion as well as intracranial vascular abnormalities such as aneurysms, arteriovenous fistulae, tumors, and parenchymal hemorrhage could be identified. Early arteriograms were crudely performed by injecting contrast agent through a needle placed directly into the cervical carotid artery. Morbidity was significant (>6%), arch lesions were frequently missed, intracranial vessels were poorly visualized, and the severity of disease often underestimated because of the inability to obtain biplane imaging. With the advent of fluoroscopy, development of overwire retrograde femoral catheterization, use of controlled volume power injection of contrast, and the development of digital substraction enhancement, morbid risks were significantly reduced (0.5% to 3%), thus improving global acceptance of arteriography as a means for evaluating the symptomatic patient.[1] The traditional role of contrast arteriography in the preoperative evaluation of patients with cerebral vascular symptoms has changed considerably as less invasive methods of arteriography have become available.

Traditional x-ray arteriograms remain the "gold standard" for high-quality imaging of the cerebral vascular system. Despite better fluoroscopy, small catheters, and digital computer enhancement, contrast arteriography is not completely safe. Although the postangiographic risks for death or stroke remain quite low (0.1% to 1%), transient morbidity is not uncommon and is most frequently associated with catheter-induced hemorrhage (2%), embolization (2%), or allergic reactions to injected contrast media (1%). Contrast arteriography is expensive and costs almost as much as carotid endarterectomy and increases the potential for global morbid injury in the surgically treated patient by as much as 25%. Despite its disadvantages, arteriography remains an important clinical tool for the diagnosis and treatment of cerebral vascular disease. Major prospective randomized clinical trials evaluating indications and outcomes for carotid endarterectomy in symptomatic and asymptomatic patients have based their conclusions on x-ray contrast arteriogram defined categories of disease. The major arguments against using arteriography for routine assessment of cerebral vascular disease continues to be risk exposure, cost, and poor patient acceptance. The use of intra-arterial digital substraction angiography (IADSA) techniques has been effective in reducing risk exposure because contrast requirements are significantly lower than for traditional x-ray arteriography and because small catheters can be used without the need for selective cannulation of the carotids. This reduces the risk for cerebral embolization and the potential ischemic brain injury. Other advantages of IADSA include short examination time, reduced cost, and the ability to obtain "road map" images of the brachial cephalic arteries. In general, IADSA is used for evaluation of the arch and cervical carotid vessels because of its high sensitivity and specificity for the detection of hemodynamically significant stenosis and complete occlusions. Standard x-ray arteriograms are usually performed when a high degree of spatial resolution is required, as is commonly the case when intracranial vascular pathology is suspected.

DUPLEX ULTRASONOGRAPHY

The need to evaluate asymptomatic high-risk patient groups more precisely, to better select symptomatic candidates for surgical therapy, and to avoid risk exposure and escalating costs associated with contrast arteriography created the impetus for developing noninvasive tests, which could be used for both screening and surveillance. The development of real-time B-mode imaging and its coupling with Doppler ultrasound analysis of blood flow resulted in duplex testing, which made it possible to evaluate physiological characteristics of arterial blood flow across the carotid bifurcation and to evaluate morphologic changes in blood vessels that occur with the development of atherosclerotic plaques. Peak systolic and end diastolic flow velocity data as well as spectral frequency changes detected at sites of stenosis have been used to create a number of disease severity scales that are based on angiographically defined levels of stenosis. Duplex imaging has proved itself to be very accurate for detecting hemodynamically significant categories of carotid disease. It can distinguish between normal and diseased carotid vessels and between hemodynamically insignificant levels of disease and high-grade stenoses. Despite this fact, duplex imaging is not capable of precisely characterizing occlusive lesions in the border zones between mild and moderate and between moderate to severe disease. Nor can it, with absolute certainty, distinguish complete occlusion from preocclusive stenosis. Duplex imaging is very operator dependent and accuracy rates vary significantly from one laboratory to another. Any single duplex estimate of vessel lumen diameter reduction may vary by ±20% from angiographically defined disease severity calculations.[2]

Another important advantage of duplex imaging is its capacity for sonographic characterization of the atherosclerotic plaque. This information has made it easier to understand the natural history of stroke by establishing a relationship between temporal and qualitative changes in plaque morphology and the development of cerebral vascular symptoms. Pathologic grading of plaques can be based on visual ratios of echolucency (hemorrhage) and echogenicity (fibrosis) and have been used by some clinicians as a means for determining which patients with asymptomatic carotid disease might be at higher risk for stroke.[3] Improvements in Duplex scanning including the use of two-dimensional real-time imaging, color-flow imaging, and the use of peak systolic flow velocity ratios between the internal and common carotid arteries have improved the accuracy and the ability of duplex imaging to distinguish critical levels of stenosis from complete arterial occlusion.[4]

Duplex imaging is cheaper than any form of arteriography—it is safe and widely available, and therefore must be considered the preferred method for diagnostic screening, postoperative surveillance, and evaluation of asymptomatic high-risk patient groups. This test is also effective as a means for identifying candidates for carotid surgery and for determining which patients may require angiographic assessment. Although duplex imaging has assumed a central role in the diagnosis and management of carotid disease, the potential for great variation in its accuracy underscores the need for standardized protocols, quality review, and professional credentialing of laboratory facilities and their technical staff.

MAGNETIC RESONANCE ANGIOGRAPHY

Magnetic resonance angiography (MRA) is a relatively new noninvasive technique that makes it possible to evaluate the structural anatomy of the arterial circulation and to acquire functional information about arterial blood flow without interventional catheterization or injection of contrast agents. In terms of clinical value, MRA occupies an intermediate ground between duplex imaging and conventional angiography. MRA uses time-of-flight (TOF) or phase contrast (PC) pulse sequences for arterial imaging. TOF image acquisition is the most commonly used technique for visualizing the peripheral and cerebrovascular circulation. This is a gradient recalled echo technique, which uses radio frequency pulses to suppress signals from surrounding soft tissue and is based on the concept that blood flowing into a given field of view (high signals) appears bright in relationship to adjacent saturated soft tissues (low signals). Blood that is outside the imaging field is fully relaxed and magnetized. As it enters the tissue volume being interrogated, it appears bright in comparison to surrounding saturated soft tissues. Advantages of TOF imaging include minimum saturation affects for normal flow velocities, short acquisition time, and increased sensitivity to the presence of low flow in the circulation. Disadvantages of TOF imaging include sensitivity to blood flow traveling in the same plane as the magnetic field (inplane flow artifacts), motion-related artifacts, and a tendency to overestimate the severity of stenosis because of flow void, which is associated with turbulent flow and intervoxel dephasing. High resolution arteriography can be obtained using two- or three-dimensional TOF techniques.

The two-dimensional TOF arteriogram is derived from a sequence of independently acquired 1.5 mm volume imaging slices that are combined to form an arteriographic projection. Three-dimensional TOF imaging uses a much thicker tissue volume slab (3.8 cm vs. 1.5 mm) and requires higher blood flow rates to be effective, but is less sensitive to intervoxel dephasing or turbulent blood flow. It is particularly well adapted for assessment of the carotid bifurcation and complex flow to the intracranial circulation. The use of two- and three-dimensional TOF imaging in a sequential multiple overlapping thin acquisition technique (MOTSA) allows for very little saturation of blood as it traverses the interrogated tissue slab with high-contrast resolution over a large field of view. This has been helpful in eliminating the problem of inplane flow defects and intervoxel dephasing associated with two-dimensional TOF imaging.

PC imaging is based on the concept that signal intensity is proportional to blood flow velocity. PC sequences can be encoded for varying flow velocities so that faster moving protons in blood accumulate greater phase shifts relative to slowly flowing blood. Flow encoding results from the application of bipolar magnetic field gradients. These gradients can be applied in any direction across the body. Proton spins moving in the direction of a bipolar magnetic field gradient will acquire a phase shift proportional to their velocity and to the gradient amplitude and duration. Advantages of PC imaging include a sensitivity to fast or slow flow based on varied velocity encoding, short scan times, and better documentation of vessel morphology with less sensitivity to complex flow pattern artifacts. Two- and three-dimensional volume acquisitions can be made, as is the case with TOF imaging. The three-dimensional PC technique effectively decreases the amount of intervoxel dephasing and improves the delineation of complex turbulent flow. Volumes of imaging data obtained in vascular structures within the tissue volume being evaluated can be processed retrospectively and projected into any desired plane, thus allowing multidimensional views of vascular structures such as aneurysms and arteriovenous malformations. Three-dimensional PC imaging can also be used to evaluate flow direction and for calculating volumetric flow through tissue slices.[5]

Perhaps the most significant improvement in MRA imaging quality has resulted from the combined use of three-dimensional TOF and paramagnetic contrast enhancement with agents such as gadolinium. Three-dimensional TOF uses a T1-weighted fast gradient echo scan, very short echo repetition times, and large flip angles to reduce background signal intensity. Gadolinium, a nonnephrotoxic heavy metal analog that is excreted by renal filtration, acts as a potent T1-relaxation agent that enhances arterial imaging by increasing the contrast between blood and surrounding soft tissues. Gadolinium is given intravenously at a rate of 1.5 to 2 ml/s (concentration 0.3 mmol/kg) over a 30-second injection period. A dose timing curve is determined before carotid imaging so that the proper timing for the arterial phase of the scan can be determined. The use of three-dimensional TOF with gadolinium contrast enhancement has resulted in significant reduction in flow-void artifacts, elimination of inplane flow defects, and improved spatial resolution. This combination has also improved overall accuracy when compared to contrast arteriography. Sensitivity ranges from 83% to 97% and specificity from 92% to 98%.[6]

DISCUSSION

The most appropriate algorithm for pretreatment evaluation of patients with symptomatic or high-risk carotid occlusive disease will vary somewhat based on available diagnostic resources. In centers where ultrasonography and high quality MRA are available, it is possible to avoid the use of contrast arteriography in up to 85% of all symptomatic patients.[7-9] Ultrasonography should be the first test performed on patients with cervical bruits or symptoms suggestive of cerebral ischemia. Doppler ultrasound can be used to establish the presence or absence of significant cervical carotid disease, to differentiate moderate from severe carotid stenosis, and to detect the presence of complete arterial occlusion. Although reports of duplex accuracy demonstrate significant variability, one meta-analysis estimates sensitivity for lesions exceeding 60% stenosis to be from 83% to 86% and specificity to be from 89% to 94%. For duplex testing to demonstrate cost-effectiveness in screening for asymptomatic carotid stenoses, its threshold specificity should exceed 91% and cost should approximate $300. Screening is more cost-efficient when performed in patient populations with high disease prevalence (>4.5%). This would suggest that if screening in asymptomatic patients is to be performed, elderly patients with cervical bruits, a history of smoking, diabetes, high serum cholesterol levels, or a family history of stroke would benefit most.[10] It is unlikely that arteriography in any form will replace duplex ultrasound for routine diagnostic screening or for postoperative assessment because of its cost-efficiency and widespread availability. Duplex ultrasound remains our screening test of choice for the detection of carotid occlusive disease. Although some centers recommend sole use of Duplex ultrasound for preoperative selection of candidates for carotid surgery, we do not universally embrace this practice.[11,12] Clinical trials, such as the North American Symptomatic Carotid Endarterectomy Trial Collaborators, European Carotid Surgery Trialists' Collaborative Group, and the Executive Committee for the Asymptomatic Carotid Atherosclerosis Study,[13-15] propose the use of endarterectomy in the treatment of patients with carotid occlusive disease based on angiographically defined criteria for significant stenosis. The exact calculation of stenosis severity with duplex is not possible. Duplex imaging remains operator dependent, and false-positive test results or inaccurate grading of disease severity are not uncommon deficiencies when bilateral severe stenosis or contralateral internal occlusion can be documented. Although we concede that duplex ultrasonography can be used in the preoperative selection of patients with focal cerebral ischemic symptoms and ipsilateral high-grade occlusive disease, we do not consider it appropriate for the routine preoperative selection of asymptomatic patients.

We prefer the combined use of duplex imaging and MRA for evaluation of symptomatic and asymptomatic patients that are suspected of having carotid occlusive disease. In symptomatic patients, we can obtain important information regarding the intracranial and vertebral circulation and can evaluate the brain for coexisting pathology. Presence of cortical ischemia, intraparenchymal hemorrhage, tumor, and aneurysms can be documented using the MR imaging technology. MRA can also be used to determine blood flow patterns within the intracranial circulation and to quantitate regional hemispheric blood flow characteristics. We have used the acetazolamide (Diamox), which is a potent cerebral vascular dilatation agent in combination with three-dimensional TOF MRA as a stress test to evaluate compensatory intracranial blood flow in patients with carotid occlusive disease. This test can be used to distinguish patients with a potential for protective collateral hemispheric flow enhancement from patients who have a maximally dilated cerebral vascular bed and who may be more susceptible to ischemic change should blood pressure or cardiac output drop.[16] This information may become important for selecting asymptomatic patients who may benefit from carotid surgery more precisely.

Pretreatment diagnostic strategies vary depending on the availability of MRA. If it is not available or if institutional standards for diagnostic accuracy of MRA have not been established, then preliminary diagnostic testing for patients with bruits or ischemic symptoms should be done with duplex ultrasonography. Symptomatic patients with duplex evidence of high-grade stenosis or possible occlusion should have intra-arterial contrast arteriography if specificity for ultrasound is less then 91% and if institutional complications for arteriography are less than 1.4%.[10] The practice of using duplex imaging as a sole preoperative diagnostic test in patients with focal hemispheric symptoms is acceptable when good quality images are obtained by skilled technicians in certified diagnostic facilities.[17] Equivocal studies, dense arterial calcification, or the presence of contralateral internal carotid artery occlusion are associated with a higher incidence of false-positive test results, and may require angiographic clarification.[18] In patients with focal symptoms of cerebral ischemia and duplex evidence of intermediate grade stenosis (peak systolic velocity < 200 cm/sec), contrast arteriography can establish disease severity precisely and determine whether surgical or medical management is most appropriate. In asymptomatic patients with high-grade stenotic disease (peak systolic velocities > 225 cm/s), institutional policy should dictate whether arteriography should be performed. Surveillance duplex imaging should be initiated for those asymptomatic patients with moderate occlusive disease.[19]

When ultrasonography and high-quality MRA are available, it should be possible to avoid the use of contrast arteriography in at least 85% of all patients. As MRA techniques are refined and new contrast agents such as gadolinium become more available for routine clinical use, it is highly probable that MRA will become the test of choice for pretreatment evaluation of patients with focal symptoms of cerebral ischemia and for the evaluation of asymptomatic patients with suspected high-grade occlusive disease. The combined use of MRA and duplex imaging has been shown to be not only cost efficient, but also extremely accurate for diagnosis and for selective surveillance.[20] This combination of tests reduces risk exposure and cost for the patient significantly. MRA is about $800 cheaper than a standard x-ray contrast arteriogram. In symptomatic patients with duplex evidence of significant carotid occlusive disease, the use of two- and three-dimensional TOF imaging protocols will identify the location and severity of carotid disease in about 90% of all symptomatic patients. In those individuals where flow void artifacts cannot be successfully interrogated with three-dimensional TOF imaging, gadolinium-contrast enhancement should be performed. The combination of two- and three-dimensional TOF evaluation with PC imaging of the intracranial circulation is the most effective means of distinguishing high-grade stenosis from complete internal carotid artery occlusion. We generally reserve the use of contrast arteriography for circumstances in which concordance between Doppler ultrasound and MRA cannot be established, intracranial vascular pathology is suspected, or duplex imaging suggests the absence of hemodynamically significant cervical carotid disease in symptomatic patients. Contrast arteriography has better spatial resolution and allows for more precise assessment of minor vessel wall pathology and small vessel disease than is possible by MRA or duplex imaging. In asymptomatic patients with cervical bruits and duplex evidence of borderline high-grade occlusive disease, we think that three-dimensional TOF with gadolinium will provide the most accurate arteriogram and allow the most probable opportunity for accurate grading of disease severity.

Although the routine use of preoperative carotid MRA has not been accepted universally, those involved in its research and development are convinced that it will become one of the most important diagnostic imaging tests for the evaluation of carotid disease. Standardized protocols for MRA carotid imaging must be established before it can become used routinely in community health care systems. It is likely that MRA will replace routine diagnostic conventional x-ray arteriography to a large extent. It is unlikely that MRA will replace duplex ultrasound for routine screening or postoperative assessment because of its cost efficiency and widespread availability. It is also unlikely that MRA will eliminate completely the use of contrast arteriograms unless spatial resolution can equal that of contrast arteriography, and real-time imaging technology can make MRA feasible for endovascular treatments such as angioplasty, thrombolysis, and thrombo-occlusion.

REFERENCES

1. Fenright E, Trader SD, Hanna GR. Cerebral complications of angioscopy for transient ischemia and stroke: predictions of risk. *Neurolgy.* 1979;29:4–15.
2. Strandness DE Jr. Carotid endarterectomy without angiography. In: Yao JST, Pearce WH, eds. *Progress in Vascular Surgery.* Stamford, CT: Appleton & Lange; 1997:99–108.
3. Langsfeld M, Gray-Weale AC, Lusby RJ. The role of plaque morphology and diameter reduction in the development of new symptoms in asymptomatic carotid arteries. *J Vasc Surg.* 1989;9:548–557.
4. Blakeley DD, Oddone EZ, Hasselblad V, et al. Noninvasive carotid artery testing: a meta-analytic review. *Ann Intern Med.* 1995;122:360–367.
5. Anderson CM, Edelman RR, Turski PA. *Clinical Magnetic Resonance Angiography.* New York: Raven Press; 1993.
6. Prince MR, Grist TM, Debatin JF. *3D Contrast MR Angiography.* Berlin: Springer-Verlag; 1997.
7. Turnipseed WD, Kennell TW, Turski PA, et al. Combined use of duplex imaging and magnetic resonance angiography for evaluation of patients with symptomatic ipsilateral high-grade carotid stenosis. *J Vasc Surg.* 1993;17:832–840.
8. Turnipseed WD, Kennell TW, Turski PA, et al. Magnetic resonance angiography and duplex imaging: noninvasive tests for selecting symptomatic carotid endarterectomy candidates. *Surgery.* 1993;114:643–649.
9. Polak JF, Kalina P, Donaldson MC, et al. Carotid endarterectomy: preoperative evaluation of candidates with combined Doppler sonography and MR angiography. *Radiology.* 1993;186:333–338.
10. Yin D, Carpenter JP. Cost-effectiveness of screening for asymptomatic carotid stenosis. *J Vasc Surg.* 1998;27:245–255.
11. Chervu A, Moore WS. Carotid endarterectomy without arteriography. *Ann Vasc Surg.* 1984;8:296–302.
12. Strandness DE Jr. Angiography before carotid endarterectomy. *Arch Neurol.* 1995;52:832–833.
13. North American Symptomatic Carotid Endarterectomy Trial Collaborators. Beneficial effect of carotid endarterectomy in symptomatic patients with high-grade carotid stenosis. *N Engl J Med.* 1991;325:445–453.
14. European Carotid Surgery Trialists' Collaborative Group. MRC European carotid surgery trial: interim results for symptomatic patients with severe (70–90%) or with mild (0–29%) carotid stenosis. *Lancet.* 1991;337:1235–1243.
15. Executive Committee for the Asymptomatic Carotid Atherosclerosis Study. Endarterectomy for asymptomatic carotid artery stenosis. *JAMA.* 1995;273:1421–1428.
16. Turski PA, Levine R, Turnipseed W, Kennell T. MR angiography flow analysis: neurovascular applications. *MRI Clin North Am.* 1995;3:541–555.
17. Moore WS, Mohr JP, Najafi H, et al. Carotid endarterectomy: practice guidelines. Report of the Ad Hoc Committee to the Joint Council of the Society for Vascular Surgery and the

North American Chapter of the International Society for Cardiovascular Surgery. *J Vasc Surg.* 1992;15:469–479.

18. Wain RA, Lyon RT, Veith FJ, et al. Accuracy of duplex ultrasound in evaluating carotid artery anatomy before endarterectomy. *J Vasc Surg.* 1998;27:235–244.
19. Turnipseed WD. Diagnosis of carotid stenosis: MRA, duplex scan, or angiography? In: Yao JST, Pearce WH, eds. *Vascular Surgery: Twenty Years of Progress.* Stamford, CT: Appleton & Lange; 1997:63–73.
20. Kent KC, Kuntz KM, Patel MR, et al. Perioperataive imaging strategies for carotid endarterectomy: an analysis of morbidity and cost-effectiveness in symptomatic patients. *JAMA.* 1995;274:888–893.

12

Choice of Imaging Techniques in
Patients with Aortic Aneurysms

Bernardo D. Martinez, MD and
Christopher K. Zarins, MD

INTRODUCTION

Until recently, direct surgical repair was the only treatment available for abdominal aortic aneurysms (AAA). The development of endovascular prostheses or stent-grafts to treat aortic aneurysms has extended the possibility of aneurysm repair to a broader range of patients, particularly patients too frail to undergo standard operative repair. Standard imaging techniques such as abdominal ultrasound, computerized tomography, and contrast angiography have been used successfully for many years to diagnose and evaluate aneurysms and to plan for open surgical repair. However, the selection of patients suitable for stent-graft repair and planning for the endovascular treatment requires more precise preoperative imaging because stent-grafts require a suitable infrarenal aortic neck for fixation and issues such as the diameter and tortuosity of the infrarenal neck and iliac arteries are critical to the successful deployment of a stent-graft.

This chapter reviews the standard imaging techniques useful in open surgical repair as well as the newer imaging techniques necessary for the evaluation and treatment of patients with endovascular stent-grafts.

STANDARD IMAGING TECHNIQUES—OPEN SURGICAL REPAIR

Open surgical repair requires a knowledge of aneurysm size and location as well as the character of branch vessels. The relationship of the aneurysm to the renal arteries as well as branch stenoses or accessory renal arteries is important in preoperative planning. Precise dimensions of the neck and iliac arteries are less important because adjustments in graft size as well as decisions on the use of a suprarenal or infrarenal clamp and placement of a tube graft or a bifurcation graft can be made intraoperatively.

Abdominal Ultrasound

Abdominal ultrasound is the most useful and cost-effective modality for evaluating AAAs. Aneurysms can be diagnosed accurately and maximum dimensions can be determined. The precise relationship to the renal artery may at times be difficult to determine, particularly in obese patients. The iliac arteries may be poorly seen. However, abdominal ultrasound is the procedure of choice for the determining aneurysm size, screening, and following patients with serial evaluations.

Computed Tomography

Computed tomography (CT scan) provides precise information regarding aortic aneurysm size, location, and extent. In combination with intravenous contrast infusion, aortic lumen and mural thrombus can be evaluated as well as the relationship of the aneurysm to the visceral and renal arteries. The presence of an inflammatory aneurysm can be identified as well as venous anomalies, such as a retroaortic renal vein. Other intra-abdominal pathology can be identified readily, and CT scanning has become the standard for precise evaluation of AAAs. However, CT scanning has the disadvantage of requiring contrast infusion, and this may limit its use in patients with renal failure.

Conventional Angiography

Conventional angiography has long been considered the "gold standard" for vascular imaging. Its use in evaluating aortic aneurysms is limited by its inability to demonstrate true aneurysm size and dimensions in patients with significant mural thrombus (Fig. 12–1). Contrast angiography is also significantly more expensive than CT, and is both invasive and uncomfortable. However, it provides the best information on the degree

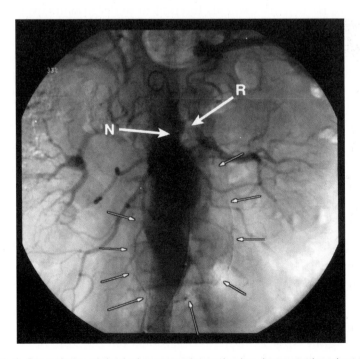

Figure 12–1. Preoperative abdominal aortography evaluation demonstrating short infrarenal neck (N) and severe left renal stenosis (R). Arrows show outer calcified borders of AAA.

of renal and visceral artery stenosis, accessory renal arteries, and the character of the iliac arteries.

NEWER IMAGING TECHNIQUES—ENDOVASCULAR REPAIR

New imaging techniques provide more precise anatomic information and are useful not only in evaluating patients for potential endovascular therapies but are also useful in helping plan open surgical repair.

Computed Axial Tomographic Angiography

Computed axial tomographic angiography involves precise timing of the intravenous contrast bolus injection such that the bolus arrives in the abdominal aorta at precisely the time that the x-ray beam is scanning the region of interest.[1,2] Continuous data collection while high density contrast is within the aorta and visceral branches allows precise depiction of aortic and branch lumen contour and artery wall dimensions. Branch vessel stenoses can readily be identified, as well as mural thrombus in the aneurysm. Transaxial cross-sectional images are displayed at 2 mm to 5 mm intervals, providing detailed information about the lumen and aortic wall as well as the size and location of the aneurysm (Figs. 12–2 and 12–3). The specific details of the visceral branches and their relationship to the aneurysm can be defined (Fig. 12–4). The infrarenal neck can be evaluated precisely, as can the common internal and external iliac arteries (Fig. 12–5). Ulceration and intramural thrombi can readily be identified (Fig. 12–6). The inferior mesenteric artery and lumbar branches can be detected, as well as double or accessory renal anatomic anomalies (Figs. 12–7 and 12–8). This modality is

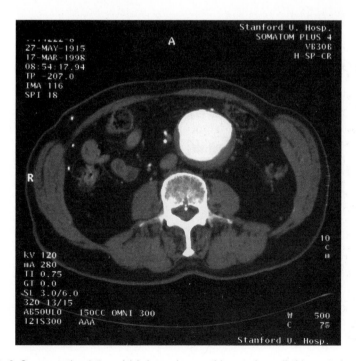

Figure 12–2. Cross-section 6.5 cm AAA. Large lumen; thin anterior wall; thin posterior organized thrombus; no calcification.

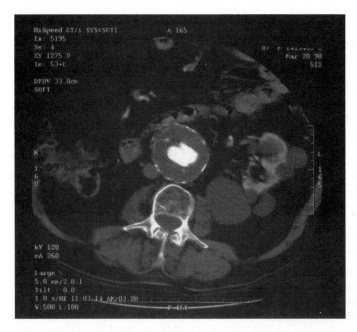

Figure 12–3. Cross-section 7.0 cm AAA. Large circular organized thrombus; moderately calcified wall.

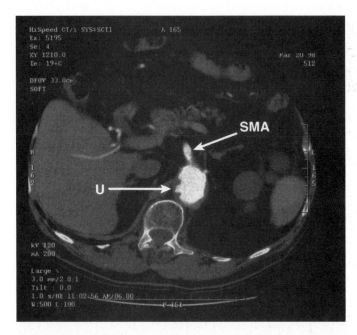

Figure 12–4. Juxtarenal 4.3 cm AAA. Cross-section below superior mesenteric artery (SMA); irregular ulcerative plaque (U).

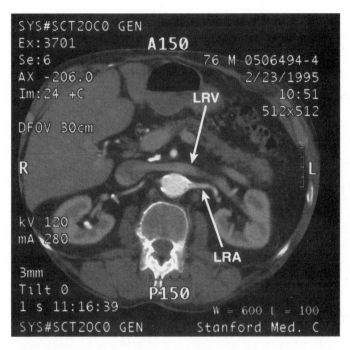

Figure 12–5. Evaluation of the neck of AAA. Cross-section of the aorta at the left renal artery origin (LRA); left renal vein (LRV).

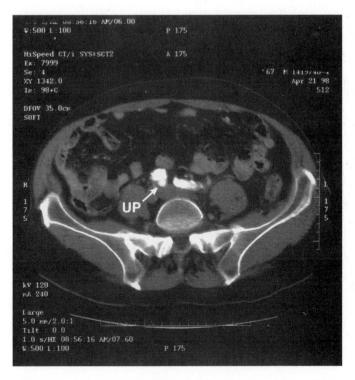

Figure 12–6. Evaluation of common iliac arteries. UP, ulcerative plaque of the right common iliac artery posteriorly.

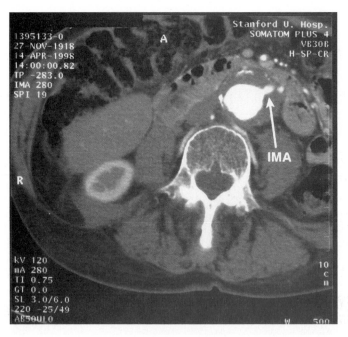

Figure 12–7. Cross-section AAA at origin of large inferior mesenteric artery (IMA).

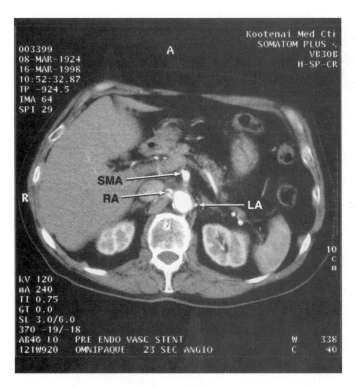

Figure 12–8. Aortic cross-section at renal level. Double right renal arteries (RA); left renal artery (LA); superior mesenteric artery (SMA).

less useful for calcific occlusive disease because the contrast density and calcification may be superimposed. CT angiography is contraindicated in patients with borderline renal dysfunction and contrast allergy.

CT Angiogram and Three-Dimensional Reconstruction

The spiral CT angiographic data acquisition is continuous and the longitudinal volumetric data can be reconstructed as three-dimensional images.[1,2] This can be displayed as maximum intensity projection (MIP), shaded surface display (SSD), or curved planer reformation (CPR). The three-dimensional images can be rotated for better visualization in areas of tortuousity.

Magnetic Resonance Angiography

The quality of imaging with magnetic resonance angiography (MRA) has improved markedly over the past several years. Two-dimensional time-of-flight (TOF) has been the standard imaging method.[3] The false-positive imaging with this technique has been significantly reduced with the use of gadolinium infusion.[4] Three-dimensional gadolinium-enhanced images now rival similar images obtained with CT angiography (Fig. 12–9).

The main indication for using MRA over CT angiography is avoidance of contrast infusion with potential renal dysfunction. Limiting factors for using MRA are implanted pacemakers and implanted orthopedic hardware; patient claustrophobia is sometimes a factor, but reduced data acquisition times have minimized this difficulty.

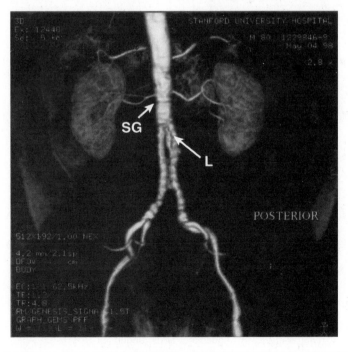

Figure 12–9. MR three-dimensional reconstruction, posterior view. Medtronic AneuRx bifurcated stent-graft (SG) shows small endoleak (L) at 1-month postoperatively. MR technique used because of transient renal dysfunction.

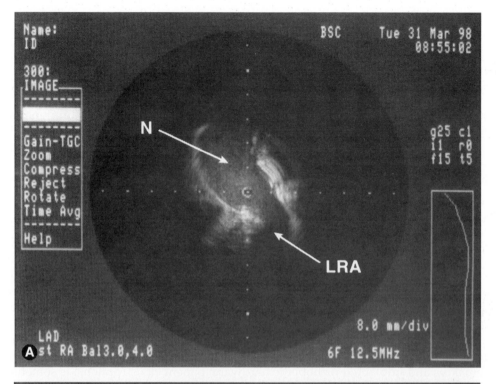

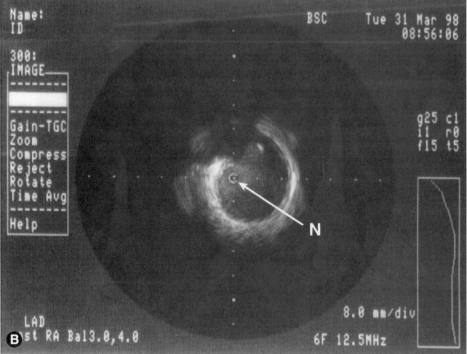

Figure 12–10. (**A–C**) The sequence of pull-back technique from preoperative IVUS evaluation is shown. Left renal artery (LRA); abdominal aortic aneurysm (AAA). (**D**) Aortogram (same patient) corroborates short and tortuous neck (8 mm) (N).

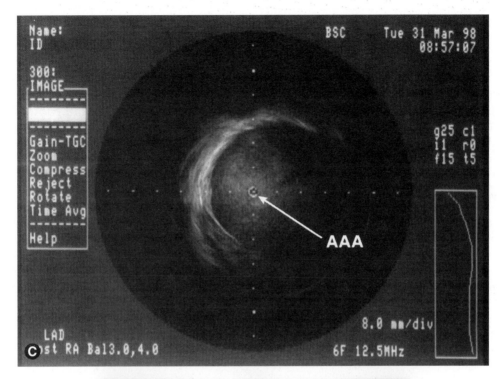

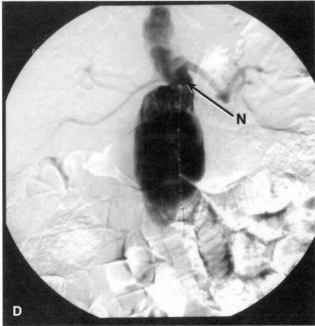

Figure 12–10. (*Continued*)

Carbon Dioxide Angiography

Carbon dioxide (CO_2) angiography is an alternative diagnostic method in patients with renal insufficiency, contrast hypersensitivity, and implanted pacemakers.[5] This technique has been used clinically in the evaluation of AAAs and aortoiliac occlusive disease. Renal and visceral arteries can be evaluated, but with less image quality than with contrast arteriography. Minor complications such as abdominal and back pain, tachypnea, and tachycardia have been reported, but CO_2 is generally well tolerated and appears to be a safe and promising vascular imaging technique in patients suffering from cardiac and renal insufficiency.

Intravascular Ultrasound

Intravascular ultrasound (IVUS) provides cross-sectional imaging data of the aortic lumen and aortic wall. It is particularly useful in evaluating the relationship of the aneurysm to the renal arteries (Fig. 12–10). IVUS can provide precise cross-sectional dimension as well as longitudinal length of the infrarenal neck (Fig. 12–11). The total length of the aneurysm and the length from the renal arteries to iliac bifurcation can be measured using a pull-back technique. This provides very important information in selecting stent-graft size prior to deployment.[6–8] IVUS is also useful to evaluate stent-graft expansion and the need for balloon angioplasty before or after stent-graft deployment.

APPLICATION OF IMAGING MODALITIES TO ENDOVASCULAR THERAPY

Patients with AAAs who are undergoing evaluation for potential stent-graft treatment are usually evaluated first with a spiral CT angiogram with 3 mm intervals. Three-dimensional image reconstruction facilitates evaluation of the infrarenal neck, renal arteries, inferior mesenteric artery, and iliac arteries (Fig. 12–12). Most endovascular stent-grafts require a minimal infrarenal neck length of 10 mm. The diameter of the infrarenal neck should be less than 28 mm. Tortuousity of the neck is an important consideration and can be evaluated with the spiral CT. The character of the infrarenal neck is assessed including the degree of calcification and ulceration or thrombus formation. The character of the celiac, superior mesenteric, and renal arteries are evaluated, as well as the presence of accessory renal arteries and patency of the inferior mesenteric artery and lumbar arteries. The size and configuration of the common iliac arteries are assessed to determine distal fixation points for the endoprosthesis. The internal iliac arteries are evaluated to rule out the possibility of aneurysm formation (Fig. 12–13). (Patients with renal dysfunction are studied with MRA rather than CT angiography.)

Patients who are found to have a satisfactory infrarenal aortic neck that is at least 1 cm in length with satisfactory iliac arteries are selected as candidates for stent-graft repair.

Further evaluation with contrast angiography can be carried out, but this is usually unnecessary if a good spiral CT scan is obtained. Contrast arteriography is obtained at the time of the endovascular procedure just prior to stent-graft deployment.[9] Intravascular ultrasound is performed just prior to stent-graft deployment to confirm transverse lumen dimension and to select the final diameter and length of the stent-graft to be used. Completion angiography is performed at the time of deployment.

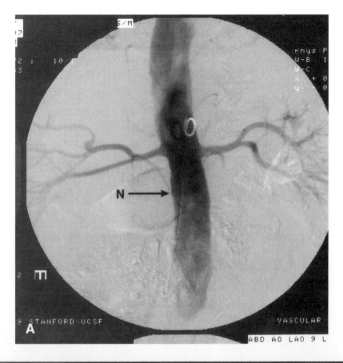

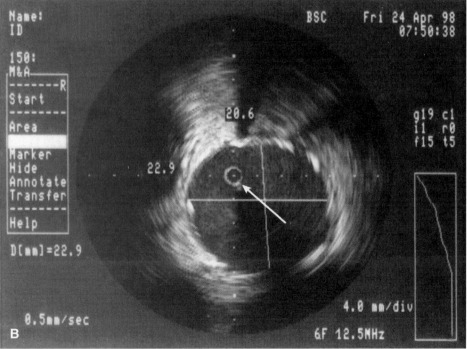

Figure 12–11. Preoperative abdominal aortogram (**A**) showing very good length neck (N) and intraoperative IVUS (*white arrow*) provides aortic neck (**B**) and iliac artery (**C**) intraluminal diameter for appropriate size selection of endovascular device.

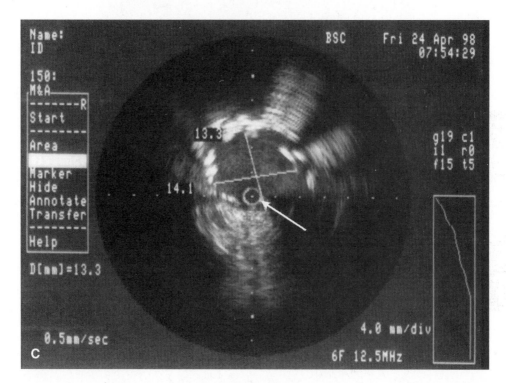

Figure 12–11. (*Continued*)

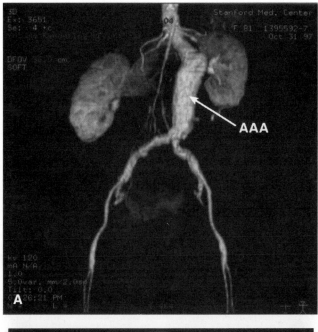

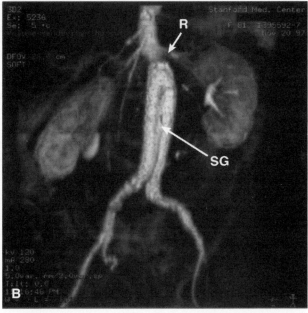

Figure 12–12. Spiral CTA—three-dimensional reconstruction. Preoperative AAA evaluation for endovascular approach (**A**). Medtronic AneuRx bifurcated stent-graft (SG). Excellent deployment below renal arteries (R) (**B**).

Postoperatively, patients are evaluated with spiral CT scanning and three-dimensional reconstruction as well as with duplex ultrasound (Fig. 12–14), which identifies endoleaks, identifies inferior mesenteric artery and lumbar branch flow, and determines the size of the abdominal aortic aneurysm reliably (Fig. 12–15). Successfully excluded aneurysms typically decrease in size, and this can be detected both with duplex ultrasound as well as CT scanning and MRA.

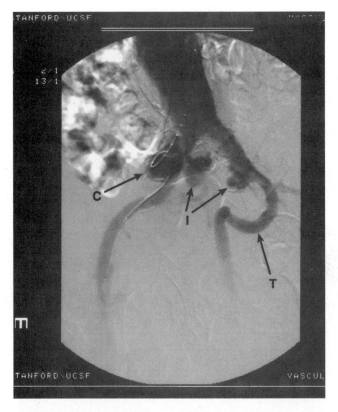

Figure 12–13. Preoperative abdominal aortogram shows AAA and right common iliac aneurysm (C), bilateral internal iliac aneurysms (I), and tortuosity in the left external iliac artery (T).

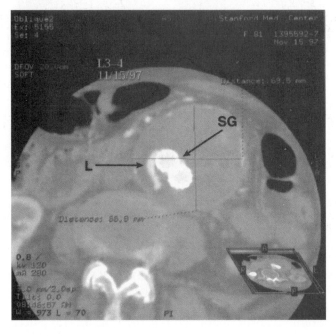

Figure 12–14. Spiral CTA—three-dimensional selective cross-sectional evaluation of endoleak (L) from stent-graft (SG) at 48 hours postoperatively.

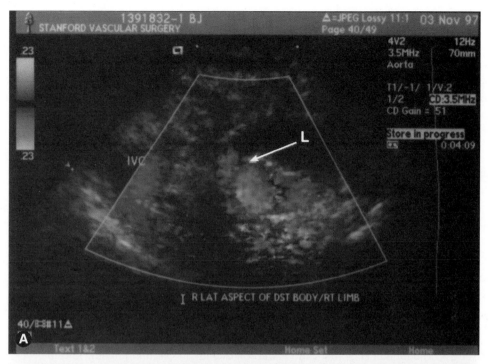

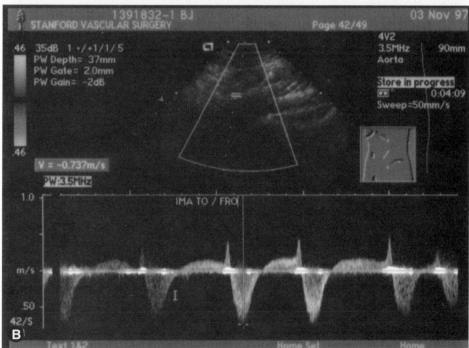

Figure 12–15. Duplex color-flow Doppler evaluation of endoleak (L) (**A**) and Doppler spectral pattern showing reversed flow (**B**) of endoleak site.

CONCLUSIONS

New imaging modalities are now available to evaluate AAAs. These imaging modalities include spiral CT angiography, three-dimensional reconstruction, MRA and IVUS. Together with color-flow duplex ultrasound, these imaging methods allow precise and comprehensive evaluation of patients with AAAs; assessment of various treatment modalities, including endovascular stent-grafting; and also allow ongoing surveillance and follow-up of patients who have undergone endovascular repair.

REFERENCES

1. Zarins CK, Krievins DK, Rubin GD. Spiral computed tomography and three-dimensional reconstruction in the evaluation of aortic aneurysm. In: Yao JST, Pearce WH, eds. *Progress in Vascular Surgery.* Stamford, CT: Appleton & Lange; 1997:117–125.
2. Beygui RE, Zarins CK. Vascular imaging. In: Greenwood G, Corson JD, Williamson RCN, eds. *Surgery.* London, England: Mosby; in print.
3. Schick F, Duda SH, Dammann F, et al. Comparison of magnetic resonance imaging methods for examination of abdominal aortic aneurysms. *Invest Radiol.* 1995;30:595–603.
4. Snidow JJ, Aisen AM, Harris VJ, et al. Iliac artery MR angiography: comparison of three-dimensional gadolinium-enhanced and two-dimensional time-of-flight techniques. *Radiology.* 1995;196:371–378.
5. Yang X, Manninnen H, Soimakallio S. Carbon dioxide in vascular imaging and intervention. *Acta Radiologica.* 1995;36:330–337.
6. White RA, Donayre C, Kopchok G, et al. Intravascular ultrasound: the ultimate tool for abdominal aortic aneurysm assessment and endovascular graft delivery. *J Endovasc Surg.* 1997;4:45–55.
7. White RA, Donayre CE, Kopchok GE. Adjunctive use of intravascular ultrasound. In: Yao JST, Pearce WH, eds. *Techniques in Vascular and Endovascular Surgery.* Stamford, CT: Appleton & Lange; 1998;7–23.
8. Lie T, Lundbom J, Hatlinghus S, et al. Ultrasound imaging during endovascular abdominal aortic aneurysm repair using the stentor bifurcated endograft. *J Endovasc Surg.* 1997;4:272–278.
9. Hodgson KJ, Mattos MA, Sumner DS. Angiography in the operation room: equipment, catheter skills, and safety issues. In: Yao JST, Pearce WH, eds. *Techniques in Vascular and Endovascular Surgery.* Stamford, CT: Appleton & Lange; 1998;25–45.
10. Queral LA. Operating room design for the future. In: Yao JST, Pearce WH, eds. *Techniques in Vascular and Endovascular Surgery.* Stamford, CT: Appleton & Lange; 1998;1–5.
11. Davis CP, Ladd ME, Romanowski BJ, et al. Human aorta: preliminary results with virtual endoscopy based on three-dimensional MR imaging data sets. *Radiology.* 1996;199:37–40.
12. Sommer T, Fehske W, Holzknecht N, et al. Aortic dissection: a comparative study of diagnosis with spiral CT, multiplanar transesophageal echocardiography, and MR imaging. *Radiology.* 1996;199:347–352.
13. Hallidy KE, Al-Kutoubi A. Draped aorta: CT sign of contained leak of aortic aneurysms. *Radiology.* 1996;199:41–43.

IV

Cerebrovascular Ischemia

13

Streamlining Hospital Care
for Patients Undergoing
Carotid Endarterectomy

M. Ashraf Mansour, MD and William H. Baker, MD

INTRODUCTION

Health care expenditure in the United States has escalated dramatically since the late 1960s. In 1960, $26.9 billion was spent on health care, a 5.1% share of the gross domestic product (GDP).[1] Despite significant efforts on the part of government and the health care industry (hospitals, health maintenance organizations [HMOs], insurers, physicians, etc.), in 1990, proportionally more dollars were spent on health care, claiming a 12.1% share of the GDP and a 26-fold increase to $697.5 billion. This alarming increase in expenditure has led government and health care providers, including physicians, to examine the methods being used to conduct business. Many initiatives to eliminate wasteful practices were initiated in the 1980s, and there may be some indication that the growth has been controlled. The latest available figures, from 1996, indicate that $1.035 trillion was spent on health care, representing 13.6% of the GDP. Some of the cost-cutting measures, rightfully or not, have been perceived by the media as excessive. This has led some legislators to mandate minimal hospital stays in certain cases, such as after mastectomy and childbirth.[2–4]

Hospitals and physicians have made great strides in their quest to cut costs and slow the health care expenditure spiral.[5–8] Many of the changes were imposed by managed care organizations.[9] Insurers as well as patients have become more cost-conscious and research both hospitals' and practitioners' cost containment histories before deciding with whom to do business. In order to survive in this competitive market, dramatic changes had to be made. Currently, insurers and managed care organizations demand advance approval for any elective operations or tests. Lengthy hospital stays are actively discouraged by controlling reimbursement. The contemporary practice of streamlining care for patients undergoing carotid endarterectomy (CEA) has focused on decreasing preoperative testing, same-day surgery admission, eliminating intensive care unit (ICU) stays for the majority of cases, and early hospital discharge. This chapter examines the evolution of these cost-cutting practices in our institution.

BUSINESS CONSIDERATIONS

To remain competitive in a changing market, surgeons and hospitals must constantly examine their diagnostic and therapeutic algorithms as well as their business practices. The implementation of diagnosis related groups (DRG) challenged both hospitals and physicians to become more cost-efficient.[5-9] The ability to provide medical and surgical services at lower cost has become a powerful marketing tool to attract prospective buyers of health care services and to recruit new patients and practice plans.

CEA is one of the most frequently performed vascular operations in the United States, with an estimated annual cost of $1.2 billion.[5-7,10] In the 1970s, it was not uncommon to have a 10-day length of stay associated with CEA. Patients were admitted routinely for the preoperative work-up, which included cerebral angiography. All patients had an obligatory 1- to 3-day stay in the ICU and were frequently kept in the hospital for a total of 5 days postoperatively.[7] Clearly, many of these practices are now considered unnecessary and wasteful. Every aspect of patient care has been scrutinized, from preoperative testing to postoperative home care. Surgeons have taken the lead in reducing costs and streamlining care without compromising patient well-being.[11]

PREOPERATIVE WORK-UP

The indications for carotid endarterectomy have slowly shifted in the last several years. Prior to the publication of the large asymptomatic carotid trials, CEA was performed mainly for symptomatic carotid stenosis.[12] Since the late 1980s, the proportion of patients with asymptomatic carotid stenosis undergoing CEA has increased.[13] In our hospital, 64% of the patients having CEAs in 1997 were asymptomatic. Most of our patients are referred by community physicians, who usually are first to obtain a carotid color-flow scan.

At the time of the first encounter, a detailed history is taken and a physical examination is performed. Patients with unstable angina or a history of congestive heart failure or poorly controlled hypertension can thus be selected for more detailed preoperative evaluation. In a review we performed in 1995, we found that preoperative cardiac work-up with a stress test or adenosine thallium was performed in 64% of patients.[14] The indications for cardiac evaluation were significant hypertension, changes in the electrocardiogram (ECG), or cardiac symptoms. Of 27 patients with reversible or nonreversible defects, 9 had cardiac catheterization, 2 patients required preoperative coronary balloon angioplasty, and 1 patient underwent a coronoray artery bypass. In 1997, only 14 (11.6%) of our symptomatic patients had preoperative adenosine thallium or cardiac catheterization.

PREOPERATIVE CAROTID STUDIES

One of the great advances in carotid surgery has been the utilization of color-flow Duplex scanning. Before its availability, patients were routinely admitted for cerebral angiography 1 or 2 days prior to surgery. Currently, most accredited vascular laboratories with experienced technicians are able to detect carotid stenosis with an accuracy exceeding 90%. This has prompted many vascular surgeons to rely on the duplex scan as the only preoperative diagnostic test.[15-19] In a prospective study by Dawson and colleagues,[15] CEA was performed on the basis of duplex scanning alone in 93% of cases.

Preoperative angiography changed the clinical management in only one patient (1.1%). Many authors have reported on the safety of performing CEA without angiography. [15-19]

CAROTID ENDARTERECTOMY

Currently, it is the rare vascular surgery patient who requires hospital admission prior to an elective operation. Consequently, the majority of our patients are admitted to the hospital 2 hours prior to the scheduled operation, having received their preoperative teaching and interview by the anesthesiologist at an earlier time. The choice of anesthetic for the operation depends on several factors, including patient and surgeon preference, cardiac status, and type and location of the lesion. Although many surgeons advocate regional anesthesia, we prefer general anesthesia for most patients. The technical details of the operation have been covered previously. Most hospitals charge patients a global fee for the use of the operating room (OR). Therefore, the opportunity to reduce OR costs significantly is virtually nonexistent. In analyzing the details of 100 consecutive CEAs, shunts were used selectively based on the carotid back pressure measured. [14] Other centers advocate the use of electroencephalograph (EEG) monitoring or transcranial Doppler during CEA, a practice that may add to the cost of the operation. The average cross-clamp time of nonshunted patients was 41 minutes. Vein patches were used in 31 patients and synthetic patches were used in 26 patients. The average OR time was 2 hours, 32 minutes. Since 1995, we have used synthetic patches for more than 97% of patients and performed intraoperative color-flow scanning for a similar proportion. Preliminary data indicate that routine patching decreases the incidence of early carotid restenosis, and intraoperative scanning has allowed us to correct technical defects prior to leaving the operating room. [20]

POSTOPERATIVE MANAGEMENT

In the late 1970s, the common practice was to admit patients to the ICU after a short stay in the recovery room following CEA. In 1992, we found that we were discharging patients routinely 1 day postoperatively, and some patients were going home directly from the ICU. We began to question the necessity for ICU admission and reviewed 100 consecutive patients undergoing CEA. [14] We also sought to find any preoperative indicators that might help us identify patients in need of ICU admission. Sixty-one men and 39 women had CEA in an 18-month period ending in June 1992. The average age was 64 (range 43–87) years. Significant preoperative risk factors included refractory hypertension (3 or more antihypertensive medications), poorly controlled hypertension (systolic BP > 170 mm Hg or diastolic BP > 100 mm Hg), recent stroke within the preceding 30 days, and significant coronary artery disease. All patients had preoperative duplex scanning and angiography was obtained in 80%. Fifty-nine patients had symptomatic carotid stenosis and 18 patients had a contralateral internal carotid artery (ICA) occlusion. General anesthesia was used in all patients. The decision to shunt was based on the carotid back pressure. Thirty-one patients had a vein patch and 26 patients received a synthetic patch. All patients were admitted to the ICU after an average of 2 hours, 30 minutes in the recovery room (range 1–9 hours). ICU monitoring included continuous systemic arterial pressure and hourly neurological checks.

Two patients had a postoperative stroke, one of whom died as a result of his stroke. The latter patient had suffered a stroke 3 weeks preoperatively and had significant hypertension. In addition, he was found to have a contralateral ICA occlusion, and he required a shunt because his stump pressure was only 25 mm Hg. Although the operation was uneventful, the patient did not wake up from anesthesia. The postoperative head CT scan showed bilateral hemispheric infarcts and the patient died quickly. At autopsy, the endarterectomy site was found to be occluded.

The other stroke occurred in a hypertensive patient with renal failure who also had a contralateral carotid occlusion. This patient was noted to have mild upper extremity incoordination in the recovery room on the side opposite the occluded ICA. Her hospital course was further complicated by poorly controlled hypertension and vein patch blowout 20 hours postoperatively. After prompt reexploration, the vein was replaced with an expanded polytetrafluoroethylene (PTFE) patch. Subsequently, she was discharged with minimal residual upper-extremity incoordination. There were two other patients who required reexploration of the neck for an expanding hematoma discovered in the recovery room within 2 hours of the operation. All four patients had significant hypertension in the recovery room requiring intravenous vasodilators for adequate blood pressure control. Each of these complications was recognized prior to transfer to the ICU.[14]

SELECTION OF PATIENTS REQUIRING ADMISSION TO THE INTENSIVE CARE UNIT

In our initial report, we found that 44 patients required some form of intervention in the ICU after a short stay in the recovery room. However, only 16 patients were truly in need of ICU-level care, which we defined as therapy or intervention not routinely administered on the ward—that is, intravenous vasoactive medications, antiarrhythmics, ventilatory support, or intensive monitoring. In this subgroup of 16 patients, 2 had a cerebrovascular accident (CVA), 2 had neck hematomas, 5 had hypertension, 5 had hypotension, and 2 had cardiac dysrhythmias. Fifteen of 16 patients (93%) who needed ICU admission were identified in the recovery room and therapy was initiated there. The remaining patient received atropine for a recurring bradyarrhythmia, which was treated initially in the recovery room. There were no postoperative myocardial infarctions (MIs) and no patient weaned from vasoactive medication in the recovery room required reinstitution of this therapy. Careful analysis revealed that only significant preoperative hypertension predicted the need for postoperative ICU admission. Age, sex, recent stroke, coronary artery disease, diabetes, operative indication, and management did not predict the need for postoperative ICU. We thus concluded from that review that the clinical course in the recovery room determined whether a patient would need ICU admission.[14]

Our findings were similar to those of O'Brien and Ricotta,[21] who reported that 18% of their patients required the ICU, 77% of whom could be selected based on their recovery room course. In their series, the stroke rate was 6.9% and the MI rate was 2.4%. Collier[22] found that only 10% of his patients required ICU admission, and, in his series, the stroke rate was 3.8%, with no postoperative MI.

The importance of hypertension as the main risk factor influencing the postoperative course has also been emphasized by others. In a report from a consortium of 11 academic medical centers, McCrory and associates[23] investigated patients who were at higher risk of postoperative stroke, MI, and death. The following risk factors were considered important: angina, MI within 6 months of operation, congestive heart failure, severe hypertension, chronic obstructive pulmonary disease, age more than 70 years, and severe obesity. In their investigation, they found that the probability of stroke, MI, and death rose from 5% in patients with no or one risk factor, to 8.7% if two to seven risk factors were present. The probability of stroke and death was 3.1% for no or one risk factor, compared to 6.3% for two or more risk factors.

Ideally, the anesthesiologist and surgeon would be able to select the patients who are most likely to require special management in the postoperative period. Assidao and colleagues[24] found that postoperative hemodynamic lability was more likely to occur in patients with poorly controlled hypertension. None of the other risk factors, such as diabetes, coronary artery disease, severity of carotid stenosis, or duration of anesthesia, had any significant influence on postoperative complications. Risk factor analysis by multivariate linear regression to identify preoperative indicators of ICU admission was performed by Lipsett and associates.[25] They found that hypertension, MI, arrhythmia, and chronic renal failure were 83% predictive for ICU stay. Only 24% of their patients were considered in the low-risk category and consequently did not require ICU monitoring.

Our initial review provided important information about the postoperative course of patients having CEA. Thus we established a protocol to identify patients in need of postoperative ICU monitoring. From January 1993 to June 1995, we had 190 patients undergoing CEA.[26] The decision to admit a patient to the ICU rested on a 1- to 3-hour stay in the recovery room. Patients who remained neurologically and hemodynamically stable in recovery went directly to the surgical ward. The indications for ICU admission were hypotension or hypertension requiring vasoactive drips, significant mental status changes, focal neurological deficit, airway compromise, or hemorrhage requiring prolonged observation or return to the operating room. None of the patients required more than a 4-hour stay in the recovery room. Seventy-nine percent of patients were transferred to the ward directly from the recovery room after an average stay of 1 hour, 59 minutes, and 88% of those patients were subsequently discharged from hospital within 24 hours. All the remaining patients, except one, were discharged within 72 hours.

There were nine postoperative complications in patients who were not admitted to the ICU. Two patients had neurological events, one had a transient ischemic attack (TIA) 6 hours postoperatively that resolved without sequelae, and one had a vertebrobasilar stroke that occurred 8 hours postoperatively. There were three patients who developed postoperative urinary retention requiring Foley catheter placement. One patient returned to the emergency department for an episode of hypoglycemia. Another patient suffered a vein patch blow-out at home on the fourth postoperative day and returned to the hospital to have a successful emergent repair. A wound infection developed in one patient, and one patient had a retinal infarction. None of the patients who were transferred directly to the ward required ICU admission or return to the OR.[26]

Thirty-nine patients (21%) required ICU monitoring. The indications for ICU admission were: hypotension (14), hypertension (14), cardiac observation (3), hematomas (2), arrhythmia (2), TIA (2), stroke (1), and respiratory distress (1). We concluded that patients who required ICU monitoring were readily identified based on their clinical course in the recovery room. We also reviewed the length of stay in the recovery room and found that it averaged 178 minutes in the first 3 years of the study, compared with 128 minutes in the last 2 years of the study, which suggests an increasing confidence in this algorithm. The estimated cost savings realized by avoidance of ICU stays were $1010 per patient (in 1994 dollars).[27]

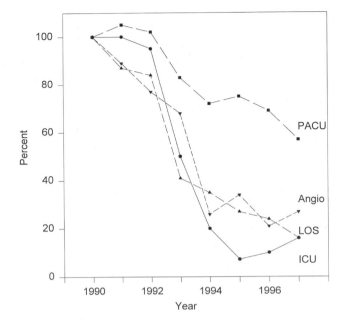

Figure 13–1. Decreased resource utilization for carotid endarterectomy at Loyola: trends from 1990 to 1997. The 1990 figures were considered the 100% benchmark. That year, all patients were admitted to the ICU after a mean of 174 minutes in the PACU, the average length of stay was 6.2 days, and 93% of patients had preoperative angiography. Angio, cerebral angiography; ICU, intensive care unit; PACU, postanesthesia recovery; LOS, length of stay.

From our two reports and other published papers on the subject, it is clear that the decision for ICU admission can be based on a short recovery room stay regardless of the patient's other comorbid factors.[8,11,21,22,26–28] By adopting this policy, we have gone from 100% ICU admissions postoperatively in the 1980s to only 7.2% admission in 1995 and 10% in 1996 (Fig. 13–1).

EARLY DISCHARGE

The postoperative hospital stay has declined considerably in the last few years. In the late 1980s, the average length of stay for carotid patients at Loyola was 6.2 days. The average length of stay continued to decline steadily at Loyola until it reached a low of 1.3 days in 1996[26,27] (Fig. 13–1). In 1997, 79% of our patients were discharged within 23 hours of operation, and in a few cases, we discharged patients 6 hours postoperatively, providing they were both neurologically and hemodynamically stable and had adequate supervision at home. In a random audit of hospital charges for patients who were discharged within 23 hours of admission for CEA, we found that the average charges were $10,725. The collective experience from several investigators, as well as our own experience, has demonstrated that extended postoperative stays are not necessary.[5–8,11,21]

POSTOPERATIVE SURVEILLANCE

There is a small but real risk of carotid restenosis in the postoperative period.[29] Early lesions that develop in the first 24 months after CEA are, for the most part, due to intimal hyperplasia and are probably benign. Recurrent lesions detected after 2 years are mostly due to atherosclerosis and may lead to symptoms.[30] Because recurrent stenosis may develop in 8% to 15% of patients, it is recommended that patient follow-up include serial color-flow scans. Postoperative carotid surveillance allows clinicians to detect recurrent stenosis that may be progressive. Ideally, patients should have a scan at 6 months; however, such a policy would be neither practical nor cost-efficient. In our laboratory, we obtain a postoperative carotid scan at 6 months, then, if the artery is normal, we obtain a yearly study.[30]

CONCLUSION

Patients with carotid artery stenosis are now being managed in a more cost-efficient manner. Wasteful practices have been eliminated from all aspects of their perioperative care, allowing for better resource allocation. Preoperative angiograms are seldom needed, postoperative ICU admission is only required in a small group, and discharge from hospital within 23 hours of admission can be anticipated in more than 70% of patients. These changes have been implemented without affecting the safety and efficacy of CEA adversely.

REFERENCES

1. Seward WF. National health expenditures. *Bull Am Coll Surg.* 1998;83:8–9.
2. Annas GJ. Women and children first. *N Engl J Med.* 1995;333:1647–1651.
3. Clark G. Model legislation would safeguard newborns. *AAP News.* 1996;12:1,4.
4. Parisi VM, Meyer BA. To stay or not to stay? That is the question. *N Engl J Med.* 1995;333:1635–1637.
5. Kraiss LW, Kilberg L, Critch S, et al. Short-stay carotid endarterectomy is safe and cost-effective. *Am J Surg.* 1995;169:512–515.
6. Luna G, Adye B. Cost-effective carotid endarterectomy. *Am J Surg.* 1995;169:516–518.
7. Maini BS, Mullins TF, Catlin J, et al. Carotid endarterectomy: a ten-year analysis of outcome and cost of treatment. *J Vasc Surg.* 1990;12:732–740.
8. Collier PE. Do clinical pathways for major vascular surgery improve outcomes and reduce costs? *J Vasc Surg.* 1997;26:179–185.
9. Aston G. Managed care cited for slowdown in spending. *AMA News.* February 2, 1998;3.
10. Stanley JC. The changing vascular surgery workforce. *Semin Vasc Surg.* 1997;10:65–71.
11. Collier PE. Fast tracking carotid endarterectomy: practical considerations *Semin Vasc Surg.* 1998;11:41–45.
12. Executive Committee for the Asymptomatic Carotid Atherosclerosis Study. Endarterectomy for asymptomatic carotid artery stenosis. *JAMA.* 1995;273:1421–1428.
13. Hertzer NR, O'Hara PJ, Mascha EJ, et al. Early outcome assessment for 2228 consecutive carotid endarterectomy procedures: the Cleveland Clinic experience from 1989 to 1995. *J Vasc Surg.* 1997;26:1–10.
14. Morasch MD, Hodgett D, Burke K, et al. Selective use of the intensive care unit following carotid endarterectomy. *Ann Vasc Surg.* 1995;9:229–234.
15. Dawson DL, Zierler RE, Strandness DE, et al. The role of duplex scanning and arteriography before endarterectomy: a prospective study. *J Vasc Surg.* 1993;18:673–683.
16. Goodson SF, Flanigan PF, Bishara RA, et al. Can carotid duplex scanning supplant arteriography in patients with focal carotid territory symptoms? *J Vasc Surg.* 1987;5:551–557.
17. Horn M, Michelini M, Greisler HP, et al. Carotid endarterectomy without angiography: the preeminent role of the vascular laboratory. *Ann Vasc Surg.* 1994;8:221–224.

18. Mattos MA, Hodgson KJ, Faught WE, et al. Carotid endarterectomy without angiography: is color-flow duplex scanning sufficient? *Surgery.* 1994;116:776–783.
19. Ricotta JJ, Holen J, Schenk E, et al. Is routine angiography necessary prior to carotid endarterectomy? *J Vasc Surg.* 1984;1:96–102.
20. Baker WH, Koustas G, Burke K, et al. Intraoperative duplex scanning and late carotid stenosis. *J Vasc Surg.* 1994;19:829–833.
21. O'Brien MS, Ricotta JJ. Conserving resources after carotid endarterectomy: selective use of the intensive care unit. *J Vasc Surg.* 1991;14:796–802.
22. Collier PE. Carotid endarterectomy: a safe cost-efficient approach. *J Vasc Surg.* 1992; 16:926–933.
23. McCrory DC, Goldstein LB, Samsa GP, et al. Predicting complications of carotid endarterectomy. *Stroke.* 1993;24:1285–1291.
24. Asiddao CB, Donegan JH, Whitesell RC, et al. Factors associated with perioperative complications during carotid endarterectomy. *Anesth Anal.* 1982;61:631–637.
25. Lipsett PA, Tierney S, Gordon TA, et al. Carotid endarterectomy—is intensive care unit necessary? *J Vasc Surg.* 1994;20:403–410.
26. Morasch MD, Hirko MK, Hirasa T, et al. Intensive care after carotid endarterectomy: a prospective evaluation. *J Am Coll Surg.* 1996;183:387–392.
27. Hirko MK, Morasch MD, Burke K, et al. The changing face of carotid endarterectomy. *J Vasc Surg.* 1996;23:622–627.
28. McConnell DB, Yeager RA, Moneta GL, et al. Just in time decision making for ICU care after carotid endarterectomy. *Am J Surg.* 1996;171:502–504.
29. Mattos MA, van Bemmelen PS, Barkmeier LD, et al. Routine surveillance after carotid endarterectomy: does it affect clinical management? *J Vasc Surg.* 1993;17:819–831.
30. Mansour MA, Kang SS, Baker WH, et al. Carotid endarterectomy for recurrent stenosis. *J Vasc Surg.* 1997;25:877–883.

14

Coronary Artery Bypass Grafting with Carotid Endarterectomy

Thomas Bilfinger, MD, Michael Petersen, MD, and John J. Ricotta, MD, FACS

The debate concerning proper treatment of patients with surgical lesions of both the coronary and extracranial carotid circulation remains unsettled. Much of this results from the devastation that either stroke or myocardial infarction (MI) can cause in the postoperative period. Stroke remains the major cause of noncardiac morbidity after coronary bypass, and MI is the major nonneurologic cause of both early and late morbidity in patients after carotid endarterectomy (CEA). For many years, physicians have ignored the multifocal nature of atherosclerotic disease, focusing only on symptomatic lesions. However, this trend has changed. Cardiac evaluation is more common in patients with peripheral vascular and cerebrovascular disease than it formerly was and increasing numbers of cardiac centers are performing routine carotid duplex screening in patients with coronary disease. As a consequence, concomitant disease is more often discovered, and its management is an increasingly important question for clinicians.

Data from New York's statewide cardiac database[1] provide interesting insights into this problem. In 1994, 18,051 patients underwent isolated coronary artery bypass grafting (CABG) in the state with a mortality rate of 2.4% for primary surgery and 4.7% for secondary operations. Of these patients, 1042 patients (5.77%) had a history of stroke and their associated operative mortality was 4.41%. Carotid–cerebrovascular disease was reported in 2100 patients (11.6%) with a mortality of 4.86%. Although new neurologic deficits were reported in only 293 patients (1.62%), associated mortality was 26.6%. It is likely that the incidence of neurologic deficits was underreported in this registry. Nonetheless, these data show that the presence preoperatively of stroke or cerebrovascular disease doubled operative mortality and was associated with similar risk to reoperative surgery. Furthermore, the occurrence of a perioperative stroke, although rare, was often fatal. These data bear eloquent witness to the importance of identifying and managing cerebrovascular disease in cardiac surgery patients.

One might ask why, given the previously mentioned data, routine screening for and treatment of carotid stenosis is not the standard of care in CABG patients. Those who minimize the importance of detecting extracranial vascular disease in this group point out the multifactorial nature of stroke after bypass and the lack of proof for the effectiveness of CEA in postoperative stroke reduction. Additional arguments are made that identification of carotid stenosis by duplex screening adds expense, and is not likely to be cost-effective because of the low overall incidence of stroke in the CABG population. The low incidence of events in the general CABG population also desensitizes many clinicians to the problem of stroke in cardiac patients because even a moderately sized clinical program (eg, 500 CABGs per year) is likely to see only a handful of strokes after bypass. Finally, many smaller centers have limited experience with combined operative management of coronary and carotid disease and have had disappointing or even disastrous results.

In sequential fashion, this chapter presents the available data on the incidence of carotid stenosis in CABG patients, the relationship of carotid stenosis and perioperative stroke, comments about the cost-effectiveness of treatment protocols, and algorithms for management of combined lesions.

INCIDENCE OF CAROTID STENOSIS IN PATIENTS WITH CORONARY ARTERY BYPASS GRAFT

Increasing data have become available on the incidence of carotid stenosis in CABG patients. As initially reported in the 1980s, the incidence of significant carotid disease detected by routine screening ranged from 3.5% to 6%.[2-13] However, this incidence has increased significantly (Table 14–1), almost certainly as a consequence of the advancing age of the coronary bypass population. Faggioli and associates[8] and Berens and associates[11] both correlated the incidence of carotid stenosis with advancing age. In reports published between 1990 and 1997, stenosis in excess of 70% was seen in 4% to 8.7% of patients. In a survey of 917 patients screened for carotid stenosis by duplex prior to CABG, a multi-institutional group [Coronary Artery Bypass Endarterectomy Se-

TABLE 14–1. INCIDENCE OF CAROTID STENOSIS IN PATIENTS WITH CORONARY ARTERY BYPASS GRAFT (CABG)

Study	Year	Number of Patients	Stenosis (%)	Incidence (%)
Mehigan et al.[2]	1977	874	>50	5.6
Turnipseed et al.[3]	1980	170	>50	11.8
Balderman et al.[4]	1983	500	>50	3.4
Barnes et al.[5]	1985	324	>50	12.3
Brener et al.[6]	1987	4047	>50	3.4
Jausseran et al.[7]	1989	210	>50	
Faggioli et al.[8]	1990	539	>50	19.9
			>75	8.7
Berens et al.[11]	1992	1087	>50	17.0
			>80	5.9
Ricotta et al.[9]	1995	1779	>50	17.5
Pillai et al[10]	1994	1603	>50	7.6
Petersen et al.[12]	1998	2500	>75	4.0
D'Agostino et al.[13]	1996	1279	>50	
CABEST[a]	1996	917	>75	7.7

[a] Unpublished data, 1996.

quencing Trials (CABEST) investigators, unpublished data, 1996] showed that 7.7% of patients had operable carotid lesions (ie, severe stenosis without occlusion) and an additional 9.9% of patients had "possible operative lesions" (equivocal duplex screening). Reported predictors of carotid stenosis include age, diabetes, female sex, left main stenosis, prior neurologic event, and peripheral vascular disease.[8,11,14] Thus, whereas the prevalence of severe carotid stenosis in the CABG population as a whole may be 5% to 10%, certain subgroups have an enriched incidence of disease. Routine screening of all coronary patients may not be cost-effective, but those with the risk factors noted previously can be expected to have a prevalence of disease high enough to warrant duplex evaluation. To this group we would also add patients with a midcervical carotid bruit, although this observation has not been borne out by prospective study.

CAROTID STENOSIS AND POSTOPERATIVE STROKE

It is clear that the majority of post-CABG strokes occur in patients without significant carotid stenosis. It is equally clear that only one-half to two-thirds of strokes in patients with carotid stenosis are ipsilateral to the stenotic artery. Data from the Coronary Artery Surgery Study indicates that most strokes occur (or are recognized) more than 24 hours after coronary bypass.[15] As stated earlier, there are many potential causes for stroke after bypass: hypoperfusion during nonpulsatile extracorporeal circulation, emboli during cannulation or clamping of a diseased aorta, changes in coagulation relevant to the bypass circuit, loss of cerebral autoregulation, and embolization from the carotid bifurcation. The association between carotid bifurcation stenosis and postoperative stroke is clear in the case of neurologically symptomatic patients, but is less clear in those with asymptomatic carotid stenoses.[16] Faggioli and associates[8] reported a 14.3% incidence of stroke in patients with asymptomatic stenosis who underwent CABG without CEA. In a separate study, Ricotta and colleagues[9] reported that the presence of a carotid stenosis of more than 50% was a most powerful predictor of postoperative stroke, increasing the risk sixfold. Others have reported similar data. In contrast, Barnes and associates[5] and, more recently, D'Agostino and colleagues[13] from the Lahey Hitchcock Medical Center reported stroke rates of less than 3% in patients with asymptomatic carotid stenoses subjected to CABG alone. However, all of these studies have been retrospective. Gerraty and coworkers[16] reported on a mixed group of vascular cardiac patients with carotid stenoses of more than 50%. There were 53 with asymptomatic stenoses (28 of which were >80%), none of whom sustained an infarct after surgery. With the exception of this report, prospective data on large populations of patients with known asymptomatic carotid stenosis who are managed by CABG alone are not available.

Carotid stenosis may have an impact on stroke rate in several ways. In some patients it is likely that there may be alterations of cerebral autoregulation or areas of hypoperfusion that may become symptomatic when patients are placed on bypass. The fact that about 20% of patients with asymptomatic carotid stenosis are known to have cerebral infarction on computed tomographic (CT) scan[17,18] suggests that this may be a more common phenomenon than one might imagine. Carotid bifurcation lesions may become a source of emboli, particularly if there are changes in the thrombophilic state of patients after bypass. Finally, carotid stenosis may simply be a marker for intracranial or arch atherosclerosis. Although there are numerous studies documenting associations between various perioperative conditions or preoperative risk factors and stroke, studies defining the nature of post-CABG stroke are surprisingly few in number. Wijdicks and Jack[19] from the Mayo Clinic reviewed CT scans of 25 patients who suffered stroke after CABG, and found that 16 were the result of hypoperfusion and were embolic in nature. The majority of these were unifocal. The only other study is from Blossom and coworkers,[20] which reviewed the CT scans of 46 patients who suffered a stroke after CABG. Emboli were the cause of stroke in 54%, while the remainder had hypoperfusion as the cause of their stroke. Excepting these two reports, detailed classification of the etiology of post-CABG stroke is nonexistent.

There appear to be several clinical scenarios in which carotid stenosis is recognized to have increased stroke risk. The first of these is the patient with symptoms referable to the carotid lesion. In these cases there is near unanimity that this lesion must be dealt with prior to or at the time of coronary bypass. The second situation is the patient with bilateral hemodynamically significant carotid stenosis, including patients with unilateral occlusion and contralateral stenosis. Data from several studies[6,21,22] indicate that these individuals are at increased risk of perioperative stroke without endarterectomy. Even physicians who object to routine screening of asymptomatic patients often favor treatment of one or both carotid lesions if bilateral stenosis is present. Here again, however, inconsistency is the rule of the day, because some groups treat one lesion whereas others may treat both, using staged followed by combined procedures. Finally, Chang and coworkers[23] have reported combining bilateral CEA with coronary bypass for management of patients with bilateral carotid disease. Predictably, none of these data are prospective or randomized.

CAROTID ENDARTERECTOMY TO PREVENT STROKE AFTER CORONARY ARTERY BYPASS GRAFT

Although there are multiple factors that contribute to stroke after CABG, carotid stenosis is one of the few that can be influenced to potentially reduce stroke risk. This provides the rationale for the continued interest in CEA as a mechanism to reduce perioperative stroke. Multiple prospective trials have demonstrated the efficacy of CEA in reducing long-term morbidity from stroke in both symptomatic and asymptomatic patients with severe carotid stenosis.[24–27] Efficacy has been demonstrated in asymptomatic patients with stenosis of more than 60% and in symptomatic patients with stenosis of more than 50%. Unfortunately, whereas long-term stroke reduction may be extrapolated from these studies, no data are available that convincingly demonstrate reduction of perioperative stroke rate in CABG patients. Brener and coworkers[6] reported a large series in which patients were screened for carotid stenosis using noninvasive tests, and subsequently patients with carotid stenosis who underwent simultaneous CEA and CABG were compared to patients who underwent CABG alone. These authors failed to demonstrate a significant reduction in perioperative stroke rate with combined procedures. This was due to a relatively high perioperative complication rate in the combined group (8.8% stroke rate) and a relatively modest number of patients—problems that continue to plague many contemporary reports. Furthermore, Brener and coworkers' reports[6] were neither prospective nor randomized, a situation that continues to apply to all recent reports. Hertzer and colleagues[21] undertook a prospective trial comparing staged, combined, and delayed CEA in patients with unilateral asymptomatic carotid stenosis. Patients were randomized according to certain prescribed rules, and only one-third of patients were able to be randomized to CEA before CABG because of the perceived severity of their coronary disease. Two-thirds of the patients were allocated randomly to combined versus delayed surgery. Only 24 patients underwent CEA followed by CABG, with one fatal stroke (4%). The combined group consisted of 71 patients in which there were two strokes and three deaths (7%). The delayed

TABLE 14–2. STROKE IN PATIENTS WITH KNOWN CAROTID STENOSIS UNDERGOING ISOLATED CABG

Study	Number of Cases	Stroke Rate (%)
Faggioli et al.[8]	28	14.3
Pillai et al.[10]	67	9.0
Turnipseed et al.[3]	20	10.0
Barnes et al.[5]	40	2.5
Brener et al.[6]	64	6.3
Ivey et al.[28]	16	0
Schultz et al.[29]	50	8.0
Hertzer et al.[21]	58	6.9[a]

[a] Stroke rate after CABG in "reverse staged" strategy.

group (58 patients) experienced two deaths (3.4%) and four strokes (6.9%) associated with the CABG, an incidence not significantly different from combined surgery ($p = .25$). However, in the overall analysis the delayed groups were significantly disadvantaged in comparison to the group undergoing combined surgery as a result of the unusually high morbidity of the subsequent CEA (1.9% mortality, 7.5% stroke). The authors noted that this increased morbidity was seen primarily in patients who had CEA prior to their initial discharge and was not evident when the secondary operation was deferred for more than 1 month. Although this report contains the only prospective randomized data currently available, the small numbers of patients, their nonuniform distribution, variations in management, and the unusual rate of complications with delayed endarterectomy prevent one from drawing definitive conclusions.

The central problem is lack of a suitable control group—that is, patients with known carotid stenosis who undergo CABG alone. There are some data that can be extracted from selected series in the literature (Table 14–2). Stroke rates in these patients are somewhat variable and likely reflect subjective criteria that were used to select these patients for nonoperative management of their carotid lesion. It is very possible that these patients may be either a high-risk or a low-risk subgroup, and therefore not comparable to those patients selected for CEA. Review of these data suggest that a post-CABG stroke rate of 6% to 8% can be expected in patients with asymptomatic stenosis subjected to CABG alone. The data from Hertzer and colleagues[21] provide some insight in this regard if the stroke risk of CABG alone in the reverse staged (ie, CABG first) group is examined. These data are particularly significant in that they

TABLE 14–3. HYPOTHETICAL MODELS OF OVERALL RISK FOR REVERSE STAGED (DELAYED CEA) STRATEGY IN CABG PATIENTS WITH SYMPTOMATIC AND ASYMPTOMATIC CAROTID STENOSIS (STROKE AND DEATH)

	CABG (%)	CEA (%)	Total (%)
Symptomatic carotid stenosis	>11.8[a]	5.8[d]	>17.6
Asymptomatic carotid stenosis (Model 1)	10.3[b]	2.3[e]	12.6
Asymptomatic carotid stenosis (Model 2)	2.7[c]	2.3[e]	5.0

[a] Assumes >6.9% stroke (Hertzer et al.[21]) and 4.9% mortality (New York State Dept. of Health[1]).
[b] Based on data from Hertzer et al.[21] for CABG alone in reverse staged group.
[c] Based on D'Agostino et al.[13]
[d] NASCET data.[24]
[e] ACAS data.[24]

TABLE 14–4. MORBIDITY OF CEA–CABG IN PATIENTS WITH SYMPTOMATIC CAROTID DISEASE

Study	Number of Patients	Stroke Rate (%)
Perler et al.[30]	16	6.3
Lubicz et al.[31]	28	7.1
Hertzer et al.[21]	158	10.0
Minami et al.[32]	50	10.0
Rizzo et al.[33]	87	9.2
Mackey et al.[34]	100	9.0

represent the only randomized allocation to a delayed strategy. As noted previously, morbidity in this group was 10.3%, with a stroke rate of 6.9%.

In the absence of hard data on sequential patients with known carotid stenosis subjected to CABG alone, one must be content with calculating a "theoretical risk" of deferred endarterectomy based on the risks of each procedure. Such a theoretical model[1] is presented in Table 14–3. Estimates of CABG morbidity for patients with symptomatic stenosis are taken from New York State data on the mortality of patients with cerebrovascular disease[1] and a minimum stroke rate equivalent to that of asymptomatic stenosis reported by Hertzer and coworkers.[21] Two estimates of morbidity in patients with asymptomatic carotid stenosis are modeled, one from the data on reverse staged patients reported by Hertzer and colleagues[21] and the second from the report from D'Agostino and coworkers.[13] The risk of subsequent CEA for symptomatic and asymptomatic stenosis is based on data from the North American Symptomatic Carotid Endarterectomy Trial[24] and the Asymptomatic Carotid Atherosclerosis Study,[27] respectively. Using this model, an overall mortality of more than 17.6% would be expected if endarterectomy is deferred in symptomatic patients. This is probably an underestimate because the stroke risk of CABG alone in symptomatic patients is unknown. The results in patients with asymptomatic stenosis are much less predictable, with the model estimating complication rates of between 6% and 12%.

Data from some published series suggest that these rates may be achievable by combined or staged (CEA first) strategies in the modern era. Data on patients with high-risk carotid lesions (ie, symptomatic or severe bilateral disease) who undergo simultaneous CEA–CABG suggest a stroke risk of approximately 5% to 15% (Tables 14–4 and 14–5). Results of series of combined procedures published since 1990 are shown in Fig. 14–1.[14,23,33,36–40] The majority of these operations were for asymptomatic stenosis. Whereas some reports continue to indicate that combined surgery is associated with high mortality, other larger series in which the majority of patients have asymptomatic unilateral stenosis suggest that this is not the case if combined surgery is done as

TABLE 14–5. MORBIDITY OF CEA–CABG IN PATIENTS WITH BILATERAL CAROTID STENOSIS

Study	Number of Patients	Stroke Rate (%)
Hertzer et al.[21]	30	16.7
Dunn[45]	52	13.5
Babu et al.[35]	10	0
Brener et al.[6]	15	0
Rizzo et al.[33]	73	5.3

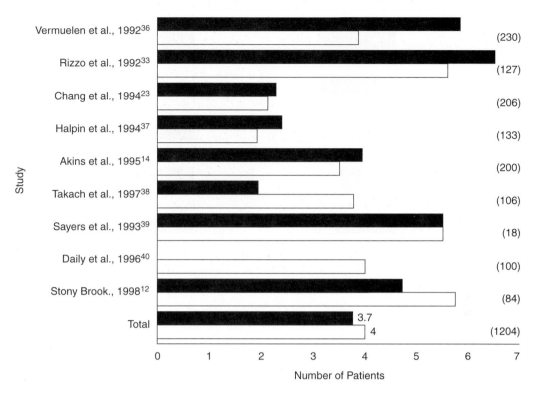

Figure 14–1. Studies showing incidence of significant carotid disease detected by routine screening, 1992–1997. Solid bars indicate stroke; open bars indicate mortality.

a routine rather than in selected patients who may be at high risk. Certainly data from Albany,[23] Massachusetts General Hospital,[14] and our own experience[12] suggest that overall morbidity and mortality in the range of 6% to 8% is realistic for combined surgery. It is apparent that these numbers are equivalent to or better than results predicted by our model for a strategy that defers CEA until after coronary revascularization. However, a definitive answer to the efficacy of CEA in reducing perioperative stroke awaits a prospective randomized trial.

SURGICAL OPTIONS FOR MANAGEMENT OF COMBINED DISEASE

There are only three options for managing patients with combined disease: (1) perform CEA at a separate operation prior to coronary bypass; (2) perform CEA at a separate operation subsequent to coronary bypass; or (3) perform the operations under the same anesthetic. The rationale for staging procedures is based on the assumption that combined surgery is associated with unacceptable levels of morbidity, which can be reduced by staged procedures. As discussed previously, the risks of deferring CEA have been difficult to quantitate. Evaluation of prior CEA is somewhat easier although still not without qualification. Several authors have reported series in which they employed both staged (CEA first) and combined strategies to manage patients with combined disease, and their data on stroke and death are presented in Figs. 14–1 and 14–2.[21,38,41,42] In each instance, there was a slightly reduced risk associated with the staged strategy. A major caveat in the interpretation of these data is the likelihood that

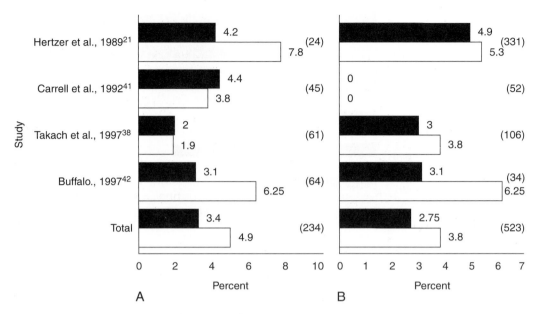

Figure 14–2. (A) Stroke and **(B)** mortality rates of selected studies concerning patients with known carotid stenosis who undergo staged (solid bar) and synchronous (open bar) CEA–CABG procedures.

these patient groups are not similar and that the staged strategy was most likely applied to the most stable patients. This presumption is supported by the observation that complication rates in these series for combined surgery exceed those in which the combined operation is performed on all eligible patients.

Brener and colleagues[22] reviewed the published English literature through 1993 concerning the management of patients with combined carotid and coronary disease. Using a meta-analysis technique, they demonstrated that there are no significant differences in the overall morbidity and mortality of the three staging strategies, with a tendency for combined surgery to have slightly better results. Performing endarterectomy first increased the cardiac risk, whereas deferring endarterectomy increased the stroke risk and minimized cardiac risk. Although interesting, this analysis is of limited value because of the wide variation of selection criteria among authors.

In addition to staging options, there are a number of options in the technical management of these patients. The senior author of this chapter has had a preference for performing endarterectomy separately prior to CABG. In this case, it has been most useful to perform the endarterectomy under cervical block anesthesia with sedation. This avoids the hemodynamic changes associated with general anesthesia, loss of homeostatic protective mechanisms, and the stimulation of endotracheal anesthesia. This option has been used routinely since the late 1980s in patients with severe coronary disease. Coronary bypass is performed shortly after CEA. In our experience, the interval has varied from 18 hours to 7 days. With this strategy for staging, overall mortality from both procedures has been 3%, and the stroke rate has been in the same range.[42] Management of bilateral lesions has been individualized. In some patients unilateral CEA is performed followed by a combined procedure. In very stable patients staged bilateral endarterectomies have been performed several days apart, then followed by CABG. In other patients, the second endarterectomy has been deferred until after CABG if the stenosis was not preocclusive and the coronary disease was critical. Flexibility in approach has been important in the absence of hard data.

Combined operations can be performed in several ways. In most cases, CEA is performed prior to cardiopulmonary bypass while the vein is being harvested. This requires a two-team approach. The advantage of this approach is that the carotid is clamped while the brain is subjected to pulsatile flow and, presumably, normal cerebral regulatory mechanisms. The wound is then packed and skin closed loosely with clips while coronary bypass is performed. A second option is to perform endarterectomy while the patient is on cardiopulmonary bypass. In most cases when this is done a side arm shunt is used to perfuse the distal carotid while endarterectomy is performed. This technique is most commonly employed when a single surgeon is performing both procedures. Finally, there have been some reports of CEA under deep hypothermia, with the purpose of providing increased cerebral protection.[43] This technique has not gained wide acceptance and provides no benefit in the routine case. Chang and coworkers[23] have reported a series of patients in whom bilateral CEAs were performed at the time of coronary bypass. Although they reported good results, this has not been the policy of most centers.

The appropriate time to wait after CABG to perform delayed CEA has not been established. The data from Hertzer and associates[21] suggest that early CEA may be associated with unacceptably high complication rates, although the reasons for this are unclear. Nonetheless, it was their recommendation that, should a decision be made to perform CABG alone, endarterectomy should be deferred for at least 1 month following CABG.

COST CONSIDERATIONS

Although cost should not be the primary factor in selecting a treatment strategy for patients with combined disease, it should be considered if equivalence between the options is demonstrated. In the current era of increased cost awareness, outcomes research, and supervision by federal and other agencies, it is necessary to review the available data pertaining to these areas of concern. Although it would appear that a combined strategy would be most cost-effective, this would apply only if morbidity and mortality were not increased. Generally, interventions that cost $50,000 or less per quality-adjusted life-year (QALY) are deemed worthwhile. Interventions that cost $50,000 to $100,000 are considered borderline; interventions that cost in excess of $100,000 are not cost-effective. If the marginal cost-effectiveness of accepted interventions is examined, we find that, for instance, CABG surgery for left main artery disease costs $6300 to $7000 per QALY (in 1993 US dollars). The costs of screening for hypertension are $12,000 to $42,600 per year of life saved (in 1993 US dollars).

According to the methodology published by Lee and associates,[44] funding and operating on patients with asymptomatic carotid stenosis fulfills the criteria for marginal effectiveness only if the procedural costs can be lowered by half. However, if patients have indications for CABG and an asymptomatic carotid stenosis, combining CABG and CEA, this appears to be a cost-effective strategy. At Stony Brook, where CABG and CEA were performed synchronously in a population of case-matched patients in whom age, sex, ejection fraction, and amount of coronary artery disease were controlled, the following costs (in 1997 US dollars) were incurred: CABG (DRG 106), $19,263; CABG and CEA, $29,288; CABG with stroke, $49,479; CABG–CEA and stroke, $38,130. Comparing synchronous CEA and CABG to isolated CEA and isolated CABG, Daily and associates[40] found a reduction in reimbursement for the hospital component of $8575 (27.1%; 1995 US dollars), in addition to an 18.21% savings in the surgical fee and a 17.6% savings in the anesthetic fee, for a total savings of $10,077 (25.3%) by performing combined operation. These numbers should be viewed critically and with reservation. The underlying assumption is that the outcomes are equal. It is the opinion of the present authors that if an institution cannot achieve combined CABG–CEA with a stroke rate of less than 6%, costs probably should not be the primary consideration. Furthermore, prospective studies on cost, including costs associated with morbidity, are clearly needed.

PATIENT EVALUATION AND SELECTION

Patient evaluation and the selection of an appropriate strategy depends on thorough assessment of cardiac and cerebrovascular risk. In data from our own institution, the State University of New York at Stony Brook, the occurrence of stroke and death after CABG was related to cardiac and hemodynamic complications more strongly than to any other factor.[12] The variation in cardiac and, to a lesser extent, cerebrovascular risk probably accounts for the large discrepancies that exist in reports of combined procedures from different centers. The centers with the worst results with combined procedures often reserve them for the highest risk patients. As noted earlier, it is generally agreed that patients with symptomatic carotid stenoses and patients with bilateral severe lesions (>80% diameter stenosis) are at the highest risk for stroke after CABG. The number of patients in this high-risk category is less than 50%, although the absolute frequency is difficult to determine. In large series where combined surgery is applied liberally, the incidence of such patients ranges from 20% to 40%. In the series reported by Brener and coworkers,[6] 25% of patients had bilateral stenoses larger than 50%, but the number with bilateral severe lesions is undoubtedly somewhat less. In the senior author's series of sequentially screened patients, 7.8% had stenoses larger than 70%, and about 15% of this group had severe bilateral disease. General experience suggests that symptomatic lesions are about three to four times less frequent than asymptomatic stenoses in CABG patients. The numbers of high-risk cardiac patients are much more common, particularly as interventional techniques and medical management have become more effective. High-risk patients include patients with left main stenosis or severe triple vessel disease (left main equivalent), unstable angina unresponsive to medical management, malignant ventricular arrhythmia, uncompensated congestive heart failure, ejection fraction less than 30%, and hemodynamic instability requiring inotropic or balloon pump support. These individuals are generally unsuitable for any operation until their coronary condition has been treated. The true size of this group depends on each physician's clinical threshold. In the study by Hertzer and associates,[21] two-thirds of patients were judged to be too unstable from the cardiac perspective to undergo a staged procedure, whereas in a series by Ricotta and colleagues[42] only one-third of patients required the combined operation. In this latter experience, staged procedures were done on urgent patients who were medically controlled with heparin and/or nitroglycerin drips in about 25% of cases. Thus, one might expect that between 40% to 60% of patients would likely fall into a high-risk category. In a prospective evaluation of 584 patients, 356 (61%) were judged to be a high cardiac risk using these criteria (CABEST investigators, unpublished data, 1996).

Once cardiac and cerebrovascular risk have been established, proper strategies for management can be developed (Fig. 14–3). To a great extent, these strategies depend on institutional experience and results. In patients with high cerebrovascular risk who are not at high cardiac risk, either a staged or combined strategy is applicable depending on local experience and results. Our theoretical model predicts that a morbidity rate

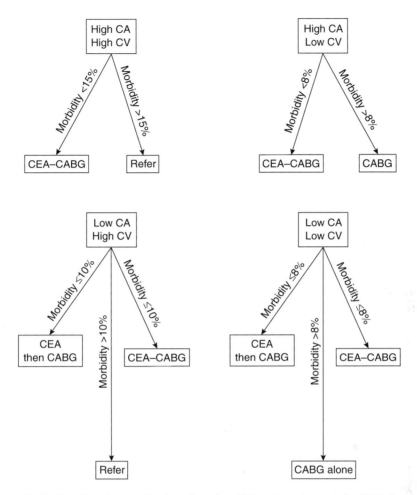

Figure 14–3. Algorithms for stratification of cardiac (CA) and cerebrovascular (CV) disease.

of 15% to 17% for combined procedures would be expected in these patients if CEA was deferred. However, it is our experience that these patients can be operated on with less than 10% risk using a staged strategy. If this is not possible using a staged or combined approach, then deferring the CABG procedure and referral to a center with a successful experience of managing these patients should be considered. In patients with high cardiac and cerebral risk, a combined operation should be undertaken. In this case a threshold complication rate of 15% to 17% is probably reasonable. Again, it is optimal to have these patients cared for by an experienced team, but this may not always be practical. This small patient group may be one in which carotid angioplasty will have a role in the future, although this is purely experimental at present. Patients need to understand that this is a serious situation no matter what strategy is applied. In patients who have unilateral asymptomatic carotid stenosis (ie, low cerebrovascular risk), there is more latitude in management. If the patient is not at high cardiac risk, at present our preference is to perform CEA either prior to or with CABG, providing the overall complication rate for these cases does not exceed the cumulative rate of 8%. Although our theoretical model suggests that complication rates of up to 12% may be acceptable, we believe that conservatism is warranted until the absolute risk of deferring CEA in a contemporary series is documented. Patients with high cardiac risk and unilateral asymptomatic carotid stenosis may be subjected to the combined operation if experience indicates acceptable complication rates. If complication rates exceed the 8% range for patients with asymptomatic unilateral stenosis, endarterectomy should be deferred until such time as the natural history of CABG alone in this population is known. In developing these guidelines it is important to understand that they differ in each case, dependent on the carotid and cerebrovascular risk, and must be developed for each institution or operative team.

CONCLUSIONS AND RECOMMENDATIONS

At present, the management of patients with combined coronary and carotid disease remains the subject of debate and is dictated by local experience and bias. Ultimate resolution of this problem will require a prospective randomized trial that characterizes the patients' cardiac and cerebrovascular risks preoperatively. At the current time we recommend that patients who have risk factors for carotid stenosis—that is, age more than 65 years, prior stroke, left main disease, peripheral vascular disease, carotid bruit, and smoking history—should be screened for the presence of carotid stenosis. This should be done to complete the overall risk assessment of the patient because carotid stenosis is a risk factor for both perioperative stroke and death. The prevalence of disease in these patient populations is sufficient to make carotid screening worthwhile.

When patients are found to have significant carotid disease they should be managed according to the algorithm we have developed. This algorithm is dictated by both the preoperative cardiac and cerebrovascular risk and the operative experience of the surgical team. As in any type of surgery, ongoing objective analysis of surgical results is of vital importance. Utilizing these algorithms, the surgeon can ensure that addition of CEA prior to or with coronary bypass will not significantly increase morbidity as compared to CABG alone, until such time as prospective data are available.

REFERENCES

1. New York State Department of Health. Coronary artery bypass surgery in New York State 1994–1996. Albany: New York State Department of Health; 1998.
2. Mehigan JT, Buch WS, Pipkin ED, et al. A planned approach to coexistent cerebrovascular disease in coronary artery bypass candidates. *Arch Surg.* 1977;112:1403–1409.
3. Turnipseed WD, Berkoff HA, Belzer FO. Postoperative stroke in cardiac and peripheral vascular disease. *Ann Surg.* 1980;192:365–368.
4. Balderman SC, Gutierrez IZ, Makula P, et al. Noninvasive screening for asymptomatic carotid artery disease prior to cardiac operation. Experience with 500 patients. *J Thorac Cardiovasc Surg.* 1983;85:427–433.
5. Barnes RW, Nix ML, Sansonetti D, et al. Late outcome of untreated asymptomatic carotid disease following cardiovascular operations. *J Vasc Surg.* 1985;2:843–849.
6. Brener BJ, Brief DK, Alpert J, et al. The risk of stroke in patients with asymptomatic carotid stenosis undergoing cardiac surgery: a follow-up study. *J Vasc Surg.* 1987;5:269–279.
7. Jausseran JM, Bergeron P, Reggi M, et al. Single staged carotid and coronary arteries surgery: indications and results. *J Cardiovasc Surg.* 1989;30:407–413.
8. Faggioli GL, Curl GR, Ricotta JJ. The role of carotid screening before coronary artery bypass. *J Vasc Surg.* 1990;12:724–731.
9. Ricotta JJ, Faggioli GL, Castilone A, et al. Risk factors for stroke after cardiac surgery. Buffalo Cardiac–Cerebral Study Group. *J Vasc Surg.* 1995;21:359–364.

10. Pillai L, Gutierrez IZ, Curl GR, et al. Evaluation and treatment of carotid stenosis in open-heart surgery patients. *J Surg Res.* 1994;56:312–315.
11. Berens ES, Kouchoukos NT, Murphy SF, et al. Preoperative carotid artery screening in elderly patients undergoing cardiac surgery. *J Vasc Surg.* 1992;15:313–323.
12. Petersen MJ, McBee CM, Bilfinger T, et al. Determinants of morbidity and mortality after combined carotid endarterectomy and open heart surgery. *Stroke.* 1998;29:269.
13. D'Agostino RS, Svensson LJ, Neumann DJ, et al. Screening carotid ultrasonography and risk factors for stroke in coronary artery surgery patients. *Ann Thorac Surg.* 1996;62:1714–1723.
14. Akins CW, Moncure AC, Daggett WM, et al. Safety and efficacy of concomitant carotid and coronary artery operations. *Ann Thorac Surg.* 1995;60:311–318.
15. Frye RL, Kronmal R, Schaff HV, et al. Stroke in coronary artery bypass grafting surgery: an analysis of the CASS experience. The participants in the Coronary Artery Surgery Study. *Int J Cardiol.* 1992;36:213–221.
16. Gerraty RP, Gates PC, Doyle JC. Carotid stenosis and perioperative stroke risk in symptomatic and symptomatic patients undergoing vascular or coronary surgery. *Stroke.* 1993;24(8):1115–1118.
17. Ricotta JJ, Ouriel K, Green RM, et al. Use of computerized cerebral tomography in selection of patients for elective and urgent carotid endarterectomy. *Ann Surg.* 1985;202:783–787.
18. Norris JW, Zhu CZ. Silent stroke and carotid stenosis. *Stroke.* 1992;23:483.
19. Wijdicks EF, Jack CR. Coronary artery bypass grafting–associated ischemic stroke. A clinical and neuroradiological study. *J Neuroimag.* 1996;6:20.
20. Blossom GB, Fietsam R Jr, Bassett JS, et al. Characteristics of cerebrovascular accidents after coronary artery bypass grafting. *Am Surg.* 1992;58:584–589.
21. Hertzer NR, Loop FD, Beven EG, et al. Surgical staging for simultaneous coronary and carotid disease: a study including prospective randomization. *J Vasc Surg.* 1989;9:455–463.
22. Brener BJ, Hermans H, Eisenbud D, et al. The management of patients requiring coronary bypass and carotid endarterectomy. In: Moore WS, ed. *Surgery for Cerebrovascular Disease,* 2nd ed. Philadelphia: WB Saunders; 1996:278–287.
23. Chang BB, Darling RC III, Shah DM, et al. Carotid endarterectomy can be safely performed with acceptable mortality and morbidity in patients requiring coronary artery bypass grafts. *Am J Surg.* 1994;168(2):94–96.
24. North American Symptomatic Carotid Endarterectomy Trial Collaborators. Beneficial effect of carotid endarterectomy in symptomatic patients with high-grade carotid stenosis. *N Engl J Med.* 1991;325:445–453.
25. MRC European Carotid Surgery Trial. Interim results for symptomatic patients with severe (70–99%) or with mild (0–29%) carotid stenosis. European Carotid Surgery Trialists' Collaborative Group. *Lancet.* 1991;337:1235–1243.
26. Hobson RN II, Weiss DG, Fields W, et al. Efficacy of carotid endarterectomy for asymptomatic carotid stenosis. *N Engl J Med.* 1986;228:221–227.
27. Executive Committee for the Asymptomatic Carotid Atherosclerosis Study. Endarterectomy for asymptomatic carotid artery stenosis. *JAMA.* 1995;273:1421–1428.
28. Ivey TD, Strandness E, Williams DB, et al. Management of patients with carotid bruit undergoing cardiopulmonary bypass. *J Thorac Cardiovasc Surg.* 1984;87:183–189.
29. Schultz RD, Sterpetti AV, Feldhaus RJ. Early and late results in patients with carotid disease undergoing myocardial revascularization. *Ann Thorac Surg.* 1988;45:603–609.
30. Perler BA, Burdick JF, Minken SL, et al. Should we perform carotid endarterectomy simultaneously with cardiac surgical procedures? *J Vasc Surg.* 1988;8:402–409.
31. Lubicz S, Kelly A, Field PL, et al. Combined carotid and coronary surgery. *Austr NZ J Surg.* 1987;57:593–597.
32. Minami K, Gawaz M, Ohlmeier H, et al. Management of concomitant occlusive disease of coronary and carotid arteries using cardiopulmonary bypass for both procedures. *J Cardiovasc Surg.* 1989;30:723–728.
33. Rizzo RJ, Whittemore AD, Couper GS, et al. Combined carotid and coronary revascularization: the preferred approach to the severe vasculopath. *Ann Thorac Surg.* 1992;52:1099–1109.
34. Mackey WC, Khabbaz K, Bojar R, et al. Simultaneous carotid endarterectomy and coronary bypass: perioperative risk and long-term survival. *J Vasc Surg.* 1996;24:58–64.

35. Babu SC, Shah PM, Singh BM, et al. Coexisting carotid stenosis in patients undergoing cardiac surgery: indications and guidelines for simultaneous operations. *Am J Surg.* 1985;150:207–211.

36. Vermuelen FEE, Hamerlijnck RPHM, Defauw JJAM, et al. Synchronous operation for ischemic cardiac and cerebrovascular disease: early results and long term follow up. *Ann Thorac Surg.* 1992;53:381–390.

37. Halpin DP, Riggins S, Carmichael JD, et al. Management of coexistent carotid and coronary artery disease. *J Cardiovasc Surg.* 1991;32:787–793.

38. Takach TJ, Reul GJ Jr., Cooley DA, et al. Is an integrated approach warranted for concomitant carotid and coronary artery disease? *Ann Thorac Surg.* 1997;64:16–22.

39. Sayers RD, Thompson MM, Underwood MJ, et al. Early results of combined carotid endarterectomy and coronary artery bypass grafting in patients with severe coronary and carotid artery disease. *J Roy Coll Surg Edin.* 1993;38:340–343.

40. Daily PO, Freeman RK, Dembitsky WP, et al. Cost reduction by combined endarterectomy and coronary artery bypass grafting. *Ann Thorac Surg.* 1997;63:516–521.

41. Carrel T, Stillhard G, Turina M. Combined carotid and coronary artery surgery: early and late results. *Cardiology.* 1992;80:118–125.

42. Ricotta JJ. Carotid endarterectomy and coronary bypass. In: Yao JST, Pearce WH, eds. *Progress in Vascular Surgery.* Stamford, CT: Appleton & Lange, 1997.

43. Kouchoukos NT, Daily BB, Wareing TH, et al. Hypothermic circulatory arrest for cerebral protection during combined carotid and cardiac surgery in patients with bilateral carotid artery disease. *Ann Surg.* 1994;219:699–706.

44. Lee PT, Solomon NA, Heidenreich PA, et al. Cost-effectiveness of screening for carotid stenosis in asymptomatic persons. *Ann Intern Med.* 1997;126:337–346.

45. Dunn EJ. Concomitant cerebral and myocardial revascularization. *Surg Clin North Am.* 1986;66:385.

15

Surgery for Asymptomatic Carotid Artery Disease

Is It Cost-Effective?

Jack L. Cronenwett, MD and John D. Birkmeyer, MD

INTRODUCTION

Natural history studies have demonstrated that a 2% to 5% annual ipsilateral stroke risk is associated with internal carotid artery (ICA) stenoses 50% or more diameter reduction, increasing with stenosis severity.[1-6] Based on excellent results following surgical treatment, carotid endarterectomy (CEA) has been recommended to prevent future stroke in asymptomatic patients with severe carotid stenosis.[7] This recommendation was confirmed by the Asymptomatic Carotid Atherosclerosis Study (ACAS) in 1995.[1] In this prospective, multicenter trial, 40- to 79-year-old asymptomatic patients with 60% to 99% ICA stenoses were randomized to receive either aggressive medical management (aspirin plus risk-factor reduction) or CEA plus medical management. Patients in the surgical group demonstrated an annual ipsilateral stroke rate of only 1% per year, compared with a 2.3% annual stroke rate under medical management ($p = 0.004$). This represented a relative stroke risk reduction of 54% by CEA, similar to the 65% relative stroke risk reduction reported in the North American Symptomatic Carotid Endarterectomy Trial (NASCET).[8] However, the absolute reduction in ipsilateral stroke risk by surgery in ACAS was only 6% after 5 years (11% medical vs. 5.1% surgical), compared with 17% stroke reduction by CEA in symptomatic patients in NASCET after only 2 years (26% medical vs. 9% surgical). Thus, although the results of NASCET were widely acclaimed, the smaller absolute benefit of CEA in ACAS led some to conclude that the expense of surgery might not be justified in asymptomatic patients. In fact, the ACAS authors noted that 19 CEAs would have to be performed to prevent 1 stroke in 5 years,[1] and the accompanying editorial concluded that this practice would not be cost-effective.[9] This conclusion is not obvious, however, because stroke is associated with high costs, and some asymptomatic patients will develop transient ischemic attacks (TIAs) during follow-up and incur or the cost of surgery anyway. To address this question more rigorously, we developed a decision analysis model to compare medical management versus CEA for asymptomatic patients with

60% to 99% ICA stenoses, using outcomes from ACAS.[10] This model allows us to determine the clinical circumstances in which endarterectomy would improve quality-adjusted life expectancy, and to calculate the cost-effectiveness of CEA in these settings.

CALCULATING COST-EFFECTIVENESS

The cost-effectiveness of a given procedure is defined as its cost divided by its benefit.[11] Typically, marginal cost-effectiveness is calculated, where the costs and benefits of two alternative strategies are compared. Thus, the cost-effectiveness ratio (C/E ratio) of Strategy A versus Strategy B is defined as

$$C/E = \frac{[\text{Cost A} - \text{Cost B}]}{[\text{Benefit A} - \text{Benefit B}]}$$

It is important for costs and benefits to be analyzed from the same perspective, which could reflect the viewpoint of the patient, the hospital, the third-party payer, or society at large.[12] Although each perspective may be relevant depending on the specific question being asked, the societal perspective is usually most relevant. As an example, a study performed from a hospital perspective might determine that early discharge of patients following vascular surgery to a rehabilitation center was very cost-effective because of reduced length of stay. However, this perspective ignores the cost of the rehabilitation, which might invalidate its conclusion from a broader, societal perspective. It is also important to recognize that charges for health care do not reflect actual costs.[13] The former is determined by the marketplace and by a variety of accounting practices that may shift cost responsibilities within an institution. Real costs are calculated by determining the actual costs of supplies, wages, utilities, and so on that are required for a specific treatment. Some analyses also include indirect costs, such as lost wages by the patient or by relatives who provide home care. Because of difficulties in estimating such indirect costs, however, most analyses include only direct costs. Unfortunately, the literature is replete with reports in which charges are used as a surrogate for costs, often in a misleading and inaccurate manner.

Measuring the benefits of health care is equally complicated because different interventions result in diverse outcomes that are difficult to compare.[14] For example, one intervention might improve survival, whereas another intervention might relieve suffering or improve well-being. The most commonly used metric to compare these different outcomes is quality-adjusted life expectancy, measured in quality-adjusted life years (QALY). This summary measurement captures the effect of an intervention on both the quantity and quality of life. To adjust absolute life expectancy for quality of life, time spent in imperfect health is multiplied by a fraction between 0 (death) and 1 (perfect health), which is determined by individuals or society to be the relative value of that health state. For example, based on interviews with patients following major stroke, it was determined that their quality of life was 40% of perfect health. Thus, if a patient lived 10 years following a major stroke, the quality-adjusted survival would be 0.40 × 10, or 4 QALYs. When comparing the cost-effectiveness of two alternative procedures, it is necessary to compare their costs, measured in dollars, and their benefits, measured in QALYs. Thus, a C/E ratio is defined in terms of dollars/QALYs. Because most people value current benefits more than remote future benefits, it is customary to discount future benefits (and costs) by approximately 5% per year.

For a rigorous cost-effectiveness analysis, it is necessary to know or to estimate the exact outcome of the treatment strategies being compared. Because this differs among individual patients and is defined by probabilities rather than precision, a decision-analysis model is used to project all of the possible treatment outcomes, their probabilities, and their associated costs. One such model, a Markov analysis, projects the outcome of a hypothetical cohort of patients from their initial health state until their death, based on the probabilities for different events as derived from the medical literature.[15] For example, a 65-year-old man with an asymptomatic carotid stenosis might live normally for 5 years, then experience a major stroke and die 5 years later (i.e., at age 75 years). The Markov analysis would calculate quality-adjusted survival for this patient based on the number of years in each health state, reducing the value of life after stroke, as noted previously. A similar patient might live 20 years with no stroke. Based on the probabilities for all of these events, the Markov analysis calculates the average quality-adjusted life expectancy for each cohort of patients with certain baseline characteristics. It also assigns a cost to each outcome and calculates the ultimate cost per QALY. Finally, this analysis compares the C/E ratio for two different strategies. The strategy that improves quality-adjusted life expectancy is preferred, and the C/E ratio determines the incremental cost for achieving that incremental benefit. Although there is no rigid definition for "cost-effective" therapy, it is generally agreed that procedures with an incremental C/E ratio of less than $20,000 per QALY are very cost-effective, whereas procedures with an incremental C/E ratio of more than $100,000 are not cost-effective.[16] In the intermediate range, many procedures are considered cost-effective, depending on a variety of factors that influence public opinion (Table 15–1).

An important benefit of decision-analysis modeling is the ability to vary the baseline assumptions about patient characteristics, outcome probabilities, or costs in order to determine whether the choice of optimal therapy is "sensitive" to these variables (*sensitivity analysis*). Thus, in formulating a decision model, the plausible range for key variables and costs is studied, which allows one to ask questions such as: What if the cost of surgery were lower? Or, what if the patient were older? This then identifies the key variables that will change the correct treatment choice, which helps physicians focus on the relevant issues for individual patients.[17]

TABLE 15–1. COST-EFFECTIVENESS OF SELECTED MEDICAL PRACTICES

Medical Practice	Cost/QALY
Treatment of mild–moderate hypertension compared with no treatment	
Propranolol	$13,000
Captopril	87,000
Hemodialysis for end-stage renal disease	53,000
Total hip replacement for severe osteoarthritis	4600
Coronary artery bypass compared to medical treatment of severe angina	
Left main disease	7000
Single-vessel disease	51,000
Transplantation compared with medical treatment	
Heart	33,000
Kidney	20,000
Treatment of hyperlipidemia with cholestyramine	189,000
Universal precautions for HIV[a] prevention in health-care workers	770,000

[a] Human immunodeficiency virus.

Cronenwett JL, Birkmeyer JD, Nackman GB, et al. Cost-effectiveness of carotid endarterectomy in asymptomatic patients. *J Vasc Surg.* 1997;25:298–309; discussion 310–311.

DEVELOPING THE DECISION MODEL

In our Markov decision-analysis model, we used the average patient characteristics and outcomes reported in ACAS.[10] Thus, for a base-case analysis, we assumed an average age of 67 years, with 66% men in the hypothetical population. We assumed that patients under medical management would receive aspirin therapy and risk-factor reduction as in ACAS, but would not undergo CEA as long as they remained asymptomatic. Unlike ACAS, but to more accurately reflect current clinical practice, we assumed that patients in the medical group would undergo CEA if they experienced a TIA or minor stroke. We assumed a 2.3% annual ipsilateral stroke rate (50% major stroke) and a 30-day stroke and death rate of 2.3% based on ACAS, which included the risk of arteriography. For patients in the medical group who developed TIAs or minor strokes and then underwent CEA, we used outcome probabilities from NASCET.[8] We calculated expected long-term survival based on ACAS results that included an excess mortality from generalized atherosclerosis, in addition to specific cerebrovascular events. We estimated the quality of life after stroke based on a published assessment in elderly patients (0.39 after first major stroke),[18] and assumed that patients with minor stroke had complete resolution by 3 months. We calculated the cost of CEA at $8500 and arteriography at $1600, based on a cost-accounting system in which both fixed hospital overhead costs and variable costs related specifically to this diagnosis were derived from our institution.[10] This calculation included an estimate of physician costs, based on current Medicare reimbursement. We estimated the cost of major stroke at $34,000 during the first year followed by $18,000 annually, based on population-based reports.[19, 20] We applied a discount rate of 5% to adjust future costs and health benefits to their present value. Further details associated with these assumptions are described in our original publication.[10]

IS ENDARTERECTOMY COST-EFFECTIVE?

For the average 67-year-old patient in ACAS, our calculations indicated that quality-adjusted life expectancy in the medical group was 7.87 QALYs versus 8.12 QALYs in the surgical group, a difference of 0.25 QALYs (3 months) in favor of surgical treatment.[10] The predicted lifetime cost was $12,407 for medical treatment and $14,448 for surgical treatment, a difference of $2041 in favor of medical treatment. Thus, the incremental cost-effectiveness ratio for surgical treatment was $2041/0.25 QALYs, or $8000 per QALY compared with medical treatment. Thus, for the average patient in the ACAS study, CEA was clearly cost-effective when compared with other commonly accepted medical practices (Table 15–1). This is because the initial cost of surgery is offset by the high cost of major stroke, and also because many medical patients develop symptoms during follow-up and then incur the cost of surgery.

A detailed analysis indicated that the majority of costs in the medical group were associated with stroke, whereas most costs in the surgical group were associated with CEA (Fig. 15–1). In the medical group, 79% of costs were attributed to the initial and subsequent care of patients with major stroke, and 15% of costs were associated with subsequent CEA for patients who became symptomatic. In contrast, 67% of total costs in the surgical group were associated with CEA, wheeras 31% of costs were associated with care for major stroke in this group. It is noteworthy that 26% of medically managed patients experienced TIAs or minor stroke during their lifetime that led to CEA (TIAs at 2.1% per year and minor stroke at 1.1% per year based on ACAS). Not surprisingly,

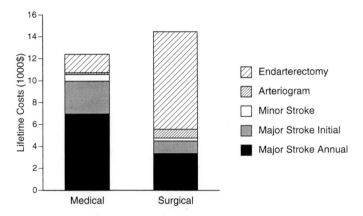

Figure 15–1. Lifetime cost estimates (discounted at 5%) for medical and surgical treatment of 67-year-old patients with 60% or more asymptomatic carotid stenosis. Medical patients experienced total costs that were $2000 less than surgical patients, heavily allocated to care after major stroke. Costs for surgical patients were influenced predominantly by initial procedural costs. (*Cronenwett JL, Birkmeyer JD, Nackman GB, et al. Cost-effectiveness of carotid endarterectomy in asymptomatic patients.* J Vasc Surg. *1997;25:298–309; discussion 310–311.*)

the proportion of patients who experience such symptoms is substantially increased for younger patients with longer life expectancy (32% for 60-year-old patients versus only 14% for 80-year-old patients). Our model predicted that these symptoms would occur at a median time of 5.5 years following initial evaluation. The cost of stroke was substantial in our model, with a projected lifetime cost of $192,000 following a major stroke. Of these costs, 30% ($57,600) were associated with care during the first year after major stroke, and 70% ($134,000) of costs were associated with chronic care of that portion of patients who remained disabled after major stroke. In the medical group, 12% of patients experienced a major stroke during their lifetime, compared with only 5% of patients in the surgical group, a risk reduction of 58%, comparable to the overall 53% ipsilateral stroke risk reduction reported in ACAS.

KEY VARIABLES THAT DETERMINE COST-EFFECTIVENESS

In order to identify relevant clinical parameters that have a major impact on cost-effectiveness, we used sensitivity analysis, as described previously. Based on a literature review using population-based studies when possible, we determined the plausible range of each variable in our model, and investigated the impact of changes in these variables on the cost-effectiveness of carotid surgery. Of all the variables, we found that life expectancy had the most significant influence on cost-effectiveness in our analysis.[10]

Age

Although age is only a proxy for life expectancy, it is the most accurate predictor in large, population-based models. For individual patients, many other variables can be used to predict life expectancy more accurately. However, in decision-analysis models, age is a useful surrogate for life expectancy, and its impact on the cost-effectiveness of CEA for asymptomatic 60% or more ICA stenosis is shown in Fig. 15–2. This demonstrates that for patients younger than approximately 70 years of age, the incremental cost of surgical treatment was less than $20,000 per QALY and clearly cost-

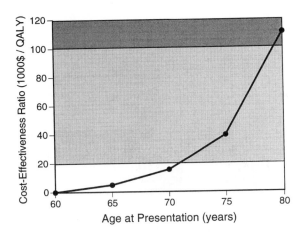

Figure 15–2. Cost-effectiveness of surgical treatment compared with medical management as a function of age in the base-case analysis of patients with 60% or more asymptomatic carotid stenosis. Shading indicates three categories of cost-effectiveness: less than $20,000 per QALY, clearly cost-effective; $20,000 to more than $100,000, intermediate cost-effectiveness; more than $100,000, not cost-effective. By these definitions, surgical treatment is cost-effective until at least age 72 and perhaps to age 79. (*Cronenwett JL, Birkmeyer JD, Nackman GB, et al. Cost-effectiveness of carotid endarterectomy in asymptomatic patients.* J Vasc Surg. *1997; 25:298–309; discussion 310–311.*)

effective. It also demonstrates that for patients younger than 60 years, surgery was "dominant" (both more effective and less expensive). The cost of surgical treatment increased exponentially for patients older than 70 years and exceeded $100,000 per QALY by age 79. This exponential increase in the cost-effectiveness ratio with increasing age is an important concept that can be attributed to decreased life expectancy in older patients, with reduced opportunity to experience the benefit of prophylactic CEA after incurring the initial cost. Thus, CEA in asymptomatic patients is unlikely to be cost-effective for patients older than 80 years of age unless they have a life expectancy much better than average, or a stroke risk much higher than average (see next section).

Stroke Risk

The second variable we identified with a major influence on cost-effectiveness is the ipsilateral stroke rate observed during medical management (Fig. 15–3).[10] It is difficult to predict the precise stroke risk for a given patient. The average estimate of 2.3% per year from ACAS is very similar to the rate of 2.4% per year for male patients in the Veterans' Administration Cooperative Study with 50% to 99% ICA stenoses.[3] It is also similar to the annual ipsilateral stroke rate of 2.3% observed during follow-up of asymptomatic patients with 50% to 79% ICA stenoses by Mansour and colleagues.[4] However, individual patient factors undoubtedly influence this result. For example, there is convincing evidence that progression of ICA stenoses during follow-up substantially increases stroke risk. In the asymptomatic patients with 50% to 79% ICA stenosis followed by Mansour and coworkers,[4] the stroke rate was only 0.23% per year if the stenosis remained stable, but fully 6.8% per year if the stenosis progressed to more than 80%. This detrimental effect of ICA stenosis progression has been noted by others.[21] Carotid ulceration and plaque composition also appear to predict stroke risk during medical management.[7] Although carotid ulceration is difficult to detect, initial reports suggest that echolucent plaque, detectable by duplex ultrasound, significantly increases

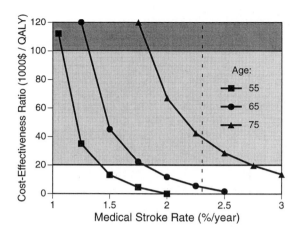

Figure 15–3. Cost-effectiveness of surgical treatment for 60% or more asymptomatic carotid stenosis as a function of ipsilateral stroke rate during medical management for three different age groups. For young patients (age 55), surgery is cost-effective even at low annual stroke risk (1.5%/year). For older patients (age 75), surgery is cost-effective only if medical stroke risk is high (> 2.5%/year). The broken line at 2.3% annual stroke risk indicates the base-case assumption based on ACAS. (*Cronenwett JL, Birkmeyer JD, Nackman GB, et al. Cost-effectiveness of carotid endarterectomy in asymptomatic patients.* J Vasc Surg. *1997;25:298–309; discussion 310–311.*)

the likelihood of future symptoms.[22] Thus, prophylactic CEA is probably not cost-effective for stable, nonprogressive ICA stenoses, but is likely to be very cost-effective for progressive stenoses even in elderly patients in whom the stroke rate during medical management exceeds 3% per year (Fig. 15–3).

Surgical Risk

The final important variable that determines the cost-effectiveness of CEA is the risk of perioperative stroke or death. For very young patients the cost of surgical treatment was less than $20,000 per QALY with perioperative event rates as high as 6% (Fig. 15–4).[10] Such a high operative stroke rate exceeds the recommended threshold for performing CEA in asymptomatic patients.[7] However, because of the long life expectancy in these young patients during medical management, this is offset by the cumulative 12% stroke rate that occurs. This makes surgical treatment cost-effective even at higher perioperative risk in younger patients. For patients older than 75 years of age, however, the cost of surgical treatment exceeds $20,000 per QALY at a perioperative event rate of only 2%, reinforcing the important influence of age on the choice of medical versus surgical treatment (see Fig. 15–4). This also emphasizes the importance of evaluating surgeon-specific outcomes when considering a recommendation for prophylactic CEA. Published guidelines suggest that CEA for asymptomatic patients should be offered only when the perioperative stroke–death rate is less than 3%,[7] which would clearly be cost-effective according to our analysis. Unfortunately, population-based studies suggest that these results are often not achieved, especially by surgeons who perform a low volume of carotid surgery.[23,24]

Cost of Stroke and Surgery

Examination of costs in our model demonstrated that only the annual cost of major stroke and the cost of CEA had a significant influence on cost-effectiveness when

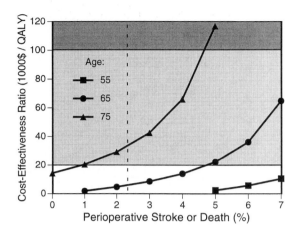

Figure 15–4. Cost-effectiveness of surgical treatment for 60% or more asymptomatic carotid stenosis as a function of perioperative stroke or death rate for three different age groups. For young patients, surgery is cost-effective even at higher operative event rates. For older patients, however, perioperative event rate must be much lower for surgical treatment to be cost-effective. The broken line at 2.3% indicates the base-case assumption for perioperative event rate based on ACAS. (*Cronenwett JL, Birkmeyer JD, Nackman GB, et al. Cost-effectiveness of carotid endarterectomy in asymptomatic patients.* J Vasc Surg. *1997;25:298–309; discussion 310–311.*)

examined over their plausible range. We created a "worst-case" scenario for surgery by combining the lowest published cost estimate for annual stroke care ($9500 per year) with the highest estimated cost for CEA ($11,600).[10] We also developed a low cost estimate (best case for surgery) using the highest cost estimate for annual stroke care ($32,000 per year) and the lowest cost estimate for CEA ($7500). As shown in Fig. 15–5, for a 70-year-old patient, the cost of surgical treatment increases from $15,000

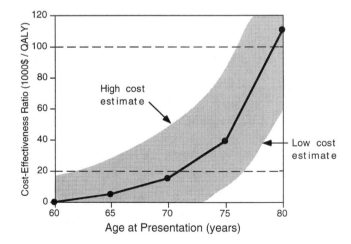

Figure 15–5. Extreme estimates (shaded range) for cost-effectiveness of surgical treatment of 60% or more asymptomatic carotid stenosis as a function of age, based on varying cost for surgical and medical care. High-cost estimate uses the lowest cost for stroke care and the highest cost for surgery. Low-cost estimate uses the highest cost for stroke care and the lowest cost for surgery. (*Cronenwett JL, Birkmeyer JD, Nackman GB, et al. Cost-effectiveness of carotid endarterectomy in asymptomatic patients.* J Vasc Surg. *1997;25:298–309; discussion 310–311.*)

per QALY (base-case assumption) to $43,000 per QALY at the high-cost estimate, a range that is still generally cost-effective compared with other medical practices (Table 15–1). At the low-cost estimate for a 70-year-old patient, surgery is dominant (both more effective and less expensive). It is apparent that major changes in the cost of stroke care or surgical treatment could have significant influences on cost-effectiveness. However, within the plausible range of these values, our overall conclusion remains unchanged—namely, that CEA is cost-effective for the average patient with asymptomatic 60% to 99% stenosis, as represented by the ACAS results. Other factors that change costs can also influence cost-effectiveness, such as arteriography. In our model, we assumed that 50% of patients would undergo arteriography, which added significant cost to the surgical group (estimated $1600).[10] If arteriography is replaced by lower cost duplex ultrasound, surgical treatment becomes more cost-effective if duplex has comparable accuracy for selecting severe ICA stenoses.

CONCLUSIONS

Our analysis indicates that CEA is cost-effective for treating asymptomatic patients with 60% to 99% ICA stenoses, assuming the outcomes reported in ACAS. This is true despite the requirement to perform 19 CEAs to prevent 1 stroke, because the high cost of stroke care compensates for the cost of surgery. The most important factor that should influence patient selection is age, because older patients with limited life expectancy have less opportunity to benefit from stroke risk reduction after CEA. Unfortunately, because carotid atherosclerosis increases as a function of age, most asymptomatic stenoses are detected in patients who are least likely to benefit from prophylactic CEA. This underscores the importance of careful patient selection, which also requires an estimate of stroke risk during medical management and an accurate understanding of surgeon-specific operative risk. More research is needed to identify risk factors, such as stenosis progression, that increase stroke risk during follow-up, and more individual outcome analysis needs to be performed by surgeons. In order to recommend CEA for appropriate asymptomatic patients, surgical stroke risk must be low, at least less than 3%, a result unlikely to be achieved by the occasional surgeon.

Cost-effectiveness analysis should not substitute for clinical judgment when recommending appropriate treatment for individual patients. However, this technique identifies the important variables, such as age and stroke risk, that should influence decision making. Overall, our results indicate that CEA is cost-effective in asymptomatic patients 75 years of age or younger with 60% or more ICA stenosis when compared with other commonly accepted medical practices. Application of this conclusion requires excellent surgical results and at least average patient life expectancy. Using these guidelines from a cost-effectiveness analysis facilitates the selection of asymptomatic patients for CEA.

REFERENCES

1. Executive Committee for the Asymptomatic Carotid Atherosclerosis Study. Endarterectomy for asymptomatic carotid artery stenosis. *JAMA.* 1995;273:1421–1428.
2. The European Carotid Surgery Trialists' Collaborative Group. Risk of stroke in the distribution of an asymptomatic carotid artery. *Lancet.* 1995;345:209–212.

3. Hobson RW, Weiss DG, Fields WS, et al. Efficacy of carotid endarterectomy for asymptomatic carotid stenosis. The Veterans Affairs Cooperative Study Group. *N Engl J Med*. 1993;328: 221–227.

4. Mansour MA, Mattos MA, Faught WE, et al. The natural history of moderate (50% to 79%) internal carotid artery stenosis in symptomatic, nonhemispheric, and asymptomatic patients. *J Vasc Surg*. 1995;21:346–357.

5. Norris JW, Zhu CZ, Bornstein NM, Chambers BR. Vascular risks of asymptomatic carotid stenosis. *Stroke*. 1991;22:1485–1490.

6. The Casanova Study Group. Carotid surgery versus medical therapy in asymptomatic carotid stenosis. *Stroke*. 1991;22:1229–1235.

7. Moore WS, Barnett HJ, Beebe HG, et al. Guidelines for carotid endarterectomy. A multidisciplinary consensus statement from the ad hoc committee, American Heart Association. *Stroke*. 1995;26:188–201.

8. North American Symptomatic Carotid Endarterectomy Trial. Beneficial effect of carotid endarterectomy in symptomatic patients with high-grade carotid stenosis. *N Engl J Med*. 1991;325:445–453.

9. Mayberg MR, Winn HR. Endarterectomy for asymptomatic carotid artery stenosis. Resolving the controversy. *JAMA*. 1995;273:1459–1461.

10. Cronenwett JL, Birkmeyer JD, Nackman GB, et al. Cost-effectiveness of carotid endarterectomy in asymptomatic patients. *J Vasc Surg*. 1997;25:298–309; discussion 310–311.

11. Finlayson SR, Birkmeyer JD. Cost-effectiveness analysis in surgery. *Surgery*. 1998;123:151–156.

12. Drummond MF, Richardson WS, O'Brien BJ, et al. Users' guides to the medical literature. XIII. How to use an article on economic analysis of clinical practice. A. Are the results of the study valid? Evidence-Based Medicine Working Group. *JAMA*. 1997;277:1552–1557.

13. Russell LB, Gold MR, Siegel JE, et al. The role of cost-effectiveness analysis in health and medicine. Panel on Cost-Effectiveness in Health and Medicine. *JAMA*. 1996;276:1172–1177.

14. Weinstein MC, Siegel JE, Gold MR, et al. Recommendations of the Panel on Cost-effectiveness in Health and Medicine. *JAMA*. 1996;276:1253–1258.

15. Beck JR, Pauker SG. The Markov process in medical prognosis. *Med Dec Making*. 1983;3: 419–458.

16. Laupacis A, Feeny D, Detsky AS, Tugwell PX. How attractive does a new technology have to be to warrant adoption and utilization? Tentative guidelines for using clinical and economic evaluations. *Can Med Assoc J*. 1992;146:473–481.

17. O'Brien BJ, Heyland D, Richardson WS, et al. Users' guides to the medical literature. XIII. How to use an article on economic analysis of clinical practice. B. What are the results and will they help me in caring for my patients? Evidence-Based Medicine Working Group. *JAMA*. 1997;277:1802–1806.

18. Gage BF, Cardinalli AB, Albers GW, Owens DK. Cost-effectiveness of warfarin and aspirin for prophylaxis of stroke in patients with nonvalvular atrial fibrillation. *JAMA*. 1995;274:1839–1845.

19. Thorngren M, Westling B. Utilization of health care resources after stroke. A population-based study of 258 hospitalized cases followed during the first year. *Acta Neurol Scand*. 1991;84:303–310.

20. Terént A, Marké LA, Asplund K, et al. Costs of stroke in Sweden. A national perspective. *Stroke*. 1994;25:2363–2369.

21. Roederer GO, Langlois YE, Jager KA, et al. The natural history of carotid arterial disease in asymptomatic patients with cervical bruits. *Stroke*. 1984;15:605–613.

22. Geroulakos G, Domjan J, Nicolaides A, et al. Ultrasonic carotid artery plaque structure and the risk of cerebral infarction on computed tomography. *J Vasc Surg*. 1994;20:263–266.

23. Fisher ES, Malenka DJ, Solomon NA, et al. Risk of carotid endarterectomy in the elderly. *Am J Public Health*. 1989;79:1617–1620.

24. Segal HE, Rummel L, Wu B. The utility of PRO data on surgical volume: the example of carotid endarterectomy. *QRB Qual Rev Bull*. 1993;19:152–157.

16

Cost-Effectiveness of Carotid Endarterectomy in the Prevention of Stroke

Sheela T. Patel, MD and K. Craig Kent, MD

INTRODUCTION

Carotid endarterectomy (CEA) is the most frequently performed peripheral vascular operation in the United States. Among Medicare patients alone, approximately 110,000 of these procedures were performed in 1996 at a cost of $2 billion. The primary objective of CEA is stroke prevention. Although in the 1980s and early 1990s there was skepticism regarding the utility of CEA in accomplishing this goal, data from the North American Symptomatic Carotid Endarterectomy Trial (NASCET)[1] and the Asymptomatic Carotid Atherosclerosis Study (ACAS)[2] have since demonstrated the efficacy of this procedure. CEA, when performed in centers of surgical excellence, can provide superior protection from stroke when compared to the best medical management in symptomatic[1] and asymptomatic[2] patients with high-grade carotid stenoses. Because stroke is the third leading cause of death in the United States and the most frequent cause of serious physical disability in adults, costing more than $30 billion a year, any technique that prevents stroke has the potential to provide tremendous economic savings for society.

Although the aforementioned randomized studies revealed a role for CEA in patients with carotid stenosis, this benefit as measured by reduction in stroke was notably different for symptomatic versus asymptomatic patients. For symptomatic patients with 70% to 99% carotid stenoses,[1] the cumulative risk of ipsilateral stroke at 2 years was 9% in those patients randomized to CEA versus 26% in patients who received optimal medical therapy, yielding a relative risk reduction of 65% and an absolute difference of 17%. In contrast, for asymptomatic patients whose carotid stenoses were greater than 60%,[2] the 5-year cumulative risk of stroke was 5.1% in patients randomized to CEA and 11% in patients who received optimal medical therapy. Although the relative risk reduction for CEA in these patients was 53%, a value comparable to that achieved in NASCET, the absolute risk reduction for asymptomatic patients was much lower, at 5.9%. In fact, the number of asymptomatic patients who require treatment by CEA to prevent one stroke in 2 years is 67. In striking contrast, only six symptomatic patients need to be treated by CEA to prevent one stroke in 2 years.

Therefore, the application of CEA to all asymptomatic patients with greater than 60% stenoses as suggested by ACAS will indeed prevent strokes, but the price for achieving this benefit is the performance of a large number of CEAs. The cost incurred by these procedures is substantial.

These findings have prompted many to question the cost-effectiveness of CEA in asymptomatic patients. Interestingly, the cost-effectiveness of CEA in symptomatic patients when compared to that of other major medical interventions such as coronary artery bypass grafting (CABG) surgery is also not known. In an environment of limited health care resources and escalating costs, it is essential that surgeons demonstrate that CEA not only improves the quantity and quality of life, but is also an appropriate allocation of society's resources.

To address the question of whether CEA is cost-effective, we have employed the technique of decision analysis.[3] The following is a description of a model we have designed to answer this question. This model not only allows determination of the cost-effectiveness of CEA, but also permits identification of the factors that have a major impact on the overall cost of this intervention.

METHODOLOGY OF COST-EFFECTIVENESS ANALYSIS

The underlying goal of a decision-analytic model is to compare both the outcomes as well as the costs associated with two interventions (e.g., CEA versus medical management of carotid stenosis). Also, when comparing two strategies of patient management, both the immediate as well as the lifetime sequelae and costs of these treatments must be considered. For example, a new antihypertensive drug may initially be more costly than the standard alternative. However, if this new drug is more effective in treating hypertension, potential late complications of hypertension such as stroke may thereby be avoided. Therefore, although the initial cost of the antihypertensive medication is higher, the lifetime cost in patients treated with this drug may be lower than conventional therapy because it diminishes costly morbidity. So goes the analysis with CEA. Although carotid surgery is obviously much more costly than medical therapy, if this intervention produces a substantial reduction in subsequent costly strokes, then the lifetime costs engendered in patients treated with CEA could potentially be less than those in patients treated medically.

If a clinical strategy produces both less morbidity and is also less costly over the lifespan of a patient compared to an alternative method of treatment, this strategy is obviously preferred. However, more often a new clinical strategy reduces morbidity but incurs a higher lifetime treatment cost compared to conventional therapy. This is frequently the case with new interventions or medications. Although it is appealing to adopt the new strategy because of its ability to reduce morbidity, the costs may be prohibitive. A cost-effectiveness analysis seeks to answer whether the reduction in morbidity produced by an intervention is "worth" the additional cost, and is therefore cost-effective.

The endpoint of a cost-effectiveness analysis is the cost per *quality*-adjusted life year (QALY) saved. This is the final common denominator that allows all medical interventions to be compared. What is measured is the extension in QALYs provided by one intervention versus another divided by the additional lifetime cost incurred by this intervention. Although the cost per QALY saved is reported in terms of the extension of life, often an intervention serves to reduce morbidity as well as to extend life. Some adjustment in life expectancy is necessary to account for patients who survive but who have a major morbidity. The mechanism by which morbidity can be translated into a reduction in life expectancy is through a value called a *quality-adjustment factor*, which is assigned for each year of survival for a patient who has a major morbidity based on the patient's perception of their quality of life with that morbidity. This quality-adjustment factor may range from 0 (death) to 1 (perfect health). For example, a patient who has a major stroke following intervention will require adjustment of his life expectancy based on the morbidity produced by the stroke. Studies investigating patient attitudes towards stroke report that most consider that the quality of life of patients with a major disabling stroke is 40% of that of patients without a stroke. In this situation, the quality-adjustment factor would be 0.4. Thus, for each year a patient with a major stroke survives, he is credited with only 4/10 of a quality-adjusted year of life.

Values for cost per QALY saved for common medical practices may range from $3800 for CABG for left main disease to $79,000 for the treatment of hypertension with captopril. Table 16–1 shows examples of cost per QALY saved for various medical interventions. Although the upper limit of what is acceptable by society remains elusive, values greater than $50,000 per QALY saved are beyond the range considered appropriate for most commonly practiced medical interventions.

The process of decision analysis can be separated into five logical steps. In the following sections, these five steps are demonstrated using as an example our analysis of the cost-effectiveness of CEA.

Step 1. Formulate a Question

In our example, we ask whether medical therapy or CEA should be chosen for a patient with a high-grade carotid artery stenosis. Because the analysis is significantly different for symptomatic versus asymptomatic disease, these two questions are analyzed separately, although the same general model applies for both.

Step 2. Create a Decision Tree

A decision tree is a structural representation of the possible strategies that can be used to treat a patient and the potential outcomes associated with each strategy. Each strategy leads to a sequence of outcomes that "branch out" to create a tree. The probability of occurrence and a cost can then be assigned to each "branch" of the decision tree. By

TABLE 16–1. COST PER QUALITY-ADJUSTED LIFE YEAR SAVED FOR SEVERAL MEDICAL PRACTICES

Intervention	Cost per QALY Saved ($)
CABG for left main disease	3800
CEA for symptomatic patients	**4100**
Elective surgery for 4 cm AAA	17,400
Heart transplantation	30,000
CEA for asymptomatic patients	**52,700**
Hemodialysis for end-stage renal disease	53,000
Captopril for hypertension	79,000
Arteriography versus duplex sonography preoperatively	99,200
Routine surveillance after CEA	125,950
Autologous blood donation for total hip replacement	260,800

QALY, quality-adjusted life year; CABG, coronary artery bypass grafting; CEA, carotid endarterectomy; AAA, abdominal aortic aneurysm.

methodically weighing all possible outcomes as well as the risks, benefits, and costs associated with each branch, the best strategy for approaching a problem can be selected in an organized and coherent manner. A clinical decision is then made by applying a logical equation instead of relying on the use of intuition.

The first portion of the decision tree used in this analysis is displayed in Fig. 16–1. There are two strategies to consider when managing a hypothetical cohort of patients who have asymptomatic high-grade carotid stenosis: CEA or optimal medical therapy. The possible 30-day outcomes for CEA or medical therapy include perfect health (i.e., no event), minor stroke, major stroke, or death. The second portion of our decision tree (after 30 days) is displayed in Fig. 16–2. This type of modeling is referred to as a *Markov process.* For the first year and for subsequent years, each member of a hypothetical cohort of patients who is treated for high-grade carotid stenosis may make transitions from one state to another. For example, a patient in perfect health may progress to a stroke or die. Such transitions from one state to another allow late events to be modeled. This decision tree, which is analogous to a sophisticated equation, is constructed on a computer using commercially available decision-analytic software.

Step 3. Assign Probabilities and Costs to the Decision Tree

The next step is to assimilate into the decision tree model the probability of each of the events as well as the cost of procedures and associated morbidities. As might be anticipated, multiple probabilities and costs are required for a complete model. For this particular model, the probability of developing a stroke following CEA or, alternatively, the probability of developing a stroke if a patient is not treated with CEA are both important variables that need to be incorporated. The procedural cost is also an important factor in the cohort of patients subjected to CEA. Stroke occurring in surgically

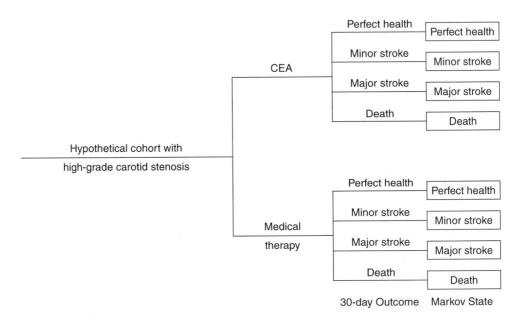

Figure 16–1. The first portion of the decision tree describes a hypothetical patient with high-grade carotid stenosis who may either undergo carotid endarterectomy (CEA) or receive medical therapy. The possible 30-day outcomes of each strategy include perfect health (no event), minor stroke, major stroke, or death. Each patient then enters a Markov state.

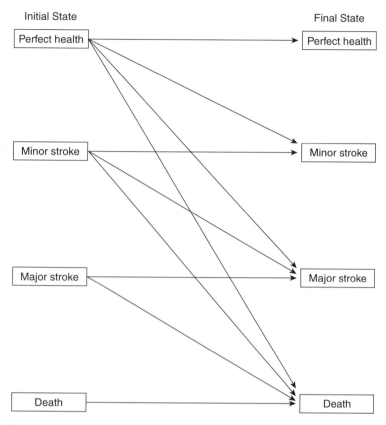

Figure 16–2. The second portion of the decision tree (post 30-day) illustrating the Markov process. Only certain transitions between health states are allowed. These transitions occur over the lifetime of the patient.

or medically treated patients must be assigned a cost. Multiple additional costs and probabilities were necessary to complete this analysis. In fact, this particular model required the assignment of 33 different variables. After realizing the multitude of factors that have an impact on the outcome of these patients, it becomes obvious why personal experience and intuition are not always sufficient to make these complex medical decisions.

Choosing the variables and costs to be included in the base-case analysis can be difficult. Both probabilities and costs may vary from one center to another. There may be controversy over the outcome of a particular strategy. For example, reports of stroke following CEA for asymptomatic disease are as low as 0% to 1% at some centers, and as high as 5% to 6% at others. Once a model has been created, data from any source can be introduced. In fact, varying the data can provide useful information about the effect that a certain variable might have on the outcome of the analysis. This process, which is described in detail later in the chapter, is termed *sensitivity analysis*. Obviously, the better the data, the more reliable the analysis. Therefore, when performing decision analysis, data from prospective randomized trials (if available) should be used preferentially over personal or center experience. In the paragraphs that follow, the important probabilities and costs that were used in our base analysis are reviewed and discussed.

The probabilities used in the decision tree for symptomatic patients were derived from NASCET (Table 16–2). The 30-day risk of stroke or death for symptomatic patients

TABLE 16–2. PROBABILITY ESTIMATES FOR PERIOPERATIVE STROKE OR DEATH AND LONG-TERM STROKE FOR SYMPTOMATIC AND ASYMPTOMATIC PATIENTS

Event	Symptomatic (NASCET) (%)		Asymptomatic (ACAS) (%)	
	Surgery	*No Surgery*	*Surgery*	*No Surgery*
Perioperative (30 days)				
Death, any cause	0.61	0.30	0.24	0.12
Major stroke	1.52	0.60	0.44[a]	0.07[a]
Minor stroke	3.66	2.42	1.01	0.17
Total	5.79	3.32	1.69[b]	0.36
Annual stroke rate (after 30 days)				
Major stroke	0.9	6.6	0.3	1.2
Minor stroke	0.9	6.7	0.3	1.1
Total	1.8	13.3	0.6	2.3

NASCET, North American Symptomatic Carotid Endartererectomy Trial; ACAS, Asymptomatic Carotid Atherosclerosis Study.
[a] Assumes that 30% of strokes are major.
[b] Excludes the five events associated with contrast arteriography.

undergoing CEA or receiving medical therapy was 5.8% and 3.3%, respectively. The ipsilateral annual stroke rate was 13.3% for symptomatic patients undergoing medical therapy and 1.8% for those undergoing CEA (87% surgical risk reduction).

The relevant probabilities for asymptomatic patients were derived from ACAS (see Table 16–2). The 30-day risk of stroke or death for asymptomatic patients undergoing CEA or receiving medical therapy was 1.7% and 0.4%, respectively. The ipsilateral annual stroke rate was 2.3% for asymptomatic patients undergoing medical therapy, and 0.6% for patients undergoing CEA (74% surgical risk reduction).

When evaluating the cost of various interventions or procedures, it is important to distinguish cost from charge or reimbursement. What hospitals or doctors charge for a particular procedure is usually irrelevant and is unrelated to what insurers pay. More importantly, what insurers pay may bear no relationship to the actual cost of an intervention. For example, Medicare reimburses a particular hospital fee for CEA. However, the procedure may actually cost less than Medicare's reimbursement in a hospital where intensive care unit (ICU) stays are eliminated and discharge is early. Conversely, in another hospital, where these cost-cutting measures have not been undertaken, the Medicare payment may be less than the hospital's actual cost.

For this analysis, the *cost* (not charge) of CEA ($11,390) was estimated from a hospital cost accounting system. The cost of resources ranging from overhead, administration, maintenance, utilities, nonprofessional and professional labor, housekeeping, pharmacy, and so on, was included in this determination. The professional fees for surgeons were derived from the Medicare reimbursement for the Current Procedural Terminology (CPT) code for CEA. The direct costs of stroke were estimated from the literature. A cost of $8550 was used for a minor stroke, reflecting the average cost per hospitalized patient for stroke. An annual cost of $730 was applied to a minor stroke to reflect outpatient care. An estimated 30% of patients surviving a major stroke will undergo inpatient rehabilitation followed by outpatient and home health care, whereas the remainder will reside in a nursing home. Under these assumptions, a cost of $47,230 was estimated for the first year after a major stroke and an annual cost of $24,820 for subsequent years. For patients who do not experience a stroke, an annual cost of $58 was assigned to reflect the cost of aspirin therapy.

Step 4. The Analysis (Base-Case)

After applying these variables, the next step is to perform a base-case analysis using cost per QALY saved as the outcome measure. Two separate analyses were employed— one for symptomatic and one for asymptomatic patients. For symptomatic patients, using data from NASCET, CEA provided a benefit of 0.35 QALYs saved compared with the best medical therapy at an additional cost of $1420, yielding a cost per QALY saved of $4100. This is a very favorable ratio, which is comparable to CABG (see Table 16–1). Alternately, CEA in asymptomatic patients, using data from ACAS, provided a benefit of 0.145 QALYs saved at an additional cost of $7648, yielding a cost per QALY saved of $52,700 (more than 13 times that for symptomatic patients). This is comparable to hemodialysis for end-stage renal disease (see Table 16–1). Therefore, although CEA for symptomatic patients with high-grade carotid stenosis is unequivocally cost-effective, CEA for asymptomatic disease may only be marginally so.

Similar analyses have been performed by others. Nussbaum and coworkers,[4] using data from NASCET, also concluded that performing CEA on symptomatic patients was economically favorable. In this analysis, CEA was found not only to extend life, but also to be less costly compared to medical management. CEA was therefore the dominant or preferred strategy. Differences between this analysis and ours were related to values chosen for the probabilities and costs. However, the conclusion of both studies was the same: CEA is extremely cost-effective in symptomatic patients.

Cronenwett and associates[5] found that CEA for asymptomatic patients was also cost-effective but with a much more attractive cost per QALY saved of $8004 (compared to the cost per QALY saved of $52,700 found in our analysis). Differences between these studies were related to both modeling [e.g., in Cronenwett's[5] analysis, patients with transient ischemic attacks (TIAs) crossed over to surgery] and values chosen for the variables (e.g., we assumed that the life expectancy of patients with carotid artery stenosis was more significantly limited due to cardiac disease than did Cronenwett et al[5]). Similar analyses have been performed by other groups and reveal ratios that are significantly less favorable (a cost per QALY saved of $247,500 was found in one analysis[6]). Although we feel comfortable concluding that CEA in asymptomatic patients is indeed cost-effective, the benefit in terms of cost may be marginal if one considers repairing all asymptomatic lesions that are of greater than 60% stenosis. Thus, there is still impetus for surgeons performing these procedures to identify ways to decrease procedural cost and increase efficacy, and thereby improve cost-effectiveness. Methods by which this can be accomplished are outlined in the following section. The difference between these various studies serves to demonstrate the extent to which the outcome of cost-effectiveness analyses are dependent on the modeling and the variables chosen.

Step 5. Test the Stability of the Base-Case Conclusion (Sensitivity Analysis)

The base-case conclusion relies on the best estimates of the probabilities and costs. However, altering a variable could potentially have a significant effect on the outcome of the analysis. Knowledge of the effect that variations in probabilities and costs have on the base-case analysis can be useful. The process of systematically changing the value of a variable is known as *sensitivity analysis*. If a base-case analysis indicates that an intervention is cost-effective, sensitivity analysis can determine under what circumstances an intervention is not cost-effective. Conversely, if an analysis suggests that a certain intervention is not cost-effective, performing sensitivity analysis might identify the circumstances under which an intervention may become an economically viable option.

In sensitivity analysis for symptomatic patients, CEA remained cost-effective despite wide variations in all of the probabilities and costs. Even if the perioperative risk was increased to as high as 17.4% (NASCET: 5.8%) or the cost of CEA increased to $20,000 (base-case: $11,390), the cost per QALY saved remained less than $50,000. However, the analysis for asymptomatic patients was highly sensitive to four variables: perioperative risk, stroke risk reduction afforded by CEA versus medical therapy, cost of CEA, and age of the patient. These same variables were also critical in the analysis performed by Cronenwett's group and are discussed in more detail next.

Perioperative Risk

The long-term benefit of CEA for high-grade asymptomatic carotid stenosis is critically dependent on the low perioperative complication rate obtained by the ACAS investigators[2] (1.7%, excluding angiographic complications). The cost-effectiveness of CEA for asymptomatic disease similarly relies on this low surgical risk. Doubling the perioperative risk from 1.7% to 3.4% increases the cost per QALY saved from $52,700 to $82,500.

In a meta-analysis of 3139 CEAs performed on asymptomatic patients, the perioperative complication rate was 3.35%.[7] A perioperative stroke and mortality rate of 4.3% was reported in the Veterans Affairs trial of asymptomatic carotid disease.[8] The use of a value this high in our analysis yielded a cost per QALY saved of $110,000. Thus, if CEA is to be cost-effective, it is imperative that centers achieve a perioperative risk for asymptomatic patients undergoing CEA that is similar to that reported in ACAS.[2] If the perioperative risk is halved from 1.7% to 0.85%, the cost per QALY saved can be reduced to $43,600.

Several studies suggest that perioperative risk is directly related to the volume of CEAs performed. In a retrospective review of CEAs performed on Medicare beneficiaries in the state of Georgia, hospitals performing less than 10 CEAs had a statistically significant higher perioperative morbidity and mortality than did hospitals with higher volumes of CEAs.[9] Perler and coworkers,[10] in a statewide analysis of 9918 CEAs, similarly noted an inverse correlation between hospital caseload and operative mortality rate, and a significantly higher neurologic complication rate in low-volume (6.1%) when compared to moderate-volume (1.3%) and high-volume (1.8%) hospitals. The experience of the surgeon is as important as hospital volume in determining perioperative outcomes. In a review of the results of 2243 CEAs, 10 surgeons who performed more than 12 CEAs per year had a statistically lower incidence of operative stroke (4.1%) compared with 21 surgeons who performed fewer procedures (7.2%). Moreover, the incidence of stroke for surgeons with additional vascular training (2.7%) was less than the stroke rate of surgeons who were not specialty trained (6.8%).[11]

In a consensus statement published by the American Heart Association, it was suggested that CEA for asymptomatic disease is indeed efficacious if the rate of stroke or death can be limited to less than 3%. In our analysis, the cost per QALY saved is $75,000 for a rate of stroke or death at this level. Thus, maintaining a rate of stroke or death in the 0% to 2% range may be necessary to allow CEA for asymptomatic carotid disease to be cost-effective.

Stroke Risk Reduction Afforded by CEA

In ACAS, the annual ipsilateral stroke rate associated with high-grade carotid stenosis treated medically is 2.3% versus 0.6% per year with CEA, yielding a surgical risk reduction of 74%. If the surgical risk reduction is only 50%, the cost per QALY saved for CEA in asymptomatic patients increases from $52,700 to $103,500. Conversely, improving the surgical risk reduction from 74% to 90% lowers the cost per QALY saved to $36,400.

Thus, patient selection is of paramount importance in determining the clinical and economic appropriateness of CEA for asymptomatic disease. If asymptomatic candidates for CEA can be identified who are at higher risk for stroke with medical treatment and thus are more likely to benefit from surgical intervention, then the cost-effectiveness of surgery for asymptomatic disease is optimized. The following factors may have some impact on the stroke risk of medically treated patients with carotid disease: degree of stenosis, plaque morphology, and sex.

Although degree of stenosis was not found to be statistically associated with stroke risk in ACAS,[2] various prior studies have suggested otherwise. In NASCET,[1] the risk reduction was greatest in patients with 90% to 99% stenosis and least in patients with 70% to 79% stenosis. An analysis of asymptomatic contralateral arteries in the European Carotid Surgery Trial (ECST)[12] revealed an annual stroke rate of 1.9 % for patients with 70% to 79% stenosis, 3.3% for patients with 80% to 89% stenosis, and 4.8% for patients with 90% to 99% stenosis. A similar gradient of stroke risk has also been reported in isolated asymptomatic disease. Norris and coworkers[13] observed an annual stroke rate of 3.3% in patients with asymptomatic carotid arteries of greater than 75% stenosis versus 1.3% in patients whose degree of stenosis was less than 75%. Progression of stenosis substantially increases stroke risk. Mansour and associates[14] observed that patients with asymptomatic carotid stenoses who progress from 50% to 79% to greater than 80% stenosis have an annual stroke rate of 6.8%, compared with 0.23% in patients with no progression. Accordingly, many surgeons now use a stenosis of greater than 80% (rather than 60%) as the threshold for intervention in asymptomatic patients with carotid disease. Because conclusive data is not yet available with regard to the benefit of this approach, it is difficult to estimate its effect on the cost-effectiveness of CEA.

Plaque morphology has been implicated as an important factor in stroke risk. There is a two- to fourfold increase in subsequent neurologic events in echolucent heterogeneous or ulcerated plaques compared with echogenic or nonulcerated plaques. Large ulcerations have been associated with a risk of stroke as high as 7.5% per year. Intraplaque hemorrhage has been postulated to cause acute luminal diameter reduction, resulting in thrombosis or intimal ulceration with embolization of debris. Although the effect of plaque morphology was not examined in ACAS,[2] forthcoming data from the Asymptomatic Carotid Surgery Trial (ACST) may clarify the influence of this variable on the risk of stroke.

Subgroup analyses in ACAS revealed that men had a 5-year relative stroke risk reduction of 66% compared to 17% for women. This observation may reflect a small sample size (568 women compared to 1091 men in ACAS) and thus a type II error. However, perioperative complication rates were much higher and the clinical course of unoperated carotid atherosclerosis appears less severe in women versus men. Schneider and associates[15] also observed that women had a trend toward greater perioperative stroke when compared to men (3.2% vs. 1.5%). However, in this study the rate of long-term freedom from stroke was virtually indistinguishable between women and men. Thus, the issue of sex dimorphism as it influences short- and long-term outcome of CEA requires further investigation.

Cost of CEA

Assigning a cost to CEA of $5000 instead of the $11,390 used in the base-case analysis lowered the cost per QALY saved for asymptomatic carotid disease from $52,700 to $8700, making CEA a much more acceptable allocation of societal resources. The value of $11,390 was derived from a hospital accounting system at a time when resource utilization was maximal and no attempts to diminish cost had been undertaken. Thus, the challenge facing vascular surgeons is to minimize the costs associated with this procedure.

Several studies have demonstrated that the costs associated with CEA can be reduced substantially without increasing surgical risk. Cost containment and optimization of resource utilization can be achieved by selective preoperative cerebral arteriography, same-day hospitalization, selective ICU admission, and shortened hospital length of stay. Many institutions have implemented clinical pathways that incorporate these cost-saving strategies to consolidate and standardize postoperative care without compromising quality (Table 16–3).[16–34] Hoyle and associates[16] reported a 29% cost reduction for CEA with the introduction of a case management protocol that avoided ICU admission and shortened hospital length of stay. Furthermore, the combined operative stroke and death rate for patients in this series was only 0.9%. Kraiss and coworkers[18] observed a more substantial 47% reduction in hospital costs associated with CEA with the use of a streamlined protocol that eliminated routine arteriography and limited ICU monitoring to high-risk patients. There were no strokes or deaths in patients treated in this manner. Thus, any means by which the cost of CEA can be reduced will make prophylactic surgery for asymptomatic disease more economically attractive.

Elimination of Routine Cerebral Arteriography. Vascular surgeons are now more frequently proceeding to CEA based on the results of noninvasive studies, thereby avoiding the costs and risks associated with cerebral arteriography. Contrast arteriography is extremely expensive. In addition to its high cost, arteriography is associated with risks related to arterial puncture, embolic complications, renal dysfunction, and contrast reactions. A substantial portion of the 30-day perioperative risk in ACAS[2] could be attributed to strokes caused by cerebral arteriography (1.2%). By avoiding routine arteriography, Hirko and associates[22] realized an average savings of 20% to 25%, which increased to almost 40% if professional fees were considered in the analysis. Even more dramatic savings were achieved by Ammar,[26] who observed a 72% reduction in charge in 230 patients attributable primarily to the elimination of routine arteriography.

Numerous centers have documented the accuracy of duplex ultrasound and magnetic resonance arteriography in detecting varying degrees of carotid stenosis. Moreover, these noninvasive modalities are free of immediate risk and produce minimal or no discomfort. It has been suggested that carotid arteriography only infrequently adds useful information to that already obtained from duplex ultrasound and/or a magnetic resonance arteriogram. Selective use of contrast arteriography appears safe and can dramatically enhance the cost-effectiveness of CEA.[35]

Selective ICU Admission. In 1991, O'Brien and Ricotta[36] first suggested the selective use of the ICU following CEA based on a retrospective review of ICU services utilized in a group of 73 patients. They found that only 18% of patients used services unique to the ICU and that the majority of these patients manifested their need for ICU services within the first 2 hours after surgery. Following the adoption of a policy of selective ICU admission, a 12.5% savings of the total hospitalization cost was realized. Hirko and coworkers[22] also found that only a short period of monitoring in the recovery room (average of 1.6 hours) was necessary to determine which patients would require the ICU. These authors were able to decrease the rate of postoperative ICU admission from 94.8% to 7.3% with no increase in morbidity or mortality. Thus, there are many studies that confirm that selective ICU admission does not result in major complications but does produce great cost savings.

TABLE 16–3. STUDIES OF CAROTID ENDARTERECTOMY UTILIZING COST-EFFECTIVE MEASURES

Source	Year of Publication	Number of CEAs	Preoperative Arteriogram (%)	Admission to ICU (%)	Average LOS (days)	Discharge on POD1 (%)	Cost CEA ($)[a]	Stroke and Death Rate (%)
Hoyle et al.[16]	1994	327	—	2	4.1	—	6879	0.9
Luna and Adye[17]	1995	65	95	2	1	—	8060	3.1
Kraiss et al.[18]	1995	18	6	22	1.3	—	5861	0
Friedman and Tortolani[19]	1995	72	47	100	1.1	88	—	0
Katz and Kohl[20]	1995	266	20	100	1.7	63	—	2.3
Gibbs et al.[21]	1995	46	—	—	2.3	—	7231	—
Hirko et al.[22]	1996	70	33	7	2	73	—	0
Kaufman et al.[23]	1996	163	64	37	3.8	50	—	4.3
Morasch et al.[24]	1996	185	35	21	—	—	—	3.2
Musser et al.[25]	1996	68	100	—	1.3	91	—	1.5
Amma[26]	1996	260	22	11	1.3	83	—	1.5
Ballard et al.[27]	1997	53	0	—	3.2	—	5534	3.8
Brothers et al.[28]	1997	68	91	—	2.2	—	7693	1
Collier[29]	1997	112	7	10	1.2	90	—	1.8
Back et al.[30]	1997	63	13	30	2	52	5699	1.6
Melissano et al.[31]	1997	380	15	2	5	—	3365	2.4
Schneider et al.[32]	1997	77	94	100	2.3	71	—	1.3
Bourke and Crimmins[33]	1998	65	2	0	—	83	—	0
Roddy et al.[34]	1998	45	11	—	2.1	—	7002	0

CEA, carotid endarterectomy; ICU, intensive care unit; LOS, length of stay; POD, postoperative day.

[a] Cost recorded only when studies report true cost (not charge).

Length of Stay.   Variations in length of hospital stay contribute significantly to health care costs. In many institutions, patients after CEA are routinely discharged on the first postoperative day with no additional mortality or morbidity. Kraiss and colleagues[18] were able to reduce the cost of CEA from $11,140 to $5861 using a streamlined protocol that allowed for a reduction in hospital length of stay from 3.1 days to 1.3 days. Although the use of local anesthesia has been proposed as a means by which length of stay can be reduced, many studies have demonstrated that after general anesthesia, patients can be discharged safely on the first postoperative day. Preoperative factors that have been found to be associated with an increased risk of complications and prolonged length of stay include advanced age, cardiac disease, and the need for postoperative anticoagulation.

Age
In sensitivity analysis, we found the cost-effectiveness of CEA in asymptomatic patients to clearly be greater in younger patients. This was related primarily to their increased life expectancy. Because the advantage in terms of stroke prevention provided by CEA accrues with time, the greater a patient's longevity, the more benefit a patient derives from this procedure. The average age of the hypothetical cohort of patients used in this model was 65 years. The cost per QALY saved for a 50-year-old patient who presents with asymptomatic carotid stenosis decreased to $33,800. Alternately, for a 75-year-old patient, this value is increased to $89,500. Cronenwett and associates[5] also observed that the cost per QALY saved of surgical treatment increased rapidly above age 70, exceeding $100,000 at age 79.

Although no randomized prospective studies have compared the outcome of CEA among different age groups, several studies have suggested an adverse impact of advanced age on perioperative morbidity and mortality. In an analysis of CEA performed in 2089 Medicare patients in New England, patients who were 80 years and older had more than four times the mortality (4.7%) of patients between 65 and 69 years (1.1%).[37] Conversely, in a report of 1160 CEAs at 12 academic medical centers, Goldstein and colleagues[38] reported no increased incidence of perioperative stroke or death among patients aged 75 years or older. Because the association between advanced age and increased perioperative risk has not been proved, this variable was not factored into our analysis. If further data prove convincingly such an association, then the cost-effectiveness of surgery in the older asymptomatic patient will become even less favorable.

CONCLUSION

With the reality of limited health care resources, it is necessary that any benefit from an intervention be achieved at reasonable cost to society. Cost-effectiveness analyses provide a cohesive mechanism for weighing and integrating the risks, benefits, and costs of medical therapies. A major limitation of cost-effectiveness analyses is their reliance on the best available data. The cost per QALY saved, which appears to be very precise, is only as reliable as the data used in its calculation, and therefore should be interpreted appropriately. Nonetheless, decision analysis is a powerful tool that is being used with increasing frequency to determine our approach to patient care.

In our analysis, the cost per QALY saved for CEA in symptomatic high-grade carotid stenosis was extremely favorable at $4100. However, the cost-effectiveness of CEA for asymptomatic high-grade carotid stenosis is marginal at best, with a cost per

QALY saved of $52,700. Only if the cost of CEA can be reduced or if subgroups of patients who have a high risk of stroke without surgical therapy can be identified will CEA for asymptomatic disease be economically appropriate. For example, the 55-year-old patient without a history of coronary artery disease who is found to have a 90% asymptomatic carotid stenosis seems to be an appealing candidate for CEA, compared to a 78-year-old patient with chronic stable angina and a 60% lesion.

Reducing the cost of CEA is of utmost importance and enhances the economic attractiveness of surgery for asymptomatic disease. This is particularly important with the emergence of carotid angioplasty and stenting (CAS), which has been advocated as a less-invasive alternative to CEA. The technical aspects of this new intervention continue to evolve, and in an early series of patients treated with CAS, an increased stroke and death rate was found when compared to CEA. A preliminary cost-effectiveness analysis performed by our group suggests that for CAS to be a cost-effective alternative to CEA, the morbidity and mortality of these two interventions need to be almost equivalent. However, this finding was dependent on CEA being performed in a cost-efficient manner. Thus, it is imperative that CEA be performed in carefully selected patients at the lowest cost and surgical risk in order to preserve its place in the treatment of carotid stenosis.

REFERENCES

1. North American Symptomatic Carotid Endarterectomy Trial Collaborators. Beneficial effect of carotid endarterectomy in symptomatic patients with high-grade carotid stenosis. *N Engl J Med.* 1991;325:443–453.
2. Executive Committee for the Asymptomatic Carotid Atherosclerosis Study. Endarterectomy for asymptomatic carotid artery stenosis. *JAMA.* 1995;273:1421–1428.
3. Kuntz KM, Kent KC. Is carotid endarterectomy cost-effective? An analysis of symptomatic and asymptomatic patients. *Circulation.* 1996;94(suppl II):II-194–II-198.
4. Nussbaum ES, Heros RC, Erickson DL. Cost-effectiveness of carotid endarterectomy. *Neurosurgery.* 1996;38:237–244.
5. Cronenwett JL, Birkmeyer JD, Nackman GB, et al. Cost-effectiveness of carotid endaterectomy in asymptomatic patients. *J Vasc Surg.* 1997;25:298–311.
6. Matchar DB, Pauk J, Lipscomb J. A health policy perspective on carotid endarterectomy: cost, effectiveness, and cost-effectiveness. In: Moore WS. *Surgery for Cerebrovascular Disease,* 2nd ed. Philadelphia: WB Saunders; 1996:680–689.
7. Rothwell PM, Slattery J, Warlow CP. A systematic comparison of the risks of stroke and death due to carotid endarterectomy for symptomatic and asymptomatic stenosis. *Stroke.* 1996;27:266–269.
8. The Veteran Affairs Cooperative Study Group. Efficacy of carotid endarterectomy for asymptomatic carotid stenosis. *N Engl J Med.* 1993;328:221–227.
9. Karp HR, Flanders D, Shipp CC, et al. Carotid endarterectomy among Medicare beneficiaries: a statewide evaluation of appropriateness and outcome. *Stroke.* 1998;29:46–52.
10. Perler BA, Dardik A, Burleyson GP, et al. Influence of age and hospital volume on the results of carotid endarterectomy: a statewide analysis of 9918 cases. *J Vasc Surg.* 1998;27:25–33.
11. Mattos MA, Modi JR, Mansour A, et al. Evolution of carotid endarterectomy in two community hospitals: Springfield revisited—seventeen years and 2243 operations later. *J Vasc Surg.* 1995;21:719–728.
12. The European Carotid Surgery Trialists Collaborative Group. Risk of stroke in the distribution of an asymptomatic carotid artery. *Lancet.* 1995;345:209–212.
13. Norris JW, Zhu CZ, Bornstein NM, Chambers BR. Vascular risks of asymptomatic carotid stenosis. *Stroke.* 1991;22:1485–1490.

14. Mansour MA, Mattos MA, Faught WE, et al. The natural history of moderate (50% to 79%) internal carotid artery stenosis in symptomatic, nonhemispheric, and asymptomatic patients. *J Vasc Surg*. 1995;21:346–357.

15. Schneider JR, Droste JS, Golan JF. Carotid endarterectomy in women versus men: patient characteristics and outcomes. *J Vasc Surg*. 1997;25:890–898.

16. Hoyle RM, Jenkins JM, Edwards WH Sr, et al. Case management in cerebral revascularization. *J Vasc Surg*. 1994;20:396–402.

17. Luna G, Adye B. Cost-effective carotid endarterectomy. *Am J Surg*. 1995;169:516–518.

18. Kraiss LW, Kilberg L, Critch S, Johansen KH. Short-stay carotid endarterectomy is safe and cost-effective. *Am J Surg*. 1995;169:512–515.

19. Friedman SG, Tortolani AJ. Reduced length of stay following carotid endarterectomy under general anesthesia. *Am J Surg*. 1995;170:235–236.

20. Katz SG, Kohl RD. Carotid endarterectomy with shortened hospital stay. *Arch Surg*. 1995;130:887–891.

21. Gibbs BF, Guzzetta VJ, Furmanski D. Cost-effective carotid endarterectomy in community practice. *Ann Vasc Surg*. 1995;9:423–427.

22. Hirko MK, Morasch MD, Burke K, et al. The changing face of carotid endarterectomy. *J Vasc Surg*. 1996;23:622–627.

23. Kaufman JL, Frank D, Rhee SW, et al. Feasibility and safety of 1-day postoperative hospitalization for carotid endarterectomy. *Arch Surg*. 1996;131:751–755.

24. Morasch MD, Hirko MK, Hirasa T, et al. Intensive care after carotid endarterectomy: a prospective evaluation. *J Am Coll Surg*. 1996;183:387–392.

25. Musser DJ, Calligaro KD, Dougherty MJ, et al. Safety and cost-efficiency of 24-hour hospitalization for carotid endarterectomy. *Ann Vasc Surg*. 1996;10:143–146.

26. Ammar AD. Cost-efficient carotid surgery: a comprehensive evaluation. *J Vasc Surg*. 1996;24:1050–1056.

27. Ballard JL, Deiparine MK, Bergan JJ, et al. Cost-effective evaluation and treatment for carotid disease. *Arch Surg*. 1997;132:268–271.

28. Brothers TE, Robison JG, Elliott BM. Relevance of quality improvement methods to surgical practice: prospective assessment of carotid endarterectomy. *Am Surg*. 1997;63:213–220.

29. Collier PE. Do clinical pathways for major vascular surgery improve outcomes and reduce cost? *J Vasc Surg*. 1997;26:179–185.

30. Back MR, Harward TRS, Huber TS, et al. Improving the cost-effectiveness of carotid endarterectomy. *J Vasc Surg*. 1997;26:456–464.

31. Melissano G, Castellano R, Mazzitelli S, et al. Safe and cost-effective approach to carotid surgery. *Eur J Vasc Endovasc Surg*. 1997;14:164–169.

32. Schneider JR, Droste JS, Golan JF. Impact of carotid endarterectomy critical pathway on surgical outcome and hospital stay. *Vasc Surg*. 1997;31:685–692.

33. Bourke BM, Crimmins DC. Overnight hospital stay for carotid endarterectomy. *Med J Aust*. 1998;168:157–160.

34. Roddy SP, O'Donnell TF, Iafrati MD, et al. Reduction of hospital resource utilization in vascular surgery: a four-year experience. *J Vasc Surg*. 1998;27:1066–1077.

35. Kent KC, Kuntz KM, Patel MR, et al. Perioperative imaging strategies for carotid endarterectomy: an analysis of morbidity and cost-effectiveness in symptomatic patients. *JAMA*. 1995;274:888–893.

36. O'Brien MS, Ricotta JJ. Conserving resources after carotid endarterectomy: selective use of the intensive care unit. *J Vasc Surg*. 1991;14:796–802.

37. Fisher ES, Malenka DJ, Solomon NA, et al. Risk of carotid endarterectomy in the elderly. *Am J Public Health*. 1989;79:1617–1620.

38. Goldstein LB, Samsa GP, Matchar DB, Oddone EZ. Multicenter review of preoperative risk factors for endarterectomy for asymptomatic carotid artery stenosis. *Stroke*. 1998;29:750–753.

V

Surgery of the
Aorta and Its
Body Branches

17

Contemporary Results of a Clamp-and-Sew Technique for Thoracoabdominal Aortic Aneurysm Repair

Richard P. Cambria, MD

BACKGROUND

Thoracoabdominal aortic aneurysm (TAA) is defined by simultaneous involvement of contiguous thoracic and abdominal aortic segments and/or aneurysm of the visceral aortic segment. This pattern of aneurysm disease is, in fact, uncommon, encompassing no more than 5% of the total spectrum of degenerative aortic aneurysm. Also distinguishing TAA from infrarenal abdominal aortic aneurysm (AAA) is the fact that up to 20% of TAAs are the sequelae of chronic aortic dissection, and there is a distinct difference in male : female sex distribution. Data from the Massachusetts General Hospital (MGH) Vascular Registry indicate that a typical 5 to 6 : 1 M : F sex predilection is noted for AAA, whereas the corresponding figure for TAA is 1 : 1.

TAA is classified according to the scheme originally devised by E. Stanley Crawford of Houston (Fig. 17–1), and considers whether the lesion is primarily a caudal extension of a descending thoracic aneurysm or a cephalad extension of total abdominal aneurysm. This classification scheme is clinically relevant because it has direct implications for both the technical conduct of operation and the incidence of perioperative complications. There is considerable variation in the overall scope of an operation required to deal with lesions within the classification of TAA. In contemporary practice, management of the type IV aneurysm should be accomplished with an overall morbidity and mortality not significantly different from that of the more routine infrarenal aneurysm[1] (Fig. 17–2). It is clear that the same cannot be said for the more extensive types I and II lesions in which resection of the entire descending thoracic aorta is required. Because graft replacement of all TAAs implies at least temporary interruption of splanchnic, renal, and, potentially, spinal cord blood flow, operative management of these lesions is potentially complicated by ischemic complications in these vascular beds, thereby increasing the overall scope and potential morbidity of the operation. Accordingly,

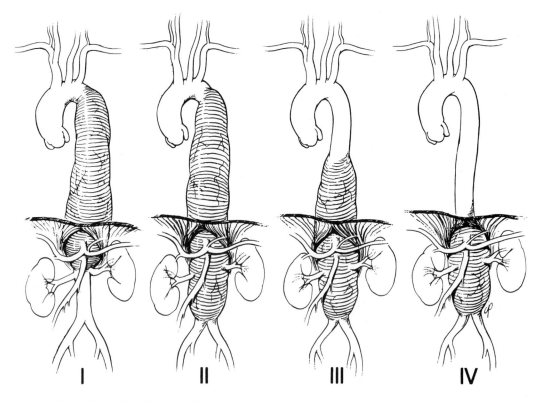

Figure 17–1. Crawford classification of extent of thoracoabdominal aortic aneurysm (TAA).

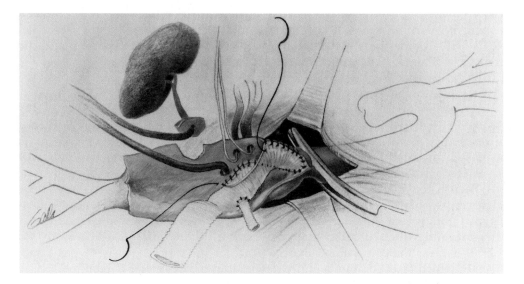

Figure 17–2. Operative approach for type IV·TAA demonstrating limited division of the diaphragm and reconstruction of the proximal aorta and visceral vessels with a single beveled proximal anastomosis. Reconstruction of the left renal artery is performed with a side-arm bypass graft. Fifty percent of type IV TAAs can be treated with this simplified approach.

acceptable surgical results with TAA repair have been achieved in most environments only since the late 1980s.

NATURAL HISTORY AND PATIENT SELECTION

Because TAA is an uncommon lesion when compared to the more routine AAA, there have been few natural history studies to guide clinical decision making, and size threshold criteria for recommending operation have only more recently been clarified. These considerations, combined with the fact that contemporary TAA repair is still accompanied by a 5% to 10% risk of major morbidity and mortality, likely account for the fact that when compared to infrarenal AAA, TAA patients are more likely to present with symptoms and to require operation in urgent or emergent circumstances. Fully 40% of patients have presented with some symptomatic manifestation prior to TAA repair, and in the majority of clinical series, urgent or emergent operation constitutes up to 20% of the experience.

Selection criteria for recommending operation are based on TAA natural history data, operative risks, and patient comorbidity considerations. Crawford and coworkers[2] reviewed an experience with 120 patients treated for ruptured TAA and noted that rupture occurred with equal frequency in the chest or abdomen, and that 80% of all aneurysms that ruptured were less than 8 cm. Furthermore, a full 13% of their patients treated had rupture occur in aneurysms less than 6 cm in diameter. Based on these data, a recommendation was made that 5 cm should be the size threshold criteria for recommendation of elective operation. However, considering the magnitude and potential morbidity of surgical repair, and the fact that the descending thoracic aorta is ordinarily larger than the infrarenal aorta in normal subjects, this recommendation appeared to this author to be overly aggressive. Studies have confirmed that in addition to the expected impact of absolute aneurysm diameter, the presence of significant chronic obstructive pulmonary disease (COPD), documented aneurysm expansion, the presence of symptoms related to the aneurysm, and possibly female sex and renal insufficiency are all markers indicating an increased risk of rupture.[3-5] The study of Juvonen and colleagues[6] also suggests that increasing patient age increases the risk of eventual rupture. This last study is particularly instructive because these authors maintained a relatively conservative 7 cm threshold for recommending operation. In their series, rupture occurred in a sobering 23% of patients under observation, obviously indicating that their 7 cm size threshold for recommending operation was overly conservative. Based on a review of the available natural history data, aneurysms less than 5 cm are thought to have a low risk of rupture and should be observed. Those between 5 and 6 cm likely have a rupture risk no higher than the overall morbidity of surgery and, accordingly, 6 cm as is used the size threshold to recommend TAA resection. The work by Perko and associates[7] demonstrated a fivefold increase in risk of rupture when thoracic–thoracoabdominal aneurysms exceeded a 6-cm size threshold. When the etiology of an aneurysm is chronic dissection or in patients with Marfan syndrome, operation should be considered when the aneurysm is a smaller size because the available literature suggests that the risk of rupture may be higher when dissection is the pathology.

THE EVOLUTION OF SURGICAL TREATMENT

The modern era in the treatment of TAA began with the pioneering work of E. Stanley Crawford of Houston, Texas. In a series of publications that laid the foundation for the widespread successful surgical management of TAA, Crawford described a simplified operative approach to these lesions using the inclusion technique, wherein visceral and intercostal vessels were reconstructed from within the aneurysm by anastomosing openings in the main Dacron graft directly to the aortic origin of the vessels (Fig. 17–3). This simplified surgical approach was a major advance compared to a multiple sidearm

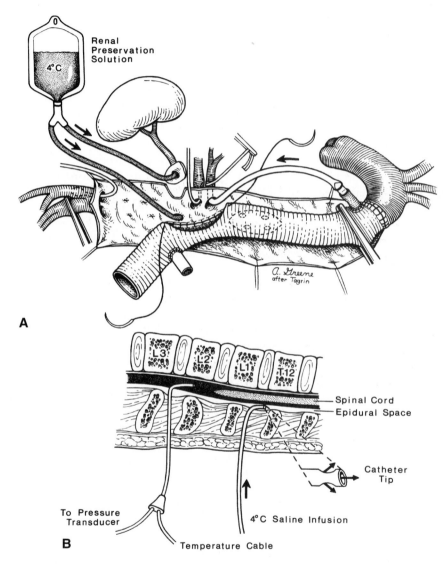

Figure 17–3. Operative approach for repair of type II TAA with a clamp-and-sew technique supplemented with regional hypothermic adjuncts for renal and spinal cord protection. (**A**) The entire aneurysm sac is continuously exposed after proximal cross-clamp application. After completion of the proximal anastomosis, pulsatile arterial perfusion is established into the mesenteric circulation via in-line mesenteric shunting into either the celiac axis (as depicted) or the superior mesenteric artery. Thereafter, critical intercostal vessels are reconstructed (dotted line), and a single inclusion button anastomosis for reconstruction of celiac, superior mesenteric, and right renal arteries is possible in the majority of cases. The left renal artery is reconstructed with a side-arm graft. (**B**) Regional spinal cord hypothermic protection is achieved via epidural cooling. A 4°C epidural saline infusion is begun in anticipation of cross-clamping. CSF temperature and pressure are monitored simultaneously with a separate intrathecal catheter. See text for details.

bypass technique. The volume of the referral practice in Houston was such that a number of surgical and nonsurgical adjuncts that continue to be applied in contemporary practice were prospectively studied by Crawford and his associates. In the course of failing to demonstrate benefit for adjuncts such as partial cardiopulmonary bypass, somatosensory evoked potentials, and cerebrospinal fluid (CSF) drainage, these investigators concluded that a simplified clamp-and-sew technique that emphasized operative expediency and simplicity without external bypasses, minimal aortic cross-clamp times, and avoidance of systemic anticoagulation because of its potential contribution to intraoperative bleeding complications produced the best results.[8,9] Crawford's summary experience in more than 1500 patients treated during the years 1960 to 1991 detailed a 10% operative mortality, a 16% rate of spinal cord ischemic complications, and an 18% perioperative renal failure rate (half of whom required perioperative dialysis).[10] Although these overall results were nothing short of spectacular considering the time interval over which they were accumulated, these investigators acknowledged that the principal complications of the operation, namely, spinal cord ischemia and renal failure, continued to occur at a distressing rate. These results created the milieu for further exploration of operative strategies driven principally by the threat of unacceptable results with spinal cord ischemic complications and perioperative renal failure. Accordingly, multiple investigators reported generally modest-size series embracing variations of a distal aortic perfusion technique.[11–13] In contemporary practice, there remains no consensus or definitive studies to indicate clear superiority for variations on the clamp-and-sew versus distal aortic perfusion techniques. Our review indicated largely equivalent results for the two approaches in a survey of the contemporary literature.[14]

The major impact on overall results was documented early to be coincident with basic tenets of improved operative technique. Using the year 1986 as a division between early and contemporary experience, greatly improved overall results were documented to be strongly correlated with decreased operative and cross-clamp times and with decreased blood turnover.[15] Although specific adjuncts have been added over the evolution of my experience, the general tenets of overall operative approach as detailed later in this chapter have not changed. In what follows, the arguments for and against the two principal variations of operation strategies are presented—namely a clamp-and-sew technique with or without adjuncts directed against the principal complications of operation versus some form of distal aortic perfusion generally carried out with a sequential clamping technique (Fig. 17–4).

PRINCIPLES OF TREATMENT

Graft replacement by a direct surgical approach is the only effective treatment for TAA. Endovascular graft placement, which has been applied to lesions isolated to the descending thoracic aorta,[16] is not applicable to TAA because of the inability to reconstruct intercostal and/or visceral vessels with this technique. Nonoperative therapy may be selected initially in very elderly patients, patients whose aneurysms are of modest size, and patients whose associated comorbid conditions make the short-term risk of surgery prohibitive or life expectancy limited to a degree that surgical treatment is not rational. Patients selected for nonoperative therapy should be treated aggressively with beta-blockade, hypertension control, and cessation of cigarette smoking. Our experience is that a majority of patients with aneurysms 6 cm or more in diameter prove fit to undergo an operation after cardiopulmonary profiling and a current assessment of renal function.

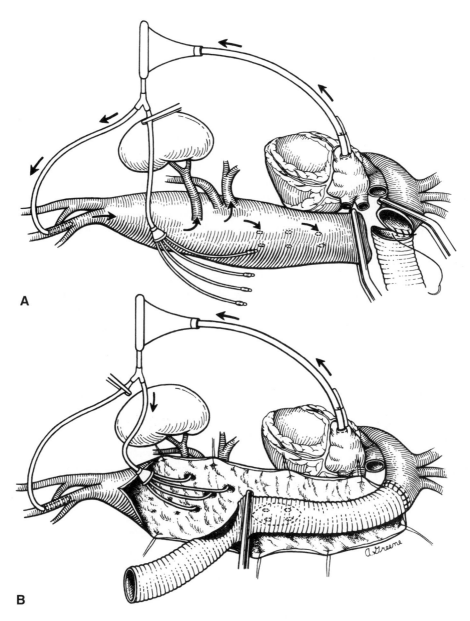

Figure 17–4. Repair of type II TAA with distal aortic perfusion via atriofemoral bypass and sequential clamping technique. (**A**) Two clamps are applied proximally and distal, retrograde, transfemoral perfusion provided to visceral, renal, and intercostal arteries during construction of the proximal aortic anastomosis. (**B**) Thereafter, the aneurysm sac is opened and visceral–renal perfusion can be provided with multiple catheter "octopus" arrangement while intercostal (dotted line) and visceral–renal artery reconstruction proceeds.

In contemporary practice, several schemes of operative management are utilized (see Figs. 17–3 and 17–4). The two general approaches involve a clamp-and-sew technique, often supplemented by adjuncts to minimize the principle complications; or the use of distal aortic perfusion usually combined with a sequential clamping technique. The rationale for distal aortic perfusion is the reduction of ischemic times to the intercostal, visceral, and renal vessels because these vascular beds are perfused during creation of the proximal anastomosis; distal perfusion has been favored for repair of isolated thoracic aneurysms. Distal aortic perfusion can be provided in either passive fashion, with an indwelling Gott shunt, or an initial right axillary to femoral bypass graft. However, partial left heart bypass techniques have been refined sufficiently that most authors who prefer distal aortic perfusion use active distal perfusion with atriofemoral bypass utilizing the Bio-Medicus pump. This centripetal, motorized pump is elegant in its simplicity, and when used with heparinized impregnated tubing can be placed without the need for systemic heparin. However, the majority of surgeons prefer at least low dose heparin if atriofemoral bypass is utilized. Our principal criticism of the atriofemoral bypass technique with sequential clamping is that it only saves the cross-clamp time required to complete the proximal aortic anastomosis, which, in our experience, has been a minimum of the overall clamp time expenditure. Following performance of the proximal aortic anastomosis, reconstruction of critical intercostal vessels and the visceral aortic segment must then proceed with distal perfusion during this stage of the operation, providing only retrograde pelvic perfusion and, at least in theory, some additional spinal cord circulation via the lateral sacral branches of the hypogastric vessels. This objection can be overcome by the use of a variety of "octopus" visceral perfusion catheter arrangements (see Fig. 17–4), which have the disadvantage of multiple catheters in the surgical field interfering with surgical exposure. The pressure–flow relationships of multiple small catheters may be difficult to overcome, and at least one study demonstrated a paradoxical detrimental effect on renal function using multiple selective visceral perfusion catheters.[17] Our current posture is in agreement with the highly selective use of atriofemoral bypass. Because its principal advantage is during the performance of the proximal aortic reconstruction, this method is used only in circumstances in which the proximal reconstruction is likely to be complex—in particular, in patients with chronic aortic dissection. In addition, atriofemoral bypass provides easily titratable mechanical unloading of the left ventricle, and this may be desirable in patients who have antecedent aortic valvular dysfunction or significant degrees of left ventricular dysfunction.

The general approach to the technical conduct of operation for TAA has continued to emphasize the principles of operative expediency and simplicity without the use of external bypasses and avoiding systemic hypothermia and heparin. The clinically significant surgical variables demonstrated to have an impact on the overall results of an operation are shown in Table 17–1.[18] Several studies[19–21] correlate urgent or emergent operations (even without TAA rupture) with poor results compared to a truly elective operation. In our own material, the influence of this clinical presentation has been paramount (more than 50% perioperative deaths occur in this category, $p < .001$), and Acher and coworkers[22] included urgent operation among variables associated with increased risk of spinal cord injury. Obviously, the urgency of operation is beyond the control of the surgeon, whereas this is not true concerning the other operative variables

TABLE 17–1. CLINICALLY SIGNIFICANT SURGICAL VARIABLES IN THORACOABDOMINAL ANEURYSM REPAIR

- Urgency of operation
- Duration $\geq$ 6 hours
- Core temperature shifts
- Blood loss
- Cross-clamp duration

listed in Table 17–1. An expedient operation is to be emphasized. We previously correlated prolonged ($\geq$ 5 hour) operations to be independently associated with an increased risk of major morbidity in abdominal aortic reconstruction [relative risk 5.11 (95% confidence interval [CI] 1.69–15.52), $p < .004$)], and prolonged operation has been independently associated with increased risk of spinal cord ischemia in our experience with TAA repair [relative risk 7.5 (95% CI 1.5–35.3) $p = .011$].[20,23] Table 17–2 shows intraoperative data from our series of TAA repairs. As anticipated, cross-clamp duration, blood turnover, and component replacement vary as a function of TAA extent, but overall operative time can be kept in the 5- to 6-hour range for most patients.[20] With use of warmed IV fluids, heated ventilation circuits, and forced-air warming covers, core temperature is maintained in the 35°C range throughout the operation.[24,25] The intuitively logical supposition that overall results will improve with decreased blood turnover and minimal cross-clamp duration has been substantiated in several reports.[10,15,26] In particular, prolonged cross-clamp duration clearly increases the risk of spinal cord ischemia complications and postoperative renal failure (Fig. 17–5).[10,26,27] These latter complications have a dominant effect on perioperative mortality.

As displayed in Fig. 17–3, our clamp-and-sew technique is used with specific regional hypothermic adjuncts for spinal cord and renal protection. A technique has been developed and applied for the provision of regional hypothermic protection to that segment of the spinal cord typically at risk for ischemic injury during TAA repair.[26] As schematized in Fig. 17–3, the system uses an iced saline epidural infusion, which provides for moderate (25° to 27°C) hypothermia to the spinal cord during the critical period when the aorta is cross clamped. Direct installation of renal preservation fluid (4°C lactated Ringers with 25 g of mannitol per liter and 1 g methylprednisolone per liter) into the renal artery ostia is performed after the aorta is opened. Initially, 250 cc of this solution is instilled into each renal artery ostium and a continuous drip of the solution is begun through size 6 French perfusion balloon-tipped catheters. Experience has shown that such an infusion results in a rapid decline of renal parenchymal temperature to 15°C after the bolus infusion. During the continuous infusion, renal core temperatures remain in the 25°C level as monitored by direct temperature probes in the renal cortex. The final adjunct in our overall approach involves in-line mesenteric shunting. As displayed in Fig. 17–3, a 10 mm Dacron sidearm graft is sewn to the main aortic graft so as to be located just beyond the region of the proximal anastomosis. A 20 to 24 French arterial perfusion cannula is attached to the sidearm graft, and immediately after performance of the proximal anastomosis, prograde pulsatile perfusion can be

TABLE 17–2. INTRAOPERATIVE DATA FOR 160 THORACOABDOMINAL ANEURYSM RESECTIONS

Variable (mean ± SD)	Types I and II TAA ($n = 75$)	Types III and IV TAA ($n = 85$)	p
Operative time (min)	323 ± 97	304 ± 109	.25
Viceral ischemic time (min)[a]	53 ± 16	41 ± 11	.001
Reperfusion of legs (min)	66 ± 24	74 ± 24	.03
Total blood transfusion (cc)[b]	3170 ± 1973	2496 ± 2376	.07
Fresh-frozen plasma (units)	6 ± 4	4 ± 4	.01
Platelets (units)	10 ± 6	6 ± 6	.01

SD, standard deviation; TAA, thoracoabdominal aneurysm.
[a] Reperfusion of celiac/superior mesenteric/right renal arteries.
[b] Sum of banked and autotransfused blood.

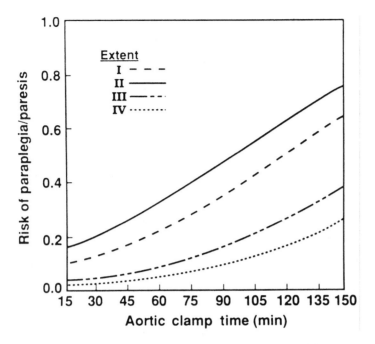

Figure 17–5. Risk of spinal cord ischemic complications as a function of TAA extent and total aortic cross-clamp duration after multivariate analysis in more than 1500 patients. Note that risk is greatest for extent II aneurysms but that for each extent the overall risk increases substantially as clamp times exceed 45 minutes. (*Reproduced with permission from Svensson LG, Crawford ES, Hess KR, et al. Experience with 1509 patients undergoing thoracoabdominal aortic operations. J Vasc Surg. 1993;17:357–370.*)

established into either the celiac axis or the superior mesenteric artery to minimize visceral ischemic time and its potential contribution to coagulopathic bleeding. Experience shows that pulsatile arterial perfusion can thus be reestablished to the mesenteric circulation within 25 minutes of initial aortic cross-clamp placement.[28] This system can be modified by using a bifurcation graft and placing a separate cannula into the left renal artery origin in patients at particular risk for perioperative renal failure.

Finally, the concept of hypothermic protection for spinal cord and visceral organs can be extended to the extreme by the use of a complete cardiopulmonary bypass technique, profound hypothermia, and circulatory arrest. Although this method has been utilized as a routine operative approach for patients with extensive TAA in at least one center,[29] the majority of surgeons avoid this technique specifically because of the potential for bleeding and pulmonary complications. Although this technique is essential for the repair of complex lesions of the ascending aorta or aortic arch, in patients with TAA, its use is only recommended in those circumstances in which proximal control and clamping of the aorta is either hazardous or not technically possible.

OPERATIVE TECHNIQUE

Irrespective of individual preferences about various technical components of the operation, the *sine qua non* for a successful technical operation is the provision of broad continuous exposure of the entire left posterolateral aspect of the aorta. Particularly in extensive type II aneurysms, maneuvers that tend to improve proximal exposure can compromise distal exposure and vice versa. The location and extent of the thoracic portion of the incision is dictated by the proximal extent of the aneurysm. The posterior portion of a standard posterolateral thoracotomy is only necessary for types I and II aneurysms. An eighth interspace thoracoabdominal incision will usually suffice for type IV aneurysms, and a double lumen tube for deflation of the left lung is generally not necessary in these cases. It is preferable to keep the abdominal portion of the incision well lateral on the abdominal wall rather than extending to the midline. This has the advantage of allowing the visceral contents to lay within the abdominal cavity, decreasing evaporative fluid and heat losses. The abdominal portion of the incision is transperitoneal, as this allows for direct inspection and assessment to the visceral circulation at the conclusion of operation.

Exposure of the left posterolateral aspect of the abdominal aorta is obtained by entering the plane posterior to the spleen, left kidney, and left colon with the electrocautery. In addition to the retroperitoneal fatty and lymphatic tissues overlying the aorta, there is a large posterior branch of the left renal vein, which typically courses across the aorta and requires division. Located topographically close to this structure is the left renal artery, and a key point in the dissection is identifying the renal artery and dissecting it back to its aortic origin. This is a convenient starting point for cephalad and caudad division of the retroperitoneal tissues over the aorta inferiorly, and division of the median arcuate ligament and diaphragmatic crura superiorly.

Management of the incision in the diaphragm can be by one of several methods (Fig. 17–6). There is little question that direct radial division of the diaphragm from underneath the costal margin to the aortic hiatus is the quickest and simplest method and affords excellent exposure. However, such radial division of the diaphragm irrevocably paralyzes the left hemidiaphragm and contributes to postoperative respiratory compromise. Some surgeons prefer a circumferential division of the diaphragm through its muscular portion leaving a few centimeters attached laterally to the chest wall. Engle and associates emphasized the benefit of preservation of the phrenic innervation of the left hemidiaphragm by dividing only a portion lateral to the phrenic nerve insertion and then taking down the muscular fibers of the diaphragmatic aortic hiatus[30] (Fig. 17–6). A large Penrose drain can thus be passed around the diaphragm pedicle for retracting superiorly and inferiorly during different stages of the subsequent reconstruction. This method has been applied liberally, particularly in patients with evidence of preoperative pulmonary compromise.

For types I and II aneurysms, proximal control of the aorta in the region of the left subclavian artery origin is necessary. Additional mobility on the vagus nerve can be obtained by dividing the nerve distal to the origin of the left recurrent nerve, which is identified and preserved. Should more proximal control be necessary, the ligamentum arteriosum is divided on the aorta. In this region, care must be taken to keep dissection directly on the underside of the aortic arch to avoid injury to the left main pulmonary artery. In patients with degenerative aneurysm, dissection in this area is generally straightforward. When chronic dissection is the pathology, the prior inflammation from the dissecting process makes dissection more difficult. The aorta is surrounded with a vessel tape on either side of the left subclavian artery, depending on the proximal extent of the aneurysm. Sufficient normal aorta should be cleared with blunt dissection on the posterior aspect of the aorta to allow room for clamp placement and an accurate proximal aortic anastomosis. External control of the left subclavian artery is not necessary, as intraluminal balloon control can be obtained if the cross-clamp needs to be placed proximal to the left subclavian artery.

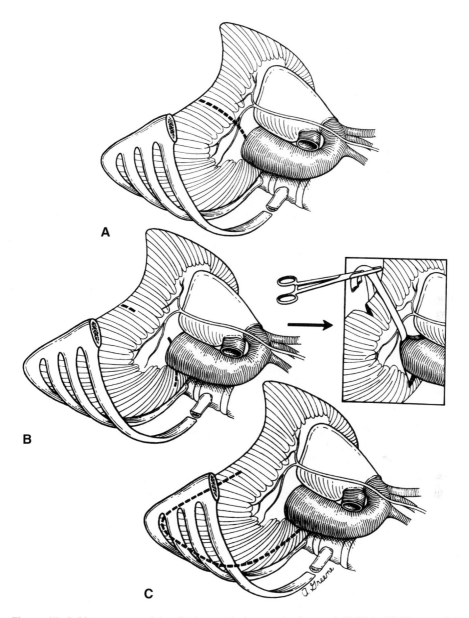

Figure 17–6. Management of the diaphragm during repair of types I–III TAA. (**A**) Direct radial division of the diaphragm provides rapid and uncompromised exposure but causes left hemidiaphragm paralysis. (**B**) Partial division under the costal margin and disassembly of the aortic hiatus allows preservation of the phrenic nerve, and the diaphragmatic pedicle can be retracted as needed with a large Penrose drain. (**C**) Circumferential division through the muscular diaphragm is time-consuming and less hemostatic, but can preserve phrenic innervation.

In cases in which the entire descending thoracic aorta is resected, the proximal intercostal vessel orifices between T_4 and T_8 are typically vigorously back-bleeding, and these are rapidly oversewn. Intercostal vessels in the critical T_9 to L_1 aortic segment are evaluated for potential reimplantation into the main body of the graft, and these vessels are balloon-occluded to both prevent back-bleeding and the negative "sump" effective on net spinal cord perfusion that can result from these vessel orifices being exposed only to atmospheric pressure.[31] The proximal aortic neck is prepared for reconstruction and we only divide the aorta circumferentially if chronic dissection of the aortic wall is present at the point that the proximal anastomosis will be carried out. Using the Creech technique with an intact posterior wall of the aorta is more expeditious and facilitates a secure proximal aortic anastomosis, which is then verified for hemostasis. A clamp is placed on the main aortic graft distal to the mesenteric shunt sidearm, flow is established in the shunt, and good perfusion to the mesentery is verified by checking for arterial back-bleeding from the other mesenteric vessel origin. Reconstruction of intercostal vessels in the T_9–L_1 segment is usually the next step in the operation. The most common technique utilized is an inclusion button anastomosis. Intercostal vessels in the region of a proximal or distal aortic anastomosis can be reconstructed by use of a long beveled suture line. Alternate methods of intercostal vessel reanastomosis include the attachment of other short sidearm grafts to the main aortic graft, or in certain cases in which the intercostal vessel origins have been rotated superiorly and to the patient's left side, it may be feasible to simply reanastomose Carrel patches of aorta containing the intercostal vessels to the main aortic graft (Fig. 17–7). Depending on the topography of intercostal vessel origins, it may be possible

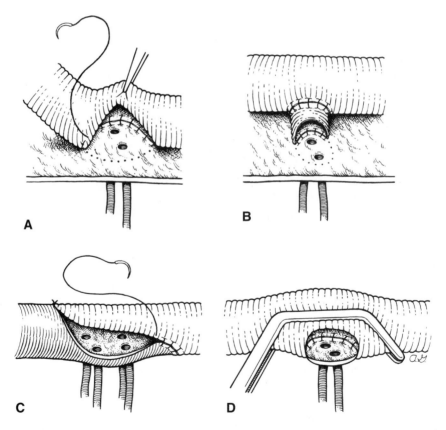

Figure 17–7. Technique for intercostal vessel reconstruction. (**A**) Inclusion button anastomosis, which is the most commonly used method. (**B**) Sidearm graft, which can be used for reconstruction after completion of the distal aortic anastomosis. (**C**) Beveled distal (or proximal) aortic anastomosis to preserve intercostal vessel origins. (**D**) Carrel patch of aorta, containing intercostal vessel origins with side-biting clamp, again facilitating repair after completion of distal aortic anastomosis.

to defer intercostal vessel reconstruction until after completion of the visceral vessel anastomosis by utilizing partial occluding clamps on the main aortic graft. Because there is the protective effect of regional spinal cord hypothermia until all aspects of the reconstruction have been completed, there is no urgency with our technique to reestablish intercostal blood flow.

Visceral and renal artery reconstruction is carried out next. Significant occlusive lesions of the right renal and superior mesenteric arteries should be treated with orifice endarterectomy. The most common method of visceral–renal artery reconstruction,

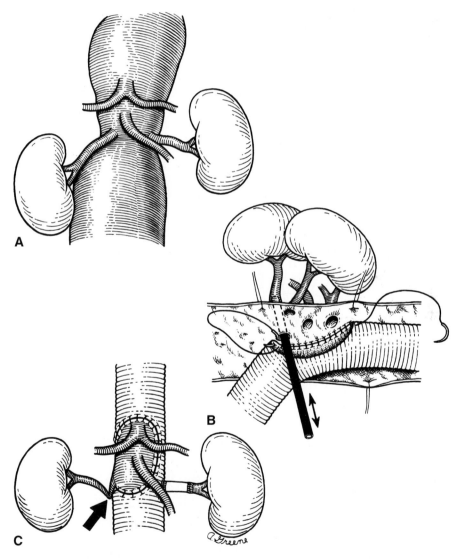

Figure 17–8. Pitfalls in right renal artery reconstruction during TAA repair. (**A**) Commonly encountered anatomy with right renal artery draping over large infrarenal component of aneurysm. (**B**) During inclusion button reconstruction of visceral–renal vessel origins, a 12 French catheter is used to stent the right renal origin as the suture line courses around it. This catheter is agitated to ensure the right renal artery origin is not compromised. (**C**) Kinking and obstruction (*arrow*) of the proximal right renal artery can result from failure to appreciate the orientation of the renal artery to the inclusion button suture line.

which has been applied in the overwhelming majority of our cases, is a single inclusion button to encompass the origins of the celiac, superior mesenteric, and right renal arteries (see Fig. 17–3). If the aneurysm is excessively large in the visceral aortic segment, wide separation of the visceral–renal ostia may necessitate multiple individual inclusion button anastomoses. By placing the graft on traction, it is usually possible to perform the posterior aspect of this suture line using single bites of the suture passing through the aorta and the Dacron graft. Suture bites should be close to the visceral vessel origins to avoid leaving too much aneurysmal aortic wall. As the posterior aspect of this suture line courses around the inferior border of the right renal artery, we exchange the 6 French perfusion catheter for a 12 French perfusion catheter to serve as a stent of sorts in the right renal artery origin. This catheter is gently agitated up and down as the suture line moves around the renal artery to ensure that the latter is not compromised

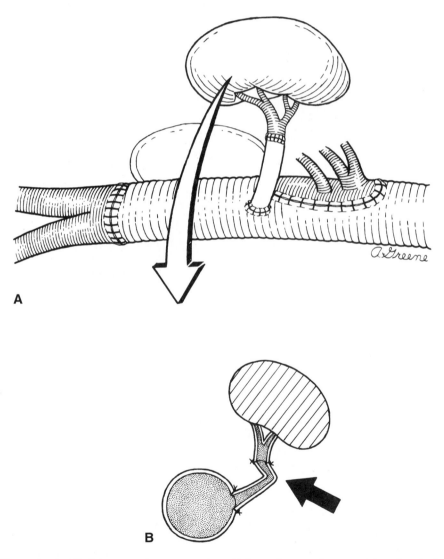

Figure 17–9. (**A**) Sidearm graft reconstruction of left renal artery. Care must be taken in the orientation of this graft because kinking and obstruction (*arrow*) can occur as the left kidney is returned to its bed (**B**), irrespective of the technique of left renal artery reconstruction.

by the suture bites as they pass outside of the aorta. In particular, the topography and course of the right renal artery should be interrogated with this indwelling catheter because in circumstances in which the right renal artery drapes over a large infrarenal component of the aneurysm, occlusion of the right renal artery is a definite technical complication of operation (Fig. 17–8).

Reconstruction of the left renal artery is now accomplished, and is performed in nearly all cases with a separate sidearm graft of 6 mm polytetrafluroethylene (PTFE). This allows a direct and deliberate anastomosis in end-to-end fashion, allowing flexibility to deal with the spectrum of occlusive lesions, multiple renal arteries, and so forth that may be encountered. As noted in Fig. 17–9, care must be taken to place this sidearm graft in an orientation where it will not kink when the left renal artery is returned to its anatomic position. Some surgeons prefer to use a single inclusion button to encompass both renal arteries along with the visceral vessels, but in our experience, this will include too great an area of aneurysmal aorta unless the aneurysm is exceedingly small in the visceral aortic segment. The clamp is then moved again to a position inferior to the origin of the left renal artery graft and the distal aortic anastomosis is carried out, completing the reconstruction. Every effort is made to perform tube-type reconstructions to the aortic bifurcation unless there is gross aneurysmal disease of the proximal common iliac arteries. Extending the reconstruction to separate iliac artery reconstructions or, indeed, tunneling to an aortofemoral graft configuration is only performed when no other technical alternative exists.

RESULTS OF SURGICAL TREATMENT

Spinal Cord Ischemic Complications

Spinal cord ischemic complications, manifested clinically as complete flaccid paraplegia or lesser degrees of lower extremity paraparesis, remain the most feared and devastating nonfatal complications of operation. A variety of surgical and adjunctive techniques notwithstanding, spinal cord ischemia remains an unsolved problem despite considerable improvements in the overall incidence of this complication. Efforts to minimize this complication have been the principal driving force in the application of the variety of general operative approaches reviewed previously. Svensson and colleagues,[10] in reviewing Crawford's experience with more than 1500 patients treated for TAA over the interval 1960 through 1991, reported a 16% incidence of lower extremity neurological deficits. Approximately one-half of these patients suffered total paraplegia without the prospect of any meaningful recovery. Patients treated for the most extensive type II TAA sustained a 31% incidence of spinal cord ischemic complications. As detailed in Table 17–3, contemporary results with variations of the clamp-and-sew technique from centers of excellence detail an approximate halving of the incidence of spinal cord ischemia detailed in Crawford's summary report.

Two factors referable to human spinal cord circulation explain the nature of ischemic risk to the spinal cord during TAA. The first of these is the vagaries of anatomy of the anterior spinal artery, which is variable both in caliber and in continuity. If the anterior spinal artery were of adequate caliber and in continuity in all individuals, there would be no risk of ischemic cord complications by clamping of the descending thoracic aorta or sacrifice of intercostal vessels. However, angiographic studies have shown that the anterior spinal artery maybe anatomically discontinuous, and the typical pattern of the anterior spinal artery is that its caliber becomes extremely narrow cephalad to its anastomosis with the greater radicular artery. Second, the human spinal cord

TABLE 17–3. OPERATIVE COMPLICATIONS IN MAJOR SERIES OF THORACOABDOMINAL AORTIC ANEURYSM REPAIR

Reference	Year of Publication	Study Interval	Number of Patients	Operative Technique	Mortality n (%)	Paraplegia/ Paraparesis n (%)	Renal Failure n (%)
Svensson et al.[10]	1993	1960–1991	1509	c/s (83%)[a]	155 (10)	234 (16)	269 (18)
Coselli and Plestis[50]	1998	1986–1997	984	c/s (72%)[a]	72 (7.3)	52 (5.2)	107 (11)
Grabitz et al.[39]	1996	1981–1995	260	c/s	37 (14.2)	39 (15)	27 (10.4)[b]
Acher et al.[19]	1998	1984–1996	217[c]	c/s	21 (9.7)	17 (7.8)	4 (3.8)[b]
Hollier et al.[51]	1992	1980–1991	150	c/s	15 (10)	6 (4)	14 (9.3)
Cambria et al.[20]	1997	1986–1997	210	c/s	17 (8)	15 (7.2)	22 (10.6)
TOTALS†	—	—	3330	—	317 (9.5)	363 (10.9)	443 (13.3)

c/s, clamp-and-sew.
[a] Balance of procedures done with atriofemoral bypass.
[b] Only those requiring dialysis.
[c] Includes some descending thoracic aneurysm repairs (Acher et al., 19%).
† Updated.

is supplied irregularly by radiculomedullary arteries. Although radicular arteries are contributed at each segmental level, only a few of these arteries actually go on to contribute medullary (i.e., actually reaching the cord) components. The thoracolumbar region is at the most risk for ischemic injury because this region is typically supplied by a single radiculomedullary artery, referred to as the *artery of Adamkiewicz* or the *greater radicular artery*. This artery enters the vertebral canal between the ninth and the twelfth thoracic vertebral segments in 75% to 80% of individuals, and angiographic studies have shown that one or more intercostal arteries can contribute to it.[32] In addition to the variations in normal anatomy reviewed previously, TAA patients may have the added variable of mural thrombus potentially obliterating many or all of the intercostal vessels. Such gradual obliteration of intercostal vessels in a chronic degenerative aneurysm serves to establish antecedent collateral circulation prior to surgical correction, and most authors agree that the risk of cord injury is considerably less in patients whose intercostal vessels in the critical T_9–L_1 zone have been obliterated by mural thrombus.[33,34] The variation in patency of intercostal vessels between degenerative and dissected aneurysms (the latter typically have multiple patent intercostals) accounts for the higher risk of cord injury in patients treated with aneurysms in which the etiology is dissection.

The pathogenesis of spinal cord injury after aortic replacement is likely multifactoral, but ultimately is a result of the ischemic insult caused by temporary or permanent interruption of spinal cord blood supply. Debate continues about the relative importance of the initial ischemic insult versus reperfusion injury. The clinical observation of delayed deficits has led some authors to speculate that swelling in the rigid bony spinal canal, accompanied by relative increases in CSF, are pathogenesis of such delayed deficits.[35] Other authors have speculated that the initial ischemic insult in the operating room creates the milieu for programmed neuronal cell death as an inevitable consequence of the intraoperative ischemic insult.[36] There is a striking correlation between perioperative hypotension and delayed onset neurological deficit, suggesting that the principal and collateral circulation to the cord may be in a delicate balance for some time after operation. Careful attention to maintain adequate perfusion pressure in the days following TAA resection is important in limiting the occurrence of delayed deficit, but other mechanisms such as thrombosis of reconstructed vessels and microembolization may contribute to the development of delayed deficits.

There is general consensus that the clinical variables of aortic cross-clamp duration, extent of TAA aneurysm, emergency operations, and operations in which dissection is the pathology increase the risks of spinal cord injury, although the last has been disputed.[10,19,21] Crawford demonstrated that for each extent of TAA, risk of spinal cord injury increased with increased duration of aortic cross-clamping[10] (see Fig. 17–5). Similarly, it has been reported that a visceral cross-clamp time longer than 60 minutes was significantly associated ($p = .02$) with ischemic cord injury.[26] Risk of cord injury clearly increases in treatment for the more extensive types I and II TAA. Svensson and coworkers[10] noted a 24% incidence of spinal cord injury in treatment of types I and II TAA as opposed to a 5.5% incidence for types III and IV TAA. Griepp and associates[37] noted that spinal cord injury increased dramatically when 10 or more pairs of intercostal vessels were sacrificed; that is, resection of the entire descending thoracic aorta was required. The circumstances of the clinical presentation have great bearing on the risk of spinal cord injury. In Crawford's experience, as reported by Svensson and colleagues,[10] spinal cord injury rates doubled in treatment for ruptured verses intact aneurysms. Cambria and colleagues[20] noted that operation for acute presentation (half for frank rupture and/or dissection) was independently associated with postoperative lower extremity neurologic deficit [relative risk 7.9 (95% CI, 1.7–37.7; p = .009)]. Acher and coworkers[22] incorporated the previously mentioned clinical variables into the formulation of a predictive model for neurological deficit after TAA repair. These authors demonstrated an excellent correlation (r = 0.997) between the predicted incidence of neurological deficits from their model and the incidence actually reported in 16 series published prior to 1993.

A variety of clinical strategies and adjuncts have been applied in an effort to prevent ischemic spinal cord injury, and these have been reviewed extensively elsewhere.[14] As displayed in Table 17–4, these methods can be divided into two general categories. The first of these is surgical or adjunctive methods designed to preserve relative spinal cord perfusion pressure. Localization techniques (preoperative angiography and intraoperative evoked potential or polargraphic) act as guides for the surgeon to preserve or reconstruct critical intercostal arteries. Evoked potential monitoring evaluates the ability of the long tracks of the spinal cord to conduct an impulse during the cross-clamp period. Variations in the latency and amplitude of recorded potentials imply ischemia of the cord. Newer techniques for evoked potential monitoring, such as direct spinal cord stimulation with epidural electrodes and motor-evoked potentials, have shown promise in both the correlation of spinal cord deficits with intraoperative evoked potential monitoring, and as a guide to the surgeon to apply intraoperative adjuncts when cord ischemia is detected with initial cross-clamping.[38,39]

The rationale for CSF pressure monitoring and drainage relates to the concept of spinal cord perfusion pressure as the subtraction product of the distal arterial pressure below the clamp and the CSF pressure.[40] Thoracic aortic clamping can result in an abrupt increase in intracerebral blood flow, which is likely the principal mechanism

TABLE 17–4. STRATEGIES TO PREVENT SPINAL CORD ISCHEMIA DURING THORACOABDOMINAL ANEURYSM REPAIR

Maintenance of Spinal Cord Blood Supply
  Identification of critical segmental (intercostal) vessels
    Preoperative selective angiography
    Intraoperative H_2 ion method
    Intraoperative evoked potential monitoring
  Shunts and bypasses—distal aortic perfusion
    Passive internal (Gott) or external (axillofemoral) shunt
    Atriofemoral or femoral–femoral bypass (partial cardiopulmonary [CP] bypass)
    Complete bypass (with or without circulatory arrest/profound hypothermia)
  CSF drainage
  Intercostal/lumbar vessel reanastamosis
  Intrathecal vasodilators
Neuroprotective Adjuncts
  Hypothermia
    Systemic
      Passive (moderate)
      Active (moderate or profound—with CP bypass)
    Regional (moderate)
      Epidural or intrathecal infusion (closed or drained)
      Isolated aortic segment perfusion
  Pharmacologic agents
    Neurotransmitter inhibition (naloxone)
    Nonspecific neuroprotective agents (steroids, barbiturates)
    Calcium channel blockers
    Oxygen free radical scavengers
    Artificial O_2 delivery (Fluosol-DA)

of the increase in CSF pressure that can accompany such clamping. However, the absolute degree of this rise is typically modest,[41] and Kazama and coworkers[42] found that CSF drainage favorably influenced spinal cord blood flow only when CSF pressure was experimentally elevated to four times baseline values. Thus, the assumptions on which the theoretical benefit of CSF drainage are based may not be valid, and several studies have failed to demonstrate any benefit.[9,43] However, elevated CSF pressure has been correlated in particular with delayed onset neurologic deficit, and many authors continue to use CSF drainage either alone or, more typically, in combination with other strategies because it is simple, safe, and its use has shown promise in a variety of experimental studies.[12,19]

In the category of maintaining spinal cord blood supply, intercostal vessel reanastomosis is the most commonly applied surgical maneuver. Most authors contend that sacrifice of critical intercostal vessels or the inability to reperfuse these arteries in a timely fashion are important factors in the pathogenesis of ischemic cord injury. Some authors have demonstrated that sacrifice of intercostal vessels in the critical T_9–L_1 zone correlate with postoperative cord injury.[26,33,34] Reattachment of critical intercostal vessels can be technically impossible in circumstances in which excessive atheroma or acute dissection surrounds the intercostal vessel origin. Intraoperatively, the surgeon typically faces the management dilemma of expending aortic cross-clamp time to reattach intercostal vessels, and because the critical intercostal zone lies in proximity topographically to the visceral aortic segment, it is generally not possible to separate reconstruction in the critical intercostal segment from the visceral aortic segment with a distal perfusion and sequential clamping technique. Some authors have suggested that expending aortic clamp time for intercostal vessel reanastomosis is a worthless maneuver, and routinely oversew or occlude all intercostal vessels, often with the use of other adjuncts directed against spinal cord ischemia.[22,37] The best documentation of the worth of intercostal vessel reattachment was provided by Grabitz and coworkers,[39] who used direct spinal cord evoked potential monitoring (scSEEP). These investigators reported increased neurological deficits when rapid loss of scSSEPs were noted after aortic cross-clamping. Furthermore, neurological outcome for each group of SSEP responses was correlated with the ability to achieve rapid return of the evoked potentials with early intercostal vessel reimplantation.[39] However, restoration of intercostal vessel perfusion maybe inadequate as a stand-alone adjunct simply because it cannot be performed rapidly enough.

Neuroprotective adjuncts are intended to increase the tolerance of the spinal cord to ischemia during the cross-clamp interval. There are two general categories of such adjuncts: hypothermia, which can be either systemic or regional; and a variety of pharmacologic agents that can be classified according to their intended mechanisms of actions: nonspecific neuroprotective agents (e.g., steroids, prostaglandins, magnesium, barbiturates); excitatory neurotransmitter inhibitors such as Naloxone; and calcium channel blockers and oxygen free radical scavengers that act at different points on the cascade of reperfusion injury. Determining the benefit of any of these agents in the clinical setting is difficult because they are typically used in combination with other strategies. The preeminent clinical experience involving this general strategy has been reported by Acher and coworkers,[19] who applied endorphin receptor blockade with Naloxone in combination with CSF drainage and a policy of routine intercostal vessel ligation. These authors have reported overall spinal cord ischemic injury rates of 3.5%, equivalent or superior to that achieved using other strategies.

The protective effect of hypothermia is presumed to be secondary to decreased tissue metabolism; however, the mechanism may be more complex, involving membrane stabilization and reduced release of excitatory neurotransmitters.[44] Oxygen requirements in central nervous system (CNS) tissue are known to decrease 6% to 7% for each degree Celsius decrement in spinal cord temperature. Hypothermia for purposes of spinal cord protection during TAA surgery can be either regional—that is, confined to the spinal cord itself—or systemic.[45–47] Regional hypothermic methods have the distinct advantage of avoiding systemic hypothermia, a concept believed to be important to the overall operative management of TAA patients. Clinical application of regional hypothermic techniques was based on convincing experimental data wherein a 100% protective effect against spinal cord injury was demonstrated. Marsala and associates demonstrated that a clinically applicable closed epidural infusion system that achieved moderate (26° to 28°C) levels of cord hypothermia could be 100% effective against spinal cord ischemia induced by double thoracic aortic clamping in a dog model.[48] We adopted this strategy and have applied it in patients since 1993.[49] The mechanics of this clinically applicable system (see Fig. 17–3) are straightforward, with an epidural catheter used for infusion of 4°C saline and a separate intrathecal catheter used to measure CSF temperature and pressure. It is necessary to maintain a continuous infusion to achieve moderate (approximately 25°C) levels of cord hypothermia and the infusion must be initiated some 45 minutes prior to the anticipated application of the cross-clamp. The principal technical limitation of the epidural infusion system is related to the fact the CSF pressures rise during the epidural infusion—averaging twice baseline in our patients—and is a matter of significant concern relative to spinal cord perfusion above the level of cooling. It is therefore necessary to maintain an arbitrary 30 to 40 mm Hg between mean arterial pressure and mean CSF pressure either by decreasing the epidural infusion rate or by increasing systemic arterial pressure. Neurological outcome in our first 70 patients treated with this method was significantly improved when compared to institutional controls operated in the 3-year period prior to adoption of the epidural cooling technique. Neurological deficits after elective resections of types I, II, and III TAAs were reduced to the 3% range in elective operations with the adjunctive use of epidural cooling.[26]

Operative Mortality and Other Major Complications

As displayed in Table 17–3, operative mortality in large clinical series averages in the 10% range[10,19,29,39,50,51]; however, other reports detail considerably higher perioperative mortality.[52,53] Not surprisingly, the circumstances of the clinical presentation are the dominant factor with respect the preoperative variables associated with operative mortality. In our material, operations for either ruptured TAA or urgent (vs. elective) operation were highly predictive ($p < .001$) of perioperative mortality. Similar data have been reported by others.[19,21,52] Some contemporary series have demonstrated an increased risk of operative mortality in elderly patients.[19,21] The presence of increasing numbers of comorbid conditions can naturally be expected to increase overall operative risk. Individual series variously demonstrate increased operative risks with patients with antecedent coronary artery disease, significant COPD, and, in particular, preoperative renal insufficiency. Stated differently, the presence of significant dysfunction in these respective organ systems clearly increases the risks of organ-specific complications after operation, which clearly have a major impact on the risk of operative mortality. In fact, aside from the dominant influence of emergency operation and TAA rupture, the major correlates of operative mortality are the major postoperative complications. Patients who sustain major neurological deficits, postoperative renal failure, and cardiopulmonary complications have a significantly increased risk of operative mortality. Cambria and associates[20] found that the risk of operative mortality was increased more than sixfold in patients with postoperative renal failure and increased by a factor of sixteen in those with paraplegia, findings similar to those of Svensson and coworkers.[10] These data emphasize the importance of minimizing such complications.

Perioperative Hemorrhage

Intraoperative bleeding complications can occur from technical mishaps or dilutional coagulopathy caused by excessive blood turnover, and previously was an important source of early mortality.[15] Blood turnover in extensive aneurysm cases is, of necessity, significant because large type II aneurysms, for example, can contain up to several liters of blood in the aneurysm sac alone. This blood is routinely returned to the patient in the form of autotransfusion, and my experience has been that roughly half the blood turnover during TAA resection is returned to the patient by autotransfusion methods. Total blood transfusion for resection of the more extensive types I and II aneurysms averages more than 3 liters, and it is not surprising that this figure varies with the extent of aortic replacement (Table 17–2). Coselli and associates[21] documented that blood and plasma transfusions increased with use of partial cardiopulmonary bypass. Anticipatory use of blood component replacement in the form of fresh-frozen plasma and especially platelet transfusions, once perfusion to the abdominal viscera and lower extremities has been restored, is an important component of avoiding coagulopathic bleeding in the operating room. With this policy, avoidance of systemic heparin, and careful attention to hemostasis throughout the course of operation, significant coagulo-pathic bleeding in the operating room has rarely been observed in contemporary practice. Considerable attention has been focused on hepatic and mesenteric ischemia as contributory or principally responsible for the development of intraoperative coagulo-pathic bleeding.[54] Significant depletion of coagulation factors that occur intraoperatively in the course of a supraceliac aortic clamp and the fact that these changes are quantita-tively more severe when compared to an infrarenal aortic cross-clamp have been docu-mented.[55] Although such coagulation factor depletion is clearly demonstrable with laboratory testing, the clinical complication of coagulopathic bleeding has been dis-tinctly uncommon. Irrespective of whether the mechanism of coagulopathic bleeding is hepatic ischemia or bacterial translocation in ischemic gut, the available experimental data and clinical observations suggest that minimizing mesenteric ischemia is an impor-tant component of avoiding coagulopathic bleeding. As displayed in Fig. 17–3, it is preferable to reestablish mesenteric perfusion by means of an in-line mesenteric shunt immediately after completion of the proximal aortic anastomosis, and it has been demonstrated that this technique can blunt the coagulation defect seen with supra-celiac clamping.[28]

Reexploration for bleeding complications had a highly significant impact on overall operative mortality in Crawford's summary experience (as reported in Svensson et al.[10]). This was required in 7% of Crawford's patients, but currently occurs in less than 3% of patients. Postoperative splenic bleeding and undetected back-bleeding from intercostal or lumbar vessels have been the principal sources of postoperative hemor-rhage. A careful search of the entire aneurysm sac for back-bleeding and lumbar and intercostal vessels after all suture lines have been completed and an aggressive posture towards splenectomy for even apparently trivial splenic tears should prevent these complications.

Respiratory Insufficiency

Despite the more evident focus on spinal cord ischemic complications and renal failure, postoperative respiratory failure is the single most common complication after TAA resection in the majority of clinical series, occurring in 25% to 45% of patients.[19,20,50] There may be confusion as to how this is defined because the term *prolonged ventilatory support* (the most common problem) may be variably interpreted. A slow wean from ventilatory support, often planned to proceed over several days, is appropriate management in certain patients after extensive TAA resection, particularly patients with baseline pulmonary insufficiency. Despite varying definitions, postoperative respiratory insufficiency is common, and the variables predictive of his complication include active cigarette smoking; baseline COPD, especially patients with significant reductions in FeV_1; and cardiac, renal, or bleeding complications.[20,56] In the circumstance of elective operation, it is vital for the patient to discontinue tobacco use for a minimum of 1 month prior to operation. Preoperative consultation with a pulmonologist for optimization of bronchodilator therapy is an important component in the management of patients with significant COPD. However, institution of preoperative steroid therapy with the intent of improving respiratory function is contraindicated because this maneuver has been shown to precipitate aneurysm rupture. It is intuitively logical that paralysis of the left hemidiaphragm by its radial division to the aortic hiatus will contribute significantly to postoperative respiratory failure. Accordingly, a diaphragm-sparing operative technique has been applied routinely in contemporary practice.

Perioperative Renal Insufficiency

Postoperative renal failure has traditionally been an important factor in the overall morbidity of extensive aortic surgery. The summary experience of Crawford reinforced this fact: Svensson and associates[10] reported that among more than 1500 patients undergoing TAA resection, significant postoperative renal failure occurred in 18% of patients, with dialysis being required in half of these. The risk of operative mortality increased fivefold in patients sustaining postoperative renal failure. Data from Kashyap and associates[27] are consistent with the significant impact of postoperative renal failure on operative mortality. More than 180 TAA operations were reviewed and it was found that in the 8% of patients who sustained significant postoperative renal failure, the risk of mortality was increased almost 10 times (odds ratio 9.2; 95% CI, 2.6–33; $p < .005$).

Postoperative renal failure, as used in this chapter, is defined as both a doubling of the baseline serum creatinine level and an absolute postoperative creatinine level of more than 3.0 mg per deciliter, a definition applied in most major clinical series. The important etiologic factors in the development of postoperative renal failure include the duration of renal ischemia, baseline renal dysfunction, cholesterol embolization from surgical manipulation of the aneurysm in the region of the renal artery orifices, and failure of a renal artery reconstruction. Transient and modest decreases in overall excretory function are the inevitable consequence of some obligatory period of renal ischemia and, in the majority of patients, this is nonoliguric and reverses rapidly with appropriate maintenance of intravascular volume. Not surprisingly, the risk of significant renal dysfunction increases as a function of total aortic cross-clamp time. In addition, virtually all reports that examine this complication have indicated that the most powerful predictive variable for the development of postoperative renal failure is the presence of preoperative renal insufficiency. An abnormal preoperative serum creatinine and a prolonged aortic cross-clamp time have been found to increase the risk of postoperative renal failure by a factor of four, findings consistent with those reported by others.[17,19,27,50] The most important maneuver to minimize the risk of postoperative renal failure is, of course, minimizing renal ischemic time. The other frequently applied intraoperative adjunct, and the one preferred on our service, is selective hypothermic renal artery perfusion as detailed previously (Fig. 17–3). Although such regional renal hypothermia is likely to be unnecessary in patients whose preoperative renal function is normal and whose renal ischemic time is less than 1 hour, it can provide a margin of safety in circumstances of either technical difficulty or prolongation of renal ischemia. An additional intraoperative adjunct employed to minimize the risk of postoperative renal failure is an aggressive posture towards the treatment of renal artery occlusive lesions.[50]

Management of perioperative renal failure is usually conservative if the patient remains nonoliguric. Patients who take diuretic medications preoperatively generally need to continue their medications in the postoperative period; renal dose dopamine infusions can also help to maintain an appropriate diuresis. It is preferable to avoid the use of hemodialysis therapy unless a clearcut indication exists on either a metabolic or blood-volume basis. Conventional hemodialysis is accompanied by a substantial risk of hemodynamic instability in the patient after TAA resection, and it has been observed that hypotension precipitates spinal cord ischemic events even weeks after surgery. The availability of continuous *veno venous* hemodialysis therapy has obviated this consideration somewhat, and provides for a smoother hemodynamic course than conventional hemodialysis. Nonetheless, the need for anticoagulation, the potential complications of vascular access devices, and the threat of hemodynamic instability make hemodialysis therapy undesirable unless it is absolutely necessary.

Late Survival

The most exhaustive review of late survival in patients after TAA resection was reported by Svensson and associates.[10] These investigators reported Kaplan Meier survival projections in the 60% range at 5 years after operation, figures almost identical with my own. These data indicate that the substantial resource investment required to bring these patients through successful operation and recovery is an appropriate expenditure of such resources. The majority of operative survivors return to their preoperative independent living status.[57] Rupture of another aneurysm accounts for approximately 10% of late deaths.[10,57] This indicates the desirability of ongoing aortic surveillance after successful operative treatment of TAA. Cardiac events are the most common source of late mortality. Similar to their negative effect on early postoperative survival, patients who sustained postoperative lower extremity neurological deficits or are converted to a dialysis dependent state have distinctly inferior late survival.[10]

SUMMARY

Considerable progress has been demonstrated in the overall results of surgical treatment for TAA. The multiplicity of surgical strategies and adjuncts applied in efforts to minimize the principle complications of operation indicate that the evolution of surgical sophistication is, as yet, incomplete. Figure 17–10 shows overall results since 1986 of operations applying the principles and techniques reviewed herein. Favorable results have been achieved with the clamp-and-sew technique, with adjuncts directed against the principle complications. Similar to the evolution of surgical treatment of infrarenal AAA, an increase in the percentage of patients treated in elective circumstances will be necessary to improve results in the future.

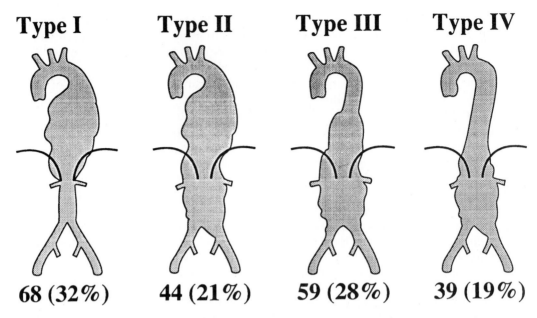

Type I   Type II   Type III   Type IV

68 (32%)   44 (21%)   59 (28%)   39 (19%)

Figure 17–10. Distribution of 210 TAA treated since 1986 and results achieved. Overall operative mortality was 8%; paraparesis/paraplegia was 7.2% with these figures being halved for patients treated in elective circumstances.

REFERENCES

1. Schwartz LB, Belkin M, Donaldson M, et al. Improvements in results of repair of type IV thoracoabdominal aortic aneurysms. *J Vasc Surg.* 1996;24:74–81.
2. Crawford ES, Hess KR, Cohen JS, Safi HJ. Ruptured aneurysm of the descending thoracic and thoracoabdominal aorta. *Ann Surg.* 1991;213:417–426.
3. Cambria RA, Gloviczki P, Stanson A, et al. Outcome and expansion rate of 57 thoracoabdominal aortic aneurysms managed nonoperatively. *Am J Surg.* 1995;170:213–217.
4. Lobato AC, Puech-Leao P. Predictive factors for rupture of thoracoabdominal aortic aneurysm. *J Vasc Surg.* 1998;27:446–453.
5. Masuda Y, Takanashi K, Takasu J, et al. Expansion rate of thoracic aortic aneurysms and influencing factors. *Chest.* 1992;102:461–466.
6. Juvonen T, Ergin MA, Galla JD, et al. Prospective study of the natural history of thoracic aortic aneurysms. *Ann Thorac Surg.* 1997;63:1533–1545.
7. Perko MJ, Norgaard M, Herzog TM, et al. Unoperated aortic aneurysm: a survey of 170 patients. *Ann Thorac Surg.* 1995;59:1204–1209.
8. Crawford ES, Mizrahi EM, Hess KR, et al. The impact of distal perfusion and somatosensory evoked potential monitoring on prevention of paraplegia after aortic aneurysm operation. *J Thorac Cardiovasc Surg.* 1988;95:357–366.
9. Crawford ES, Svensson LG, Hess KR, et al. A prospective randomized study of cerebrospinal fluid drainage to prevent paraplegia after high risk surgery on the thoracoabdominal aorta. *J Vasc Surg.* 1991;13:36–46.
10. Svensson LG, Crawford ES, Hess KR, et al. Experience with 1509 patients undergoing thoracoabdominal aortic operations. *J Vasc Surg.* 1993; 17:357–370.
11. Frank S, Parker S, Rock P, et al. Moderate hypothermia, with partial bypass and segmental sequential repair for thoracoabdominal aortic aneurysm. *J Vasc Surg.* 1994;19:687–697.
12. Safi H, Hess KR, Randel M, et al. Cerebrospinal fluid drainage and distal aortic perfusion: reducing neurologic complications in repair of thoroacoabdominal aortic aneurysms, type I and type II. *J Vasc Surg.* 1996;23(2):223–228.

13. Schepens M, Defauw J, Hamerlijnck R, Vermeulen F. Use of left heart bypass in the surgical repair of thoracoabdominal aortic aneurysms. *Ann Vasc Surg.* 1995;9:327–335.

14. Cambria RP, Giglia J. Prevention of spinal cord ischemic complications after thoracoabdominal aortic surgery. *Europ J Vasc Endovasc Surg.* 198;15:96–109.

15. Cambria R, Brewster D, Moncure A, et al. Recent experience with thoracoabdominal aneurysm repair. *Arch Surg.* 1989;124:620–624.

16. Dake MD, Miller DC, Semba CP, et al. Transluminal placement of endovascular stent-grafts for the treatment of descending thoracic aortic aneurysms. *N Engl J Med.* 1994;331:1729–1734.

17. Safi HJ, Harlin SA, Miller CC. Predictive factors for acute renal failure in thoracic and thoracoabdominal aortic aneurysm surgery. *J Vasc Surg.* 1996;24:338–345.

18. Wirthlin DJ, Cambria RP. Surgery-specific considerations in the cardiac patient undergoing non-cardiac surgery. In: Eagle KA (ed). *Progress in Cardiovascular Diseases.* Philadelphia, PA: WB Saunders; 1998;453–468.

19. Acher CW, Wynn MM, Hoch JR, Kranner PW. Cardiac function is a risk factor for paralysis in thoracoabdominal aortic replacement. *J Vasc Surg.* 1998;27:821–830.

20. Cambria R, Davison J, Kenneth JK, et al. Thoracoabdominal aneurysm repair: perspectives over a decade with the clamp-and-sew technique. *Ann Surg.* 1997;226:294–305.

21. Coselli JS, LeMaitre SA, Poli de Figueiredo L, Kirby RP. Paraplegia after thoracoabdominal aortic aneurysm repair: is dissection a risk factor? *Ann Thorac Surg.* 1997;63:28–36.

22. Acher CW, Wynn MM, Hoch JR, et al. Combined use of cerebral spinal fluid drainage and naloxone reduces the risk of paraplegia in thoracoabdominal aneurysm repair. *J Vasc Surg.* 1994;19:236–248.

23. Cambria RP, Brewster DC, Abbott WM, et al. The impact of selective use of dipyridamole–thallium scans and surgical factors on the current morbidity of aortic surgery. *J Vasc Surg.* 1992;15:43–51.

24. Bush HJ, Hydo LJ, Fischer E, et al. Hypothermia during elective abdominal aortic aneurysm repair: the high risk of avoidable morbidity. *J Vasc Surg.* 1995;21:392–400.

25. Frank SM, Fleisher LA, Breslow MJ, et al. Perioperative maintenance of normothermia reduces the incidence of morbid cardiac events. A randomized clinical trial. *JAMA.* 1997;227:1127–1134.

26. Cambria RP, Davison JK, Zannetti S, et al. Clinical experience with epidural cooling for spinal cord protection during thoracic and thoracoabdominal aneurysm repair. *J Vasc Surg.* 1997;25:234–243.

27. Kashyap VS, Cambria RP, Davison JK, L'Italien GJ. Renal failure after thoracoabdominal aortic surgery. *J Vasc Surg.* 1997;26:949–957.

28. Cambria RP, Davison JK, Giglia JS, Gertler JP. Mesenteric shunting decreases visceral ischemic time during thoracoabdominal aneurysm repair. *J Vasc Surg.* 1998;27:745–749.

29. Kouchoukos N, Daily BB, Rokkas CK, et al. Hypothermic bypass and circulatory arrest for operations on the descending thoracic and thoracoabdominal aorta. *Ann Thorac Surg.* 1995;60:67–77.

30. Engle J, Safi HJ, Muller CC, et al. The impact of diaphragm management on prolonged ventilator support following thoracoabdominal aortic repair. *J Vasc Surg.* (in press).

31. Wadouh F, Arndt C, Oppermann E, et al. The mechanism of spinal cord injury after simple and double aortic cross-clamping. *J Thorac Cardiovasc Surg.* 1986;92:121–127.

32. Savader SJ, Williams GM., Trerotola SO, et al. Preoperative spinal artery localization and its relationship to postoperative neurologic complications. *Radiology.* 1993;189(1):165–171.

33. Safi HJ, Miller III CC, Carr C, et al. Importance of intercostal artery reattachment during thoracoabdominal aortic aneurysm repair. *J Vasc Surg.* 1998;27:58–68.

34. Svensson LG, Hess KR, Coselli JS, Safi HJ. Influence of segmental arteries, extent and atriofemoral bypass on postoperative paraplegia after thoracoabdominal aortic operations. *J Vasc Surg.* 1994;20:255–262.

35. Safi HJ, Miller CC, Azizzadeh A, et al. Observations on delayed neurologic deficit after thoracoabdominal aneurysm repair. *J Vasc Surg.* 1997;26:616–622.

36. Rokkas CK, Kouchoukos NT. Profound hypothermia for spinal cord protection in operations on the descending and thoracoabdominal aorta. *Semin Thorac Cardiovasc Surg.* 1998;10:57–60.

37. Griepp RB, Ergen MA, Galla JD, et al. Looking for the artery of Adamkiewicz: a quest to minimize paraplegia after operations for aneurysm of the descending thoracic and thoracoabdominal aorta. *J Thorac Cardiovasc Surg.* 1996;112:1202–1215.

38. deHaan P, Kalkman CJ, De Mol BA, et al. Efficacy of transcranial motor-evoked myogenic potentials to detect spinal cord ischemia during operations for thoracoabdominal aneurysms. *J Thorac Cardiovasc Surg.* 1997;113:87–101.

39. Grabitz K, Sandmann W, Stuhmeirer K, et al. The risk of ischemic spinal cord injury in patients undergoing graft replacement for thoracoabdominal aortic aneurysms. *J Vasc Surg.* 1996;23(2):230–240.

40. Blaisdell FW, Cooley DA. The mechanism of paraplegia after temporary aortic occlusion and its relationship to spinal fluid pressure. *Surgery.* 1962;57:351–355.

41. Berendes J, Bredee J, Schipperheyn J, Mashhour Y. Mechanism of spinal cord injury after cross-clamping of the descending thoracic aorta. *Circulation.* 1982;66 Suppl1:112–116.

42. Kazama S, Masaki Y, Maruyama S, Ishihara A. Effect of altering cerebrospinal fluid pressure on spinal cord blood flow. *Ann Thorac Surg.* 1994;58:112–115.

43. Murray MJ, Bower TC, Oliver WCJ, et al. Effects of cerebrospinal fluid drainage in patients undergoing thoracic and thoracoabdominal aortic surgery. *J Cardiothorac Vasc Anesth.* 1993;7:266–272.

44. Rokkas C, Cronin C, Nitta T, et al. Profound systemic hypothermia inhibits the release of neurotransmitter amino acids in spinal cord ischemia. *J Thorac Cardiovasc Surg.* 1995;110:27–35.

45. Berguer R, Porto J, Fedoronko B, Dragovic L. Selective deep hypothermia of the spinal cord prevents paraplegia after aortic cross-clamping in the dog model. *J Vasc Surg.* 1992;15:62–72.

46. Rokkas C, Sundaresan S, Shuman TA, et al. Profound systemic hypothermia protects the spinal cord in a primate model of spinal cord ischemia. *J Thorac Cardiovasc Surg.* 1993;106:1024–1035.

47. Salzano R, Ellison LH, Altonji PF, et al. Regional deep hypothermia of the spinal cord protects against ischemic injury during thoracic aortic cross-clamping. *Ann Thorac Surg.* 1994;57(1):65–70.

48. Marsala M, Vanicky I, Galik J, et al. Panmyelic epidural cooling protects against ischemic spinal cord damage. *J Surg Res.* 1993;55:21–31.

49. Davison J, Cambria R, Vierra D, et al. Epidural cooling for regional spinal cord hypothermia during thoracoabdominal aneurysm repair. *J Vasc Surg.* 1994;20:304–310.

50. Coselli JS, Plestis KA. Thoracoabdominal aortic aneurysm repair in patients with visceral artery occlusive disease. *J Vasc Surg.* (in press).

51. Hollier L, Money SR, Naslund TC, et al. Risk of spinal cord dysfunction in patients undergoing thoracoabdominal aortic replacement. *Am J Surg.* 1992;164:210–213.

52. Cox GS, O'Hara PJ, Hertzer N, et al. Thoracoabdominal aneurysm repair: a representative experience. *J Vasc Surg.* 1992;15:780–788.

53. Gilling-Smith GL, Worswick OL, Knight PF, et al. Surgical repair of thoracoabdominal aortic aneurysm: 10 years experience. *Brit J Surg.* 1995;82:624–629.

54. Cohen JR, Angus L, Asher A, et al. Disseminated intravascular coagulation as a result of supraceliac clamping: implications for thoracoabdominal aneurysm repair. *Ann Vasc Surg.* 1987;1:552–557.

55. Gertler JP, Cambria RP, Laposata M, Abbott WM. Coagulation changes during thoracoabdominal aneurysm repair. *J Vasc Surg.* 1996;24:936–945.

56. Money SR, Rice K, Crockett D, et al. Risk of respiratory failure after repair of thoracoabdominal aortic aneurysms. *Am J Surg.* 1994;168:152–155.

57. Schepens MA, Dekkar E, Hanerlijnck RP, Vermeulen FE. Survival and aortic events after graft replacement for thoracoabdominal aortic aneurysm. *Cardiovasc Surg.* 1996;4:713–719.

18

Treatment Options for Aortoiliac Occlusive Disease

David C. Brewster, MD

The infrarenal abdominal aorta and iliac arteries are among the most common sites of chronic atherosclerosis in patients with symptomatic occlusive disease of the lower extremities. Because arteriosclerosis is frequently a generalized process, obliterative disease in the aortoiliac segment frequently coexists with disease below the inguinal ligament.[1] Despite its widespread nature, however, aortoiliac disease is usually segmental in distribution and therefore amenable to effective treatment. Even in patients with multilevel disease, successful correction of hemodynamically significant inflow disease frequently provides adequate revascularization of the extremities and satisfactory clinical relief of ischemic symptoms. Careful assessment of the adequacy of arterial inflow is also of crucial importance even in patients whose principle disease is infrainguinal in location, in order to ensure that effective and durable results of distal arterial reconstruction are obtained. For all of these reasons, management of aortoiliac disease is an important component in the day-to-day clinical practice of all vascular surgeons.

Since introduction of initial methods of revascularization by means of homografts and endarterectomy in the early 1950s, a wide variety of therapeutic options have been developed and advocated for management of aortoiliac disease. These can be categorized broadly as anatomic or direct reconstructive procedures on the aortoiliac vessels, so-called extra-anatomic or indirect bypass grafts, which avoid normal anatomic pathways; and various nonoperative catheter-based endoluminal therapies, which emphasize treatment of occlusive lesions via a remote, often percutaneous, access site to the arterial system. Although the availability of these numerous alternative therapies is certainly beneficial, enabling the surgeon to select a procedure appropriate to the individual anatomy and risk status of each patient, decision making is frequently complex and difficult. Substantial differences in reported early and late results of alternative methods has contributed to confusion. Purported benefits and advantages, particularly of endoluminal techniques, have been accentuated by the explosive growth of cost and length-of-stay (LOS) considerations and the implication by some that less invasive treatment is inherently superior. Indeed, determination of what is the best treatment option for aortoiliac disease represents one of the most controversial areas of contemporary vascular surgery practice.

It is important to emphasize at the onset that little truly definitive data on these topics exists. There are few prospective randomized comparative studies with adequate control of the complex variables involved. Personal bias, previous surgical training, and prior individual experience remain important factors in decision making. In addition, the need to individualize each decision, as dictated by specific anatomic distribution of disease and operative risk considerations unique to every patient, means by definition that there is not a single optimal procedure. The best procedure will, and likely should, vary from patient to patient.

DIRECT ANATOMIC METHODS

Endarterectomy vs. Grafting

Although aortoiliac endarterectomy was frequently employed in the early era of aortic reconstruction,[2-4] it is rarely utilized by most vascular surgeons in current practice. The principal potential benefit of endarterectomy is avoidance of use of prosthetic grafts with their possible complications of dilation, infection, anastomotic aneurysm, or other degenerative problems. However, these are all fortunately relatively unusual problems, especially with the improved quality of modern vascular grafts. Endarterectomy is also advocated by some as more likely to improve sexual potency in male patients by more effectively improving hypogastric artery blood flow. However, this has not been demonstrated in any study, and the more extensive dissection in the region of the aortic bifurcation required in endarterectomy seems likely to result in a higher incidence of neurogenic problems and ejaculatory disturbance.

Endarterectomy may be utilized for localized disease confined to the distal aorta, aortic bifurcation, and common iliac arteries. In such patients, the long-term patency is excellent and equivalent to graft procedures.[4-7] However, it has been well documented that more extensive endarterectomy extending into the external iliac arteries or beyond does not have the same durability and patency as bypass grafting.[5,8] Because localized aortoiliac disease most amenable to endarterectomy is encountered in only 5% to 10% of patients requiring aortic reconstruction,[1] the vast majority of patients with more extensive disease are not suitable for endarterectomy and are better treated by graft insertion.

In addition, since the late 1980s, use of PTA, stent insertion, atherectomy, and other endoluminal procedures for relatively localized aortoiliac disease has further encroached on cases formerly considered for possible conventional endarterectomy. Finally, endarterectomy is acknowledged to be a technically demanding procedure. Although a few centers continue to perform an adequate number of aortoiliac endarterectomy procedures for trainees to feel comfortable with the technique, most vascular surgeons trained within the past several decades have little to no training or experience with this method.

For these reasons, bypass grafting has become the standard method of direct surgical repair for occlusive disease in almost all patients. Endarterectomy remains possibly useful for a small number of patients with localized disease, particularly very young patients with an expected life span of 20 to 30 years in whom a higher incidence of possible graft-related late problems might be anticipated, or in patients who may have an increased risk of infection with a nonautogenous reconstruction.[9]

Aortofemoral Graft

Since the pioneering development of a fabric arterial graft by Voorhees[10] and the initial use of prosthetic aortic grafts in the 1950s,[11,12] extensive clinical experience has clearly established aortobifemoral (ABF) grafts as the gold standard in the treatment of aorto-iliac disease. Subsequent refinements in operative techniques, improvement in prosthetic graft and suture materials, and, in particular, striking advances in preoperative evaluation, intraoperative anesthetic management, and postoperative supportive care have all contributed to steadily improving outcome and generally excellent results attainable in current contemporary practice.[5,13–18] The major reasons for the primary role of ABF are its well-documented durability (long-term patency), superior functional results (hemodynamic improvement, symptom relief, and limb salvage), and wide applicability to most patterns of aortoiliac disease. Principal emphasis is appropriately placed on long-term patency rates of 85% to 90% at 5 years and 75% to 80% at 10 years, results unmatched by other methods. In current practice, elective mortality rates of approximately 1% to 2% in appropriately selected patients, with low early and late complication rates, are currently obtained at many experienced centers. For all of these reasons, the results of ABF are indeed the yardstick to which competitive methods of revascularization must be justifiably compared.

Although the indications for and basic principles of ABF have become fairly standardized and well accepted, differences of opinion persist regarding certain technical aspects of the procedure and some remain topics of intense debate.[19] Such areas include the configuration of the proximal anastomosis (end-to-end vs. end-to-side), how often and by what specific technique profundaplasty ought to be combined with ABF, when concomitant distal bypass should be performed, and what type of prosthetic graft should be employed. Needless to say, definitive answers to these controversies are not available, but opinions and bias abound.

Proximal Anastomosis.   In my view, end-to-end anastomosis is generally preferable, principally due to superior hemodynamic characteristics and lack of competitive flow with the diseased but patent native aortoiliac system.[20] Such considerations have led to better long-term patency of end-to-end grafts in some series,[5,21] but other studies have not demonstrated any differences in late patency rates between the two anastomotic configurations.[22–25]

End-to-side graft anastomosis appears to be potentially advantageous in certain anatomic patterns of disease.[20] Specifically, it is the simplest method of preserving flow in a patent inferior mesenteric artery (IMA) or clinically significant accessory renal arteries arising from the infrarenal aortic segment. Most often, the choice of end-to-side anastomosis is used when the surgeon wishes to preserve pelvic blood flow in patients with extensive occlusive disease in both external iliac arteries that precludes retrograde pelvic perfusion.

Role of Profundaplasty.   Establishment of adequate graft outflow at the level of the femoral anastomosis has been documented to be clearly of paramount importance to both early and late graft patency and the hemodynamic results of revascularization in terms of symptom relief.[5,13,22,26,27] The fact that 50% or more of patients undergoing ABF have multilevel disease underscores the crucial role of adequate profunda flow.[20,28–30] It is imperative that any profunda stenosis be identified and corrected. Whether correction of profunda origin disease is best achieved by a long beveled hood of the graft tip, by separate patch profundaplasty employing prosthetic or autogenous tissue material, or, indeed, if formal profunda endarterectomy is also required is of less importance than the basic principle of ensuring a reliable outflow tract.

The importance of this tenet has raised the question of whether some form of profundaplasty should be done in all patients having aortofemoral grafts. Some authors have suggested that the mere existence of an occluded superficial femoral artery (SFA) in itself causes a "functional" profunda stenosis approximating a 50% diameter reducing lesion, even in the absence of actual orificial disease of the profunda.[31] However, the bulk of evidence suggests that "routine" profundaplasty, by whatever method, in all such patients does not improve the hemodynamic result or late patency of the graft.[22] Therefore, anastomosis to the common femoral artery is acceptable unless some actual proximal profunda disease is evident at the time of graft implantation. Although profunda disease may develop in later years in some patients, this may subsequently be dealt with more easily if the deep femoral artery has not been previously dissected and reconstructed.

Management of Multilevel Disease.   A common dilemma in patients with multilevel disease (MLD) is whether proximal revascularization alone will suffice. Although it is generally accepted that 75% to 80% of these patients are improved by a properly performed aortic procedure, many series have documented that from 25% to 33% of patients with MLD fail to have sufficient relief of ischemic symptoms and may require later infrainguinal procedures.[28] If such patients could be identified preoperatively, it would often be logical and beneficial to perform simultaneous inflow and outflow revascularization. Accurate prediction remains elusive, however, and no single reliable indicator has been determined. Nonetheless, several criteria exist that together usually enable the surgeon to make this clinical judgment.

Factors to be considered include demonstration of only modest degrees of proximal inflow disease, particularly in the presence of obviously extensive and hemodynamically severe infrainguinal disease, and a small or diffusely diseased profunda femoris, not suitable for profundaplasty and likely to provide an inadequate collateral runoff tract to the lower extremity. Most important is the degree of distal ischemia. If the foot is severely ischemic, as with ischemic necrosis or digital gangrene likely to require local amputation, it is clear that maximal revascularization is often mandated if limb salvage is to be attained.

In these circumstances, synchronous proximal and distal reconstruction seems both desirable and appropriate, avoiding the difficulties and possible complications of later groin reoperation for staged bypass and providing the best chance of relief for ischemic symptoms or salvage of the threatened limb. The frequency of combined operation appears to be increasing significantly in contemporary practice.[32] The use of two surgical teams can reduce additional operative time considerably, and thereby minimize the increased risk that was often cited in earlier years as an important reason to avoid simultaneous proximal and distal bypass in favor of a staged approach.

The Best Graft.   Although standard fabric prosthetic grafts have generally performed well for aortofemoral reconstruction, numerous modifications in graft material (Dacron vs. PTFE, etc.), methods of fabrication (knitted vs. woven, external vs. double velour, porosity differences, etc.), and additions of various biologic coatings (collagen, gelatin, albumin) to the graft have been devised. Such alterations have been designed with the hope of improving the performance and characteristics of the graft: patency, durability, healing, resistance to infection, reduced blood loss, and improved handling features. Various claims concerning the benefits of one type of graft over another have been made, but it is often difficult to discern science from salesmanship.

One may currently conclude that no single large caliber prosthesis is clearly superior for aortic reconstruction. Patency seems generally equivalent in the aortic position, so a choice should be based on other considerations, such as handling properties, infectivity, reduction of blood loss, and ease of reoperation (dissection, thrombectomy, or thrombolysis). Objective scientific evaluation of these qualities is difficult. Ultimately, cost rather than such subjective and subtle attributes may determine the choice.

Irrespective of the exact type of graft material and fabrication, the use of a proper-sized graft is important. Previously, many surgeons employed grafts that were too large in comparison to the size of outflow tract vessels, which tended to promote sluggish flow in graft limbs and deposition of excessive laminar pseudointima in the prosthesis. This in turn may often have a propensity to later fragmentation or dislodgment, leading to occlusion of one or both limbs of the graft. For occlusive disease, a 16 × 8 mm bifurcated graft is most often employed, with no hesitation to use a 14 × 7 mm or even smaller prosthesis when appropriate, as is frequently the case in some female patients with hypoplastic aortas. The limb size of such grafts most closely approximates the femoral arteries of patients with occlusive disease, or more particularly the size of the profunda femoris, which often remains as the only outflow tract. In addition, it is now well recognized that many Dacron prosthetic grafts have a tendency to dilate 10% to 20% when subjected to arterial pressure.[33] Selection of a smaller graft size helps compensate for this.

The Best Approach.   Since the late 1980s, there has been a reawakening of enthusiasm for a retroperitoneal (RP) approach for aortic surgery. In addition to some potential technical considerations, advocates have claimed possible physiological advantages such as less cardiac stress, reduced pulmonary disturbance, decreased ileus, and lessened third-space fluid losses.[34]

Most such data has related to aneurysm repair, however, and most of the suggested benefits have not been documented conclusively. Indeed, no significant outcome differences were found in a randomized prospective study examining this issue.[35] Although perhaps advantageous for certain complex aortic disease, in my opinion, routine use of an RP approach for all cases of conventional aortofemoral grafting for standard aortoiliac occlusive disease cannot be recommended. A major drawback is that positioning often makes adequate exposure of the right femoral artery and graft tunneling to the right groin difficult, particularly in the obese patient. Access to the right renal artery is poor, and if control and possible repair of the right iliac artery may be necessary, this is often quite difficult with a left flank approach.

However, an RP approach may certainly be advantageous in certain circumstances, often related to technical issues.[35,36] Multiple previous intra-abdominal surgical procedures, prior aortic surgery, or other forms of hostile abdominal pathology are examples. If significant juxta- or pararenal disease requires repair, or concomitant left renal artery revascularization or other visceral artery repair is necessary, an RP approach may be quite helpful. For most cases of ABF graft for occlusive disease, however, I certainly prefer the standard midline transabdominal route.

ALTERNATIVES TO DIRECT AORTIC REVASCULARIZATION

Despite the well-documented durability, effectiveness, and increasing safety of ABF, which have justifiably established it as the gold standard of revascularization for aorto-iliac occlusive disease, it is paradoxical that one of the most successful procedures in vascular surgical practice is being utilized less frequently in current day practice. Increasing use of alternative therapies, particularly catheter-based endoluminal modalities such as percutaneous transluminal angioplasty (PTA) in place of ABF grafting for treatment of symptomatic aortoiliac disease is attributable to several factors. Changing patient demographics and patient profiles are apparent to all practitioners; patients in current practice are, indeed, often older and sicker. Results of alternative methods have also improved as these techniques undergo further evolution and refinement. In addition, the less invasive nature of these procedures has great patient appeal and is part of the considerable momentum towards minimally invasive care in all spheres of surgical practice. The potential advantages of alternative therapies are indeed attractive: reduced risk, reduced hospital stays, quicker recovery, and the perceived cost advantages stemming from these characteristics.

Nonetheless, it is important to recognize possible disadvantages of these methods as well. They are almost certainly less durable than ABF grafts, often less effective in terms of incomplete revascularization, and generally less broadly applicable to patients with common (i.e., extensive) patterns of disease. All of these potential deficiencies may blunt possible cost benefits. In fact, the cost-effectiveness of many of these methods as compared to conventional treatment remains unproved.

Extra-Anatomic Grafts

Since their introduction in the early 1960s for management of difficult and often desperate technical problems usually related to infection or failure of previous grafts, use of a variety of extra-anatomic bypasses has increased to include wider application in patients perceived to be at high risk for conventional ABF grafts or for patients with more limited disease not otherwise suitable for PTA or stents. In these circumstances, the goal is to achieve revascularization by means of grafts that utilize remote, frequently subcutaneous, pathways and can be performed with potentially lower morbidity and mortality.

Whether such reconstructive options represent reasonable alternatives to ABF grafts in a greater number of patients remains ill-defined at present.[19,37] Currently, most debate centers on two areas: the most appropriate management of unilateral iliac disease and the possible expanded role of axillofemoral (Ax-Fem) grafts suggested by reported improved results.[38–40]

As is the case with consideration of the role of PTA, a considerable part of uncertainty regarding these issues is related to substantial variations in reported long-term effectiveness of these surgical alternatives. For example, a review of the literature reveals 3- to 5-year patencies of Ax-Fem grafts ranging from 10% to 85%.[19] This is due in part to inconsistencies of reporting methods in some earlier series, which reported secondary rather than primary patency rates, as well as the confounding influence of combining results of grafts used in differing clinical settings. As emphasized by Rutherford and coworkers,[37] the results of extra-anatomic grafts are quite different in patients with good versus poor runoff (SFA status) or when used as primary procedures versus reoperative reconstruction for failure of prior grafts. Thus, a more detailed consideration of specific clinical indications and anatomic patterns of disease is necessary to more accurately predict likely outcome and attain a perspective on the application of such methods.

Although aortoiliac disease is generally a diffuse process eventually involving both iliofemoral (IF) arterial segments, it is not uncommon that patients will manifest largely unilateral symptoms, with a normal femoral pulse and absence of ischemic symptoms in the contralateral limb. In this setting, the question frequently arises as to whether a conventional ABF graft should be done or a more limited reconstruction aimed at treatment of only the symptomatic side. Femorofemoral (FF) and IF bypass are the most commonly employed surgical alternatives to ABF grafts in these circumstances. Although endarterectomy may also be performed for relatively localized unilateral iliofemoral disease, this has been large supplanted in the current era by PTA and stenting.

Both FF and IF bypass can provide highly satisfactory long-term patency and relief of ischemic symptoms in properly selected patients, particularly when adjunctive profundaplasty is also carried out when indicated.[41–46] IF grafts may have somewhat better late patency rates, and also the additional advantage of avoiding surgery and possible complications on the opposite asymptomatic limb.[39,45-47] However, FF bypass is generally easier, involves less dissection, and therefore has a lower morbidity risk. FF grafts can also be used for patients with common iliac artery occlusion or heavy calcification, which preclude IF bypass and carry the least risk of postoperative disturbance of sexual function, which may be a consideration even in the patient whose risk is low.

Nonetheless, the patency rate of either alternative is less than that of ABF, and the hemodynamic performance of extra-anatomic grafts such as FF bypass often inferior.[48] Furthermore, use of unilateral reconstructions may lead to the later need for operation on the contralateral side due to progressive disease in the aorta or opposite iliac artery. Although the frequency of this event is quite variable in the literature, ranging from 5% to 38% of patients in differing series, it is a consideration perhaps favoring ABF in a young patient at low risk.[38] ABF grafts also do not appear to be as adversely influenced by the presence of runoff disease or limb-salvage indications for operation as do extra-anatomic reconstructions.[37] Thus, for older patients with significant comorbid conditions, use of FF or IF bypass to treat unilateral iliac disease is often a practical choice. In my view, in young, low-risk patients, ABF graft is still preferred in most instances.

Even more controversial is the claim that contemporary results of Ax-Fem bypasses have improved dramatically and are now essentially equivalent to those achieved by conventional ABF grafts. Since the introduction of axillounifemoral and axillobifemoral grafts in the 1960s, nearly all vascular surgeons have recognized the utility of such extra-anatomic alternatives for specific indications, usually involving infection, obviously hostile intra-abdominal pathology, or truly prohibitive risk patients. However, it was generally agreed that Ax-Fem grafts represented a compromise selection, trading inferior long-term durability and less comprehensive hemodynamic improvement for a lower morbidity and mortality risk.

This view has been challenged by the report of Passman et al.[40] from Portland. These authors described results of a prospective concurrent comparison of 117 Ax-Fem and 139 ABF grafts during the 6-year period from 1988 to 1993. Patients were not randomized, however, and procedure choice was made by each surgeon based on assessment of surgical risk. Patients undergoing Ax-Fem grafts were older, had more comorbid conditions, and were operated on for limb salvage indications more often. Although 5-year primary patency (80% ABF, 75% Ax-Fem) and operative mortality (<1% ABF, 3.4% Ax-Fem) results favored the conventional ABF procedure, these differences were not statistically significant. Major postoperative complications were noted to be more frequent following ABF (ABF 20.9%, Ax-Fem 10.3%, $p < .05\%$). No significant difference in 5-year limb salvage rates was detected. Not unexpectedly, 5-year patient survival was significantly inferior for Ax-Fem bypass (45% Ax-Fem, 72% ABF). These results prompted Passman et al.[40] to question the prevailing opinion that ABF constitutes the gold standard for inflow revascularization.

Passman et al.[40] stress that the modern-day results of ABF grafts in the patient population currently requiring surgical revascularization for aortoiliac disease are largely unknown. They emphasize that many older series that are frequently employed for reference standards included a high percentage of patients operated on for claudication alone, and with relatively localized disease, more favorable circumstances often treated today by other modalities such as PTA, and so on. Furthermore, they note other reported series that also describe improved results of Ax-Fem bypass.[49,50]

Prior studies comparing concurrent Ax-Fem and ABF graft results are retrospective, but all have shown superior patency results of the traditional anatomic reconstruction.[19]

TABLE 18–1. PROHIBITIVE RISK FACTORS: INDICATIONS FOR AXILLOBIFEMORAL BYPASS

1. Cardiac: Recent myocardial infarction, intractable heart failure, significant angina pectoris
2. Renal: Chronic azotemia or creatinine clearance <40 mL/mm
3. Pulmonary: Severe emphysema (dyspnea at rest, O_2 dependence or FEV_1 <1 L/s)
4. Morbid obesity: (<45 kg or <100% above ideal body weight)
5. Uncontrolled malignancy or other systemic disease with limited life-expectancy (<2 yr)

Reprinted with permission from Rutherford RB. Choosing between options for aortoiliac disease: a management algorithm. *Semin Vasc Surg.* 1994;7:60–63.

There are no prospective, randomized trials to provide definitive data. Neither is there data to suggest that current results of ABF in today's patient population are necessarily inferior to those previously published, one of the principle assumptions made by Passman and coworkers.[40] Finally, their improved results need to be validated by other studies. At present, I would agree that Ax-Fem grafts currently should be regarded as acceptable alternatives for inflow operation, with specific advantages and disadvantages, and may be more liberally applied in current practice for appropriate clinical indications (Table 18–1) without undue concern about poor long-term results. However, in my opinion, they are not equivalent in durability or efficiency as ABF grafts, and remain a second choice.

CATHETER-BASED THERAPIES

Iliac PTA and Stents

Although some of the decrease in frequency with which ABF grafting is performed is attributable to increased use of extra-anatomic surgical bypass, it is clear that the major impact has been the marked increase in the use of iliac PTA and acceleration of this trend by the rapid growth of intraluminal stents used in conjunction with balloon angioplasty.

Two carefully performed studies by Johnston and coworkers[51,52] have done much to assess results of iliac PTA objectively and indicate when this may be considered a reasonable alternative to conventional surgical repair. Results of their prospective study of 667 iliac PTA procedures demonstrated that chances of long-term success can be predicted accurately depending on four key variables: indication, site, severity, and runoff. In the most favorable circumstances, that of a localized common iliac stenosis in a patient with claudication alone and good runoff, a 3-year success rate of 68% was noted. Conversely, for common or external iliac occlusion in patients with limb-threatening ischemia and poor runoff, a successful result was noted in only 10% to 20% of patients. Overall, the 3-year success rate of iliac PTA determined in the Toronto experience was approximately 60%, certainly considerably inferior to that routinely achieved in all surgical series.

A true comparison of iliac PTA with ABF graft is difficult, as the anatomy (distribution and extent) and severity of disease are usually quite different in patients selected for each method of management. Little randomized prospective data exists. In one study by Wilson et al.[53] comparing patients with limited disease suitable for treatment by either modality, the overall cumulative long-term success rate favored surgery (81% vs. 62% success rate at 3 years). This statistically significant difference between surgery and PTA was due almost entirely to the initial failure rate of PTA (15.5%) rather than late PTA failures. In fact, if early PTA failures are excluded, the durability of the two methods appeared equivalent. In a similar randomized prospective trial by Holm et al.[54] in Sweden, immediate and 1-year results of PTA and surgery were equivalent, and PTA patients had a significantly shorter hospital stay. It is important to note, however, that only patients who could be treated by both methods were included, constituting only 5% of the total number of patients treated during the study period.

It appears reasonable to conclude at present that iliac PTA does have an established and valuable role in the treatment of selected patients with aortoiliac disease, and should be considered as potential primary therapy if the chances of long-term success are good. Proper criteria for its use have been fairly well established, and emphasize principally localized disease, ideally short stenotic lesions in the common iliac arteries. Iliac PTA for focal iliac disease is also a valuable adjunct when combined with distal surgical procedures in appropriate patients with multilevel occlusive disease.[55,56] Given these indications, iliac PTA may be a reasonable alternative to ABF graft or related surgical procedures in perhaps 10% to 15% of patients with aortoiliac disease. Alternatively, PTA may have a role to extend indications for intervention in patients with milder symptoms who would not normally be considered for surgical therapy. Although long-term clinical success even in these favorable subsets of patients appears to be less than with surgical reconstruction, the likely benefits in terms of decreased morbidity and probable cost savings may well justify its use in these circumstances.

Whether stents can improve late results of iliac PTA and thereby extend indications for its use to include more aggressive catheter-based treatment of a greater proportion of patients with more extensive aortoiliac disease (longer diseased segments, multiple lesions, total occlusions) remains much more unsettled, and thus the topic of considerable current debate and controversy. Selective use of stents may well improve early results of PTA in some cases if inadequate hemodynamic improvement is attributable to technical factors leading to insufficient recanalization, such as "elastic recoil" of dilated segments or localized dissections of dilated plaques which produce flow obstruction.[57] However, if a poor hemodynamic result reflects diffuse disease or multiple "subcritical" serial lesions, the benefit of stenting is less well established.

Richter et al.[58] have reported preliminary results in several abstracts of a widely cited prospective randomized study comparing balloon angioplasty and stenting for iliac artery disease; however, a detailed publication has not currently become available, despite widespread claims of superior results with stents. The interim data suggest a clear advantage for the routine use of stents, with a 92.7% 5-year clinical success rate for iliac stenting as compared to 69.7% for PTA alone. However, final conclusions as to the validity of the study and general application of its findings must await detailed publication. This example serves to emphasize the need for properly reported detailed analysis of long-term results that is imperative for informed decision making.

Finally, potential application of aggressive PTA and covered stents (endoluminal stent-grafts) have been suggested as an alternative treatment method for aortoiliac occlusive disease. In two separate studies, Marin and colleagues[59,60] have described the biggest experience with these procedures, which can potentially manage more extensive, long-segment disease. In addition, such an approach may lend itself well to a combined approach in conjunction with conventional infrainguinal bypass procedures in management of patients with extensive multilevel arterial disease. Although their results and other experience mostly in European centers has been encouraging, more experience and data are necessary before such an approach may be widely recommended for most patients.

At present, caution concerning overzealous application of stenting and broadening of indications for iliac PTA seems warranted. Although effective for localized disease, most patients with symptomatic aortoiliac disease severe enough to merit revascularization have more diffuse patterns of disease that are generally best corrected from a long-term perspective by surgical bypass procedures. Although appealing because of its expediency and potentially lower morbidity, the inferior durability of PTA and possible need for multiple reinterventions must be also considered. Potential cost advantages of minimally invasive treatments in general are diminished if frequent reinterventions are required, and cost–benefit analysis must therefore recognize the additional expense of repeat procedures and not simply initial therapy—a concept of "lifetime treatment cost." It is also clear that increased use of stenting to treat more extensive disease requires deployment of multiple stents; at $600 to $1000 per stent, it is obvious that insertion of four or five stents in a single patient largely offsets any procedural cost advantages. The same is even more true for costly endoluminal stent-graft devices. In addition, although failure of PTA generally is thought to seldom preclude or complicate later surgical revascularization, deployment of multiple stents throughout the aortoiliac system may indeed make subsequent operation more difficult or hazardous.

Finally, it seems certain that expanded use of endoluminal modalities to treat more extensive and complex disease will undoubtedly require increased procedure time, need for additional medical and ancillary personnel, and more sophisticated equipment, all factors that diminish cost advantages of less invasive therapies.

Current Perspective

It is clear that no single option for inflow revascularization is optimal in all instances. In every patient, a decision about which method is the best choice is made by consideration of several factors. Primarily, these include the extent and distribution of disease and the anticipated risk of the possible alternatives that might be employed. The likely success of various methods in terms of hemodynamic improvement, symptom relief, and sustained patency can usually be predicted with relative accuracy, and such estimates must be judged in the context of patient age, expected length of survival, and the specific clinical needs of each patient. Durability must often be balanced against the possible advantages of safety and expediency.

Alternative therapies have a well-established role in the management of occlusive disease of limited extent or lesser severity, and in the treatment of patients with adverse technical challenges or high operative risk for conventional direct aortic reconstruction. However, for the majority of patients with diffuse aortoiliac occlusive disease, ABF grafts remain the most durable and functionally effective means of revascularization and should continue to be rightfully regarded as the gold standard or basis of comparison to which other options must be properly compared. It is worth remembering that as the availability and results of alternative techniques have improved, so too has the safety of standard repair. Indeed, the very definition of a "high-risk" patient is currently much more indistinct than in previous eras. No doubt the future will bring new advances in alternative methods, but it is hoped that properly designed and performed randomized studies, outcome assessment, and cost–benefit analyses will help clarify their role. The need for such data is quite evident; without it, one of the most effective and beneficial procedures that vascular surgeons have to offer may be inappropriately abandoned due to the seductive guises of "less is best."

In the final analysis, the alternatives for inflow revascularization may not be as competitive with one another as first seems apparent. Each has its own specific advantages and disadvantages, and when used in appropriate circumstances, can give excellent results (Figs. 18–1 and 18–2).[61] Indeed, it is this very broad spectrum of options

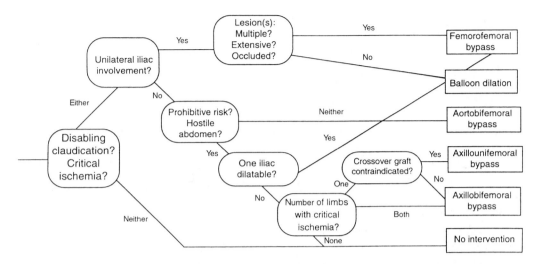

Figure 18–1. Algorithm for initial management of aortoiliac occlusive disease. (*Reprinted with permission from Rutherford RB. Choosing between options for aortoiliac disease: a management algorithm.* Semin Vasc Surg. *1994;7:60–63.*)

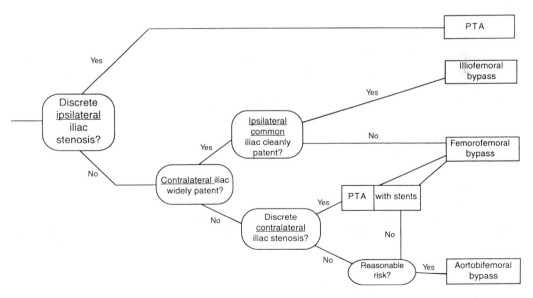

Figure 18–2. Management algorithm for unilateral symptomatic iliac occlusive disease. (*Reprinted with permission from Rutherford RB. Choosing between options for aortoiliac disease: a management algorithm.* Semin Vasc Surg. *1994;7:60–63.*)

that makes treatment of aortoiliac occlusive disease one of the most successful areas of current vascular practice.

REFERENCES

1. Brewster DC. Clinical and anatomic considerations for surgery in aortoiliac disease and results of surgical treatment. *Circulation.* 1991;83(Suppl I):I42–I52.
2. Wylie EJ. Thromboendarterectomy for arteriosclerotic thrombosis of major arteries. *Surgery.* 1952;32:275–290.
3. Barker WF, Cannon JA. An evaluation of endarterectomy. *Arch Surg.* 1953;66:488–495.
4. Darling RC, Linton RR. Aortoiliofemoral endarterectomy for atherosclerotic occlusive disease. *Surgery.* 1964;55:184–194.
5. Brewster DC, Darling RC. Optimal methods of aortoiliac reconstruction. *Surgery.* 1978; 84:739–748.
6. Inahara T. Evaluation of endarterectomy for aortoiliac and aortoiliofemoral occlusive disease. *Arch Surg.* 1975;110:1458–1464.
7. van den Akker PJ, van Schilfgaarde R, Brand R, et al. Long-term results of prosthetic and nonprosthetic reconstruction for obstructive aorto-iliac disease. *Eur J Vasc Surg.* 1992;6:53–61.
8. Crawford ES, Manning LG, Kelly TF. "Redo" surgery after operations for aneurysm and occlusion of the abdominal aorta. *Surgery.* 1977;81:41–52.
9. Ehrenfeld WK, Wilber BC, Olcott CN, Stoney RJ. Autogenous tissue reconstruction in the management of infected prosthetic grafts. *Surgery.* 1979;85:82–92.
10. Voorhees AB Jr, Jaretzki A III, Blakemore AH. Use of tubes constructed from Vinyon "N" cloth in bridging arterial defects: preliminary report. *Ann Surg.* 1952;135:332–336.
11. Edwards SW, Lyons C. Three years' experience with peripheral arterial grafts of crimped nylon and teflon. *Surg Gynecol Obstet.* 1958;107:62–68.
12. DeBakey ME, Cooley DA. Clinical application of a new flexible knitted Dacron arterial substitute. *Am Surg.* 1958;24:862–869.
13. Brewster DC, Cooke JC. Longevity of aortofemoral bypass grafts. In: Yao JST, Pearce WH, eds. *Long-Term Results in Vascular Surgery.* East Norwalk, CT: Appleton & Lange; 1993:149–161.
14. Malone JM, Moore WS, Goldstone J. The natural history of bilateral aortofemoral bypass grafts for ischemia of the lower extremities. *Arch Surg.* 1975;110:1300–1306.
15. Crawford ES, Bomberger RA, Glaeser DH, et al. Aortoiliac occlusive disease: factors influencing survival and function following reconstructive operation over a twenty-five year period. *Surgery.* 1981;90:1055–1067.
16. Szilagyi DE, Elliott JP Jr, Smith RF, et al. A thirty-year survey of the reconstructive surgical treatment of aortoiliac disease. *J Vasc Surg.* 1986;3:421–436.
17. Nevelsteen A, Wouters L, Suy R. Aortofemoral Dacron reconstruction for aortoiliac occlusive disease: a 25 year survey. *Eur J Vasc Surg.* 1991;5:179–186.
18. Poulias GE, Doundoulakis N, Prombonas E, et al. Aorto-femoral bypass and determinants of early success and late favorable outcome: experience with 1000 consecutive cases. *J Cardiovasc Surg.* 1992;33:664–678.
19. Brewster DC. Current controversies in the management of aortoiliac occlusive disease. *J Vasc Surg.* 1997;25:365–379.
20. Brewster DC. Direct reconstruction for aortoiliac occlusive disease In: Rutherford RB, ed. *Vascular Surgery.* 4th ed. Philadelphia: WB Saunders; 1995:766–794.
21. Pierce GE, Turrentine M, Stringfield S, et al. Evaluation of end-to-side v. end-to-end proximal anastomosis in aortobifemoral bypass. *Arch Surg.* 1982;117:1580–1588.
22. Rutherford RB, Jones DN, Martin MS, et al. Serial hemodynamic assessment of aortobifemoral bypass. *J Vasc Surg.* 1986;4:428–435.
23. Ameli FM, Stein M, Aro L, et al. End-to-end versus end-to-side proximal anastomosis in aortobifemoral bypass surgery: does it matter? *Can J Surg.* 1991;34:243–246.

24. Dunn DA, Downs AR, Lye CR. Aortoiliac reconstruction for occlusive disease: comparison of end-to-end and end-to-side proximal anastomoses. *Can J Surg.* 1982;25:382–384.
25. Melliere D, Labastie J, Becquemin J-P, et al. Proximal anastomosis in aortobifemoral bypass: end-to-end or end-to-side? *J Cardiovasc Surg.* 1990;31:77–80.
26. Bernhard VM, Ray LI, Militello JP. The role of angioplasty in the profunda femoris artery in revascularization of the ischemic limb. *Surg Gynecol Obstet.* 1976;142:840–844.
27. Malone JM, Goldstone J, Moore WS. Autogenous profundaplasty: the key to long-term patency in secondary repair of aortofemoral graft occlusion. *Ann Surg.* 1978;188:817–823.
28. Brewster DC, Perler BA, Robison JG, Darling RC. Aortofemoral graft for multilevel occlusive disease: predictors of success and need for distal bypass. *Arch Surg.* 1982;117:1593–1600.
29. Martinez BD, Hertzer NR, Beven EG. Influence of distal arterial occlusive disease on prognosis following aortobifemoral bypass. *Surgery.* 1980;88:795–805.
30. Hill DA, McGrath MA, Lord RSA, et al. The effect of superficial femoral artery occlusion on the outcome of aortofemoral bypass for intermittent claudication. *Surgery.* 1980;87:133–136.
31. Berguer R, Higgins RF, Cotton LT. Geometry, blood flow, and reconstruction of the deep femoral artery. *Am J Surg.* 1975;130:68–73.
32. Dalman RL, Taylor LM Jr, Moneta GL, et al. Simultaneous operative repair of multilevel lower extremity occlusive disease. *J Vasc Surg.* 1991;13:211–221.
33. Nunn DB, Carter MM, Donahue MT, et al. Postoperative dilation of knitted Dacron aortic bifurcation graft. *J Vasc Surg.* 1990;12:291–297.
34. Sicard GA, Reilly JM, Rubin BG, et al. Transabdominal versus retroperitoneal incision for abdominal aortic surgery: report of a prospective randomized trial. *J Vasc Surg.* 1995;21: 174–183.
35. Cambria RP, Brewster DC, Abbott WM, et al. Transperitoneal versus retroperitoneal approach for aortic reconstruction: a randomized prospective study. *J Vasc Surg.* 1990;11:314–325.
36. Shepard AD, Tollefson DFJ, Reddy DJ, et al. Left flank retroperitoneal exposure: a technical aid to complex aortic reconstruction. *J Vasc Surg.* 1991;14:283–291.
37. Rutherford RB, Patt A, Pearce WH. Extra-anatomic bypass: a closer view. *J Vasc Surg.* 1987;6:437–446.
38. Piotrowski JJ, Pearce WH, Jones DN, et al. Aortobifemoral bypass: the operation of choice for unilateral iliac occlusion? *J Vasc Surg.* 1988;8:211–218.
39. Harrington ME, Harrington EB. Options in the management of unilateral iliac occlusive disease. *Semin Vasc Surg.* 1994;7:45–53.
40. Passman MA, Taylor LM Jr, Moneta GL, et al. Comparison of axillofemoral and aortofemoral bypass for aortoiliac occlusive disease. *J Vasc Surg.* 1996;23:263–271.
41. Brener BJ, Brief DK, Alpert J, et al. Femorofemoral bypass: a twenty-five year experience. In: Yao JST, Pearce WH, eds. *Long-Term Results in Vascular Surgery.* East Norwalk, CT: Appleton & Lange; 1993:385–393.
42. Kalman PG, Hosang M, Johnston KW, Walker PM. The current role for femorofemoral bypass. *J Vasc Surg.* 1987;6:71–76.
43. Harrington ME, Harrington EB, Haimov M, et al. Iliofemoral versus femorofemoral bypass: the case for an individualized approach. *J Vasc Surg.* 1992;16:841–854.
44. Kalman PG, Hosang M, Johnston KW, Walker PM. Unilateral iliac disease: the role of iliofemoral bypass. *J Vasc Surg.* 1987;6:139–143.
45. Perler BA, Burdick JF, Williams GM. Femoro-femoral or iliofemoral bypass for unilateral iliac reconstruction. *Am J Surg.* 1991;161:426–430.
46. Ng RLH, Gillies TE, Davies AH, et al. Iliofemoral versus femorofemoral bypass: a 6-year audit. *Br J Surg.* 1992;79:1011–1013.
47. Association Universitaire de Recherche en Chirugie, Ricco J-B. Unilateral iliac artery occlusive disease: a randomized multicenter trial examining direct revascularization versus crossover bypass. *Ann Vasc Surg.* 1992;6:209–219.
48. Schneider JR, Besso SR, Walsh DB, et al. Femorofemoral versus aortobifemoral bypass: outcome and hemodynamic results. *J Vasc Surg.* 1994;19:43–57.
49. El-Massry S, Saad E, Sauvage LR, et al. Axillofemoral bypass with externally supported, knitted Dacron grafts: a follow-up through twelve years. *J Vasc Surg.* 1993;17:107–115.

50. Wittens CHA, Van Houtte HJKP, Van Urk H. European prospective randomized multicentre axillobifemoral trial. *Eur J Vasc Surg.* 1992;6:115–123.
51. Johnston KW, Rae H, Hoss-Johnston SA, et al. Five-year results of a prospective study of percutaneous transluminal angioplasty. *Ann Surg.* 1987;206:404–413.
52. Johnston KW. Iliac arteries: reanalysis of results of balloon angioplasty. *Intervent Radiol.* 1993;186:207–212.
53. Wilson SE, Wolf GL, Cross AP. Percutaneous transluminal angioplasty versus operation for peripheral arteriosclerosis: report of a prospective randomized trial in a selected group of patients. *J Vasc Surg.* 1989;9:1–9.
54. Holm J, Arfvidsson B, Jivegad L, et al. Chronic lower limb ischemia. A prospective randomized controlled study comparing the 1-year results of vascular surgery and percutaneous transluminal angioplasty (PTA). *Eur J Vasc Surg.* 1991;5:517–522.
55. Brewster DC, Cambria RP, Darling RC, et al. Long-term results of combined iliac balloon angioplasty and distal surgical revascularization. *Ann Surg.* 1989;210:324–331.
56. Brewster DC. The role of angioplasty to improve inflow for infrainguinal bypasses. *Eur J Vasc Surg.* 1995;9:262–266.
57. Becker GJ. Intravascular stents: general principles and status of lower extremity arterial applications. *Circulation.* 1991;83(Suppl I)I22–I36.
58. Richter GM, Roeren T, Brado M, Noeldge G. Further update of the randomized trial: iliac stent placement versus PTA-morphology, clinical success rates, and failure analysis. *JVIR.* 1993;4:30.
59. Marin ML, Veith FJ, Cynamon J, et al. Initial experience with transluminally placed endovascular grafts for the treatment of complex vascular lesions. *Ann Surg.* 1995;222:449–469.
60. Marin ML, Veith FJ, Sanchez LA, et al. Endovascular aortoiliac grafts in combination with standard infrainguinal arterial bypasses in the management of limb-threatening ischemia: preliminary report. *J Vasc Surg.* 1995;22:316–324.
61. Rutherford RB. Choosing between options for aortoiliac disease: a management algorithm. *Semin Vasc Surg.* 1994;7:60–63.

19

Management Options for Atheroembolization

Richard R. Keen, MD and James S. T. Yao, MD, PhD

Atheroembolization, the proximal to distal movement of arterial wall plaque and thrombus within the arterial circulation, is one of the most challenging clinical problems encountered in the care of patients with peripheral vascular disease.[1] Spontaneous atheroembolization can be very difficult to diagnose early in its course unless the clinician has a high index of suspicion. The primary physician often fails to recognize the protean or even paradoxical characteristics of atheroemboli in these patients. The skin discoloration of livedo reticularis can be subtle (Fig. 19–1). The discordant physical findings of strongly palpable pedal pulses immediately proximal to seemingly ischemic digits usually are not reconcilable except to the physician who entertains the diagnosis of atheroemboli (see Fig. 19–1). The result of the failure to recognize these often subtle clues is a pathologic condition the diagnosis of which is often delayed. This delay in the diagnosis of distal atheroembolic events from proximal arterial sources can result in repeated embolic episodes and severe, irreversible ischemia.[2,3] The eventual outcome of untreated atheroembolization is loss of visceral organ function, extremity amputation, or both, depending on the location of the proximal arterial source and the target vessels in which the atheroemboli lodge.[4]

Vascular operations[5] and interventional procedures performed by the vascular specialist[6,7] can also trigger massive atheroembolization. The initial personal satisfaction that accompanies the completion of a vascular operation or endovascular procedure can be overshadowed very quickly by the necessity of treating the unexpected catastrophe of massive atheroembolization.[8,9] A greater number of atheroembolic complications appear to follow endovascular operations, with one study reporting a 27% incidence of atheroemboli during endovascular aortic graft placement.[10] The growth in the number of endovascular procedures probably has resulted in an increase in both the true incidence of atheroembolization[11] and in the recognition of this clinical entity.

This chapter discusses the natural history of atheroembolization and the physical findings characteristic of microemboli and macroemboli. Our experience with the imaging techniques that are safest and most efficient for localizing the source of atheroemboli and the methods available for treating the ischemic complications of atheroembolization are reported. The operative procedures and endovascular interventions that can be used to treat the source of the atheroemboli are discussed. Finally, techniques

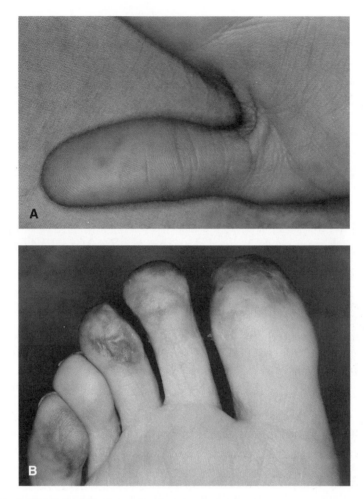

Figure 19–1. (A) Livedo reticularis in a 34-year-old woman with microemboli to her left thumb from her subclavian artery. **(B)** Blue toes caused by shaggy aorta syndrome.

we have found useful in decreasing the incidence of iatrogenic atheroembolization are reviewed.

NATURAL HISTORY

Untreated spontaneous atheroembolization and untreated iatrogenic atheroemboliza-tion have poor outcomes because of the high incidence of recurrent embolization that takes place if the source is not treated promptly.[2,4,12] The first suggested association between a severely diseased thoracic or abdominal aorta and recurrent, episodic distal embolization was made in 1945 by Flory, the pathologist in 1945.[13] While performing autopsy studies, Flory recorded evidence of massive, repeated embolic events that eventually caused multiple organ failure, muscle necrosis, and death. The first large series documenting recurrent atheroembolic events was made by Karmody in 1976, when he described the blue toe syndrome in 31 patients with lower extremity ischemia secondary to atheroemboli originating from an ulcerated aortic or superficial femoral artery lesion. Among five patients who did not undergo an operation to treat the superficial femoral artery lesion, four of five patients (80%) had recurrent embolic events and three of five patients (60%) lost a limb.[2] In 1979, Kempczinski described repeated atheroembolic events in four patients with emboli originating from aortic pathology. Persistent atheroembolization occurred despite treatment with aspirin or warfarin.[3] Hollier et al.[12] observed that the 5-year survival was less than 10% in patients with an aortic source of atheroembolization who did not undergo operative treatment. The poor outcome observed in untreated atheroembolization makes the early diagnosis of atheroembolization as the cause of either extremity ischemia or visceral organ dysfunction essential for its successful management and optimal outcomes.

Physical Findings

Atheroemboli can vary in size from as small as 100 μm (microemboli) to as large as 1 cm (macroemboli). The symptoms experienced by the patient and the physical findings observed by the physician vary depending on the size of the emboli. A single patient can experience a combination of both micro- and macroembolization.[4] The diagnosis of either type of atheroembolization can be missed if the clinician does not have a high index of suspicion.

Macroscopic atheroemboli present as acute arterial occlusions. In this setting of acute limb ischemia, the diagnosis of macroembolization *per se* is not as difficult as the recognition that the source of the embolus is not cardiac, but rather a proximal large artery. In cases of acute arterial occlusion, atheroembolization should be suspected and the search for a proximal arterial source for emboli should be initiated when atrial fibrillation is absent and when the transthoracic echocardiogram is without evidence of valvular abnormalities. Transesophageal echocardiography (TEE) can be helpful not only in ruling out evidence of atrial or ventricular mural thrombus but also in the diagnosis of a shaggy thoracic aorta as the source of atheroemboli.[14]

The diagnosis of atheroembolization due to microscopic emboli to an extremity is dependent on recognizing its characteristic physical appearance. Microemboli are made up of cholesterol crystals, fibrinoplatelet aggregates, or thrombus. These microemboli occlude terminal arterioles in digits and subcutaneous tissues, resulting in focal areas of dermal cyanosis and ischemia. This violaceous skin discoloration is called *livedo*, derived from the Latin root meaning "black and blue." The smallest microemboli cause areas of poorly perfused skin to be intermixed with areas of normal dermal perfusion. These focal areas of cyanosis and capillary dilation appear either as a weblike network of erythema (livedo reticularis) or as scattered purplish discoloration (blue toe syndrome). Livedo reticularis is a pathognomonic sign of diffuse microembolization.

Microscopic atheroemboli usually cause an exquisite tenderness and pain in the region that sustains an embolic shower. Tenderness occurs because of a localized inflammatory response. Cholesterol crystals that lodge in small arterioles trigger a focal vasculitis, characterized by foreign body giant cells, granulocyte infiltration, and necrotizing angiitis.[15,16] Because this tenderness suggests an inflammatory condition, the blue toes and livedo reticularis due to emboli can be misdiagnosed as a dermatitis or a primary vasculitis.

Digital pressures and Doppler waveforms obtained in the noninvasive vascular lab also can be useful in determining that ischemia is the cause of tender, discolored digits as opposed to other causes of livedo. When encountering blue, ischemic digits in the setting of palpable pedal or wrist pulses, the findings of tender and painful digits or the lack thereof can help the clinician confirm or exclude the diagnosis of microembolization. For example, the blue toes in diabetic or nondiabetic patients with chronic digital ischemia usually are not tender. The only common exception is in the setting of localized infection. A skin biopsy may provide a definitive diagnosis of cholesterol microembolization.[17]

Aortic aneurysms[18] and aneurysms of larger arteries such as the subclavian, femoral, and popliteal arteries can manifest themselves with distal embolization. Although abdominal aortic aneurysms that embolize appear to present most commonly with symptomatic microembolization, subclavian and popliteal aneurysms that embolize seem to present with more occult symptoms.[19] It is not unusual for patients with subclavian[20] or popliteal artery aneurysms[21] to present with nearly complete obliteration of the distal arterial circulation and an otherwise unremarkable history and paucity of physical findings other than the aneurysm and profound distal ischemia. One possible explanation for the lack of hyperesthesia and tenderness in patients with peripheral aneurysms may be the difference in the nature of the emboli that originate in peripheral and aortic sources. The embolic debris that originates from aortic sources is more commonly cholesterol. The luminal thrombus that embolizes from extremity aneurysms does not appear to promote the same type of vasculitic response that is seen with the cholesterol embolization from aortic sources.

NORTHWESTERN UNIVERSITY EXPERIENCE WITH ATHEROEMBOLIZATION

We have reported our experience in more than 100 patients with atheroemboli.[4]

Demographics

Our population of 141 patients with atheroemboli had a mean age of 62 years and ranged from 32 to 90 years in age. Our patients were 70% men and 30% women. Risk factors for atheroemboli did not appear to differ from those for vascular disease in general: 74% of patients were smokers, 46% were hypertensive, and 22% were diabetics.

Types of Emboli

Microemboli were more common than macroemboli. Microemboli alone were seen in 45% of patients, whereas macroemboli, defined as emboli large enough to occlude named extremity arteries, occurred in 39% of patients. A combination of macro- and microemboli occurred in 16% of patients.

Targets of Embolization

The lower extremities were the most common targets of atheroemboli. Renal atheroemboli occurred in 11% of patients. Renal biopsy and eosinophilia may help differentiate renal failure due to myoglobinuria from that induced by atheroemboli.[22]

Sources of Atheroemboli

The abdominal aorta was the most common source of atheroemboli. Among 107 patients with extremity or visceral atheroemboli, aortoiliac occlusive disease was responsible in 56 patients (52%). Small aortic aneurysms caused embolization in 21 patients (20%). Femoral artery stenoses, the cause of the classic "blue toe syndrome," were responsible for only 11% of atheroembolic events. Since the time of our original study, we have noticed that in black patients a higher percentage of atheroembolic events, approximating 30%, originate from femoral and popliteal artery stenoses. This demographic variable may explain the discrepancy between our data from Northwestern and that reported by others, including Fisher et al.[23] and Karmody et al.,[2] both of whom reported that femoral artery pathology was responsible for 23 of 31 (74%) of all atheroembolic events. When one includes shaggy thoracoabdominal aorta (8%) and degenerating bypass grafts (7%), we found that atherosclerotic disease proximal to the inguinal ligament accounted for more than 80% of all atheroembolization. Because many current vascular imaging techniques suitable for evaluating the thoracic and abdominal aorta [such as computed tomography (CT), magnetic resonance imaging (MRI), and TEE] were not available at the time of these other studies, the true frequency of aortic pathology as the source of atheroembolization was probably underreported in previous studies.

Only small aortic aneurysms appear to embolize. The mean diameter of 21 infrarenal aneurysms that embolized was 3.5 cm.[4] The increased blood flow velocity seen in small versus large aortic aneurysms appears to increase the incidence of embolic events in the abdominal aorta, just as an increased flow velocity increases the incidence of embolic events in the carotid distribution.

Upper extremity sources and targets of atheroembolization are much less frequent. Thirty of our 141 patients had atheroembolism due to subclavian, axillary, or brachial artery pathology. The thoracic outlet syndrome was responsible for about 50% of the upper extremity atheroemboli.[4] As many as 70% of upper extremity aneurysms present with atheroembolization.[20]

Imaging Techniques to Identify the Embolic Source

The initial extremity pulse examination guides the strategy for performing diagnostic imaging tests to localize the source of emboli. All patients presenting with a new pulse deficit should undergo two-dimensional echocardiography to rule out a cardiac source of the macroembolus because the heart remains the source for the majority of all macroemboli. The first localizing test for patients who present with a new pulse deficit and have an echocardiogram that is negative for a source of emboli is an aortic angiogram with extremity run-off. The majority of all patients with atheroembolization (55%) present with a pulse deficit. We used arteriography as a localizing test in more than 80% of our patients, making arteriography the most common test performed to localize the atheroembolic source. Arteriography has the advantage of both localizing the responsible arterial source and providing anatomic detail of the distal arterial circulation such that appropriate intervention can be initiated to treat the ischemic extremity.

The strategy for localizing the atheroembolic source in the minority of patients who present with microemboli alone (intact extremity pulses) is different from the strategy used when a pulse deficit is found. Because the axial arterial circulation is patent, there is no longer a need for arteriography to obtain a map of the extremity run-off. Because the most frequent source of microemboli is the abdominal or thoracic aorta, the best diagnostic test would be noninvasive but still provide enough detail of the aortic luminal surface to permit recognition of an atheroembolic source.

For these reasons, contrast-enhanced CT of the abdominal and thoracic aorta should be the first localizing test performed in patients with the stigmata of microemboli (blue toes or livedo reticularis) and intact extremity pulses. CT provides excellent detail of the aortic luminal thrombus. The characteristic appearance of lesions that undergo atheroembolization can be recognized with CT, and CT imaging can diagnose a small aortic aneurysm, aortoiliac occlusive disease, a shaggy thoracic aorta, or an aortic ulcer.[24] Intravenous iodinated contrast medium is essential to delineate the blood–aortic lumen interface. Obtaining an optimally timed CT scan that provides adequate detail of both the thoracic and abdominal aortas with a single contrast injection is difficult, so we perform separate contrast bolus injections for the thoracic and abdominal aortas in order to obtain sufficient detail of both regions. The characteristic image on CT scan in patients with atheroembolization from an aortic source is an irregular or star-shaped thrombus within the aortic lumen (Fig. 19–2).

Contrast-enhanced CT usually is the only test performed prior to treating the embolic source in many patients with microemboli. Two-dimensional echocardiography is not helpful in localizing the source of microemboli because the microemboli that

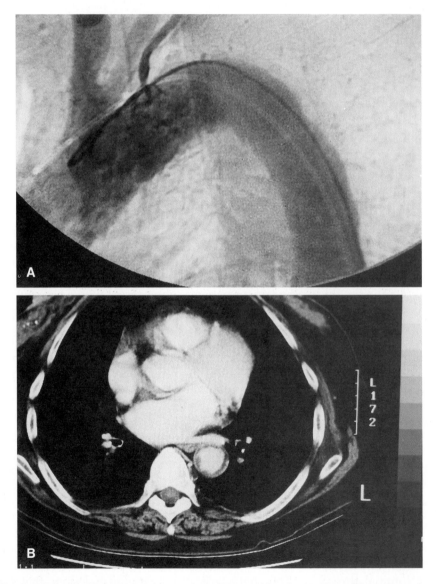

Figure 19–2. (A) Thoracic arteriogram in a 67-year-old patient with a diffuse visceral and lower extremity microembolization demonstrates an irregular luminal surface. **(B)** Computed tomography (CT) image of the thoracic aorta in the same patient also demonstrates a "shaggy aorta."

cause blue toes or livedo reticularis are not known to originate in the heart. Echocardiography is probably helpful only in assessing cardiac function in this group of patients.

In patients with microembolization alone, arteriography usually is unnecessary and often dangerous. Contrast-enhanced CT of the aorta can delineate the blood–thrombus interface just as well as thoracic or abdominal aortography without provoking an additional atheroembolic shower that arterial catheterization could produce. For patients with a shaggy aorta or a small aortic aneurysm that is lined with thrombus, the risk of the catheter acting as a "Roto-Rooter" and inducing an embolic shower is real.[6] In our study of atheroembolization, arteriography triggered the initial atheroembolic event in 17% of patients.[4] Arteriography can be undertaken if CT imaging is inconclusive or nondiagnostic. There may be no safe arteriographic approach for patients who present with microembolization. For patients with bilateral lower extremity microembolization in whom arteriography truly is required, an axillary as opposed to a femoral access is probably safer.

TEE and MRI of the thoracic aorta can be important localizing tests[1,14] that are especially helpful in patients with renal insufficiency because nephrotoxic contrast is not required for adequate imaging.

Duplex ultrasonography can be useful in confirming accelerated luminal velocities in stenosed peripheral vessels, in defining ulcerated plaques with thrombus, and in diagnosing extremity aneurysms with intraluminal thrombus. We have found duplex scanning to be very helpful for localizing or confirming femoral and popliteal artery pathology. Duplex scanning has limited utility in localizing subclavian aneurysms or iliac stenoses as embolic sources because of technical difficulties in performing duplex imaging of intrathoracic and pelvic arteries.

MANAGEMENT OPTIONS IN ATHEROEMBOLIZATION

Nonoperative Treatment

Patients with atheroembolization may experience tremendous morbidity if they do not undergo an operative intervention directed at the embolic source. Excessive rates of limb loss, renal failure, and death have been reported in small but consistent natural history studies performed by Karmody and associates,[2] Kempczinski,[3] and Hollier and associates.[12] Although this patient group sometimes appears to manifest enough comorbidities to make even the most aggressive vascular specialist proceed with trepidation, the vascular surgeon must remember that untreated atheroembolism engenders a uniformly worse prognosis.

The management of atheroembolization includes the methods and procedures useful in treating extremity ischemia secondary to the emboli and the operations and interventions that are available for the definitive treatment of the embolic source. The procedures utilized for the management of severe extremity ischemia are those of standard practice and include anticoagulation with intravenous heparin. Our experience with heparin has been that it does not appear to initiate or trigger further atheroembolization, so it can be used to prevent thrombus propagation and improve extremity perfusion. These findings with heparin differ markedly from our experience[4] and that of others[25,26] with warfarin, which has been shown to be a causative agent in atheroembolization. Because of our favorable outcomes using intravenous heparin, we have begun to use low molecular weight heparin in outpatients with atheroembolization whose operation for treating an atheroembolic source needs to be postponed. We only use warfarin with caution in these patients when anticoagulation with warfarin is mandated by a separate medical condition.

Thrombolytic Therapy

Following diagnostic arteriography in patients with macroemboli, thrombolytic therapy should be considered as a first-line treatment, as it would be in any other patient with an acute arterial occlusion. The role for thrombolytic therapy in the initial management of acute arterial occlusions secondary to macroemboli is probably no different than its role in the care of any other patient with acute limb ischemia, but an increased risk of iatrogenic complications should be entertained. Thrombolytic therapy can provoke atheroembolization both with arterial catheterization[27] and without.[28]

Thrombolytic agents do not dissolve atherosclerotic plaque or microscopic cholesterol crystals, so the role of thrombolytic therapy in the management of microembolization is limited to cases in which the embolic debris is thrombus. Indeed, thrombolytic therapy has been shown to be beneficial in the management of extremity ischemia caused by emboli from subclavian (Fig. 19–3) and popliteal artery aneurysms,[21] in which the embolic material is predominantly thrombus.

Percutaneous Interventions

The success of percutaneous transluminal angioplasty (PTA) in the management of atherosclerotic lesions in the iliac arteries has made it the preferred approach for treating focal arterial occlusive disease in this location. PTA with stent placement can be considered in selected patients with focal iliac artery ulcerated plaques that are the source of atheroemboli. We have used PTA and stent placement for the treatment of atheroembolic iliac artery lesions in sexually active men with emboli originating from ulcerated plaques in the left common iliac artery (Fig. 19–4). This approach using PTA markedly diminishes the risk of sexual dysfunction in male patients that accompanies open operative iliac artery endarterectomy. Compared to operative iliac artery endartectomy and patching, the complication rate in iliac artery PTA and stenting, including iliac artery rupture, dissection, and distal embolization, is higher.[4,29] A primary patency rate for iliac artery stenting of only 61% at 18 months and 55% at 24 months,[29] combined with the risk of embolization with stenting and the excellent results with iliac artery endarterectomy, dissuades us from using PTA and stents as the primary treatment in other patient groups with iliac artery atheroembolism.

The superficial femoral and above-the-knee popliteal arteries are other frequent locations for atheroembolic disease that tempt percutaneous interventionalists. However, the increased risk of triggering further embolization by passing guidewires and balloons over unstable plaques and thrombus in small caliber arteries is real, as was demonstrated in trials of carotid artery PTA and stent placement.[30] The long-term results of percutaneous angioplasty and stent placement for atheroembolic disease in the superficial femoral artery has yet to be determined. One report documented a 1-year primary patency rate of 22% when PTA and stents were used in the primary treatment of long segment superficial femoral artery disease.[31] However, we observed no early failures with superficial femoral and popliteal artery endarterectomy performed for atheroembolism.[4] These data suggest that the results of PTA and stenting for superficial femoral artery atheroembolism will probably be found to be markedly inferior to those results obtained with operative endarterectomy and patch angioplasty. It may be difficult to justify the use of PTA and stenting for superficial femoral artery atheroembolism outside the setting of a clinical trial.

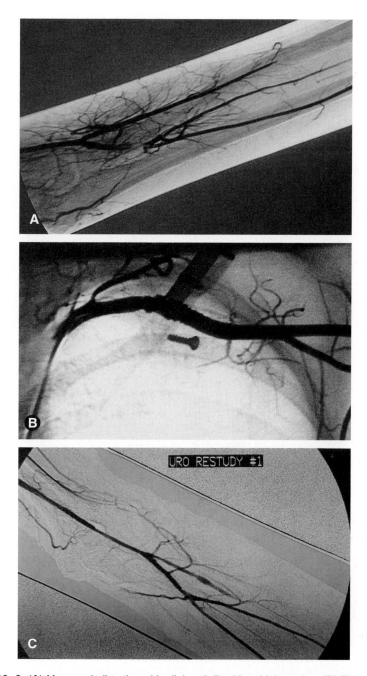

Figure 19–3. (A) Macroemboli to the midradial and distal brachial arteries. **(B)** The source of macroemboli is the left subclavian artery. **(C)** Successful thrombolysis of the embolus to the left brachial artery. The radial artery did not reopen with thrombolytic therapy.

Operative Management

The surgical options for treating atheroembolic sources include direct endarterectomy and patch of the artery, replacement of the artery with an autogenous or prosthetic bypass graft, and extra anatomic reconstruction with exclusion of the proximal source of emboli.[32]

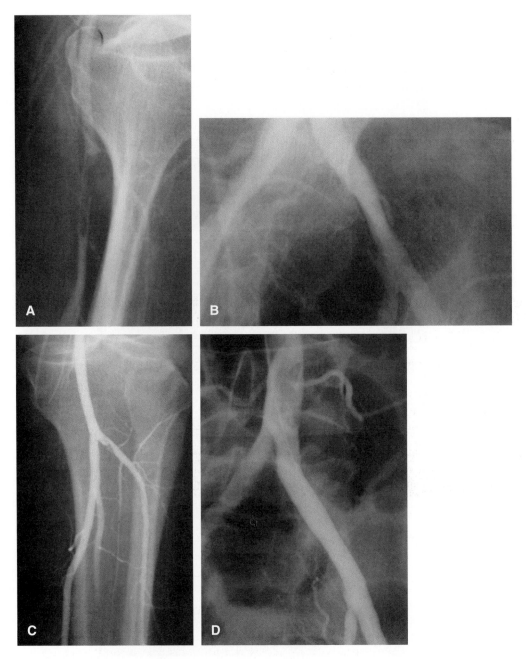

Figure 19–4. (A) Macroembolus to the below-the-knee popliteal artery. **(B)** The macroembolus originated from an ulcerated plaque in the left common iliac artery. **(C)** Successful treatment of the popliteal artery occlusion with thrombolytic therapy. **(D)** Percutaneous transluminal angioplasty (PTA) and stenting of the source of macroemboli in the left common iliac artery.

We reported our series of 141 patients with visceral, upper extremity, or lower extremity atheroemboli.[4,19] Only 25 patients did not undergo an operation, either because of medical unfitness or patient refusal. Among the remaining 116 patients who received operations, 86 patients had operations or visceral or lower extremity atheroemboli and 30 patients had operations for upper extremity atheroemboli. Arterial complications of the thoracic outlet syndrome causing emboli in 16 patients were reported separately.[19] Our study focused on 100 remaining patients who underwent operations to treat an atheroembolic source.

Aortic operations were the most common type performed. Among the 63 patients who underwent operations on the abdominal aorta or iliac arteries, aortofemoral bypass was performed in 26 patients, aortoiliac bypass was performed in 10 patients, aortic tube grafts were placed in 16 patients, and endartectomy and patch of the aorta was undertaken in 5 patients. Iliac artery endarterectomy and patch was performed in 6 patients.

We observed that three distinct patterns of aortoiliac disease were responsible for atheroemboli: (1) aortoiliac occlusive disease; (2) small aortic aneurysms with basically normal iliac arteries; and (3) small aortic aneurysms accompanied by iliac artery occlusive disease. Aortoiliac occlusive disease was the most common. Neither large aortic aneurysms nor iliac artery aneurysms were found to be associated with atheroembolization. Perhaps in these latter two types of aortic disease, the significantly decreased intra-arterial blood flow velocity that results from a markedly increased aortic or iliac artery diameter does not generate sufficient kinetic energy to dislodge luminal thrombus. A narrower arterial diameter has been shown to be clearly associated with an increased risk of atheroemboli within the carotid circulation. Hollier and coworkers[12] were able to demonstrate that by decreasing the mean aortic blood flow velocity with axillofemoral bypass, atheroembolism from shaggy aortas ceased. This finding suggests that changes in the intra-arterial blood flow velocity and shear stress, in addition to the nature and stability of the plaque, are important factors that influence the incidence of atheroembolization.

Extra-anatomic reconstructions, including both axillofemoral bypass and cross-femoral bypass, were performed in six patients. Infrainguinal arterial reconstructions (including common femoral, superficial femoral, and popliteal arteries), endarterectomy and patch, and femoropopliteal and femorotibeal artery bypasses were completed in 17 patients (17%). Overall, local endarterectomy with patch was performed in 22 patients (22%) and bypass grafts were placed in 78 patients (78%).

Operative treatment resulted in a 30-day mortality of 4%. All of the mortality occurred in patients undergoing operations for aortic disease, with no mortality or significant morbidity in the 31 patients with extremity operations. Cumulative survival probabilities were 89% at 1 year and 73% at 5 years. Careful review of the thoracic and abdominal CT scans of 7 patients who died within 6 months of their operation revealed that recurrent embolization was possible from residual suprarenal aortic thrombus that had not been removed at the time of the initial operation. In retrospect, 12 patients had residual suprarenal aortic thrombus and 5 patients sustained recurrences from this untreated disease. The time of the recurrence was between 1 and 8 months following the operation, and 4 of the 5 patients were taking warfarin at the time of the recurrent event. Only 1 of 82 patients not taking warfarin sustained a recurrent atheroembolic episode. Thus, the failure to completely eliminate suprarenal aortic thrombus and postoperative warfarin treatment appear to be significant risk factors for recurrent atheroembolism. In terms of managing these patients with extensive aortic thrombus, complete removal of all aortic thrombus, if practical, appears to be the best option. Extra-anatomic reconstruction is an additional option and is superior to nonoperative treatment with warfarin anticoagulation. Visceral atheroembolization contributed to 6 of the 7 mortalities that occurred within 6 months, and led to temporary or permanent hemodialysis in 10 of 11 patients who sustained renal atheroemboli.

There is significant risk of intraoperative embolization to the viscera, trunk, or extremities in operations performed for atheroemboli of the abdominal aorta. In our series, 7 of 63 patients (11%) who underwent aortoiliac reconstructions experienced intraoperative atheroembolic events, despite the knowledge that the indication for operative intervention was atheroembolization. This high rate of intraoperative embolization draws attention to the fact that vascular procedures can easily turn arterial wall atheroemboli *in situ* into distal emboli if certain precautions are not observed.

Intraoperative embolization from the aorta can occur during mobilization and manipulation of the aorta, and the initial placement and subsequent release of the proximal aortic clamp.[5] To minimize the chances of embolization occurring during the dissection, control of the arteries can be obtained without encircling them with vascular loops. In addition, the distal aorta or iliac arteries should be clamped prior to clamping the proximal aorta. If thrombus is noted on CT to extend up to or proximal to the renal arteries, the renal arteries should be temporarily occluded prior to proximal aortic clamping.[33] In order to decrease the attendant morbidity of any proximal or distal atherosclerotic debris that may have become dislodged during clamping for the operative repair, all clamped arteries should be flushed or irrigated with heparinized saline prior to restoring arterial flow. At the time of unclamping, an attempt should be made to direct the initial arterial flow into the hypogastric circulation. If the external and internal iliac arteries are not clamped separately, the hands of an assistant can be applied with force to both groins directly over the common femoral arteries, acting to temporarily occlude these arteries and direct blood flow down the hypogastric arteries.

In our series, postoperative leg amputations were required in 9 patients and toe amputations were performed in an additional 10 patients. Healing of distal gangrenous lesions that are due to atheroemboli can be very difficult. We have used Silvadene as a topical agent. Lumbar sympathectomy has been proposed as an additional technique that may improve distal perfusion and enhance healing in these patients.[3,34]

COMMENT

Operations for atheroembolization should be performed in the majority of patients with this challenging problem. An overall low morbidity and mortality can be expected if the characteristics of atheroembolism are recognized and the diagnosis is made early in its course. The embolic source needs to be localized promptly but carefully, and the operative strategy is directed at eliminating or excluding the source of the emboli.

REFERENCES

1. Keen RR, Yao JST. Experience in the management of atherosclerotic emboli. In: Yao JST, Pearce WH, eds. *The Ischemic Extremity*. Norwalk CT: Appleton & Lange; 1995:313–323.
2. Karmody AM, Powers SR, Monaco VJ, et al. "Blue-toe" syndrome: an indication for limb salvage surgery. *Arch Surg.* 1976;3:1263–1268.
3. Kempczinski RF. Lower-extremity arterial emboli from ulcerating atherosclerotic plaques. *JAMA.* 1979;241:800–810.
4. Keen RR, McCarthy WJ, Pearce WH, et al. Surgical management of atheroembolization. *J Vasc Surg.* 1995;21:773–781.

5. Keen RR, Yao JST. Aneurysms and embolization: detection and management. In: Yao JST, Pearce WH, eds. *Aneurysms: New Findings and Treatments.* Norwalk CT: Appleton & Lange; 1994:305–313.

6. Gaines PA, Kennedy A, Moorehead P, et al. Cholesterol embolization: a lethal complication of vascular catheterization. *Lancet.* 1988;1:168–170.

7. Karalis DG, Quinn V, Victor MF, et al. Risk of catheter-related emboli in patients with atherosclerotic debris in the thoracic aorta. *Am Heart J.* 1996;131:1149–1155.

8. Keen RR, Yao JST. Atheroembolism—diagnosis and management of the blue toe syndrome. In: Perler BA, Becker GJ, eds. *A Clinical Approach to Vascular Intervention.* New York: Theime; 1998:203–210.

9. Parodi JC. Endovascular repair of abdominal aortic aneurysms and other arterial lesions. *J Vasc Surg.* 1995;21:549–555.

10. Marin ML, Veith FJ, Cynamon J, et al. Initial experience with transluminally placed endovascular grafts for the treatment of complex vascular lesions. *Ann Surg.* 1995;222:449–469.

11. Thompson MM, Smith J, Naylor AR, et al. Microembolization during endovascular and conventional aneurysm repair. *J Vasc Surg.* 1997;25:179–186.

12. Hollier LH, Kazmier FJ, Ochsner J, et al. "Shaggy" aorta syndrome with atheromatous embolization to visceral vessels. *Ann Vasc Surg.* 1991;5:439–444.

13. Flory CM. Arterial occlusions produced by emboli from eroded aortic atheromatous plaques. *Am J Pathol.* 1945;21:549–565.

14. Wiet SP, Pearce WH, McCarthy WJ, et al. Utility of transesophageal echocardiography in the diagnosis of disease of the thoracic aorta. *Vasc Surg.* 1994;20:613–620.

15. Richards AM, Elliot RS, Kanjuh VI, et al. Cholesterol embolism: a multiple disease masquerading as polyarteritis nodosa. *Am J Cardiol.* 1965;5:696–707.

16. Cappiello RA, Espinoza LR, Adelman H, et al. Cholesterol embolism: a pseudovasculitic syndrome. *Semin Arthritis Rheum.* 1989;18:240–246.

17. Dahlberg PJ, Frecentese DF, Gogbill TH. Cholesterol embolism: experience with 22 histologically proven cases. *Surgery.* 1989;105:737–746.

18. Baxter BT, McGee GS, Flinn WR, et al. Distal embolization as a presenting symptom of aortic aneurysms. *Am J Surg.* 1990;160:197–201.

19. Durham JR, Yao JST, Pearce WH, et al. Arterial injuries in the thoracic outlet syndrome. *J Vasc Surg.* 1995;21:57–70.

20. Mesh CL, Yao JST. Upper extremity bypass: five-year follow-up. In: Yao JST, Pearce WH, eds. *Long-Term Results in Vascular Surgery.* Norwalk CT: Appleton & Lange; 1993:353–365.

21. Giddings AEB. Influence of thrombolytic therapy in the management of popliteal aneurysms. In: Yao JST, Pearce WH, eds. *Aneurysms: New Findings and Treatments.* Norwalk CT: Appleton & Lange; 1994:493–508.

22. Kasinath BSM, Corwin HL, Bidani AK, et al. Eosinophilia in the diagnosis of atheroembolic renal disease. *Am J Nephrol.* 1987;7:173–177.

23. Fisher DF Jr, Clagett GP, Brigham RA, et al. Dilemmas in dealing with the blue toe syndrome: aortic versus peripheral source. *Am J Surg.* 1984;148:836–839.

24. Rubin BG, Allen BT, Anderson CB, et al. An embolizing lesion in a minimally diseased aorta. *Surgery.* 1992;112:607–610.

25. Bruns FJ, Segel DP, Adler S. Case report: control of cholesterol embolization by discontinuation of anticoagulant therapy. *Am J Med Sci.* 1978;275:105–108.

26. Hyman BT, Landas SK, Ashman RF, et al. Warfarin-related purple toes syndrome and cholesterol microembolization. *Am J Med.* 1978;82:1233–1237.

27. Bhardwjah M, Goldweit R, Erlebacher J, et al. Tissue plasminogen activator and cholesterol crystal embolization. *Ann Intern Med.* 1989;11:687–688.

28. Pettelot G, Bracco J, Barrillon D, et al. Cholesterol embolization: unrecognized complication of thrombolysis. *Circulation.* 1998;197:1522.

29. Ballard J, Sparks S, Taylor F, et al. Complications of iliac artery stent deployment. *J Vasc Surg.* 1996;24:545–555.

30. Jordan W, Schroeder P, Fisher W, et al. A comparison of angioplasty with stenting versus endarterectomy for the treatment of carotid artery stenosis. *Ann Vasc Surg.* 1997;11:2–8.

31. Gray BH, Sullivan TM, Childs MB, et al. High incidence of restenosis/reocclusion of stents in the percutaneous treatment of long-segment superficial femoral artery disease after suboptimal angioplasty. *J Vasc Surg.* 1997;25:74–83.
32. Kaufman JL, Saifi J, Chang BB, et al. The role of extraanatomic exclusion bypass in the treatment of disseminated atheroembolism syndrome. *Ann Vasc Surg.* 1990;4:260–263.
33. Starr DS, Lawrie GM, Morris GC Jr. Prevention of distal embolism during arterial reconstruction. *Am J Surg.* 1979;138:764–769.
34. Kazmier FJ. Shaggy aorta syndrome and disseminated atheromatous embolization. In: Bergan JJ, Yao JST, eds. *Aortic Surgery.* Philadelphia: WB Saunders; 1989:189–194.

20

Management of Visceral Artery Aneurysm

Sandra C. Carr, MD and William H. Pearce, MD

INTRODUCTION

Aneurysms of the visceral arteries (VAA) are an uncommon but potentially lethal form of vascular disease. These lesions are rare, with an incidence of 0.01% to 0.2% in routine autopsies, but are being diagnosed with increasing frequency in the aging population.[1] The most commonly involved vessels include the splenic, hepatic, superior mesenteric, and celiac arteries in decreasing order of frequency. Although splenic artery aneurysms have been the most common visceral artery aneurysms encountered, hepatic artery aneurysms are being diagnosed and reported with increasing frequency in the more current series.[2] The gastric–gastroepiploic, jejunal–ileal–colic, pancreatoduodenal–pancreatic, gastroduodenal, and inferior mesenteric arteries are less often involved.

The earliest report of a VAA was in 1770 by Beaussier,[3] who first reported a splenic artery aneurysm while injecting the aorta and femoral veins of a 60-year-old female cadaver for anatomic demonstration. In 1834, Jackson[4] first published a case of hemobilia caused by a hepatic artery aneurysm with intrabiliary rupture. In 1871, Quincke[4] described the "classic" triad of abdominal pain, hemobilia, and obstructive jaundice with hepatic artery aneurysm. In 1881, American President James A. Garfield died from a ruptured splenic artery aneurysm 2 months after being shot in the abdomen by an assassin.[5] In 1953, DeBakey and Cooley[6] reported the first successful resection of a superior mesenteric artery aneurysm. Before 1960, only a few reports of VAA with high mortality rates had been published. Over the next few decades, reports of these lesions increased in number. In 1970, Stanley and associates[7] reviewed the literature concerning 1098 visceral artery aneurysms published at that time. Since then, the number of reported cases has increased dramatically, with more than 2400 cases reported in the literature.[8]

In the past, most VAAs were discovered at autopsy, with rupture often being the cause of death. In 1986, Stanley and coworkers[9] noted that nearly 22% of all reported VAAs presented as clinical emergencies, including 8.5% that resulted in death. Today, with the routine use of computed tomography (CT) and angiography, many aneurysms are being discovered in the asymptomatic state. The increasing use of diagnostic and therapeutic percutaneous angiographic and biliary procedures has led to the detection of an increasing number of VAAs. Despite these advances, the majority of VAAs still present with rupture, emphasizing the need for aggressive diagnosis and treatment of these rare vascular lesions.[10]

Although the various types of VAA have many features in common, the etiology, presentation, and natural history of the disease differ. Thus, the splenic, hepatic, superior mesenteric, celiac, gastric–gastroepiploic, jejunal–ilial–colic, pancreatoduodenal–pancreatic–gastroduodenal, and inferior mesenteric artery aneurysms are discussed separately.

SPLENIC ARTERY ANEURYSMS

Traditionally, splenic artery aneurysm (SAA) has been thought to be the most common of VAA (Fig. 20–1). SAA is reported as an incidental finding in 0.78% of arteriograms and can be found in 0.1% to 10.4% of autopsies.[11] SAAs are usually saccular and commonly occur at bifurcations. About 70% of SAAs are solitary, and most of the multiple aneurysms are small and saccular.[12] About 44% are located in the midportion of the artery, whereas approximately 35% are located distally. Most SAAs (72%) are true aneurysms. The mean age of patients with SAA at presentation is 52 years, with a range of 2 to 98 years. SAA occurs more frequently in women (66%) than in men (34%).[2]

Several etiologies for SAA have been proposed. SAA has been associated with multiparity in females. Forty-five percent of female patients with SAA have had six or more pregnancies, 88% have had two or more pregnancies, and 98% have had at least one pregnancy.[5] In a report by Trastek and associates,[13] women who were pregnant at the time of diagnosis of SAA had an average of 4.5 previous pregnancies. The pathogenesis of SAA in pregnant women is thought to depend on hemodynamic and hormonal factors. In addition to the increased blood flow to the spleen during pregnancy, it is

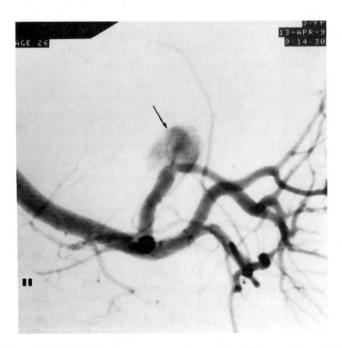

Figure 20–1. Splenic artery aneurysm (*arrow*) in a 26-year-old woman.

possible that estrogen, or the hormone relaxin (which is secreted during the last trimester of pregnancy), has some effect on the elastic support of the arteries.[14] In addition to pregnancy, portal hypertension is another condition associated with the development of SAA. Thirty-four percent of SAA are found in patients with portal hypertension.[2] In patients with portal hypertension being evaluated with angiography, 7% to 20% have been found to have evidence of an SAA.[1,11] The development of SAA in patients with portal hypertension and splenomegaly is thought to be a consequence of a hyperkinetic state in the spleen. These same hemodynamic factors may also account for the increasing recognition of SAA in patients following orthotopic liver transplantation. Fibromuscular dysplasia (FMD) is the etiology in 13% of SAA.[2] Aneurysms of the splenic artery may occur in association with FMD of the renal arteries, with 4% of patients with renal artery FMD having concomitant SAA. Both splenic and intracerebral artery aneurysms are frequent in patients with medial dysplasia.[15] Approximately 10% of SAA are found in patients with pancreatitis.[2] In these patients, an aneurysm may form as a result of the inflammatory process eroding into the adjacent vessel wall. These aneurysms are often located in the pseudocyst wall formed weeks after acute inflammation, or may present as part of chronic pancreatitis.

Most patients with SAA are asymptomatic, but some may have symptoms of vague left upper quadrant or epigastric pain, sometimes with radiation to the left subscapular region. The abdominal pain is worsened with acute expansion or rupture and may be accompanied by hypotension, diaphragmatic irritation, and diaphoresis.[16] Forty-six percent of patients with SAA present with abdominal pain, and 6% complain of back pain.[2] Patients may also present with hypotension or gastrointestinal bleeding. Aneurysm rupture often presents with hemorrhage initially confined to the lesser sac. Exsanguinating hemorrhage follows as blood escapes through the foramen of Winslow into the peritoneal cavity. This "double rupture" phenomenon was first described in 1930 by Brockman.[16] SAA may present with gastrointestinal (GI) hemorrhage after rupture into the GI tract, which occurs in approximately 13% of cases.[2] In patients with pancreatitis, rupture may occur into an adjacent pseudocyst. Rupture can also occur into the pancreatic duct, splenic vein, retroperitoneum, stomach, colon, or pancreas.

The reported risk of rupture of SAA is low in cases not associated with pregnancy. Early reports documented a 10% risk of rupture for SAA, but contemporary reports suggest that rupture rates are closer to 2%.[17] However, the mortality rate associated with aneurysm rupture is significant, 36%.[11] The presence of an SAA in a woman of childbearing age represents a serious and potentially life-threatening condition. Approximately 95% of SAA diagnosed during pregnancy present with rupture, the majority during the last trimester. Rupture during pregnancy is accompanied by a maternal mortality rate of 70% and a fetal death rate of 95%.[9] Treatment of SAA is therefore indicated in pregnant patients or in women of childbearing age who might become pregnant. Treatment is also indicated in patients with symptomatic or enlarging lesions. Aneurysm size greater than 2.5 cm has been considered a relative indication for therapy. There is some evidence that small asymptomatic SAA in older patients may be observed safely.[10]

HEPATIC ARTERY ANEURYSMS

Although splenic artery aneurysms have traditionally been thought to be the most common of the visceral artery aneurysms, hepatic artery aneurysms (HAA) have been more frequently reported. This trend is thought to be partially due to the increasing use of percutaneous diagnostic and therapeutic biliary procedures. During these procedures, injury to the intrahepatic branches of the hepatic artery can result in pseudoaneurysm formation. A second factor that may account for the increasing number of HAA reported may be the increased use of CT scanning following blunt liver trauma, which has led to increased detection of posttraumatic pseudoaneurysms of the intrahepatic arterial branches. Nearly 50% of all HAA reported since the late 1980s are false aneurysms of the intrahepatic portions of the hepatic artery.[11] This is in contrast to the older data, wherein approximately 80% of HAA were extrahepatic in location.[15] More recent data states that approximately 66% of HAA are extrahepatic. The majority of these aneurysms (91%) are solitary. Forty-seven percent are located in the right hepatic artery, 22% in the common hepatic artery, 16% in the proper hepatic artery, and 13% in the left hepatic artery.[2] Rarely, aneurysms may involve the cystic artery. The mean age of patients with HAA is 52 years, with a range from 2 to 93 years.[2]

Although infection was the most common cause of HAA in the past, mycotic aneurysms currently account for only 4% of HAA.[2] Aneurysms of traumatic etiology may be caused by major crush injury, penetrating wound, or as a result of surgery. An increasingly common source of iatrogenic injury is the percutaneous placement of a transhepatic biliary drainage catheter for relief of benign or malignant biliary obstruction. Periarteritis nodosa, FMD, and other arteriopathies have also been known to cause HAA. An increasing number of aneurysms have been discovered following orthotopic liver transplantation. HAA have also been seen following cholecystectomy and acute or chronic pancreatitis.

Patients with HAA may present with right upper quadrant pain or epigastric pain, which sometimes mimics the symptoms of pancreatitis. The pain may radiate to the back or to the right shoulder, and is usually unrelated to meals. Fifty-five percent of patients with HAA present with abdominal pain, and 46% present with GI hemorrhage or hemobilia. Rarely, a large HAA may obstruct the biliary tract, leading to jaundice. The "classic" triad of pain, hemobilia, and obstructive jaundice is seen in only one-third of patients.[4,12]

In up to 80% of patients with HAA, rupture of the aneurysm is the reason for first medical consultation, when patients present with pain or hemorrhage. Rupture of HAA occurs with equal frequency into the peritoneal cavity or into the biliary tract. Rupture may also occur into the duodenum, gallbladder, portal vein, or stomach. The overall mortality of HAA is high, approaching 35%.[9] Because of the tendency of these aneurysms to rupture and cause hemorrhage and because of the high mortality rates associated with rupture, most HAA should be treated aggressively, even if asymptomatic.

SUPERIOR MESENTERIC ARTERY ANEURYSMS

Superior mesenteric artery (SMA) aneurysms are rare, comprising between 5% and 8% of all VAA.[18] These aneurysms may be saccular or fusiform, and are most often located within the first 5 cm of the SMA.[19,20] Sixty-three percent of patients with SMA aneurysms are male, with a mean age of 52 years, and range from 13 to 87 years (Fig. 20–2).[19]

In the past, the majority of SMA aneurysms were mycotic. Most of these were secondary to subacute bacterial endocarditis caused by nonhemolytic *Streptococcus*. Currently, approximately 31% of SMA aneurysms are thought to be of infectious origin.[19] SMA aneurysms can also be found in patients with FMD, polyarteritis nodosa, pancreatitis, biliary disease, or may occur as a result of dissection. True aneurysms of the SMA in patients with atherosclerotic disease are being reported with increasing frequency.

The majority of SMA aneurysms (90%) are symptomatic. Abdominal pain is the most common symptom, occurring in 67% of patients.[19] This pain may be intermittent

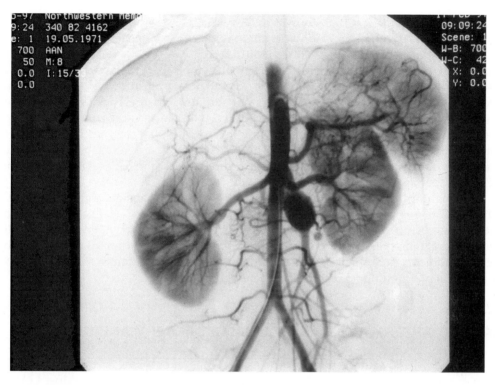

Figure 20–2. Superior mesenteric artery aneurysm in a 25-year-old female who presented with complaints of abdominal pain in the third trimester of pregnancy.

and is usually located in the upper abdomen or epigastrium. Some patients may present with symptoms suggestive of chronic mesenteric ischemia. Twenty-seven percent of patients have an abdominal mass, which may be tender, mobile, or pulsatile in nature.[11,19] Other symptoms include fever, nausea, emesis, GI hemorrhage, hemobilia, jaundice, and chronic anemia.[11]

Rupture of SMA aneurysms occurs in up to 50% of patients.[8,12,18] Rupture is usually followed by acute, massive retroperitoneal, intrabdominal, or GI bleeding. SMA aneurysm rupture often results in shock and sudden death. Expansion of the aneurysm accompanied by dissection or propagation of intraluminal thrombus may occlude collateral flow, leading to intestinal infarction. The mortality rate following SMA aneurysm rupture is 30%.[11] Because complications from this disease can lead to mesenteric infarction and because the natural history of these lesions appears to be progressive expansion and rupture, intervention is indicated in essentially all lesions, even if asymptomatic.

CELIAC ARTERY ANEURYSMS

Aneurysms of the celiac artery (CAA) are rare, representing only 4% of all VAA.[15,20] Prior to 1950, most CAA were secondary to syphilis. Today, most of these lesions are associated with atherosclerotic disease or medial degeneration, and approximately 14% are mycotic.[2,11] Other causes of CAA include poststenotic dilation, trauma, and reentry from aortic dissection. Fifty-five percent of CAA are true aneurysms. CAA are slightly more common in males, who comprise 66% of cases. The mean age of patients with

CAA is 56 years, with a range from 18 to 86 years.[2] These lesions are often associated with aneurysms in other locations; with abdominal aortic aneurysm (AAA) present in 20% of patients, and other VAA in up to 40%.[20]

Approximately 75% of patients reported are symptomatic at the time of diagnosis. Abdominal pain is the most common symptom, occurring in 69%.[2,11] Some patients may complain of epigastric abdominal pain radiating to the back, whereas others describe vague abdominal pain that is associated with nausea and vomiting. The pain is sometimes exacerbated with meals, mimicking intestinal angina. Nearly 30% of patients have a palpable abdominal mass, and 37% have an abdominal bruit on physical exam.[20] Involvement of adjacent organs may result in GI hemorrhage (sometimes associated with hemoptysis) or obstructive jaundice.

The natural history of CAA appears to be one of expansion and rupture, with some reports citing a risk of rupture to be approximately 13%.[11] The mortality rate with rupture is very high, reported to be 100% in one series,[11] and is often complicated by intestinal infarction. Currently, intervention is recommended for all aneurysms that are symptomatic. Treatment is also recommended for asymptomatic CAA discovered as an incidental finding, except in the very high risk patient.

GASTRIC ARTERY AND GASTROEPIPLOIC ARTERY ANEURYSMS

Gastric artery (GA) and gastroepiploic artery (GEA) aneurysms account for only 4% of all VAA. GA aneurysms are 10 times more frequent than the GEA. Most GA and GEA aneurysms are solitary. These aneurysms are more common in men, with a male to female ratio of 3:1. Most patients are in the sixth or seventh decade of life. GA and GEA aneurysms are often the result of an inflammatory process, such as pancreatitis. Aneurysms may also occur in patients with FMD, atherosclerotic disease, or in patients with vasculitis associated with autoimmune disease.[9]

Although a few GA and GEA aneurysms are discovered during angiography for other diseases, 90% of patients present emergently with rupture. About two-thirds of these ruptured aneurysms cause upper GI bleeding, whereas the remainder rupture into the peritoneal cavity.[12] Hemobilia can occur following rupture of left GA aneurysms. Rupture of GA and GEA aneurysms is often accompanied by exsanguinating hemorrhage, with a 70% mortality rate. Of patients who present emergently, 70% have GI bleeding and 30% have life-threatening intraperitoneal hemorrhage.[12] Because of the serious complications associated with aneurysm rupture, aggressive treatment is recommended for nearly all GA and GEA aneurysms.

JEJUNAL, ILEAL, AND COLIC ARTERY ANEURYSMS

Aneurysms of the jejunal, ileal, and colic arteries represent only 3% of all VAA.[1] These aneurysms are usually solitary and small in diameter, from several millimeters up to 15 mm. Jejunal aneurysms are more common, followed by aneurysms of the middle colic and ileal arteries. Patients with aneurysms of the jejunal, ileal, or colic arteries are usually in the seventh decade of life, with men and women being affected equally. The mean age of these patients is 55 years, with a range from 19 to 70 years.[19] Pathogenic processes associated with jejunal, ileal, and colic aneurysms include medial degenerative diseases, trauma, periarteritis nodosa, and atherosclerotic disease. Often these aneurysms may be associated with bacterial endocarditis and streptococcal bacteremia.

Seventy percent of jejunal, ileal, and colic aneurysms are symptomatic at the time of diagnosis. Patients may present with abdominal pain (87%), GI hemorrhage or hemobilia, or a tender abdominal mass.[9,19] Fifty-two percent of patients initially present with shock. Patients may also have complaints of nausea and emesis, or jaundice.[9,19] Most jejunal, ileal, and colic artery aneurysms are discovered during exploratory celiotomy for GI or intraperitoneal bleeding. The frequency of rupture of these SMA branch aneurysms is unknown and is not predicted by the size of the aneurysm. Although the risk of rupture is thought to be low, the mortality rate with rupture is 20%, supporting an aggressive treatment of these aneurysms.[9]

PANCREATODUODENAL, PANCREATIC, AND GASTRODUODENAL ARTERY ANEURYSMS

Aneurysms of the pancreatic (PA) and pancreatoduodenal arteries (PDA) represent only 2% of all VAA. Gastroduodenal artery (GDA) aneurysms account for an additional 1.5%.[9] These aneurysms occur more frequently in men (68%) than in women (32%). The mean age of patients is 48 years, and range from 22 to 78 years.[19] Many of these aneurysms are associated with pancreatitis, which leads to periarterial inflammation or vessel erosion from an adjacent pseudodcyst. Approximately 60% of GDA and 30% of PDA aneurysms are related to pancreatitis.[9] GDA and PDA aneurysms have also been reported in association with celiac artery occlusive disease. The development of aneurysms in patients with occlusive disease may be a consequence of the increased flow present in the collateral vessels (Fig. 20–3).[21]

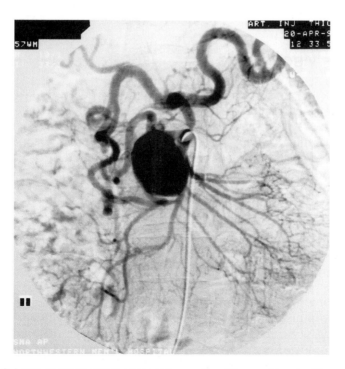

Figure 20–3. Large gastroduodenal artery aneurysm in a 57-year-old male. The patient has a chronic occlusion of the proximal celiac artery with the development of an aneurysm in an enlarged collateral vessel. The patient was treated surgically with a saphenous vein graft bypass to the celiac artery and ligation of the vessels feeding the aneurysm.

Because of this relationship to pancreatitis, most patients (80%) with PA, PDA, and GDA aneurysms have symptoms of abdominal pain and discomfort. As these aneurysms frequently erode into an adjacent portion of the GI tract, more than 50% of patients have evidence of GI hemorrhage. Between 14% and 31% of patients have jaundice at the time of presentation, which may be a result of the underlying pancreatic or biliary tract disease often seen with these aneurysms.[11,19] Up to 68% of PA, PDA, and GDA aneurysms are ruptured at the time of presentation.[11] Rupture may occur into the retroperitoneum, into the free peritoneal cavity, or into an adjacent viscus. These aneurysms may also erode into the portal vein, or into the biliary tract, resulting in hemobilia. The mortality rate accompanying rupture is high, nearly 50%.[9] Thus, intervention is usually indicated and sometimes involves operative treatment of the associated pancreatitis or pseudocyst.

INFERIOR MESENTERIC ARTERY ANEURYSMS

Aneurysms of the inferior mesenteric artery (IMA) are the most rare of all VAA. Discussions of their clinical presentation and therapy are almost anecdotal. The etiology of IMA aneurysms is varied, with lesions being due to medial degeneration, atherosclerosis, and mycotic causes. The majority of patients with IMA aneurysms (88%) are men. The mean age at presentation is 53 years, and range from 22 to 79 years.[19]

Many patients with IMA aneurysms (50%) present with symptoms of abdominal pain or a palpable abdominal mass (50%).[19] The natural history and rupture rate of IMA aneurysms is undefined. It has been suggested that all mycotic lesions and large IMA aneurysms be treated.

DIAGNOSIS OF VISCERAL ARTERY ANEURYSMS

In many cases, the diagnosis of a VAA can be suspected on the abdominal plain film. As many of these aneurysms have secondary calcification, a characteristic curvilinear "eggshell" pattern may be seen in the epigastrium, right or left upper quadrant. About two-thirds of SAA have this finding, localized to the left upper quadrant. A rim of calcification in the right upper quadrant seen on plain abdominal x-ray or a smooth filling defect in the duodenum seen on GI contrast studies may suggest an HAA.[12,22]

Many VAA are discovered incidentally during routine abdominal ultrasonography for unrelated symptoms. Abdominal ultrasound done to evaluate right upper quadrant pain may demonstrate an adjacent mass with an arterial flow pattern. The lesion appears as an isolated hypoechogenic nodule or an anechoic cystic mass. The connection of the mass with the feeding artery and the presence of calcifications can help to make the diagnosis. Color-flow duplex can be an useful adjunct, especially in intrahepatic lesions.[23,24]

Computed tomography has become a useful diagnostic modality for these lesions (Fig. 20–4). The administration of intravenous contrast often demonstrates the vascular nature of a mass. Not only are intact aneurysms well demonstrated, but ruptured aneurysms also produce characteristic findings. A contained hematoma within the lesser sac is often found with ruptured SAA before the blood escapes through the foramen of Winslow into the peritoneal cavity.[25] Other CT findings include a retroperitoneal hematoma or enhancing mass with extravasation of contrast. Ultrasound and CT,

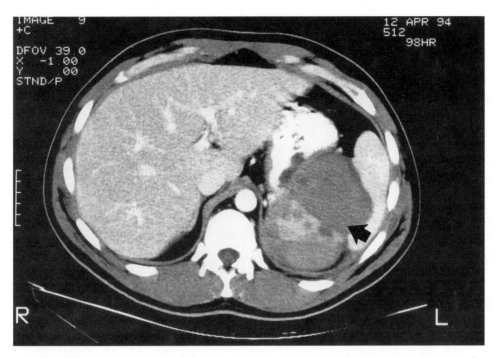

Figure 20–4. Adominal CT scan demonstrating a splenic artery aneurysm in a 26-year-old male patient.

however, frequently may be misleading. Although the diagnosis of an aneurysm is suggested by these noninvasive imaging modalities, the artery of origin is not always clear and angiography is often required to plan for treatment. Newer noninvasive imaging modalities, such as spiral CT angiography with three-dimensional reconstruction, can give detailed anatomic information and may identify the vessel of origin.[26,27]

Magnetic resonance imaging (MRI) has been used to diagnose VAA (Fig. 20–5). The presence of a central flow void and surrounding thrombus are characteristic. A high T_1 signal within a mass suggests thrombosis of an aneurysm. MRI and magnetic resonance angiography (MRA) may be able to identify larger aneurysms and their artery of origin. Aneurysms of the smaller branch vessels and small aneurysms less than 5 mm diameter are not well seen.[22] Evolving MRI techniques using gadolinium enhancement and breath holding maneuvers provide more anatomic detail and may allow for better imaging of VAA and the visceral arterial anatomy.

Although plain films, ultrasound, CT, and MRI studies can often suggest a VAA, contrast angiography is usually necessary to confirm the diagnosis and define the visceral arterial anatomy. Arteriography is currently the method of choice for diagnosis and is recommended for all elective cases. Biplanar angiography with selective injection is needed to define the extent of the aneurysm, visualize collateral vessels, define the distal vasculature, and exclude the presence of associated aneurysms. SAA, for example, are multiple in 20% of cases. This is especially important in the visceral arteries as there is a lot of anatomic variation. For example, angiography is very important for the evaluation of anatomic variations of the hepatic artery origins. Not only can angiography establish an accurate diagnosis and define the arterial anatomy, but it also provides the opportunity for transcatheter treatment of some of these lesions.

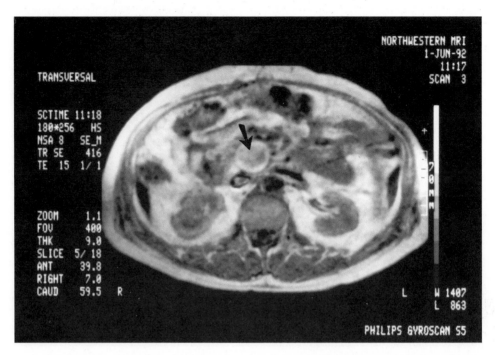

Figure 20–5. MRI demonstrating an aneurysm of the gastroduodenal artery in a 57-year-old male.

TREATMENT OPTIONS

The main methods of therapy for VAA include surgery and transcatheter occlusion of the aneurysm. Surgical treatment of VAA usually involves ligation or resection of the aneurysm with or without vascular reconstruction. Surgical options differ somewhat for each type of VAA. Angiographic embolization has been used for several years in patients with VAA who are poor surgical risks. Greater experience with the techniques of transcatheter embolization has made this an option for primary treatment of some types of aneurysms. The process involves selective catheterization of the involved vessel, followed by injection of Gelfoam particles or steel coils. Detachable balloons have been used as an alternative.

Splenic Artery Aneurysms

Surgical therapy for SAA usually consists of splenectomy and removal of that portion of the splenic artery containing the aneurysm. Exposure of SAA is usually obtained through the lesser sac. In most cases proximal and distal splenic artery control can be obtained and the aneurysm can be excised. Proximal SAA may be treated with proximal and distal ligation with or without aneurysmectomy, with preservation of the spleen. Because of excellent collateral flow in most patients, it is usually not necessary to revascularize the spleen. The extensive blood supply from the stomach through the short gastric arteries usually prevents infarction in most cases. In cases in which extensive dissection of the pancreas or adjacent structures is required, aneurysm exclusion with ligation of contributing vessels is appropriate. Pseudoaneurysms associated with pancreatitis may be more safely treated by arterial ligation from within the aneurysm, especially if the lesion is located in the midportion of the splenic artery or is embedded in the pancreas. Pseudoaneurysms of the distal splenic artery that are embedded in the pancreas may require distal pancreatectomy along with aneurysm resection.[14]

Laparoscopic ligation has also been reported for SAA with good results. Both the supine and lateral approaches have been described. The supine approach involves an initial trocar for the laparoscope, inserted at the umbilicus. Two 12-mm trocars are placed at the right and left midclavicular lines in the midabdomen for insertion of instruments and staplers. A 5-mm trocar is placed at the right hypochondrium for retraction by the assistant. The lateral approach, described by Leung and associates,[29] is performed with the patient in a lateral decubitus position with the left side up. A 12-mm port is inserted in the left subcostal region at the midclavicular line for introduction of the laparoscope. Two additional 12-mm ports are inserted in the left anterior axillary line and in the left midaxillary line at the level of the umbilicus. The EndoGIA is used to transect the ligated splenic artery.[14,28–31]

Transcatheter embolization of SAA is a treatment modality that has been used with increasing frequency since the late 1980s. Treatment involves occlusion of the splenic artery itself or direct embolization of the aneurysm. Multiple coils placed into the neck of the lesion cause thrombosis of the aneurysm and the more proximal splenic artery. Modern coaxial microcatheter techniques make it possible in some cases to fill the aneurysm with coils and maintain flow in the main splenic artery, thus preserving the spleen.[14,32,33]

There are few guidelines on what to do in the event of an SAA identified during pregnancy. Options include elective surgery during the second trimester and elective cesarean section with operative treatment of the aneurysm at the same time. Because of the high risk of rupture during the third trimester, observation of SAA in obstetric patients is not recommended.[14,16]

Hepatic Artery Aneurysms

Appropriate treatment of HAA requires detailed angiographic characterization of hepatic artery blood flow. Treatment depends on the location of the aneurysm within the hepatic artery. Aneurysms of the proximal hepatic artery (proximal to the gastroduodenal artery) can be treated by excision or by exclusion without reconstruction. There is usually sufficient collateral circulation through the SMA to the gastroduodenal artery. In distal lesions or in those involving the gastroduodenal artery, revascularization may be necessary.[22] When revascularization is necessary, autogenous tissue is the conduit of choice for most VAA, although prosthetic grafts have been used. Reconstruction may take the form of aortohepatic artery bypass, splenohepatic anastomosis, or interposition grafting with reimplantation of the gastroduodenal artery. For intrahepatic artery aneurysms, surgical correction may require hepatic resection of the area involving the aneurysm or simple ligation of the involved artery before it enters the liver parenchyma. Exposure of some aneurysms of the hepatic artery may be difficult due to the close relationship of this artery to the bile duct and portal vein. With large aneurysms and arteries associated with signficant inflammation, proximal and distal control may be more easily obtained by opening the aneurysm and controlling feeding vessels from within the sac. Patients presenting with aneurysm rupture with shock are more vulnerable to hepatic ischemia following ligation of an HAA. Hepatic artery ligation done in the presence of hypotension or hepatocellular damage is associated with a higher incidence of hepatic necrosis. Some authors have recommended that vascular reconstruction be attempted after aneurysm resection in all patients with extrahepatic lesions. When reconstruction is not possible, ligation should be done as close to the porta hepatis as possible in an attempt to spare collateral flow to the liver.[1,11,34,35]

Successful percutaneous embolizaton of an HAA was first reported in 1977. Transcatheter embolization of these lesions has increased tremendously since the late 1980s and is thought to be the treatment of choice for many HAA. Currently, approximately 37% of HAA are treated with percutaneous embolization.[2] An advantage of selective arterial embolization is its precision in limiting hepatic devascularization. Percutaneous embolization has become the preferred treatment by many for posttraumatic pseudoaneurysms of the hepatic artery and especially for intrahepatic lesions. Using a percutaneous transhepatic route, distally located aneurysms may be better accessed, especially in patients with tortuous proximal vessels (Fig. 20–6). It is important to thrombose the vessel as distally as possible, as embolization of a more proximal vessel feeding the aneurysm may result in incomplete thrombosis and recurrence.[1,11,22]

Superior Mesenteric Artery Aneurysms

Superior mesenteric artery aneurysms are usually treated operatively through a transmesenteric or retroperitoneal approach. Transmesenteric exposure can be obtained by dissection at the base of the transverse colon mesentery. Alternatively, exposure of the proximal SMA can be obtained by a retroperitoneal route using medial visceral rotation.[11] Simple ligation of vessels entering and exiting the aneurysm has been successful in 30% of reported cases. Collateral flow from the celiac axis through the inferior pancreaticoduodenal artery or from the IMA through the middle colic artery may be adequate to prevent mesenteric ischemia. Aneurysmectomy with reconstruction is most often necessary, especially if there is doubt about sufficient collateral circulation. With proximal SMA lesions, the proximal anastomosis is to the aorta, using operative techniques similar to those used with mesenteric occlusive disease. If the aneurysm is not

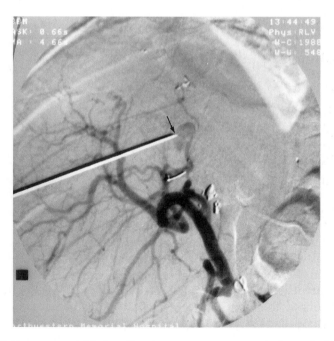

Figure 20–6. Recurrence of this hepatic artery aneurysm occurred after embolization of the right hepatic artery. Successful thrombosis was obtained after a combined percutaneous transhepatic and transarterial approach. Note needle (*arrow*) approaching the aneurysm for direct occlusion.

mycotic, either autogenous or prosthetic material may be used. In patients with infected aneurysm or intestinal ischemia, autogenous bypass or reimplantation of the SMA into the adjacent aorta are appropriate alternatives. If the very proximal SMA is normal, an interposition graft of autogenous tissue can be used to reconstruct the vessel following aneurysm excision (Fig. 20–7). Endoaneurysmorrhaphy is a possible alternative, especially with saccular aneurysms.[9,12,18,20]

The availability of wires and catheters for superselective catheterization has permitted precise localization and treatment of aneurysms of the SMA and its branches. Several centers have used these techniques to treat large aneurysms by filling the aneurysm itself, or by occluding only the neck of the lesion, thus avoiding bowel ischemia. Submucosal aneurysms and small aneurysms that are difficult to access surgically may be candidates for transcatheter embolization,[36] which may be an alternative treatment in patients who are not good surgical candidates (i.e., hostile abdomen) or patients who have failed surgical treatment. However, because of the risks of intestinal infarction, transcatheter embolization is not often used for the treatment of SMA aneurysms.

Celiac Artery Aneurysms

Most CAA can be approached operatively through a transabdominal incision with medial visceral rotation. Alternatively, the celiac artery may be approached through the lesser sac.[11] For CAA, aneurysmectomy with arterial reconstruction is the preferred treatment. Aneurysm resection is followed by aortoceliac bypass using autogenous or prosthetic conduit originating from the supraceliac aorta. Although celiac artery ligation

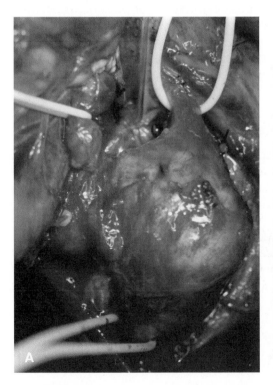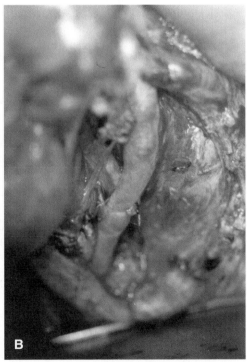

Figure 20–7. A superior mesenteric artery aneurysm in a young female patient was treated with resection of the aneurysm and revascularization with a saphenous vein interposition graft. (**A**) Vessel loops are placed around the proximal SMA, the middle colic artery, and a large branch of the SMA. (**B**) The aneurysm was resected and the interposition graft is shown.

can be done if adequate collateral circulation to the foregut is demonstrated, this carries the risk of hepatic necrosis, especially in patients with shock or preexisting liver disease. Aneurysmorrhaphy for discrete saccular lesions is an alternative.[9,11,20]

Gastric–Gastroepiploic and Pancreatoduodenal–Pancreatic–Gastroduodenal Artery Aneurysms

Gastric artery and GEA aneurysms that occur in an extragastric location may be treated successfully with ligation, sometimes accompanied by aneurysm excision. Intramural lesions are best excised with the involved portion of the stomach. With pancreatic, PDA, and GDA aneurysms, simple ligation of the proximal and distal vessels is often difficult because of multiple communicating vessels. The aneurysm may be opened and suture ligation of entering and exiting vessels can be accomplished from within the aneurysm. Generally, treatment in these patients involves obliteration of the aneurysm and treatment of any associated pathology. Treatment of pseudoaneurysms secondary to pancreatic pseudocysts often involves drainage of the pseudocyst as well, usually internal drainage. Small aneurysms of the PDA embedded in the mid- or distal region of the pancreas may require pancreatic resection.[9,11,20]

Because many patients with these aneurysms have severe underlying medical conditions, often severe pancreatitis, the operative mortality rates associated with aneurysm repair remain high, up to 13%.[11] There has been an increasing number of patients treated with percutaneous embolization. As many as 15% of patients are treated with transcatheter techniques.[11] Multiple communicating vessels present a challenge to embolization, as recanalization or incomplete thrombosis of the aneurysm may occur. Many of these lesions are treated using a staged approach with multiple embolization attempts. Percutaneous puncture combined with transarterial embolization may be required to achieve complete thrombosis.[10] As many patients presenting with these aneurysms have severe concomitant illnesses, transcatheter embolization may prove to be an increasingly attractive therapeutic option.[1]

Mesenteric Branch Artery Aneurysms

Aneurysms of the mesenteric branch vessels are usually treated with arterial ligation, aneurysmectomy, and resection of ischemic bowel segments. As with other VAA, a search for multiple branch vessel aneurysms is appropriate. MA aneurysms can be treated with ligation with or without revascularization, depending on the status of the intestinal circulation. Nonruptured aneurysms are most often treated with aneurysmectomy. Ruptured jejunal, ileal, colic, and IMA aneurysms are often accompanied by a large hematoma in the mesentery. These cases are frequently complicated by mesenteric venous stasis and ischemic bowel segments. Because of the significant risk for bowel ischemia, transcatheter embolization has had a limited role in the treatment of these lesions.

NORTHWESTERN EXPERIENCE

Since 1980, 37 patients were diagnosed with 46 VAA at Northwestern Memorial Hospital in Chicago, Illinois. Four patients had multiple aneurysms. There were 22 SAA, 10 HAA, 4 SMA, 2 GD, 3 CAA, 2 left gastric, 1 pancreaticoduodenal, 1 jejunal–ileal, and 1 IMA aneurysms. There were 20 men and 17 women whose ages ranged from 26 to 85 years, with a mean of 60 years (Table 20–1).

Nearly 50% of the VAA diagnosed were located in the splenic artery. Causes included atherosclerosis (6), infection (3), hypersplenism (2), pancreatitis (2), trauma (1), connective tissue disease (1), and unknown (7). None of the patients treated at this hospital were pregnant. Four patients (18%) presented with acute rupture of the aneurysm and underwent emergent celiotomy. Nine aneurysms (41%) were found incidentally during evaluation for concomitant disease. Seven of the 22 cases of SAA were treated with splenectomy, most of which were done emergently for ruptured aneurysms. Eleven aneurysms were treated with surgery, three underwent embolization, and eight were observed. Patients who were observed included three women (60 to 65 years of age) with small (less than 2 cm) aneurysms. Other reasons for observation included metastatic cancer and advanced age. There was one death due to SAA rupture in a woman with connective tissue disease and acute pancreatitis. The patient died with a ruptured SAA before any surgical therapy could be attempted.

In this series, 10 patients (22%) were found with HAA; six were intrahepatic and four were extraphepatic. Most HAA (four patients) were caused by trauma. Other associated conditions included atherosclerosis, aortic dissection, infection, pancreatitis, and portal hypertension. HAA were associated with the placement of biliary stents for obstructive jaundice as a result of malignant disease in two patients. The majority of aneurysms were symptomatic at the time of treatment, including six that presented with rupture (60%). The most common symptoms were abdominal pain and hemobilia. Three aneurysms were discovered during ultrasound done for suspected cholelithiasis. Five patients with HAA were treated with transcatheter embolization. Surgical treatments included ligation, excision with saphenous vein interposition graft, and hepatic lobectomy in a patient with multiple intrahepatic aneurysms. One patient who refused surgery was observed.

There were four SMA aneurysms and three CAA. SMA aneurysms were mycotic (two), associated with portal hypertension (one), and of unknown etiology (one). CAA was associated with atherosclerosis (one), infection (one), and of unknown etiology (one). Although none of the SMA or CAA presented with rupture, the majority (57%) were symptomatic at presentation. Seventy-five percent of patients with SMA aneu-

TABLE 20–1. DISTRIBUTION AND CLINICAL PRESENTATION OF VISCERAL ARTERY ANEURYSMS

Aneurysm Location	Mean Age (yr)	M:F	Asymptomatic (no.)	Symptomatic Without Rupture (no.)	Ruptured (no.)
Splenic (22)	60	6:16	40.9% (9)	40.9% (9)	18.2% (4)
Hepatic (10)	63	9:1	30.0% (3)	10.0% (1)	60.0% (6)
Superior mesenteric artery (4) and celiac (3)	56	4:3	43.0% (3)	57.0% (4)	0.0% (0)
Other Gastroduodenal (2) Left gastric (2) Pancreatoduodenal (1) Jejunal–ileal (1) Inferior mesenteric (1)	54	3:4	28.6% (2)	57.1% (4)	14.3% (1)
Total of 46 aneurysms			37.0% (17)	39.1% (18)	23.9% (11)

Reprinted with permission from Carr SC, Pearce WH, Vogelzang RL, et al. Current management of visceral artery aneurysms. *Surgery.* 1996;120(4):627–634.

TABLE 20–2. RESULTS OF THERAPY FOR VISCERAL ARTERY ANEURYSMS

Treatment (no.)	Complications (no.)	Outcome	Deaths (no.)
Surgical (17)	Splenic abscess (2) Failure to thombose (1)	Successfully treated percutaneously	0
Embolization (12)[a]	Focal splenic infarction (1) Recurrent bleeding (2)	Resolved without treatment Successfully treated percutaneously	0
Observation (9)		None became symptomatic during follow-up	Splenic artery aneurysm rupture (1)

[a] One patient was treated with surgery followed by transcatheter embolization.

Reprinted with permission from Carr SC, Pearce WH, Vogelzang RL, et al. Current management of visceral artery aneurysms. *Surgery.* 1996;120(4):627–634.

rysms were symptomatic, with complaints of abdominal pain. The majority of patients with these aneurysms underwent operative repair with saphenous vein interposition and ligation of the vessels feeding the aneurysms in one patient. One patient with multiple previous abdominal procedures and severe portal hypertension was treated with transcatheter embolization.

Two patients in this series had aneurysms of the GD artery. One of these was secondary to iatrogenic trauma associated with insertion of an infusion pump for chemotherapy to treat metastatic colon cancer. Two left GA aneurysms and one jejunal–ileal artery aneurysm were mycotic in origin. One IMA aneurysm was found in a patient with portal hypertension. Most of these patients were symptomatic (57%) with complaints of abdominal pain. One patient with a GDA aneurysm presented with rupture. Two patients were treated primarily with transcatheter embolization. One of the surgically treated aneurysms underwent ligation. The one patient with the GDA associated with chronic occlusion of the proximal celiac artery was treated operatively with saphenous vein bypass of the occluded celiac artery and ligation of the vessels feeding the large GDA aneurysm. Postoperatively, the GDA aneurysm recurred. The patient was then treated with a combined percutaneous and transarterial embolization procedure, which resulted in successful thrombosis of the aneurysm.

The results of therapy for VAA are summarized in Table 20–2.

COMMENTS

Visceral artery aneurysms are rare but clinically important lesions. With the increasing use of CT and angiography, many aneurysms are being discovered prior to rupture or thrombosis. Improvements in CT and MRI technology have led to the increased detection of VAA in patients being evaluated for abdominal pain or other disease. At this time, angiography remains the method of choice to determine the extent of an aneurysm, to define the anatomy of the collateral circulation, and to identify multiple aneurysms.

Most VAA, even if asymptomatic, require some form of therapy to prevent the complications of rupture or end-organ ischemia. Surgical options include splencecomy with removal of the aneurysm, aneurysm exclusion with ligation, excision with or without vascular reconstruction, and ligation of the vessels entering and exiting the aneurysm. As laparoscopic technology continues to improve, more aneurysms may be amenable to laparoscopic ligation. Transcatheter embolization of VAA is becoming an important treatment for many aneurysms as it offers several advantages. This is particularly true with the widespread use of microcatheter techniques for aneurysm exclusion or primary aneurysm thrombosis. Advantages include precise localization of the aneurysm, assessment of collateral flow, lower risk for patients who are not good candidates for surgery, and easier approach to aneurysms for which surgical exposure would be difficult.

REFERENCES

1. Røkke O, Søndema K, Amundsen S, Bjerke-Larsen T, et al. The diagnosis and management of splanchnic artery aneurysms. *Scan J Gastroenterol.* 1996;31:737–742.
2. Shanley CJ, Shah NL, Messina LM. Common splanchnic artery aneurysms: splenic, hepatic, and celiac. *Ann Vasc Surg.* 1996;10(3):315–322.
3. Beaussier M. Sur un aneurisme de l'arteeere splenique dont les parois se sont ossifiees. *J Medical Toulouse.* 1770;32:157.
4. Psathakis D, Muller G, Noah M, Diebold J, et al. Present management of hepatic artery aneurysms. *Vasa.* 1992;21(2):210–215.
5. McGinnis HD, Deluca SA. Splenic artery aneurysms. *Am Fam Physician.* 1993;47(5):1119–1202.
6. DeBakey ME, Cooley DA. Successful resection of mycotic aneurysm of the superior mesenteric artery. *Am Surgeon.* 1953;19:202.
7. Stanley JC, Thompson NW, Fry WJ. Splanchnic artery aneurysms. *Arch Surg.* 1970;101: 689–697.
8. Kanazawa S, Inada H, Murakami T, et al. The diagnosis and management of splanchnic artery aneurysms: report of 8 cases. *J Cardiovasc Surg.* 1997;38:479–485.
9. Stanley JC, Wakefield TW, Graham LM, Whitehouse WM, et al. Clinical importance and management of splanchnic artery aneurysms. *J Vasc Surg.* 1986;3(5):836–840.
10. Carr SC, Pearce WH, Vogelzang RL, McCarthy WJ, et al. Current management of visceral artery aneurysms. *Surgery.* 1996;120(4):627–634.
11. Messina LM, Shanley CJ. Visceral artery aneurysms. *Surg Clin North Am.* 1997;77(2):425–442.
12. Jorgensen BA. Visceral artery aneurysms. *Danish Med Bull.* 1985;32:237–242.
13. Trastek VF, Pairolero PC, Joyce JW. Splenic artery aneurysms. *Surgery.* 1982;91:694–699.
14. Hallett JW Jr. Splenic artery aneurysms. *Semin Vasc Surg.* 1995;8(4):321–326.
15. Graham LM, Mesh CL. Celiac, hepatic, and splenic artery aneurysms. In: Ernst CB, Stanley JC, eds. *Current Theory in Vascular Surgery.* St. Louis, MO: Mosby-Yearbook; 1995:714–718.
16. Holdsworth RJ, Gunn A. Ruptured splenic artery in pregnancy. A review. *Br J Obstet Gynaecol.* 1992;99:595–597.
17. Mattar SG, Lumsden AB. The management of splenic artery aneurysms: experience with 23 cases. *Am J Surg.* 1995;169:580–584.
18. Lindberg CG, Stridbeck H. Aneurysms of the superior mesenteric artery and its branches. *Gastrointest Radiol.* 1992;17:132–134.
19. Shanley CJ, Nikhil LS, Messina LM. Uncommon splanchnic artery aneurysms: pancreaticoduodenal, gastroduodenal, superior mesenteric, inferior mesenteric, and colic. *Ann Vasc Surg.* 1996;10(5):506–515.
20. Graham LM, Rubin JR. Visceral artery aneurysms. In: Strandness DE, Breda A, eds. *Vascular Diseases: Surgical and Interventional Therapy.* New York: Churchill Livingstone; 1994:811–821.
21. Paty PSK, Cordero JA, Darling RC, Chang BB, et al. Aneurysms of the pancreaticoduodenal artery. *J Vasc Surg.* 1996;23:710–713.
22. Lumsden AB, Mattar SG, Allen RC, Bacha EA. Hepatic artery aneurysms: the management of 22 patients. *J Surg Res.* 1996;60:345–350.
23. Warshauer DM, Keefe B, Mauro MA. Intrahepatic hepatic artery aneurysm: computed tomography and color-flow Doppler ultrasound findings. *Gastrointest Radiol.* 1991;16:175–177.
24. Bret PM, Bretagnolle M, Enoch G, Partensky C, et al. Ultrasonic features of aneurysms of splanchnic arteries. *J Assoc Can Radiol.* 1995;36:226–229.

25. Brunet WG, Greenberg HM. CT demonstration of a ruptured splenic artery aneurysm. *J Comput Assist Tomogr.* 1991;15(1):177–178.
26. Watanabe Y, Sato M, Abe Y, et al. Three-dimensional arterial computed tomography and laparoscope-assisted splenectomy as a minimally invasive examination and treatment of splenic aneurysms. *J Laparaendosc Adv Surg Tech.* 1997;7(3):183–186.
27. Cikrit DF, Harris VJ, Hemmer CG, et al. Comparison of spiral CT scan and arteriography for evaluation of renal and visceral arteries. *Ann Vasc Surg.* 1996;10:109–116.
28. Matsumoto K, Ohgami M, Shirasugi N, Nohga K, et al. A first case report of the successful laparoscopic repair of a splenic artery aneurysm. *Surgery.* 1997;121:462–464.
29. Leung KL, Kwong KH, Tam YH, Lau WY, et al. Laparoscopic resection of splenic artery aneurysm. *Surg Endosc.* 1998;12:53.
30. Hashizume M, Ohta M, Ueno K, Okadome K, et al. Laparoscopic ligation of splenic artery aneurysms. *Surgery.* 1993;11(1):352–354.
31. Saw EK, Ku W, Ramachandra S. Laparoscopic resection of a splenic artery aneurysm. *J Laparoendosc Surg.* 1993;3(2):167–171.
32. Reidy JF, Rowe PN, Ellis FG. Technical report: splenic artery aneurysm embolization—the preferred technique to surgery. *Clin Radiol.* 1990;41(4):281–282.
33. Tarazov PG, Polysalov VN, Ryzhkov VK. Transcatheter treatment of splenic artery aneurysms: report of two cases. *J Cardiovasc Surg.* 1991;32:128–131.
34. Salo JA, Aarnio PT, Jarvinen AA, Kivilaakso EO. Aneurysms of the hepatic arteries. *Am Surgeon.* 1989;55(12):705–709.
35. Blue JM, Burney DP. Current trends in the diagnosis and treatment of hepatic artery aneurysms. *Southern Med J.* 1990;83(8):966–969.
36. Ku A, Kadir S. Embolization of a mesenteric artery aneurysm: case report. *Cardiovasc Intervent Radiol.* 1990;13:91–92.

21

Surgical Options in the Treatment of Renovascular Hypertension and Renal Failure

James C. Stanley, MD

Treatment options available to surgeons when undertaking operations for renovascular hypertension with or without renal failure vary depending on the character of the underlying renal artery disease, the presence or absence of coexistent aortic disease, and the overall health of the patient, especially their cardiac status. The indications for surgical intervention for renovascular hypertension have become relatively well established,[1,2] whereas the role of surgical treatment for renal failure secondary to ischemic nephropathy remains less well defined.[3–6]

Operative therapy of renal artery occlusive disease has become standardized since the late 1970s.[7–14] The importance of a carefully performed initial operation deserves emphasis, in that reoperation carries a relatively high risk of nephrectomy.[15] When comparing surgical treatment options to alternative therapies, such as percutaneous angioplasty with stents or long-term drug administration, it is important to relate each therapy to the specific disease states being treated. The three principal renovascular occlusive diseases—arteriosclerosis, arterial fibrodysplasia, and developmental lesions—usually involve distinctly different surgical interventions, and discussion of these treatment options must be individualized.

RENAL ARTERY ARTERIOSCLEROTIC OCCLUSIVE DISEASE

Arteriosclerotic occlusive disease of the renal arteries is usually a manifestation of systemic disease, with 65% of these stenoses representing aortic spillover lesions. An additional 30% of arteriosclerotic stenoses occur as focal eccentric or concentric narrowings limited to the proximal 1.5 cm of the renal artery. The remaining 5% occur as isolated narrowings within the segmental arteries, most often in patients with diabetes mellitus.

Arteriosclerotic renal artery occlusive lesions are amenable to four principal means of endarterectomy, including aortorenal endarterectomy through an axial aortotomy, aortorenal endarterectomy through the transected infrarenal aorta, direct renal artery endarterectomy, and eversion endarterectomy of the transected renal artery with its subsequent aortic reimplantation. The specific intervention performed depends on the extent and character of aortic and renal artery disease, and in some circumstances the necessity to perform a concomitant aortic reconstruction.

The operative exposure of the renal arteries for a transaortic endarterectomy usually involves an anterior approach through the base of the mesocolon and root of the mesentery. However, when undertaking a unilateral direct renal artery endarterectomy, an extraperitoneal approach is favored, with medial visceral rotation of the colon and foregut structures. In either case, the patient is placed supine on the operating table and a rolled blanket is placed transversely under the lower back to accentuate the patient's lumbar lordosis and enhance visualization of the retroperitoneal structures. A transverse supraumbilical abdominal incision is preferred, being extended from the contralateral anterior axillary line to the ipsilateral posterior axillary line. The small bowel is displaced from the abdominal cavity in a bowel bag and the transverse colon is retracted into the upper abdomen with the aid of fixed retraction. The ligament of Treitz is divided and the duodenum is then mobilized, being retracted superiorly to the right. The retroperitoneum over the infrarenal aorta is incised and dissection is continued to the level of the renal vein, which is mobilized by ligating and transecting contributory adrenal, gonadal, and lumbar veins.

The renal artery is skeletonized from its aortic origin for 3 to 4 cm, well beyond the obvious distal extent of atherosclerotic plaque. Small nonparenchymal branches, such as those to the adrenal gland, must be transected and ligated close to the main renal artery. This mobilization is time consuming, but is necessary to facilitate easy eversion of the renal artery during the endarterectomy.

The aorta is dissected about its circumference from 3 or 4 cm below the renal arteries to above the superior mesenteric artery (SMA). This requires incision of dense surrounding neural and fibrous tissue and division of the periaortic diaphragmatic crus perpendicular to its fibers and the aorta. Transection of the crus using the electrocautery usually prevents muscular bleeding. Ligation and transection of lumbar arteries may facilitate the aortic dissection, although these vessels are usually occluded temporarily with microvascular clamps.

Renal artery exposure for a direct unilateral endarterectomy is usually achieved in a different manner, by an extraperitoneal approach similar to the conventional medial visceral rotation used for aortorenal bypass. Patient positioning and the abdominal incision is the same as for other revascularizations, but the renal arteries are approached by reflection of the colon and foregut structures to the contralateral side. The renal vein is mobilized from the vena cava to the renal pelvis, including transection of its contributory venous branches. The renal artery is then dissected from its aortic origin to a point well beyond the obvious atherosclerotic plaque.

Before occluding the aorta or renal arteries, systemic anticoagulation is established with intravenous administration of heparin, 150 units/kg. Mannitol, 12.5 g in an average adult, is administered intravenously at the same time to induce a diuresis. Following restoration of renal blood flow, the heparin anticoagulation is reversed with the intravenous administration of 1.5 mg of protamine sulfate for each 100 units of heparin given earlier. These drug interventions are common to all renal artery reconstructive procedures undertaken in adults. The four specific forms of endarterectomy differ in their performance and they are discussed separately.

Transaortic Renal Artery Endarterectomy Through an Axial Aortotomy

This is a commonly performed method of restoring renal blood flow in cases of bilateral arteriosclerotic occlusive disease of the renal artery ostia (Fig. 21–1).[12,16,17] The aorta is

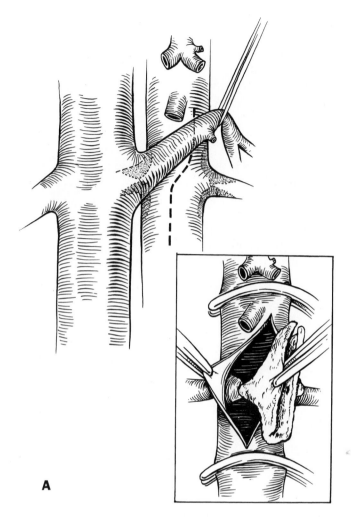

A

Figure 21–1. (**A**) Technique of transaortic renal artery endarterectomy using an axial aortotomy, extending from the level of the superior mesenteric artery to the infrarenal aorta. Transaortic renal artery endarterectomy; preoperative (**B**) and postoperative (**C**) arteriographic studies. (*From Stanley JC, Messina LM, Wakefield TW, Zelenock GB: Renal artery reconstruction. In: Bergan JJ, Yao JST, eds.* Techniques in Arterial Surgery. *Philadelphia: WB Saunders; 1990:247–263.*)

clamped above the SMA and below the renal artery origins after microvascular clamps have been applied to the renal arteries to prevent embolization of aortic debris into the kidney. The superior mesenteric artery is usually dissected 1 to 2 cm beyond its origin and is also occluded with a microvascular clamp.

An axial aortotomy is made, extending from the left anterolateral side of the aorta adjacent to the superior mesenteric artery to the anterior midline between the renal arteries, terminating 2 to 3 cm below the renal vessels. An endarterectomy plane is developed between the diseased and more normal outer aortic media. This dissection is extended circumferentially, and the plaque is transected just below the SMA orifice. Renal artery endarterectomy is accomplished by maintaining gentle traction on the renal artery extension of the aortic plaque while the everted renal artery wall is pushed away from the lesion. A well-defined end point is usually established with feathering

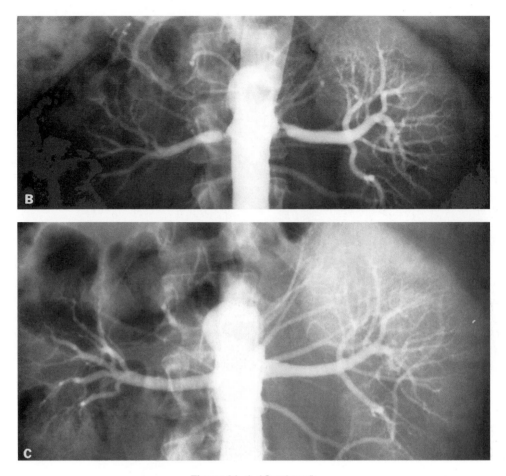

Figure 21–1. (*Continued*)

of the distal plaque onto the distal renal artery. If an intimal flap is suspected, a separate axial renal artery incision should be made beyond the plaque end point, followed by tacking of the distal plaque and closure of the renal artery. The later frequently requires closure with a vein patch. The aortotomy is subsequently closed with a continuous 4-0 cardiovascular suture following vigorous saline irrigation of the endarterectomized aortic segment and renal arteries. The aortic and renal artery clamps are then removed and antegrade flow to the kidneys is reestablished.

Transaortic endarterectomy is best undertaken when disease is limited to the proximal renal artery. Poststenotic dilation in these circumstances is indicative of relative ease in obtaining a well-defined endarterectomy end point. Transaortic renal artery endarterectomy through an axial aortotomy is particularly useful in managing disease of multiple renal arteries, which would otherwise require a complex reconstruction if conventional bypass procedures were undertaken. Documentation of normal renal artery blood flow following endarterectomy may be accomplished by Doppler ultrasonography, but intraoperative duplex scanning is more likely to reveal important defects warranting correction.[18] Postoperative arteriography more precisely confirms the adequacy of the revascularization and can serve as the basis for further clinical follow-up, but may not be cost-justified.

Transaortic Renal Artery Endarterectomy Through the Transected Infrarenal Aorta

In patients undergoing concomitant aortic reconstruction, renal artery endarterectomy is performed in a different manner (Fig. 21–2).[12,19] In these instances the initial dissection of the aorta and renal arteries is undertaken as previously described. However, rather than performing an axial aortotomy, the aorta is transected just below the renal arteries. The aorta may or may not then be transposed anterior to the renal vein. Endarterectomy of the diseased aorta and everted renal arteries is undertaken through the divided aorta. Subsequently, the aortic reconstruction is completed in a conventional manner, with restoration of kidney blood flow usually reestablished after the proximal aortic graft anastomosis by occluding the prosthesis and removing the proximal aortic clamp before completing the distal aortic, iliac, or femoral graft anastomoses.

Direct Renal Artery Endarterectomy

In select patients without extensive aortic atherosclerosis, especially in patients with unilateral proximal lesions with involvement of early branchings, direct renal artery endarterectomy may be preferred (Fig. 21–3).[12] The renal artery is most often exposed by an extraperitoneal approach. In these cases a direct anterior renal arteriotomy is

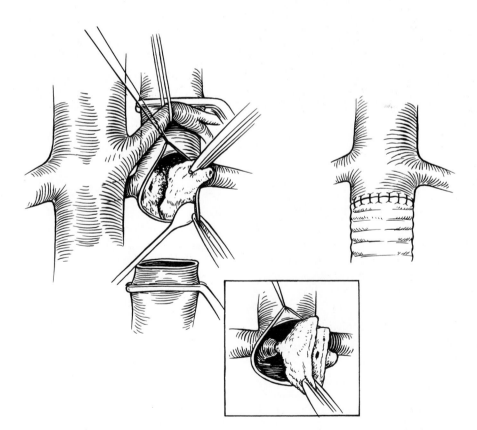

Figure 21–2. Technique of transaortic renal artery endarterectomy through a transected aorta undertaken in association with aortic reconstruction for aneurysmal or occlusive disease. (*From Stanley JC, Messina LM, Wakefield TW, Zelenock GB: Renal artery reconstruction. In: Bergan JJ, Yao JST, eds.* Techniques in Arterial Surgery. *Philadelphia: WB Saunders; 1990:247–263.*)

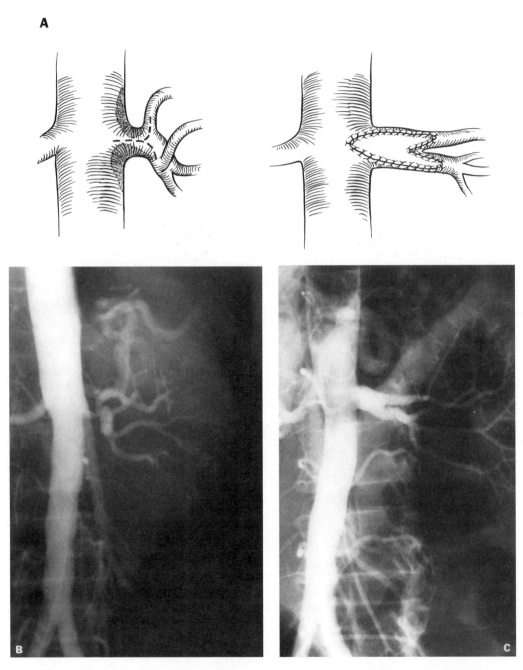

Figure 21–3. (**A**) Technique of direct renal artery endarterectomy with patch graft arterial closure. Direct renal artery endarterectomy with patch graft arterial closure; preoperative (**B**) and postoperative (**C**) arteriographic studies. (*From Stanley JC, Messina LM, Wakefield TW, Zelenock GB: Renal artery reconstruction. In: Bergan JJ, Yao JST, eds.* Techniques in Arterial Surgery. *Philadelphia: WB Saunders; 1990:247–263.*)

performed, being extended for a short distance onto the aorta. The direct endarterectomy is followed by either a simple primary closure or patch graft closure of the arteriotomy. Although this approach may also be applicable to bilateral renal artery disease, closure of lengthy renal artery incisions often requires time-consuming placement of a patch graft. If the stenotic disease on both sides is not preocclusive with prior development of collateral vessels to the kidney, ischemic renal injury may follow prolonged interruption of renal blood flow while completing such a patch closure of the arteriotomy.

Renal Artery Endarterectomy and Aortic Reimplantation

Some patients may have arteriosclerotic disease limited to a single vessel orifice with no involvement of the opposite renal artery and an aorta free of obvious arteriosclerosis. In such a case the artery may be transected and ligated at its origin, with aortic reimplantation of the renal artery after an eversion endarterectomy. In an occasional patient with multiple renal arteries to a kidney, including one that is free of disease, the diseased renal artery may be reimplanted beyond its arteriosclerotic lesion onto the adjacent undiseased renal artery. Aortic clamping required of an aortorenal endarterectomy or aortorenal bypass is avoided in this setting.

Aortorenal Bypass

Arteriosclerotic renal artery disease is often treated using a reversed autogenous saphenous vein or synthetic aortorenal graft.[12,20] Operative exposure is similar to that of a direct renal endarterectomy, with a retroperitoneal approach and medial visceral rotation of the colon and foregut structures, providing direct access to the renal pedicle and aorta. Careful retraction of the overlying renal vein and initial isolation of the artery in its midportion proceeding toward the aorta is recommended. In certain patients with right-sided ostial atherosclerosis, it is possible to retract the vena cava laterally and dissect the proximal renal artery beyond the site of obstruction without the necessity for an extraperitoneal exposure of the distal renal artery.

The aortotomy for origination of the graft in these patients should be performed cautiously so as not to create a plane within the atherosclerotic aortic media that might result in a later dissection. Similarly, sutures for the graft-to-aortic anastomosis should be carefully placed so as to coapt diseased intimal and medial tissues together. Details regarding graft positioning and anastomoses are similar to those discussed in the section on fibrodysplastic disease.

Splenorenal, Hepatorenal, and Iliorenal Bypasses

In circumstances of marginal cardiac function or when aortic disease exists, such that aortic clamping for endarterectomy or creation of an aortic orifice for a renal bypass graft might prove hazardous, an indirect reconstruction arising from the splenic, hepatic, or iliac arteries should be considered.[21-23] When undertaking a splenorenal or hepatorenal bypass it must first be documented by an appropriate imaging study that the proximal celiac artery does not have an occlusive lesion that would perpetuate the hypertensive state following the reconstruction.

Splenorenal bypass usually involves direct end-to-end anastomosis of the splenic artery to the renal artery (Fig. 21–4). Occasionally this nonanatomic reconstruction may necessitate placement of an interposition vein graft between the splenic and renal arteries. Exposure of the left renal artery is similar to that previously described for a direct renal artery endarterectomy or an aortorenal bypass. The exposure of the splenic artery may be undertaken directly through the base of the mesentery and mesocolon,

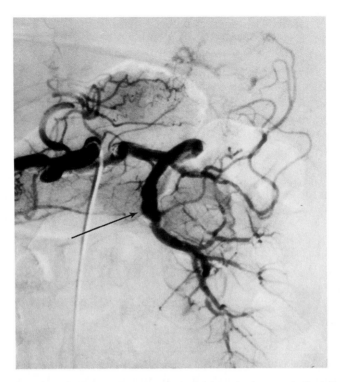

Figure 21–4. Splenorenal bypass, with anastomosis of the splenic artery to the left renal artery, in an end-to-end fashion. (*From Stanley JC, Messina LM: Renal revascularization for recurrent pulmonary edema in patients with poorly controlled renovascular hypertension and renal insufficiency. In: Veith FJ, ed.* Current Critical Problems in Vascular Surgery. *Vol. 5. 1993:309–315, St. Louis, Missouri, Quality Medical Publishing.*)

but such is fraught with bleeding from small vessels and limitations in the length of splenic artery easily dissected. The preferred approach to the splenic artery is one through the retroperitoneum following medial mobilization of the colon. The splenic artery usually lies within a few centimeters of the left renal artery and is easily palpated as it courses adjacent to the pancreas. Many splenic arteries are tortuous and heavily calcified. Because of the latter it may be difficult to mobilize the splenic artery extensively for the anastomosis to the renal artery without buckling or kinking the former vessel, and care in its positioning before completing an anastomosis is very important. The splenic and renal arteries or an interposition vein graft (if used) should be spatulated so as to create an ovoid anastomosis in performing these reconstructions.

Hepatorenal bypass usually requires interposition of a vein graft originating from the distal common hepatic artery in an end-to-side manner and anastomosed to the renal artery in an end-to-end fashion. Exposure of the right renal artery is similar to that for a direct endarterectomy or bypass procedure, with the dissection extending somewhat further toward the renal parenchyma so as to allow upward mobilization of the artery. Exposure of the hepatic artery is through the lesser sac, with dissection of this artery continuing distally until the gastroduodenal artery is identified and encircled with a vessel loop. In a similar fashion the more distal common hepatic and proper hepatic arteries are also dissected about their circumference and encircled with vessel loops. An inferior arteriotomy is usually made in the distal common hepatic artery, or occasionally at the origin of the gastroduodenal artery, which may be transected. The vein graft is anastomosed to this site using a fine cardiovascular suture. The graft is then carried behind the duodenum and anastomosed to the mobilized renal artery. In some patients, the gastroduodenal artery may be freed from surrounding tissues and anastomosed directly to the transected renal artery. Synthetic grafts should not be used in these procedures because of their proximity to the duodenum. Some patients have enough length of the right renal artery so as to perform a direct reimplantation into the hepatic artery (Fig. 21–5).

An iliorenal bypass using either vein or synthetic grafts should be considered in certain patients with a hostile upper abdomen that precludes a conventional aortorenal reconstruction or a nonanatomic splenorenal or hepatorenal bypass. The origin of these bypasses from the anterior surface of the proximal common iliac artery is often possible, where this vessel is usually free of calcific atherosclerotic plaque. These grafts are positioned in the retroperitoneum along side the aorta with a gentle curve at the level of the kidney, where they are anastomosed to the renal artery in an end-to-end fashion. Because dissection in the region of a previous aortic graft anastomosis may lead to

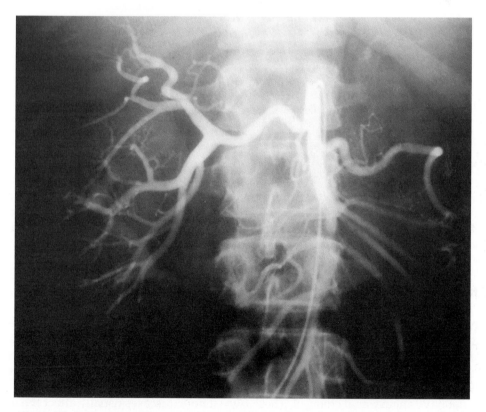

Figure 21–5. Hepatorenal bypass, with implantation of the right renal artery into an aberrant hepatic artery arising from the superior mesenteric artery, in an end-to-side fashion. (*From Stanley JC, Messina LM. Renal revascularization for recurrent pulmonary edema in patients with poorly controlled renovascular hypertension and renal insufficiency. In: Veith FJ, ed.* Current Critical Problems in Vascular Surgery, *Vol. 5. 1993:309–315, St. Louis, Missouri, Quality Medical Publishing.*)

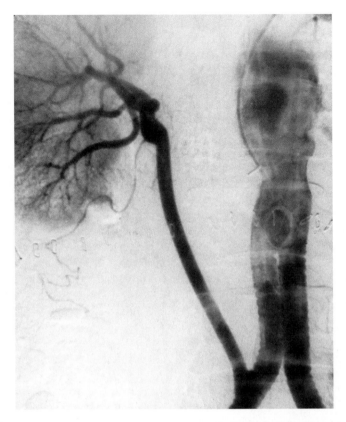

Figure 21–6. Postoperative arteriographic appearance of an ePTFE conduit taken from the limb of a previously placed Dacron aortobifemoral graft to the renal artery. (*From Messina LM, Zelenock GB, Yao KA, Stanley JC. Renal revascularization for recurrent pulmonary edema in patients with poorly controlled hypertension and renal insufficiency: a distinct subgroup of patients with arteriosclerotic renal artery occlusive disease. J Vasc Surg. 1992:15:73–82.*)

troublesome complications, patients with prosthetic grafts, such as aortofemoral bypass conduits, should have their renal graft originate from the limbs of these former conduits rather than from the proximal infrarenal aorta or graft body itself (Fig. 21–6).

RENAL ARTERY FIBRODYSPLASTIC OCCLUSIVE DISEASE

Arterial fibrodysplasia is a common cause of renal artery stenotic disease in hypertensive adult women.[24] Dysplastic lesions are categorized as to the dominant area of the vessel affected: medial fibrodysplasia, perimedial dysplasia, and intimal fibroplasia. Medial fibrodysplasia, usually presenting as serial stenoses with intervening mural aneurysms, is the most common lesion, followed by perimedial dysplasia, which is similar but does not have aneurysmal changes. These two stenotic diseases usually affect the more distal main renal artery, with extension into segmental vessels noted in 20% of cases. Renal revascularization is often complex in this group of patients.

Surgical exposure is particularly important in the treatment of fibrodysplastic stenoses. Preference is given to the use of a transverse supraumbilical abdominal incision extending from the contralateral anterior axillary line to the ipsilateral posterior axillary line, in which the rectus muscles and the oblique muscles are transected. A transverse abdominal incision provides a distinct technical advantage in the greater ease of handling instruments parallel to the longitudinal axis of the renal artery during complex procedures. Alternatively, midline vertical incisions are favored by some. The intestines are usually displaced outside the confines of the abdominal cavity.

Aortorenal Bypass

The right renal vascular pedicle and aorta are usually exposed through an extraperitoneal approach. The lateral parietes are incised from the hepatic flexure to the cecum, following which the overlying right colon, duodenum, and pancreas are reflected medially using an extended Kocher-like maneuver. The renal vein is retracted after being dissected carefully from surrounding tissues, with small branches such as those to the adrenal gland ligated and transected. This allows easy dissection of the underlying renal artery. Initial dissection of the midportion of the renal artery is less likely to result in troublesome injury to small hilar arterial and venous branches. Certain intimal lesions of the proximal right renal artery may be exposed at their origin by dissection between the aorta and the vena cava.

The left renal vessels are exposed using a similar extraperitoneal approach, with medial reflection of the viscera, including the left colon. Such an approach to the mid- and distal renal vessels is much better than exposure gained directly through an incision in the posterior retroperitoneum at the root of the mesocolon and mesentery. Adequate exposure of the left renal artery also requires mobilization of the overlying renal vein, which is facilitated by ligation and transection of its gonadal and adrenal branches.

The infrarenal aorta is dissected around its circumference for 4 to 5 cm below the origin of the renal arteries. A side-biting vascular clamp is used to partially or totally occlude the aorta after the patient is systemically anticoagulated with heparin. A lateral or anterolateral aortotomy is created, with its length approximately two to three times the graft diameter. It is unnecessary to excise an ellipse of aortic tissue, although some prefer use of an aortic punch to create a circular aortotomy.

The saphenous vein is the preferred conduit for most reconstructions in this patient population (Fig. 21–7). The vein should be removed carefully, with a branch included at its caudal end whenever possible. The adjacent walls of this branch and the parent vein are incised so that a common orifice is created. The generous circumference created by this "branch patch" lessens the likelihood of anastomotic narrowing and allows for a relatively perpendicular origin of the vein graft from the aorta. The vein graft-to-aortic anastomosis is fashioned using 4-0 or 5-0 cardiovascular suture. In some patients the hypogastric artery is used rather than saphenous vein, and in these circumstances, the branches of this vessel are similarly incised so as to create a larger orifice for anastomosis to the aorta.

The most direct route for an aortorenal graft to the right kidney is in a retrocaval position originating from a lateral aortotomy. However, some grafts are less likely to kink when arising from an anterolateral aortotomy, from which they pass in an antecaval route, then posteriorly to the renal vessels. The choice of antecaval or retrocaval positioning of grafts must be individualized. Grafts to the left kidney are almost always positioned beneath the left renal vein. The aortic clamp should remain in place during completion of the renal anastomosis. It is considered unwise to place an occluding clamp directly on the vein graft, which might be injurious and contribute to later development of a graft stenosis.

The proximal renal artery is clamped, transected, and ligated in preparation for performance of the renal anastomosis after the graft has been anastomosed to the aorta. A diuresis should be established with administration of Mannitol before interrupting

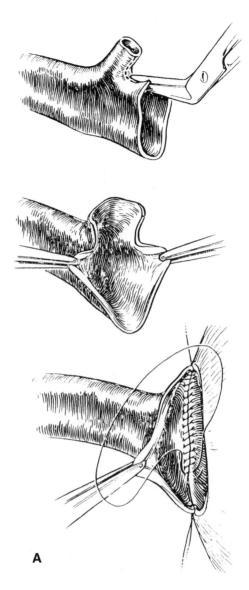

A

Figure 21–7. (A) Technique of end-to-side graft-to-aorta anastomosis following creation of a common orifice between a branch lumen and the central lumen of the saphenous vein. (*From Stanley JC, Messina LM. Renal artery fibrodysplasia and renovascular hypertension. In: Rutherford RB, ed.* Vascular Surgery, *3d ed. Philadelphia: WB Saunders; 1989:1258.*) **(B)** Postoperative arteriographic documentation of perpendicular origin of reversed saphenous vein graft from aorta, following "branch patch" maneuver. (*From Stanley JC, Messina LM, Wakefield TW, Zelenock GB. Renal artery reconstruction. In: Bergan JJ, Yao JST, eds.* Techniques in Arterial Surgery, *Philadelphia, WB Saunders; 1990:247–263.*)

renal blood flow. Preformed collateral vessels usually provide sufficient blood flow to maintain kidney viability during renal artery occlusion. Microvascular Heifetz clamps, developing noninjurious tensions from 30 to 70 gm, are used in preference to conventional macrovascular clamps or elastic slings for occluding the distal renal vessels. Because of their very small size, these microvascular clamps have the additional advantage of not obscuring the operative field.

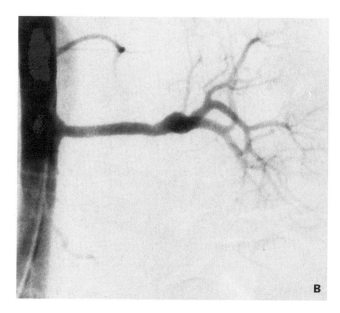

Figure 21–7. (*Continued*)

The graft-to-renal artery anastomosis is performed in an end-to-end fashion, being facilitated by spatulation of the graft posteriorly and the renal artery anteriorly (Fig. 21–8). The latter allows visualization of the artery's interior, so that inclusion of its intima with each stitch is easily assured. Stay sutures are placed through the apex of each spatulation to the tongue of the opposite vessel. In large vessel reconstructions, the anastomosis is completed using a continuous suture of 5-0 or 6-0 cardiovascular suture. In smaller arteries, 6-0 or 7-0 cardiovascular sutures are interrupted to lessen the risk of purse-string anastomotic narrowing. The spatulated anastomoses created in this manner are ovoid and are less likely to develop strictures as they heal.

Treatment of stenotic disease affecting multiple renal arteries or segmental branches may require separate implantations of the renal arteries into a single conduit (Fig. 21–9). In some circumstances it may be easier to perform side-to-side anastomoses of the diseased arteries initially, followed by an anastomosis of the graft to this common orifice (Fig. 21–10). *Ex vivo* repairs with bench construction of diseased vessels is appropriate when complex segmental renal artery fibrodysplasia is not amenable to conventional *in situ* revascularization techniques.[25–27]

Once the aortic and renal anastomoses are completed and the vascular clamps are removed, restoring antegrade renal blood flow, and the heparin anticoagulation is reversed with intravenous protamine. The adequacy of the reconstruction is then assessed using duplex scanning or a directional Doppler.

Arterial Reimplantation

Implantation of an affected artery beyond its diseased segment into an adjacent normal artery in an end-to-side manner is occasionally possible in treating select segmental or multiple renal artery stenoses. This usually involves implantations into first- or second-order branches of the renal artery, but implantation into the main renal artery may be undertaken if such can be performed without tension on the vessels. Aortic reimplanta-

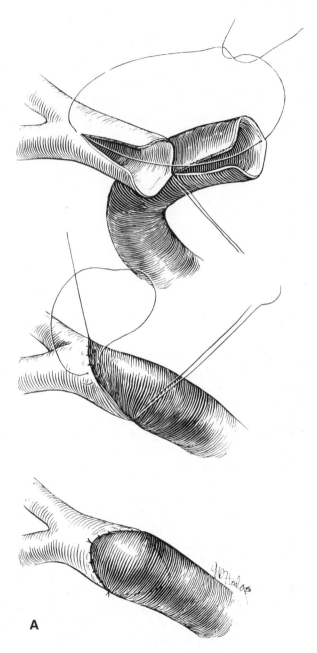

A

Figure 21–8. (A) Technique of end-to-end, vein graft-to-renal artery anastomosis following spatulation of the artery anteriorly and vein posteriorly. (*From Ernst CB, Fry WJ, Stanley JC. Surgical treatment of renovascular hypertension: revascularization with autogenous vein. In: Stanley JC, Ernst CB, Fry WJ, eds.* Renovascular Hypertension. *Philadelphia: WB Saunders; 1984:281.*) (**B**) Ovoid appearance of reversed saphenous vein–segmental renal artery anastomosis during immediate postoperative period. (*From Fry WJ, Ernst CB, Stanley JC, Brink BE. Renovascular hypertension in the pediatric patient. Arch Surg. 1973:107:692–698.*)

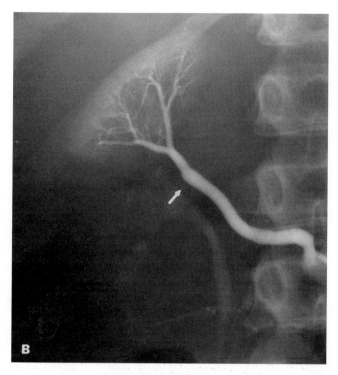

Figure 21–8. (*Continued*)

tion is occasionally possible in the management of proximal intimal lesions at the renal artery's origin. In dealing with these lesions, the renal artery should be transected beyond the orificial stenosis, then spatulated both anteriorly and posteriorly to provide a greater circumference for the end-to-side reimplantation. In the case of aortic reimplantation, it may be necessary to mobilize the kidney to reduce tension on the reimplanted renal artery.

Operative Dilation

Arterial dilation, alone or as an adjunct to conventional bypass procedures, may occasionally be used for treatment of select intraparenchymal intimal and medial fibrodysplastic stenoses.[12] This operative treatment has been supplanted in most cases by percutaneous balloon angioplasty. When undertaken, the renal artery is exposed in a manner similar to that already noted, the patient is systemically anticoagulated with heparin, and spherical- or cylindrical-tipped rigid dilators are advanced through a transverse arteriotomy in the main renal artery to the area of stenosis.

Dilators should be lubricated with heparinized blood to lessen intimal drag and endothelial cell injury. Stenotic lesions are progressively dilated in increments of 0.5 mm, with careful advancement of increasingly larger dilators. Dilators having a diameter greater than 1.0 mm larger than the normal proximal artery should not be used. Intraluminal operative dilation of fibrodysplastic renal artery stenoses using standard axial balloon catheters has certain advantages, but should only be undertaken when high-resolution fluoroscopic imaging is available.

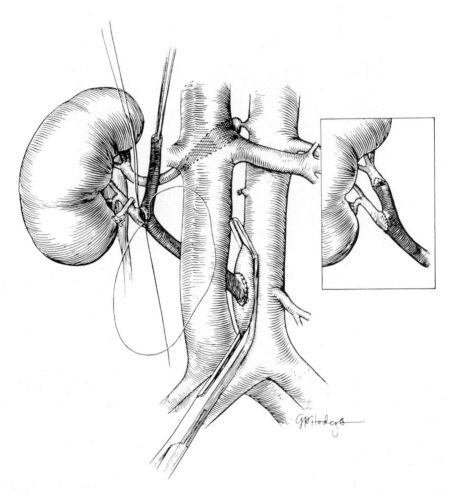

Figure 21–9. Technique of revascularization of multiple renal arteries, with subsequent anastomoses of vessels to the graft. (*From Ernst CB, Fry WJ, Stanley JC. Surgical treatment of renovascular hypertension: revascularization with autogenous vein. In: Stanley JC, Ernst CB, Fry WJ, eds.* Renovascular Hypertension. *Philadelphia: WB Saunders; 1984:283.*)

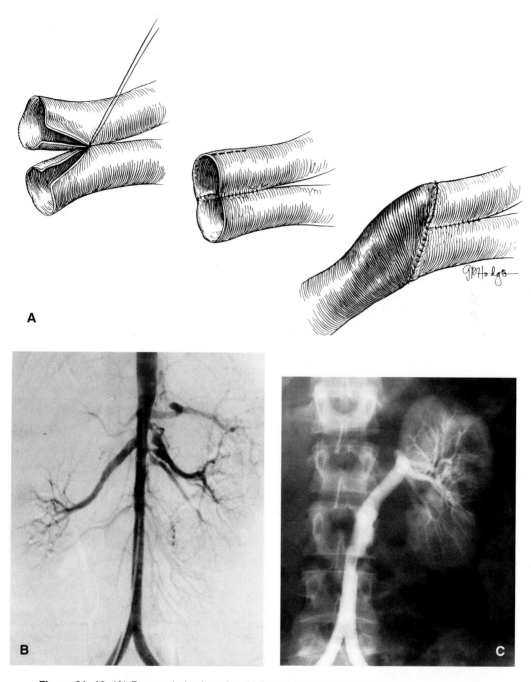

Figure 21–10. (**A**) Revascularization of multiple renal arteries with side-to-side anastomoses of affected vessels followed by anastomosis of vein graft to their common orifice. (*From Ernst CB, Fry WJ, Stanley JC. Surgical treatment of renovascular hypertension: revascularization with autogenous vein. In: Stanley JC, Ernst CB, Fry WJ, eds.* Renovascular Hypertension. *Philadelphia: WB Saunders; 1984:284.*) Preoperative (**B**) and postoperative (**C**) arteriograms of this type repair, with three vessels joined together prior to being anastomosed to a vein graft. (*From Stanley JC, Fry WJ. Pediatric renal artery occlusive disease and renovascular hypertension. Etiology, diagnosis and operative treatment.* Arch Surg *1981:116:669–676.*)

DEVELOPMENTAL OCCLUSIVE DISEASE

Developmental renal artery occlusive disease is an uncommon but important cause of blood pressure elevations in pediatric-aged patients.[28,29] The underlying renal artery stenoses are often complex and represent a heterogeneic group of diseases that must be accounted for when undertaking operative therapy. Atypical medial–perimedial dysplasia, affecting the origin of the artery, often with secondary intimal fibroplasia, exists in nearly 90% of these affected children. Nearly 40% of these renal artery lesions are bilateral. Coexistence of abdominal aortic coarctations is common, as are concomitant celiac and superior mesenteric artery narrowings.

A supraumbilical transverse abdominal incision with medial visceral rotation allows wide exposure of the renal vasculature and abdominal aorta in these young patients. In most children the intestines are eviscerated during operation, although in older children the bowel may simply be displaced to the opposite side of the abdomen. Dissection initially involves freeing the renal vein from adjacent tissues and retracting it superiorly. The proximal renal artery is dissected before mobilizing the more peripheral artery to lessen the risk of inadvertent injury to its small distal branches. The infrarenal aorta is dissected circumferentially. In cases of ostial renal artery occlusive disease, the aortorenal junction is dissected from surrounding tissues. Before aortic or renal artery occlusion in children, systemic anticoagulation is achieved with the intravenous administration of heparin 150 units/kg, and a diuresis is established, being facilitated by administration of Mannitol 0.17 gm/kg. At the conclusion of the arterial reconstruction, the heparin anticoagulation is reversed with intravenous protamine 1.5 mg/100 units of previously administered heparin.

Reimplantation

Reimplantation of the normal distal renal artery into the aorta or an adjacent renal artery after being transected beyond an ostial stenosis has become favored over an aortorenal bypass in children (Figs. 21–11 and 21–12).[29] The transected normal renal artery is spatulated arteriorly and posteriorly to create a generous anastomotic patch. An aortotomy, or arteriotomy on an adjacent renal artery, being twice the diameter of the renal artery to be reimplanted, ensures creation of a sufficiently large anastomosis. Renal artery implantation into the superior mesenteric artery is another option in these children (Fig. 21–13). Anastomoses in this age group are usually performed by use of interrupted monofilament suture depending on the size and age of the patient, with a continuous suture applicable to older patients undergoing larger renal–aortic anastomoses.

Aortorenal Bypass

The internal iliac artery has often been used in performing an aortorenal bypass in pediatric patients with developmental stenoses (Fig. 21–14).[12,29] As in the adult, the excised internal iliac artery should include a branch at its distal end that allows creation of a branch-patch orifice by incising the crotch between the branch and the trunk of the artery. Synthetic grafts, because of their potential infectivity and technical limitations in fashioning small anastomoses, and vein grafts, which commonly undergo aneurysmal dilation in children, are not favored for pediatric renal artery reconstructive procedures. If, under mitigating circumstances, a bypass must be constructed in a child with a vein graft, the conduit should be encircled with a Dacron mesh similar to that used to reinforce umbilical vein grafts.[30]

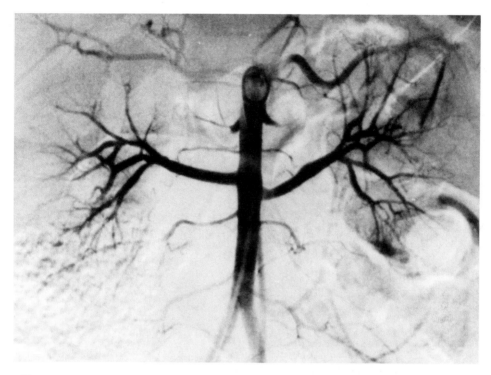

Figure 21–11. Aortic reimplantation of main renal arteries, beyond orificial stenoses. (*From Stanley JC, Zelenock GB, Messina LM, Wakefield TW. Pediatric renovascular hypertension: a thirty-year experience of operative treatment.* J Vasc Surg. *1995:21:212–227.*)

Distal renal artery-to-graft anastomoses are completed in an end-to-end manner, after spatulation of both the renal artery and the graft to increase the anastomotic circumference. Three or four running monofilament sutures are used in a discontinuous manner to allow for later growth of these anastomoses. Interrupted sutures are used in vessels 2 mm or less in diameter. If stenoses affect multiple renal arteries, the transected vessels may be anastomosed to each other to form a common orifice that then can be anastomosed to an aortorenal iliac artery graft. Parenthetically, it should be noted that splenorenal bypasses for these children are in disfavor, because of early thromboses and problems associated with the later evolution of celiac artery stenotic disease.

Thoracoabdominal Aortoaortic Bypass

A thoracoabdominal aortoaortic bypass with an expanded Teflon or fabricated Dacron prosthesis in conjunction with renal artery bypass used to be the most common operation performed for abdominal aortic narrowings and concomitant renal artery stenoses in these patients.[28] Extraperitoneal reflection of the abdominal viscera provides generous access to the proximal abdominal aorta and its renal branches in this setting. In the past, the renal artery grafts often originated from the thoracoabdominal prosthesis. However, the normal distal aorta is a better graft site of origin, because late anastomotic narrowings are less likely with autologous arterial-to-aortic anastomoses than with anastomoses to a synthetic prosthesis.

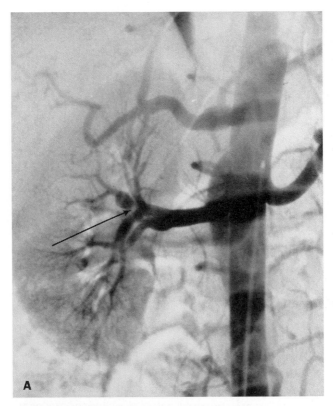

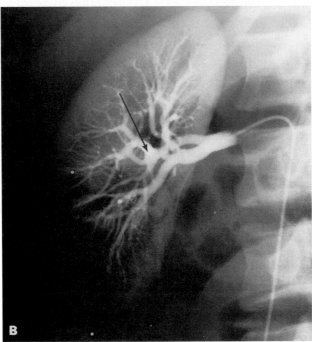

Figure 21–12. Reimplantation of segmental renal artery beyond a stenosis at its origin (**A**) on to an adjacent segmental vessel (**B**). (*From Stanley JC, Zelenock GB, Messina LM, Wakefield TW. Pediatric renovascular hypertension: a thirty-year experience of operative treatment.* J Vasc Surg. *1995:21:212–227.*)

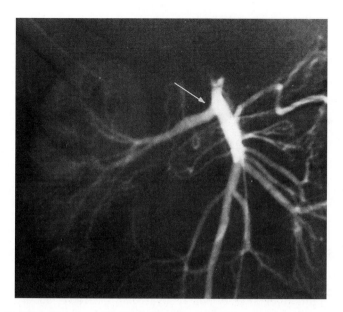

Figure 21–13. Reimplantation of right renal artery to superior mesenteric artery in an end-to-end fashion. (*From Stanley JC, Zelenock GB, Messina LM, Wakefield TW. Pediatric renovascular hypertension: a thirty-year experience of operative treatment. J Vasc Surg. 1995:21:212–227.*)

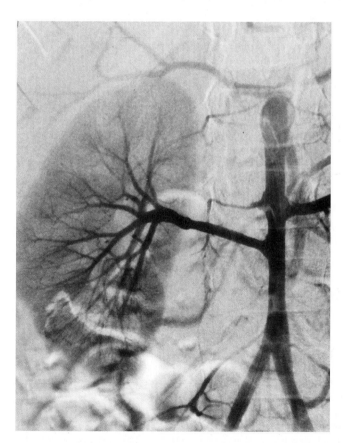

Figure 21–14. Aortorenal bypass with internal iliac artery graft. (*From Stanley JC, Zelenock GB, Messina LM, Wakefield TW. Pediatric renovascular hypertension: a thirty-year experience of operative treatment. J Vasc Surg. 1995:21:212–227.*)

Primary Patch Aortoplasty

A primary patch aortoplasty using a Teflon patch combined with reimplantation of the renal arteries into the normal distal aorta is currently preferred over a thoracoabdominal bypass and individual grafts to the renal arteries for most combined pediatric renal artery and aortic reconstructions.[29] The patch should be large enough so as not to be constrictive as the patient grows into adulthood. Avoidance of competitive parallel flow in the aorta and thoracoabdominal bypass, absence of multiple grafts to the kidneys, and performance of fewer anastomoses represent advantages of the patch aortoplasty–renal artery implantation technique.

REFERENCES

1. Stanley JC. Surgical treatment of renovascular hypertension. *Am J Surg*. 1997;174:102–110.
2. Stanley JC. Evolution of surgery for renovascular occlusive disease. *Cardiovasc Surg*. 1994;2:195–202.
3. Hallet JW, Fowl R, O'Brien PC, et al. Renovascular operations in patients with chronic renal insufficiency: do the benefits justify the risks? *J Vasc Surg*. 1987;5:622–627.
4. Hansen KJ, Thomason RB, Craven TE, et al. Surgical management of dialysis-dependent ischemic nephropathy. *J Vasc Surg*. 1995;21:197–211.
5. Messina LM, Zelenock GB, Yao KA, et al. Renal revascularization for recurrent pulmonary edema in patients with poorly controlled hypertension and renal insufficiency: a distinct subgroup of patients with arteriosclerotic renal artery occlusive disease. *J Vasc Surg*. 1992;15:73–82.
6. Whitehouse WM Jr, Kazmers A, Zelenock GB, et al. Chronic total renal artery occlusion: effects of treatment on secondary hypertension and renal function. *Surgery*. 1981;89:753–763.
7. Cambria RP, Brewster DC, L'Italien G, et al. Simultaneous aortic and renal artery reconstruction: evolution of an eighteen-year experience. *J Vasc Surg*. 1995;21:915–925.
8. Dean RH, Krueger TC, Whiteneck JM, et al. Operative management of renovascular hypertension. Results after a follow-up of fifteen to twenty-three years. *J Vasc Surg*. 1984;1:234–242.
9. Hansen KJ, Starr SM, Sands RD, et al. Contemporary surgical management of renovascular disease. *J Vasc Surg*. 1992;16:319–331.
10. Kent KC, Salvatierra O, Reilly LM, et al. Evolving strategies for the repair of complex renovascular lesions. *Ann Surg*. 1987;206:272–278.
11. Stanley JC, Ernst CB, Fry WJ. Surgical treatment of renovascular hypertension: results in specific patient subgroups. In: Stanley JC, Ernst CB, Fry WJ, eds. *Renovascular Hypertension*. Philadelphia: WB Saunders; 1984:363–371.
12. Stanley JC, Messina LM, Wakefield TW, et al. Renal artery reconstruction. In: Bergan JJ, Yao JST, eds. *Techniques in Arterial Surgery*. Philadelphia: WB Saunders; 1990:247–263.
13. Stanley JC, Whitehouse WM Jr, Graham LM, et al. Operative therapy of renovascular hypertension. *Br J Surg*. 1982;69(Suppl):S63–S66.
14. Stoney RJ, DeLuccia N, Ehrenfeld WK, et al. Aortorenal arterial autografts. Long-term assessment. *Arch Surg*. 1981;116:1416–1422.
15. Stanley JC, Whitehouse WM Jr, Zelenock GB, et al. Reoperation for complications of renal artery reconstructive surgery undertaken for treatment of renovascular hypertension. *J Vasc Surg*. 1985;2:133–144.
16. Clair DG, Belkin M, Whittemore AD, et al. Safety and efficacy of transaortic renal endarterectomy as an adjunct to aortic surgery. *J Vasc Surg*. 1995;21:926–934.
17. Dougherty MJ, Hallett JW Jr, Naessens J, et al. Renal endarterectomy vs. bypass for combined aortic and renal reconstruction: is there a difference in clinical outcome? *Ann Vasc Surg*. 1995;9:87–94.
18. Hansen KJ, O'Neil EA, Reavis SW, et al. Intraoperative duplex sonography during renal artery reconstruction. *J Vasc Surg*. 1991;14:364–374.

19. Stoney RJ, Messina LM, Goldstone J, et al. Renal endarterectomy through the transected aorta: a new technique for combined aortorenal atherosclerosis—a preliminary report. *J Vasc Surg.* 1989;9:224–233.

20. Ernst CB, Stanley JC, Fry WJ. Multiple primary and segmental renal artery revascularization utilizing autogenous saphenous vein. *Surg Gynecol Obstet.* 1973;137:1023–1026.

21. Chibaro EA, Libertino JA, Novick AC. Use of the hepatic circulation for renal revascularization. *Ann Surg.* 1984;199:406–411.

22. Khauli RB, Novick AC, Ziegelbaum M. Splenorenal bypass in the treatment of renal artery stenosis: experience with 69 cases. *J Vasc Surg.* 1985;2:547–551.

23. Moncure AC, Brewster DC, Darling RC, et al. Use of the splenic and hepatic arteries for renal revascularization. *J Vasc Surg.* 1986;3:196–203.

24. Stanley JC, Wakefield TW. Arterial fibrodysplasia. In Rutherford RB, ed. *Vascular Surgery,* 4th ed., Philadelphia: WB Saunders; 1995:264–265.

25. Brekke IB, Sodal G, Jakobsen A, et al. Fibromuscular renal artery disease treated by extracorporeal vascular reconstruction and renal autotransplantation: short- and long-term results. *Eur J Vasc Surg.* 1992;6:471–476.

26. Jordan ML, Novick AC, Cunningham RL. The role of renal autotransplantation in pediatric and young adult patients with renal artery disease. *J Vasc Surg.* 1985;2:385–392.

27. VanBockel JH, vanSchilfgaarde R, Felthuis W, et al. Long-term results of *in situ* and extracorporeal surgery for renovascular hypertension caused by fibrodysplasia. *J Vasc Surg.* 1987;6:355–364.

28. Stanley JC, Graham LM, Whitehouse WM Jr, et al. Developmental occlusive disease of the abdominal aorta, splanchnic and renal arteries. *Am J Surg.* 1981;142:190–196.

29. Stanley JC, Zelenock GB, Messina LM, et al. Pediatric renovascular hypertension: a thirty-year experience of operative treatment. *J Vasc Surg.* 1995;21:212–227.

30. Berkowitz HD, O'Neill JA Jr. Renovascular hypertension in children: surgical repair with special reference to the use of reinforced vein grafts. *J Vasc Surg.* 1989;9:46–55.

VI

Limb Ischemia Due to Infrainguinal Arterial Occlusive Disease

22

Using Low Molecular Weight
Heparin for Anticoagulation After
Lower Extremity Arterial Bypass

Walter J. McCarthy III, MD
and William D. McMillan, MD

INTRODUCTION

The use of anticoagulation after lower extremity arterial bypass remains controversial, and debate continues even after decades of clinical experience. Although there has never been an appropriate prospective randomized trial comparing anticoagulation to no treatment for patients who have had various types of arterial bypass reconstructions, there is literature on this subject. As part of this chapter the arguments based on a few fairly convincing publications are discussed for the reader. The central theme of the presentation, however, is the route for converting a patient to full anticoagulation with Coumadin using low molecular weight heparin (LMWH). Traditionally, this has been accomplished using intravenous unfractionated heparin as a bridge to full anticoagulation with Coumadin. With the availability of several LMWH products, these new medications have simplified this conversion to Coumadin anticoagulation. Although vascular surgeons debate the merits of anticoagulation after lower extremity bypass, in most practices anticoagulation is recommended at least for some patients, particularly subsets of patients with all prosthetic bypass, reconstructions. After outlining the arguments supporting anticoagulation for some patients after lower extremity bypass, the details of a case control study performed to investigate LMWH for this purpose is reviewed.

JUSTIFICATION FOR ANTICOAGULATION

It is usually taught that technical defects are the most common cause of early failure after femorodistal arterial bypass grafting. Because of such difficulties as graft twisting, kinking of the graft in tunnels, anastomotic narrowing, intimal flaps, and retained vein valves among others, these defects certainly may cause early graft occlusions. Stept and coauthors[1] reviewed the topic of early graft occlusion and found that pure technical defects were responsible for only 14.5% of the early graft occlusions in their series of 849 cases of femorodistal bypass. They also found that embolization was the cause of early failure in 9.7% of cases and inadequate arterial run-off was responsible in 11.3%. Interestingly, it seems that inadequate anticoagulation was clearly the cause in 16% of their failures, and in 48% the cause of early graft failure could not be identified. However, after thrombectomy and empiric anticoagulation, almost all of these grafts went on to long-term success. Therefore, one may surmise that in 64% of the graft failure patients empiric anticoagulation may have prevented the early thrombosis in the first place. This particular series may be somewhat biased because almost every operation included a completion arteriogram, which allows the detection of most technical errors before the patient leaves the operating room. In addition, the series included many patients with distal grafting to vessels below the knee and also utilized a high percentage of prosthetic grafts as conduit.

To assess the utility of anticoagulation following reverse saphenous vein grafting, Kretschmer and coauthors[2] compiled a prospective randomized study including 88 patients. These reconstructions included only saphenous vein and no prosthetic material and were placed either to the above- or below-the-knee popliteal position. During the second postoperative week, patients received either Dicoumarol (42 patients) or no anticoagulation (46 patients). Heparin was not used in the immediate postoperative period. The main follow-up of this group at the time of report was 30 months, during which time 19 patients had died, but none of the deaths were attributed to the anticoagulation therapy. These authors were able to show a definite trend in favor of the anticoagulation group and updated their work in 1995,[3] at which point they had been able to randomize 175 patients. In this most recent series they showed that graft failure occurred in 15 of 66 patients treated with anticoagulation, compared to 27 of the 64 control patients ($p < .01$). They also showed that the limb loss was decreased, in that 4 of 66 in the anticoagulated group lost lower extremities as compared to 13 in the control group ($p < .012$). They evaluated a secondary endpoint of mortality and showed that in the anticoagulated group only 29 of 66 died, as compared to 39 of 64 in the control cohort ($p < .029$). This study is of general interest in the argument in favor of anticoagulation, although surgical practice in the United States is generally not to anticoagulate patients who have femoropopliteal saphenous vein bypass grafts, unless there are unusual circumstances.

Edmonson and coauthors[4] report an instructive trial from the Thrombosis Research Institute in London related to LMWH. They randomized patients who were to undergo lower extremity bypass grafting to receive long-term LMWH or aspirin plus dipyridamole. The patients were to have treatment for 3 months. Follow-up was out to 12 months, and the mean follow-up of the study was about 10.5 months. This study included prosthetic and vein grafts—in fact, 75% of the grafts were prosthetic. The surgical reconstructions were 68% above-the-knee popliteal, 27% below-the-knee popliteal, and only 4% to tibial vessels. The overall Kaplan–Meier evaluation showed a significant advantage in the LMWH group for the combined series. However, subgroup analysis showed that the entire benefit seemed to lie among the patients undergoing bypass for limb salvage. In the limb salvage group, the patency for the anticoagulated group was 81.5% at 12 months as compared to 45.3% in the aspirin-dipyridamole group for a $p = .0007$. It is interesting to remember that the patients were treated with their various anticoagulation agents only for the first 3 months after bypass, and yet the benefit continued throughout the entire follow-up. The authors concluded an enthusiastic endorsement in that only 18% of their graft patients on LMWH failed at 1 year, as compared to 55% of patients using only aspirin and dipyridamole.

As a counterpoint to papers supporting anticoagulation after certain types of femoral infrainguinal bypass, Arfvidsson and coauthors[5] have come to an opposite conclusion. Their study, published in 1990, randomized all patients from their unit selected for femoral bypass, with randomization taking place just before the time of operation. All patients received postoperative unfractionated heparin for 3 to 5 days; the treatment group received long-term anticoagulation with Coumadin. Of the 116 patients randomized, all but 9 bypasses were to the popliteal, either above-the-knee (34%) or below-the-knee (66%). Thus, only 9 patients had distal anastomoses below the popliteal. In addition, only 29% of the grafts were with PTFE material, the others being with saphenous vein (42%) or an endarterectomy technique (29%). Their 3-year Kaplan–Meier plots showed strikingly similar patency between the control and treatment groups of roughly 75%, 60%, and 44% at 1, 2, and 3 years, respectively.

Morever, 13% of the treatment patients required hospitalization for bleeding complications sometime during follow-up. Interestingly, patients who had graft occlusion during the first 14 days were excluded from long-term follow-up. The authors conclusions are that from their experience, patients with femoral reconstruction should not be anticoagulated with Coumadin over the long term. We might counter in saying that their study included few patients one would expect to have had early postoperative patency difficulties, patients with prosthetic graft material placed below the knee and particularly to tibial vessels, and hardly focused on tibial reconstruction procedures at all. In addition, patients with early failures were excluded. The paper does make a strong argument that routine femoropopliteal bypass grafting may not be enhanced by long-term anticoagulation.

USING LOW MOLECULAR WEIGHT HEPARIN AS A BRIDGE TO ANTICOAGULATION

With this background and acknowledging that there are no wholly convincing randomized studies that apply to prosthetic bypass grafting below the knee, the following policy was established at Northwestern University. When prosthetic material is included in the femoral reconstruction and the distal extent of that bypass is below the knee, the patient is maintained on heparin after the operation, then converted to long-term anticoagulation with Coumadin if anticoagulation is compatible with reasonable medical safety. This would include any femoral to below-the-knee popliteal PTFE bypass graft, or any more complicated configurations, including PTFE material to the tibial vessels or composite–sequential bypass grafting to the tibial vessels. Patients with a totally venous conduit reconstruction are anticoagulated in the same way only if they have had multiple failures of bypass grafting or the distal anastomosis is to a particularly compromised run-off artery or the vein graft material itself is compromised. Thus, all venous reconstructions are not routinely anticoagulated, regardless of the location of their distal anastomosis. Occasionally patients who have failed a bypass graft reconstruction on Coumadin anticoagulation are treated after a subsequent reconstruction using Coumadin plus aspirin.

Many recent studies have suggested that subcutaneous LMWH is a safe and effective alternative to intravenous heparin to treat deep venous thrombosis and even pulmonary embolism. Realizing that some patients on the collective vascular service at Northwestern were delayed in their discharge home because their prothrombin time was not adequate to allow discontinuation of intravenous heparin, the following study was envisioned.[6] Our hypothesis was that LMWH and IV heparin would be equally effective in preventing postoperative bypass graft thrombosis while effective Coumadin anticoagulation was being established. We also felt that the rate of postoperative hematoma formation would be equal or even perhaps reduced with LMWH. As end points, we speculated that LMWH would reduce hospital lengths of stay and also reduce the number of coagulation monitoring studies required before discharge. The reason for this is that LMWH is not usually evaluated with any particular laboratory monitoring value, such as the activated partial prothromboplastin time used with the parent unfractionated heparin compound.

To study this problem we used a nonrandomized case control method in which historical controls were compared to the treatment group. During a 32-month period at Northwestern Memorial Hospital, 361 infrainguinal bypass procedures were performed, including 76 that were infrageniculate and included PTFE graft material for limb salvage. Seven patients were actually excluded from this group of 76 because we felt they had an absolute indication for IV heparin including ventricular thrombus (1 patient), prosthetic heart valve (2 patients), cardiac dysrhythmia (2 patients), and documented hypercoagulable syndromes (2 patients). Therefore, 68 patients who had 69 bypass procedures make up the study group. All patients were given 5000 units of IV heparin in the operating room before the application of vascular clamps. The study group of 28 grafts receiving LMWH (Lovenox, Rone-Poulenc Rore, Collegeville, PA) were operated on between October 2, 1994, and February 1, 1996. Each received 60 mg of the LMWH administered subcutaneously twice a day, with the first dose given in the recovery room. The control group, which was anticoagulated with IV heparin, included 41 consecutive patients operated on between June 1, 1993, and October 1, 1994. This control group had postoperative IV heparin to maintain a partial thromboplastin time of 55 to 75 sec. In both groups the initial dose of warfarin was given the evening of the first day after surgery, and the anticoagulation with warfarin was established with an international normalization ratio of 2.0 to 3.0.

All 76 patients had saphenous vein inadequate to complete an entirely autologous bypass graft. There were similar numbers of patients in each group with foot ulceration, gangrene, and rest pain. Patients were also evenly matched comparing the number of patients requiring secondary procedures and patients requiring different types of foot amputation during the same hospitalization. All bypass grafts in the entire group used the femoral artery as their inflow source.

There were not significant differences in the morbidity between groups (IV heparin 19%; LMWH 11%; p = NS). The mortality rates were also similar (IV heparin 2.5%; LMWH, 4%; p = NS). One patient in the LMWH group died of a hemorrhagic stroke on postoperative day 30 after having been converted to warfarin and having been off the LMWH for 3 days. Another patient in the IV heparin group died of a ruptured thoracic aneurysm on postoperative day 14, 6 days after a conversion to oral warfarin.

The postoperative graft thrombosis rate was remarkably low, with only one patient overall (in the IV heparin group) requiring thrombectomy of a composite sequential graft on postoperative day 3. Hematoma formation requiring reoperation was noticed in two patients (7%) from the LMWH group and 5 patients (12.5%) from the IV heparin group.

There were significant differences in the length of postoperative stay and the number of coagulation monitoring studies performed between groups. The main postoperative hospital stay for the LMWH group was 7.2 days (SD, ±3.7 days) and patients with IV heparin required an average of 9.5 days (SD, ±3.3 days) (p < .008). Also, the number of coagulation monitoring studies required before conversion to warfarin in patients with LMWH was significantly less (8.2 ± 4.2) when compared to the IV heparin group (22.0 ± 7.7) (p < .0001).

SUMMARY

Clearly, the exact indications for long-term anticoagulation after femoropopliteal or distal bypass are not established by prospective randomized trials.[7,8] However, when anticoagulation seems appropriate, this study, which is preliminary in nature and not randomized, suggests that LMWH is safe and effective when compared to IV heparin for the conversion of patients to oral anticoagulation after distal bypass grafting. The use of LMWH seems to reduce the length of hospital stay required and also the number of monitoring studies involved in the anticoagulation of patients. As a cautionary note, work has documented postoperative paraspinal bleeding related to spinal anesthetic techniques in patients who have received LMWH, and this may constitute a real contraindication to LMWH use. In addition, patients who are in renal failure do not manage LMWH in a predictable manner and may also be inappropriate for this medication. However, most patients who require anticoagulation after femoral bypass can be managed conveniently and safely using LMWH as a bridge to full anticoagulation with Coumadin.

REFERENCES

1. Stept LL, Flinn WR, McCarthy WJ, Bartlett ST, et al. Technical defects as a cause of early graft failure after femoro-distal bypass. *Arch Surg.* 1987;122(5):599–604.
2. Kretschmer G, Wenzl E, Piza F, Polterauer P, et al. The influence of anticoagulant treatment on the probability of function in femoropopliteal vein bypass surgery: analysis of a clinical series (1970–85) and interim evaluation of a controlled clinical trial. *Surgery.* 1987;102(3): 453–459.
3. Kretschmer GJ, Holzenbein T. The role of anticoagulation in infrainguinal bypass surgery. In: Yao JST, Pearce WH, eds. *The Ischemic Extremity: Advances in Treatment.* East Norwalk CT: Appleton & Lange, 1995:447–454.
4. Edmonson RA, Cohen AT, Das SK, Wagner MB, et al. Low-molecular weight heparin versus aspirin and dipyridamole after femoropopliteal bypass grafting. *Lancet.* 1994;344:914–918.
5. Arfvidsson B, Lundgren F, Drott C, Schersten T, et al. Influence of coumarin treatment on patency and limb salvage after peripheral arterial reconstructive surgery. *Am J Surg.* 1990;159:556–560.
6. McMillan WD, McCarthy WJ, Lin SJ, Matsumura JS, et al. Perioperative low molecular weight heparin for infrageniculate bypass. *J Vasc Surg.* 1998;25:5;796–801.
7. Clagett GP. Antithrombotic therapy for lower extremity bypass. *J Vasc Surg.* 1992;15:873–875.
8. Clagett GP, Krupski WC. Antithrombotic therapy in peripheral arterial occlusive disease. *Chest.* 1995;108(4):431S–433S.

23

Management of Inguinal Wound Healing

Complications of Inguinal Wounds

Jonathan B. Towne, MD and Douglas A. Coe, MD

The inguinal region is vulnerable to wound healing complications following vascular surgical reconstruction. The femoral neurovascular bundle is placed subcutaneously without adjacent muscles to protect it when there is skin breakdown, which often results in problems in the relatively avascular subcutaneous tissue, which is quite prone to infection or necrosis. The groin is also a major lymphatic terminus receiving lymphatic channels from the buttocks, lower abdominal wall, and leg. Because many patients undergoing lower limb vascular surgery have either ulcerations or wounds on their feet, there is an increased presence of bacteria in the draining lymph fluid, that can serve as a source of infection. A third factor that makes groin wounds prone to wound healing complications is the fact that, particularly in obese people, the groin skin usually is covered by the overlying paniculus, which often creates a warm moist environment which is ideal for bacterial overgrowth.

Three different types of vascular procedures are performed on the groin. The first uses the groin as outflow source for intra-abdominal prosthetic bypasses. More commonly, these are done in the treatment of abdominal aortic aneurysm and, less frequently, with the evolution of iliac angioplasty for straightforward aortofemoral bypasses. The second group consists of a variety of repairs for lower limb bypass using autogenous material. Because there is an inherent resistance of infection with autogenous material the risk of graft infection is less but not nonexistent. Finally, the groin can be the site of artificial prosthetic materials used either for patch angioplasties in the groin or for the inflow of prosthetic femorodistal bypasses. This chapter deals with the variety of wound healing complications in the groin discussing the etiology and outlining the treatment options.

THE DRAINING GROIN WOUND

Drainage of the groin wound early in the postoperative period is often the result of divided lymphatics that have not sealed. These complications are a common problem in patients who have undergone kidney transplantation, presumably caused by an increase in lymph drainage from placement of the doner kidney in the lower quadrant. The problems caused by a lymph leak were documented in a series of 126 consecutive patients, reported by Reifsnyder and coworkers,[1] who underwent *in situ* bypasses of the lower extremity. Risk factor analysis demonstrated that the development of a postoperative lymph leak was significantly related to the subsequent wound infections. In an animal model, Rubin and colleagues[2] demonstrated that lymphatics contaminated with bacteria resulted in positive blood and graft cultures. Experimentally, transsection of lymphatics at the graft site in the presence of a distal infection leads to significantly more graft infections compared to lymphatic ligation and exclusion. Lymphatic bacterial transport contributed to the graft infection both from direct seeding and transmission of bacteria to the blood leading to seeding of the graft.

TREATMENT

Because of the relationship of lymph leak with subsequent significant wound infections, these patients should be treated very aggressively. Our initial plan is to paint the wound with Betadine and apply a tight dressing. Antibiotics, usually cephalosporins, are given and the patient is placed on bed rest. If the wound continues to drain for longer than 72 h, the patient should be returned to the operating room and the wound explored. The offending lymphatic often can be identified and suture ligated. Autogenous tissue should be placed over the graft and the wound closed in layers. A subcutaneous drain, well separated from the arterial prosthesis, is then brought out through a separate stab hole. Placement of the drain allows the skin incision to heal. This technique is generally successful in controlling the wound drainage and, more importantly, prevents the secondary infection of the lymphatic cavity.

LYMPHOCELE

Patients who develop lymphoceles following groin surgery are followed expectantly. If the lymphoceles increase in size with time, they should be explored operatively and treated as noted previously in the leaking wound. Likewise, if they come into communication with the groin wound and begin to leak they should also be explored. Small- to moderate-size lymphoceles that are away from the incision and do not involve the graft can be followed, and many times they will slowly resolve with time. Lymphoceles also can be treated operatively if they become large or uncomfortable for the patient, or if it distends the groin suture wound, should be treated operatively as well. The injection of isosulfan blue into the foot prior to the operation helps in identifying lymphatic channels that feed the lymphocele. The use of duplex ultrasound can clearly identify the lymphocele and determine if it is adjacent to the prosthesis. Lymphoceles that are in close proximity to the vascular prosthesis are best drained surgically in order to prevent any possible secondary infection of the vascular graft. When the lymphocele is well separated from the vascular prosthesis, sclerotherapy using powdered tetracycline can be used. Powdered tetracycline mixed with sterile saline and injected into the lymphocele, will often sclerose a lymphocele.[3] The most important factor in dealing with lymphatic problems of the groin is prevention by doing meticulous dissection, with ligation of any lymphatic channels that are noted during vascular exposure. In particular, if a lymph node is inadvertently bisected during the dissection, both halves should be suture ligated.

CLASSIFICATION OF GROIN WOUND COMPLICATIONS

Patients with wound complications are classified using the modification by Wengrovitz and associates[4] of the Szialgyi[5] system developed for grading wound complications after prosthetic arterial reconstruction. These were: Class I—wound edge skin necrosis or lymphatic leak treated with parenteral antibiotics. Class II—wound infections or necrosis involving the subcutaneous tissue. Class III—invasive wound infections to the depth of the wound about the graft.

TYPE OF CLOSURE

There are many divergent views as to the effect of the type of closure on ultimate healing of both groin and leg incisions. It is the authors' bias that the surgical skill and technique of the closure rather than the particular technique is what influences results most favorably. On our surgical service, the most senior surgeon closes the groin. When the surgical team begins to attend to the wound closure technique, operative results always improve. In a prospective study of different techniques at skin closure, Murphy and coworkers[6] randomized patients between subcuticular, interrupted nylon, continuous nylon, or metallic clip closure. They noted no significant differences between the treatment groups, emphasizing that meticulous closure is the most important determinant in avoiding groin wound complications.

INCIDENCE OF INFECTION

The incidence of infrainguinal bypass graft infection ranges from 1.5% to 12% for prosthetic grafts and up to 1.7% for autogenous grafts.[7,8] Several important risk factors predispose to subsequent graft infection. Wound healing complications such as skin or subcutaneous tissue necrosis, cellulitis, hematoma, or lymphatic leak increases the risk of subsequent graft infection significantly, and can occur in up to 44% of infrainguinal bypass procedures.[9] In a study assessing risk factors for primary graft infections, Edwards and colleagues[10] identified postoperative wound infection as the primary predisposing factor in 33% of subsequent graft infections. Likewise, Cherry and coworkers[11] reviewed 39 cases of infrainguinal graft infections and found that postoperative wound infection occurred in 28% of cases. The presence of a groin incision greatly increases the risk of both wound and graft infections. In a study of 2411 consecutive prosthetic arterial reconstructions, 3.5% of 489 femoroperipheral reconstructions developed graft infection, which occurred only when a groin incision had been used.[12] Other risk factors for infectious complications include emergency bypass procedures and the need for early reoperation for graft thrombosis or bleeding. In a review of their arterial graft infections, Hoffert and associates[7] found that 50% of conduit infections had required early reoperation for postoperative hematoma formation, and in the series reported by Kent and coworkers[9], infectious complications were associated with emergent operations in 13% of cases.

Multiple factors predispose to wound infections and relate to specific patient characteristics. In a review of 126 consecutive patients who underwent *in situ* vein bypass, Reifsnyder and colleagues[1] found that early graft revision (<4 days) and the presence of a lymph leak significantly increased the risk for postoperative wound infection. However, factors such as age, race, diabetes, duration of operation, and presence of gangrene or ulceration did not significantly influence the incidence of infectious complications in that series. Wengrovitz and coworkers[4] retrospectively studied 163 subcutaneous saphenous vein bypasses and found on regression analysis that chronic steroid use, ipsilateral ulceration, and pedal bypasses predicted an increased incidence of wound infection. They also identified female sex, diabetes, use of continuous incisions, and procedures for limb salvage as factors associated with wound complications in their group of patients.

The natural history of graft infection depends partly on the timing of presentation, which has a widely variable interval between implantation and recognition of the infection. Multiple studies have indicated that wound and graft infections tend to occur early. In the study performed by Lorentzen and coworkers[12], 85% of graft infections occurred in the first 30 days. Likewise, Liekweg and coworkers[13] reported that 85% of groin wound infections in their series presented within 5 weeks of the initial operation. However, graft infection may not become clinically evident for months to years after placement. Early graft infections are usually easily identified due to associated wound complications and signs of systemic inflammation. Graft infections that present in a delayed fashion, however, usually do not present with signs of sepsis and are associated with more nonspecific symptoms.

Morbidity and mortality associated with graft infection depends not only on the timing of presentation, but also on microbiology, graft location, and method of treatment. Unrecognized or inadequately treated infrainguinal graft infection has a mortality rate ranging between 0% and 22% and results in amputation in between 8% and 53% of cases, with one series reporting an amputation rate of 79%.[5,14,15]

PATHOPHYSIOLOGY

The primary cause of infectious wound or graft complications involves contamination at the time of surgery. Contamination can occur when the graft contacts the skin and from breaks in surgical technique. Emergent operations potentially increase the risk for infectious complications because of lack of attention to sterile technique and possibly due to immunologic status of the stressed patient. Early reoperation also increases the risk of infection secondary to increased exposure of the graft to potential contamination and from any retained thrombus or debris, which can serve as potent culture media. In addition, factors such as prolonged operative times and extended preoperative hospitalization are thought to contribute to risk of wound and graft infection. Levy and coworkers[16] prospectively obtained skin flora cultures in patients undergoing lower extremity revascularization[16] on the day of admission, the day of surgery, and 5 days postoperatively. They demonstrated that patients enter the hospital colonized with slime-producing coagulase-negative staphylococci and that strains shift from predominantly susceptible to predominantly resistant species.

Colonization of native artery can be a source of graft contamination. Macbeth and colleagues[17] cultured arterial specimens and surrounding tissue (as controls) from patients undergoing clean, elective prosthetic arterial reconstructions.[17] Forty-three percent of arterial segments were culture positive with *Staphylococcus epidermidis* as the most common isolate, whereas all controls were sterile. Correlation of culture data to subsequent suture line disruption in infected grafts at their institution revealed that positive arterial cultures were associated with disruption in 57% of cases, whereas there were no anastomotic disruptions in patients with negative arterial cultures. Durham and associates[18] corroborated this data with a 43% culture-positive rate and noted that graft infections occurred only in culture-positive arteries. In addition, they found that positive arterial cultures had no predictive value regarding graft infection at initial operations, but that positive arterial cultures were associated with eventual graft infection in 28% of patients undergoing subsequent vascular reconstructions.

Another potential source of graft infection is from hematogenous or lymphatic seeding from remote sites of infection or colonization. Experiments in dogs have demonstrated intravenous infusion of 10^7 colony-forming units of *Staphylococcus aureus* produce clinical graft infection in nearly 100% of animals in the early postoperative period.[19] The lymphatic system has also been implicated in the pathogenesis of graft infection originating from a distal septic focus such as an infected ischemic foot ulcer by both hematogenous spread and from direct seeding of the graft. Experimentally, transection of lymphatics at the graft site in the presence of a distal infection leads to significantly more graft infections compared to lymphatic ligation and excision.[2] Lymphatic bacterial transport can contribute to graft infection both from direct graft seeding and from transmission of bacteria to the blood, leading to hematogenous seeding of the graft.

The propensity for a graft to become infected decreases with time due to development of a pseudointimal layer and incorporation within surrounding tissues, but the graft can remain at significant risk for as long as a year after implantation. Even years after implantation, the graft can be seeded by bacteremia, thought to be due to an incomplete pseudointimal lining. To what extent this mechanism contributes to the pathogenesis of graft infection in humans is unknown, but bacteremia has been associated with such procedures as central venous or bladder catheterization, GI endoscopy, dental or genitourinary instrumentation, and in patients harboring remote infections such as pneumonia, endocarditis, and distal foot infections.

The potential for graft infection is also influenced by the patient's immunocompetence and immune factors associated with the graft itself. The sequence of events involved with vascular graft infection is initiated by adhesion of bacteria to the graft surface. Subsequent colonization and biofilm production leads to activation of the host's immune response producing an inflammatory reaction involving perigraft tissues and the graft–artery anastomosis.[20] Prosthetic materials initiate an inflammatory response characterized by an acidic, ischemic environment that is inhibitory to normal host defenses and antibiotic activity, further promoting bacterial replication. Autogenous grafts, however, develop rich microvascular connections and are thereby much more resistant to bacterial growth and subsequent infection. Patients with impaired immunocompetence, such as those with malnutrition, malignancy, chemotherapy, chronic steroid use, and chronic renal failure, are potentially at increased risk of infectious complications due to inadequate host defense.

The degree to which the previously mentioned sequence of events occurs also depends in large part on the bacterial species and the characteristics of the graft material. The virulence of coagulase-positive staphylococci is enhanced by release of exotoxin and an extracellular mucin that protects the organism against antibiotics, antibodies, and phagocytes.[21] In addition, bacterial adhesion to graft materials is related to physical characteristics of the graft. Bacterial adherence to dacron has been shown to be 10 to 100 times greater than to polytetrafluoroethylene (PTFE).[22] This interaction is particularly important in less virulent strains responsible for delayed infection. Organisms such as

S. epidermidis reside in the interstices of the graft and produce an extracellular glycocalyx biofilm that provides an excellent protective environment for persistent growth.

The site of contamination and subsequent infection usually starts at one point along the course of the graft and can involve either the body of the graft or the anastomotic region. If the process is able to decompress through a sinus tract to the skin, the infection can remain localized. If, however, external drainage does not occur, infected fluid tracks along the course of the graft in the potential space between the conduit and perigraft tissues to involve the entire conduit. If anastomotic involvement ensues, destruction of the involved artery will occur, leading to disruption of the anastomosis with pseudoaneurysm formation.

MICROBIOLOGY

The bacteriology of graft infections has changed and is influenced by multiple factors. Most infections are due to bacteria, but other microorganisms have been recovered including fungi and, in aortic grafts, mycobacteria and mycoplasma.[23,24] In the past, *Staphylococcus aureus* was the predominant pathogen and was isolated in up to 50% of cases. More recently, graft infections due to *S. epidermidis* and gram-negative bacteria have increased in frequency. Specimen acquisition and culture technique has a significant impact on the species recovered. Sampling error can occur when lower numbers of bacteria are present despite gross clinical signs of infection. In particular, delayed infections due to *S. epidermidis* and other coagulase-negative staphylococci are frequently associated with negative culture results.[25]

The timing of graft infection has significant implications as to the bacteriology involved in the process. Early infections (infections that present within four months of surgery) are associated with particularly virulent strains of bacteria, with *S. aureus* being the most prevalent. These bacteria produce exotoxin and enzymes that enhance its virulence and induce an intense local and systemic inflammatory response. Although less common, gram-negative organisms such as *Proteus, Klebsiella,* and *Enterobacter* can also be responsible for early graft infections. *Pseudomonas,* an aerobic gram-negative rod, is a particularly aggressive pathogen and is frequently associated with anastomotic breakdown with bleeding.

Delayed graft infections (those presenting months to years after implantation) are usually associated with less virulent bacteria. *Staphylococcus epidermidis* and other coagulase-negative organisms have limited ability for tissue invasion and generally require the presence of a foreign body for prolonged survival.[26] Colonization by coagulase-negative staphylococci is confined to a perigraft biofilm, which contains a relatively low concentration of organisms. However, with time, the biofilm is recognized by the host's defenses and produces an inflammatory response with tissue-damaging effects. The process is insidious with few signs of systemic inflammation (fever, leukocytosis), but is capable of anastomotic disruption with pseudoaneurysm formation or development of cutaneous fistulas.

Acquisition of bacteria from graft and wound infections is necessary to guide subsequent antibiotic therapy. Studies often demonstrate a significant incidence of negative cultures despite convincing evidence of infection. This can be due to absence of tissue invasion, presence of a surface biofilm, low numbers of organisms, and concomitant antibiotic use. Virulent strains of bacteria (coagulase-positive staphylococci, gram-negatives) are easily recovered due to invasion of the bloodstream and more advanced tissue invasion. However, coagulase-negative staphylococci do not infiltrate tissues to the same extent and often are missed on routine swab culture; more sensitive techniques are required for their isolation. One such method involves submersion of a portion of several different regions of the graft and surrounding tissue in broth media with disruption of the graft, using either mechanical grinding or ultrasonication. This disperses the organisms in the media for increased bacterial growth despite negative Gram stain and routine culture results.[25] In addition, there should be communication between the surgeon and the microbiology laboratory regarding the clinical situation and potential suspected pathogens.

PRESENTATION

Presentation of graft infection ranges from deceptively subtle signs and symptoms to massive infection with life-threatening systemic sepsis or hemorrhage. Peripheral infections are generally easier to diagnose than their intracavitary counterparts, but prompt diagnosis and treatment is necessary if subsequent morbidity and mortality are to be avoided.

Wound healing complications such as hematoma, lymphocele, or tissue necrosis usually precede deeper involvement. Timing of infection determines to a large extent how the process presents. Early graft infections usually present in conjunction with wound infection and are associated with signs of systemic sepsis including fever, leukocytosis, and bacteremia. The initial presenting sign of graft infection in up to a quarter of patients is anastomotic disruption with potential exsanguinating hemorrhage.[10] Groin wounds are most commonly involved, and the majority of patients presenting with graft infection at the groin present with overt signs of wound sepsis with abscess formation, cellulitis, sinus tract development, or graft exposure. Less commonly, deeper infection may be heralded by distal petechiae from septic microembolization, graft thrombosis, or a pulsatile mass over an anastomotic site. These infections tend to occur within the first weeks of surgery and are generally associated with coagulase-positive staphylococci or virulent Gram-negative organisms.

The diagnosis of delayed graft infection is more difficult due to the less virulent nature of the causative organisms and the presence of a perigraft biofilm. Involvement can occur anywhere along the graft but most commonly occurs at femoral anastomoses. Systemic signs are usually absent, although the patient may complain of malaise, localized pain, and tenderness. Commonly, there is inflammation of perigraft tissues with erythema of the overlying skin, a palpable perigraft inflammatory mass, or a cutaneous sinus tract. Many of the superficial signs are temporarily improved with systemic antibiotics, only to return with cessation of therapy.

Laboratory studies in patients with suspected infrainguinal graft infections are nonspecific and frequently of little assistance in confirming the diagnosis. Leukocytosis with a left shift is common in patients presenting with early wound and graft infection, but may be normal in delayed infections. Likewise, the erythrocyte sedimentation rate (ESR) is elevated, but is a nonspecific finding. Blood cultures should be obtained but can be negative in a significant number of documented infections. Urinalysis should be performed, and culture data should be obtained from other sites such as foot and surgical wound drainage to rule out other sources of infection.

DIAGNOSIS

Ultrasonography

Duplex ultrasonography has great utility in the evaluation of patients with suspected graft infection, and is considered by some to be the initial diagnostic modality of choice.[27] It is particularly useful in the evaluation of pulsatile masses and can differentiate perigraft fluid collections and hematomas from pseudoaneurysms with a high degree of accuracy.[28] If an abnormal fluid collection is identified, aspiration under ultrasound guidance can be performed (Figs. 23–1 and 23–2; see color insert). Graft incorporation can be determined and vessel patency is easily confirmed using color flow and spectral analysis.

The advantages of this modality include its widespread availability, which does not involve radiation exposure or the use of intravenous contrast. It is noninvasive and easily portable, which make it useful in the initial evaluation of critically ill patients. Scan quality is technician dependent and intra- and interexaminer studies may not be consistent. Furthermore, ultrasound is unable to differentiate infected from sterile fluid collections and tissue plane resolution is inferior to that of other imaging modalities.

Computed Tomography

Although computed tomography (CT) scanning is more commonly used in the evaluation of suspected intra-abdominal graft infection, it has utility in diagnosing peripheral graft infections as well. As with ultrasonography, CT can identify abnormal fluid collections and the presence of anastomotic pseudoaneurysms (Fig. 23–3). CT-guided needle aspiration can be performed if an abnormal fluid collection is identified. In addition, the entire length of the conduit can be examined, and vessel patency can be determined. However, CT is superior to ultrasound in defining various characteristics of the inflammatory process. Loss of normal tissue planes and presence of air around the graft, indicative of soft-tissue inflammation, are among the CT criteria for graft infection[29] and are more clearly visualized by CT when compared to ultrasound. Unlike

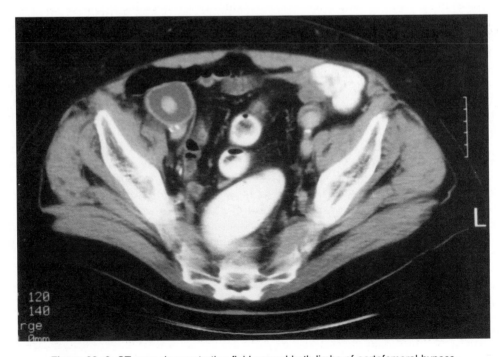

Figure 23–3. CT scan demonstrating fluid around both limbs of aortofemoral bypass.

ultrasonography, CT is not technician-dependent and has higher consistency with sequential scans.

Magnetic Resonance Imaging

Magnetic resonance imaging (MRI) is a relatively new modality for assessment of patients with possible graft infection. Most studies evaluating the efficacy of MRI in diagnosing graft infection have been with caviteric prostheses in which it has a reported overall accuracy of 88% to 94%.[30] Criteria for graft infection are similar to those of CT scan and include identification of abnormal perigraft fluid collections and loss of normal tissue planes around the graft. However, MRI has several advantages over CT scanning. First, MRI has the ability to reconstruct images in multiple planes, thereby providing better visualization of the extent of the infectious process. Second, intravenous contrast is not required to determine vessel patency due to a black "flow void" created by flowing blood on the MR image. Finally, MRI is thought by some clinicians to be more sensitive in revealing small fluid collections and soft-tissue changes due to better resolution between tissue and fluid densities.[30]

Disadvantages of MRI include its inability to differentiate infected from sterile fluid collections and the inability of differentiating perigraft gas from calcium. At present, image acquisition times are relatively long and MR-guided aspiration is cumbersome. Furthermore, the technology is costly and not universally available, and there exists a population of patients who are unable to tolerate the procedure.

Functional Imaging

Radionuclide scans using [111]Indium-labeled leukocytes and polyclonal immunoglobulin G have an adjunctive role in the diagnosis of vascular graft infection. They cannot be performed in the early postoperative period due to nonspecific uptake of signal by healing tissues. A study by Sedwitz and coworkers[31] reported a sensitivity of 100% but a specificity of 50% and an accuracy of 53% for detecting wound complications. A negative scan was reliable in ruling out an infectious process in this series. LaMuraglia and colleagues[32] studied 25 patients suspected of having graft infection using [111]Indium-labeled human IgG and reported a sensitivity of 93%, a specificity of 100%, and an accuracy of 96%. IgG scans are generally preferred over leukocyte scans because of the absence of red cell and platelet labeling and lack of exposure of the staff to blood products. Currently, functional imaging is best utilized in conjunction with anatomic imaging to better determine the location and extent of infection.

Contrast Angiography

Angiography provides little diagnostic information when evaluating a patient for graft infection, but is vital for planning therapeutic strategies. Angiograms demonstrate vessel occlusion and pseudoaneurysms, but these are also well demonstrated using duplex ultrasound and CT scanning. The utility of angiography comes in assessing the proximal and distal vascular tree for subsequent arterial reconstruction.

MANAGEMENT

General Principles

The basic goals of therapy in patients with lower extremity graft infection are the eradication of infection and the maintenance of adequate distal perfusion. Management in these patients must be highly individualized, and is dependent on factors such as the severity of the patient's clinical presentation (anastomotic hemorrhage, hemodynamic instability, signs of systemic sepsis), the extent and microbiology of the infection, the type of graft, patient comorbidity, and status of the patient's native vasculature. All surgical options should be considered, but the axiom "life over limb" must always be observed when formulating the therapeutic plan.

Initial treatment involves a thorough history and physical examination to determine the acuity of the patient's illness. Patients who present in shock due to sepsis or hypovolemia from hemorrhage require expeditious evaluation and initiation of treatment. Aggressive resuscitative efforts with blood and fluid volume in an intensive care setting is imperative in these critically ill patients. Broad-spectrum antibiotics are started early in the patient's initial hospital course, and development of a surgical strategy can proceed during the initial resuscitative period.

For patients who present with less acute symptomatology, time exists to thoroughly evaluate and optimize the patient's comorbid conditions in preparation for surgery. Again, broad-spectrum antibiotics should be started and then tailored based on sensitivity results from wound or aspiration culture. Imaging studies should be performed concomitantly to determine the nature, extent, and location of the infectious process. Finally, frank discussions with the patient regarding potential surgical options, morbidity, and mortality should also take place.

Wound Infection

Wound infection after infrainguinal arterial reconstruction is common and can occur in up to 44% of procedures.[9] Risk factors and classification of wound infection are discussed previously and impact on subsequent treatment. Classes I and II infections are considered "minor" and generally respond to operative debridement, local wound care, and intravenous antibiotics. Class III wounds with graft exposure are of more concern and are associated with more conduit complications. The prime management objectives of these wounds are early surgical debridement, drainage of any clinically significant fluid collections, and conformation of autogenous tissue coverage.[33] Ouriel and colleagues[8] managed wounds in 16 patients with exposed autogenous vein grafts with local wound care and delayed autogenous tissue coverage until adequate granulation had developed. They reported hemorrhage or thrombosis in 56% of cases managed in this manner. Alternatively, Reifsnyder and colleagues[1] described their experience with wound complication management with *early* operative debridement, autogenous tissue coverage when indicated, three times daily dressing changes and parenteral antibiotics in 55 wound infections, 13 of which were graft-threatening. This management protocol resulted in no deaths, no limb loss, and universal graft salvage. There must be a high index of suspicion of graft involvement in any wound infection, and early surgical inspection to rule out graft involvement is required if overt conduit infection is to be avoided.

Prosthetic Graft Infection

Treatment options for prosthetic graft infection include total graft excision, excision with *in situ* revascularization, excision with extra-anatomic reconstruction, and graft preservation techniques using aggressive debridement, autogenous tissue coverage, and local wound care. Graft excision is generally required if any of the following conditions exist: (1) signs of systemic sepsis; (2) anastomotic disruption with hemorrhage; (3) presence of Gram-negative organisms on culture; (4) involvement of the entire graft; and (5) associated graft thrombosis. In these situations, removal of the entire graft is essential if the infection is to be cleared. Attempts at graft preservation in this setting almost always results in recurrence or progression of the infection with the risk of systemic toxicity and delayed exsanguinating hemorrhage.

It is uncommon to remove the infected prosthesis without the need to revascularize. If the conduit was previously occluded or the original procedure was performed for claudication, collateral development may have occurred to a sufficient degree to prevent limb-threatening ischemia and immediate revascularization may not be required. Generally, if ankle Doppler signals are absent at the time of surgery, critical ischemia with its associated increase in morbidity and limb loss can be anticipated if revascularization is not performed.

If the indications for graft excision do not include anastomotic bleeding or overwhelming systemic toxicity, and distal revascularization is required, staged surgical therapy can be done by first performing the revascularization followed by graft excision several days later. Morbidity and mortality can be reduced and lower extremity ischemia is avoided using this technique. However, if the patient presents with hemorrhage or septic shock, control of bleeding and graft excision are the initial priorities and staged operations are not recommended. The conduit of choice for arterial reconstruction is autogenous vein or endarterectomized iliac or superficial femoral artery. Autogenous tissue is frequently unavailable in these patients, in which case prosthetic reconstruction using PTFE through remote and noninfected tissue planes should be performed.

Early graft infections are usually associated with more severe complications such as anastomotic bleeding or sepsis, complex wound infections, and particularly virulent bacterial pathogens (Gram-negative aerobes, coagulase-positive staphylococci) and therefore almost always require excision. Principles of graft removal include excision of the entire graft, wide debridement and irrigation of the surrounding tissues, closure of arteriotomies and arterial stumps with monofiliment suture, and aggressive antibiotic therapy. In addition, patients with questionable limb viability should be started on systemic heparin anticoagulation.

Graft infections that occur months to years after implantation are generally indolent, less extensive, and present with vague signs and symptoms. The infecting organisms are most commonly mucin-producing strains of *S. epidermidis,* although other coagulase-negative staphylococci can be isolated using appropriate techniques. In these cases, if the infection is localized and pseudoaneurysm or graft thrombosis has not occurred, graft preservation may be attempted. This therapy entails: (1) repeated, aggressive *surgical* debridement; (2) autogenous tissue coverage; (3) local wound care with dressing changes; and (4) long-term intravenous antibiotics. Several studies have reported successful graft preservation in more than 90% of cases, with significantly better limb salvage using this strategy and recommend this treatment in selected PTFE graft infections.[11,14,34]

Another method of treating delayed prosthetic graft infection caused by coagulase-negative staphylococci is excision with *in situ* replacement using autogenous or PTFE conduits. As with graft preservation treatment, the patient cannot be septic or present with hemorrhage. Essential components of *in situ* graft replacement include perioperative vancomycin, exclusion of virulent Gram-negative bacteria on culture, wide debridement and irrigation of perigraft tissue and anastomotic sites, and rotational muscle flap coverage. Towne and coworkers[35] reported results of this treatment in 20 patients with prosthetic graft infection, including both aortic and infrainguinal conduits. Coagulase-negative staphylococci were isolated in 17 (85%) cases. In this series, all wounds healed, all grafts remained patent, there was no limb loss, and all replacement grafts remained well incorporated. *In situ* replacement of biofilm graft infections is effective for treating localized graft healing problems, but because of the indolent nature of this type of infection, subsequent infection of previously uninvolved graft segments can occur.

Autogenous Graft Infection

The incidence of confirmed lower extremity autogenous graft infection is exceedingly low and often goes unreported in large series. Autogenous grafts are much more resistant to infection, but irreversible graft damage can ensue, particularly if Gram-negative pathogens are involved. Management objectives are the same as those with prosthetic graft infections: complete resolution of the infectious process and preservation of distal perfusion.

As with prosthetic graft infections, graft excision is usually required if the infection manifests as systemic toxicity, graft thrombosis, anastomotic disruption with bleeding or pseudoaneurysm formation, or if Gram-negative bacteria are involved. In these situations, reconstruction using either *in situ* replacement or extra-anatomic bypass can be utilized. However, if the infection is localized and anastomoses are intact in a patent conduit, graft preservation procedures as described previously can be attempted with favorable results.[36]

REFERENCES

1. Reifsnyder T, Bandyk D, Seabrook G, Kinney E, et al. Wound complications of the *in situ* vein bypass technique. *J Vasc Surg.* 1992;15:843–850.
2. Rubin JR, Malone JM, Goldstone J. The role of the lymphatic system in acute arterial prosthetic graft infections. *J Vasc Surg.* 1985;2:92–98.
3. Canon L, Walker AJ. Sclerotherapy of a wound lymphocele using tetracycline. *Eur J Vasc Endovasc Surg.* 1997;14(6):505.
4. Wengrovitz M, Atnip RG, Gifford RRM, Neumyer MM, et al. Wound complications of autogenous subcutaneous infrainguinal arterial bypass surgery: predisposing factors. *J Vasc Surg.* 1990;11:156–163.
5. Szilagyi DE, Smith RF, Elliot JP, Vrandecic MP. Infection in arterial reconstruction with synthetic grafts. *Ann Surg.* 1972;176:321–333.
6. Murphy PG, Tadros E, Cross ES, et al. Skin closure in the incidence of groin wound infection: a prospective study. *Ann Vasc Surg.* 1995;9:480–482.
7. Hoffert PW, Gensler S, Haimovici H. Infection complicating arterial grafts. *Arch Surg.* 1965;90:427–435.
8. Ouriel K, Geary KJ, Green RM, DeWeese JA. Fate of the exposed saphenous vein graft. *Am J Surg.* 1990;160:148–150.
9. Kent KC, Bartek S, Kuntz KM, Anninos E, et al. Prospective study of wound complications in continuous infrainguinal incisions after lower limb arterial reconstruction: incidence, risk factors, and cost. *Surgery.* 196;119:378–383.
10. Edwards WH Jr, Martin RS III, Jenkins JM, Edwards WH Sr. Primary graft infections. *J Vasc Surg.* 1987;6:235–239.
11. Cherry KJ Jr, Roland CF, Pairolero PC, Hallet JW Jr, et al. Infected femorodistal bypass: is graft removal mandatory? *J Vasc Surg.* 1992;15:295–305.
12. Lorentzen JE, Nielsen OM, Arendrup H, Kimose HH, et al. Vascular graft infection: an analysis of sixty-two graft infections in 2411 consecutively implanted synthetic vascular grafts. *Surgery.* 1985;98:81–86.
13. Liekweg WG Jr, Greenfield LJ. Vascular prosthetic infections: collected experience and results of treatment. *Surgery.* 1977;81:335–342.

14. Calligaro KD, Westcott CJ, Buckley RM, Savarese RP, et al. Infrainguinal anastomotic arterial graft infections treated by selective graft preservation. *Ann Surg.* 1992;216:74–79.

15. Kikta MJ, Goodson SF, Bishara RA, Meyer JP, et al. Mortality and limb loss with infected infrainguinal bypass. *J Vasc Surg.* 1987;5:566–571.

16. Levy MF, Schmitt DD, Edmiston CE, Bandyk DF, et al. Sequential analysis of staphylococcal colonization of body surfaces of patients undergoing vascular surgery. *J Clin Microbiol.* 1990;28:664–669.

17. Macbeth GA, Rubin JR, McIntyre KE Jr, Goldstone J, et al. The relevance of arterial wall microbiology to the treatment of prosthetic graft infections: graft infection vs. arterial infection. *J Vasc Surg.* 1984;1:750–756.

18. Durham JR, Malone JM, Bernhard VM. The impact of multiple operations on the importance of arterial wall cultures. *J Vasc Surg.* 1987;5:160–169.

19. Moore WS. Experimental studies relating to sepsis in prosthetic vascular grafting. In: Duma RJ, ed. *Infections of Prosthetic Heart Valves and Vascular Grafts.* Baltimore: University Park Press, 1977:267–285.

20. Bandyk DF, Bergamini TM. Infection in prosthetic vascular grafts. In: Rutherford RB, ed. *Vascular Surgery.* 4th ed. Philadelphia: WB Saunders, 1995:588–603.

21. Dougherty SH, Simmons RL. Infections in bionic man: the pathophysiology of infections in prosthetic devices—part II. *Curr Prob Surg.* 1982;19:269–318.

22. Schmitt DD, Bandyk DF, Pequet AJ, Towne JB. Bacterial adherence to vascular prostheses: a determinant of graft infectivity. *J Vasc Surg.* 986;3:732–740.

23. Doscher W, Krishnasastry KV, Deckoff SL. Fungal graft infections: case report and review of the literature. *J Vasc Surg.* 1987;6:398–402.

24. Dale BAS, McCormick JStC. *Mycoplasma hominis* wound infection following aortobifemoral bypass. *Eur J Vasc Surg.* 1991;5:213–14.

25. Bergamini TM, Bandyk DF, Govostis D, Vetsch R, et al. Identification of *Staphylococcus epidermidis* vascular graft infections: a comparison of culture techniques. *J Vasc Surg.* 1989;9:665–670.

26. Geary KJ, Tomkiewicz ZM, Harrison HN, Fiore WM, et al. Differential effects of a gram-negative and a gram-positive infection on autogenous and prosthetic grafts. *J Vasc Surg.* 1990;11:339–347.

27. O'Brien T, Collin J. Prosthetic vascular graft infection. *Br J Surg.* 1992;79:1262–1267.

28. Polak JE, Donaldson MC, Whittemore AD, Mannick JA, et al. Pulsatile masses surrounding vascular prostheses: real-time US color flow imaging. *Radiology.* 1989;170:363–366.

29. Haaga JR, Baldwin N, Reich NE, Beven E, et al. CT detection of infected synthetic grafts: preliminary report of a new sign. *Am J Radiol.* 1978;131:317–320.

30. Auffermann W, Olofsson PA, Rabahie GN, Tavares NJ, et al. Incorporation versus infection of retroperitoneal aortic grafts: MR imaging features. *Radiology.* 1989;172:359–362.

31. Sedwitz MM, Davies RJ, Pretorius HT, Vasquez TE. Indium 111-labeled white blood cell scans after vascular prosthetic reconstruction. *J Vasc Surg.* 1987;6:476–481.

32. LaMuraglia GM, Fischman AJ, Strauss HW, Keech F, et al. Utility of the Indium 111-labeled human immunoglobulin G scan for the detection of focal vascular graft infection. *J Vasc Surg.* 1989;10:20–28.

33. Gordon IL, Pousti TJ, Stemmer EA, Connolly JE, et al. Inguinal wound fluid collections after vascular surgery: management by early reoperation. *South Med J.* 1995;88:433–436.

34. Perler BA, Vander Kolk CA, Dufresne CR, Williams GM. Can infected prosthetic grafts be salvaged with rotational muscle flaps? *Surgery.* 1991;110:30–34.

35. Towne JB, Seabrook GR, Bandyk D, Freischlag JA, et al. *In situ* replacement of arterial prosthesis infected by bacterial biofilms: long-term follow-up. *J Vasc Surg.* 1994;19:226–235.

36. Calligaro KD, Veith FJ, Schwartz ML, Savarese RP, et al. Management of infected lower extremity autologous vein grafts by selective graft preservation. *Am J Surg.* 1992;164:291–294.

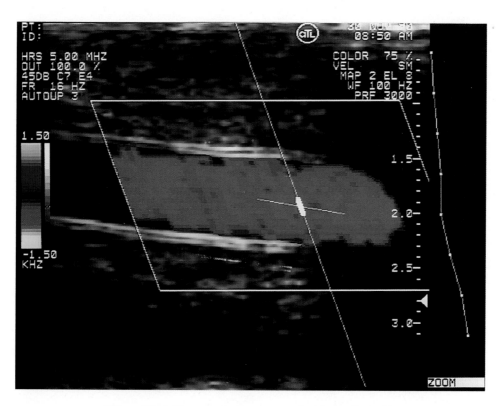

Figure 23–1. Normal color-flow image of postoperative graft.

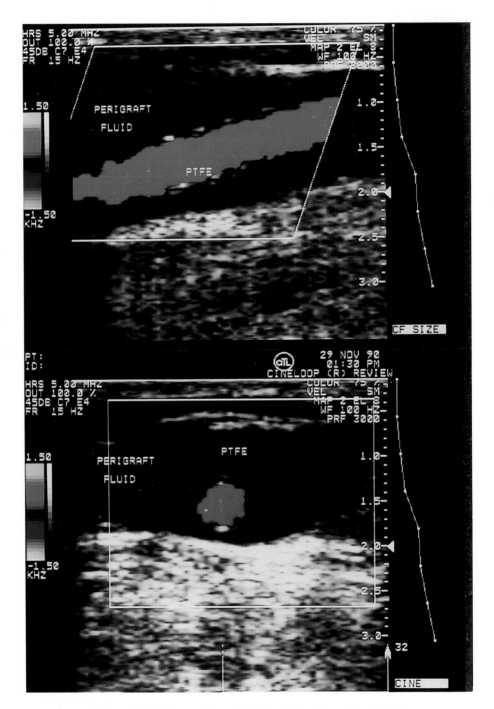

Figure 23–2. Cross-section of PTFE graft showing perigraft fluid.

24

Nonoperative Management of Femoropopliteal Occlusive Disease

Lloyd M. Taylor, Jr., MD, Gregory L. Moneta, MD, and John M. Porter, MD

Symptoms of lower extremity ischemia are important to patients because of their immediate effects and, importantly, because of their implied threat. Few patients afflicted are unaware of the risk of amputation, and few medical outcomes are more feared. How many practitioners have not heard "Doctors, I would rather die than lose my leg," or its equivalent? Given this potential dire outcome, patients and physicians alike trend toward definitive remedies, frequently surgical. Yet in truth, most individuals with femoropopliteal occlusive disease are asymptomatic or minimally symptomatic, and even patients with more significant symptoms face little actual threat of limb loss. For most patients, the condition is chronic and amenable to nonoperative management with an excellent anticipated outcome. A brief description of nonoperative management of femoropopliteal occlusive disease forms the basis for this chapter. The subjects discussed include epidemiology, natural history, patient evaluation, and nonoperative treatment including smoking cessation and exercise and pharmacological management.

EPIDEMIOLOGY

A number of population studies using noninvasive testing have shown that the vast majority of persons with atherosclerotic lower extremity arterial occlusive disease (abbreviated as *peripheral arterial disease,* PAD) are asymptomatic. The examples included in Table 24–1 include ratios of symptomatic to asymptomatic persons ranging 1:1.8 to 1:5.3.[1-4] The incidence of PAD affecting the lower extremities ranged from 2.2% of a population aged 38 to 82 years to 17% of a population aged 55 to 70 years, emphasizing the rapid increase in prevalence of PAD with increasing age. At present, only about 100,000 operations for treatment of lower extremity ischemia are performed annually in the United States.[5] Clearly, a large majority of persons with PAD are currently treated nonoperatively.

TABLE 24–1. INCIDENCE OF PAD IN VARIOUS POPULATIONS DETERMINED BY OBJECTIVE TESTING

Reference	Country	Population (years)	With PAD (%)	Symptomatic/ Asymptomatic Ratio
Debacker, 1979[1]	Belgium	40–60	4	1 : 4.4
Schroll, 1981[2]	Denmark	60	14	1 : 2.8
Criqui et al., 1985[3]	United States	38–82	2.2	1 : 5.3
Fowkes et al., 1991[4]	Scotland	55–74	17	1 : 1.8

NATURAL HISTORY OF LOWER EXTREMITY ISCHEMIA

Risk Factors for PAD

The familiar risk factors for atherosclerotic coronary heart disease, including diabetes, cigarette smoking, hypertension, lipid abnormalities, plasma fibrinogen levels, and elevated plasma homocysteine levels, have each been shown to also be related to presence of PAD (Table 24–2).

Associated Coronary and Carotid Artery Disease

Hertzer and colleagues[6] performed coronary arteriography in 1000 consecutive patients before elective vascular surgery. Angiographically identifiable coronary atherosclerosis was detected in 90% of all patients scheduled for operation to treat claudication (381 of the 1000 patients), only 47% of whom had clinical history or electrocardiographic findings of coronary disease,[7] emphasizing the asymptomatic nature of a considerable portion of the coronary disease identified angiographically. No currently utilized screening test has accuracy greater than 90%. This means that screening tests for coronary artery disease are not necessary in PAD patients; its presence can be assumed.

The Asymptomatic Carotid Atherosclerosis Study[8] showed benefit when patients with greater than 60% internal carotid artery stenosis were treated by endarterectomy. Because of this the number of PAD patients who have asymptomatic carotid artery stenoses is quite relevant to their treatment. Ahn and coworkers[9] noninvasively examined 78 patients with PAD who had no clinical evidence of carotid artery disease. They found 16% to 50% stenosis of the internal carotid artery in 33% of the patients, greater than 50% stenosis in 14% of the patients, and greater than 75% stenosis in 5% of the patients. Asymptomatic patients in our practice who were examined prior to bypass

TABLE 24–2. EXAMPLES OF INCREASE IN RELATIVE RISK OF PAD ASSOCIATED WITH VARIOUS RISK FACTORS FOR ATHEROSCLEROSIS

Reference	Country	Risk Factor	Relative Risk of PAD (95% CI)
Murabito et al., 1997[75]	United States	Diabetes	2.6 (2.0–3.4)
Fowkes et al., 1992[76]	Scotland	Smoking	3.7 (1.7–8.0)
Bowlin et al., 1994[77]	??	Cholesterol	2.05 (1.44–2.91)
Fowkes et al., 1992[76]	Scotland	Triglycerides	1.7 (1.3–2.1)
Cheng et al., 1997[78]	??	Lipoprotein (a)	2.0
Clarke et al., 1991[79]	United States	Homocysteine	22.3 (1.9–inf.)

surgery for PAD had stenoses greater than 60% in at least one caroid artery 15% of the time.[10]

These studies and others confirm that PAD is accompanied by similar disease in the coronary and cerebral beds. As with PAD, much of the coexisting disease is asymptomatic. Generally, increasing severity of PAD is accompanied by increasing severity of coronary and cerebral atherosclerosis.

Progression of PAD

As mentioned previously, a large majority of objectively diagnosable PAD remains asymptomatic. In various studies 50% to 90% of patients with hemodynamic changes sufficient to cause intermittent claudication did not describe this symptom to their physicians.[11,12] One explanation is that patients accept increasing difficulty walking as a normal consequence of aging. In one prospective study, two-thirds of patients with arteriographically proved PAD denied claudication,[13] which is a relative symptom that in order to exist requires that patients must have significant arterial obstruction and they must also exercise sufficiently to induce relative muscle ischemia.[4] The normal lower extremity arterial tree has a vast capacity to increase flow in response to exercise, and most sedentary individuals rarely stress this capacity. It is possible for increasing arterial obstruction to result in a tremendous amount of lost capacity to increase flow without an individual so affected ever becoming symptomatic. Different studies have found widely different ratios of symptomatic to asymptomatic PAD. Logically, claudication was more frequent in a study of farm workers[14] than in office workers,[12] probably because the more active workers required greater physical capacity.

The most feared consequence of PAD is progression to need for amputation. Historical studies of claudication convincingly demonstrated that this is unusual. Boyd prospectively followed 1440 patients with intermittent claudication for 10 years; only 12.2% required amputation.[15] In the Framingham study, 1.6% of claudicators followed for 8.3 years required amputation.[16]

Cigarette smoking is the most important risk factor for progression of disease. Severity of PAD as assessed by symptoms, angiography,[17] or noninvasive segmental pressure measurements is also important.[18,19] Diabetes was identified as having a higher likelihood of progression to gangrene and limb loss in some studies[11,20] but not in others.[7,19]

Survival of Patients with PAD

Patients with PAD have shortened survival compared to age-matched controls. Mortality rates for patients with claudication at 5, 10, and 15 years are 30%, 50%, and 70%, respectively, significantly in excess of patients observed in control groups.

Long-term survival of PAD patients is related to the severity of ischemia. Accordingly, 5-year survival ranges from 87% of patients with claudication treated nonoperatively[21] to 80% of patients with claudication treated by operation,[22] to 48% of patients with limb-threatening ischemia treated by operation,[23] to 12% of patients who had reoperative surgery for limb-threatening ischemia.[24] McDermott and coworkers[25] demonstrated that mortality risk for PAD patients can be stratified by ABI, just as by severity of symptoms. Continued cigarette smoking, diabetes, and the presence of symptomatic coronary and cerebrovascular disease have been identified as independent risk factors associated with an increased risk of mortality exceeding that predicted for the entire group of claudicators.

Limb-Threatening Ischemia

Clinically, limb-threatening ischemia includes rest pain, ulceration, and gangrene. Ischemic rest pain is burning, dysesthetic pain worse in the forefoot and toes and worse at night when the patient is recumbent. Rest pain is lessened by placing the foot dependent, presumably from the increase in arterial pressure resulting from gravity. Ischemic ulcerations are minor traumatic lesions that fail to heal and enlarge because of inadequate blood supply. Gangrene occurs when arterial perfusion is so inadequate that spontaneous necrosis occurs in the most poorly perfused areas.

Ultimate need for amputation is the inevitable outcome assumed by many in patients with unrelieved limb-threatening ischemia. In fact, the true prognosis for limb loss in patients with limb-threatening ischemia is not known with certainty. Progressive gangrenous changes and continuous ischemic rest pain unrelieved by dependency are unstable conditions associated with rapid progression to limb loss. In contrast, some patients have episodes of typical nocturnal ischemic rest pain that is easily relieved by limb dependency, and maintain this stable symptom complex for months or even years. In some patients, minor improvements in perfusion from specific hemorrheologic drugs may be sufficient to prevent progressive ischemia leading to limb loss.[26] One important report documented long-term improvement in limbs with advanced ischemia without specific therapy.[27] Clearly, controlled studies are needed to show therapeutic benefit from any treatment method in patients with limb-threatening ischemia.

One 1982 trial randomized 22 patients with arterial ischemic ulcers to placebo or prostaglandin treatment. Forty percent of the ulcers healed in the placebo group.[28] Another study of 120 patients reported 49% of ischemic ulcers healed and 80% of rest pain improved in the placebo group.[29] Similar findings from other studies of patients with ischemic rest pain and gangrenous ulcers suggest spontaneous improvement in 25% to 50% of patients.[30,31]

The anticipated survival of patients with limb-threatening ischemia is short, and death is at least as frequent as limb loss: both occur with alarming rapidity. Randomized trials of drug therapy for limb-threatening ischemia demonstrated that one-half of placebo treated patients had died or had amputation within 6 months.[30,32,33,34]

PATIENT EVALUATION

Lower extremity ischemia is especially suited to objective noninvasive vascular laboratory evaluation, which may be thought of as an extension of the physical examination. The authors perform noninvasive laboratory examinations on patients with chronic lower extremity ischemia as part of the initial patient evaluation. Testing includes pulse palpation and recording analog Doppler waveforms over the femoral, popliteal, and pedal arteries. Segmental pressure indices at the upper thigh, above-the-knee, below-the-knee, ankle, and great toe levels are also determined. Patients with incompressible vessels are examined with plethysmographic recordings and toe reactive hyperemia testing. Toe photoplethysmography is used to detect obstructive disease below the ankle, as is frequently present in diabetic patients. Patients with claudication are examined by having them walk on a treadmill followed by measurement of ankle pressure recovery times. These vascular laboratory data serve as a baseline against which to judge progression of disease as well as to evaluate future changes in symptoms or response to treatment. It is our practice to obtain carotid artery duplex scanning in PAD patients without symptoms of carotid artery disease, if they would be candidates for carotid endarterectomy for asymptomatic disease as directed by the ACAS study.[8]

NONOPERATIVE TREATMENT

Cessation of Smoking

The direct relationship between tobacco and PAD is well known. Ninety-eight to 99% of all patients who complain of intermittent claudication[35,36] and an equally high percentage of patients undergoing lower extremity amputation for ischemia are smokers.[37] Cigarette smoke contains more than 3000 different substances.[38] Many of these components of tobacco smoke have been demonstrated to affect each of the important components of the atherosclerotic process adversely, as outlined in Table 24–3.

Smokers have chronic vasoconstriction and hypertension, probably as a result of the nicotine in tobacco smoke. The carbon monoxide component of tobacco smoke has an adverse effect on claudication. Aronow and associates[39] demonstrated an immediate, significant decrease in treadmill walking in claudicators who breathed air containing 50 ppm of carbon monoxide.

Cessation of all tobacco use is the essential first step in nonoperative treatment of PAD. When taking the patient's history, questions such as "Do you still smoke?" or "How much do you smoke?" effectively convey that smoking is part of the problem, in contrast to the more neutral (and more typically asked) "Do you smoke?" All smokers are aware of an adverse health influence, but most associate tobacco use with pulmonary disease, specifically lung cancer. The increased risks of myocardial infarction and stroke[40,41] are less well recognized. Only 37% of smokers with PAD recognized an association with smoking in the study by Clyne and colleagues.[42] Patients must be informed clearly and unequivocally that smoking is the most important correctable cause of their disease. An unwavering recommendation that PAD patients totally cease tobacco use in all forms must be repeated at every patient encounter. Kirk and associates[43] found that strong and repeated advice by physicians to cease smoking resulted in abstinence by 37% of smokers with PAD.

For most smokers, tobacco use represents a powerful chemical addiction, defined by Pollin[44] as the "inability to discontinue smoking despite awareness of the medical consequences." Patients able to cease smoking on being informed of the importance

TABLE 24–3. ADVERSE EFFECTS OF TOBACCO SMOKING ON COMPONENTS OF ATHEROGENESIS

I. Endothelial effects
  A. Increased endothelial denudation[85]
  B. Increased endothelial cell turnover[85]
  C. Decreased endothelial cell prostacyclin production[86]
II. Platelet effects
  A. Increased platelet count[50]
  B. Increased platelet aggregation[87]
  C. Increased platelet adhesiveness[88]
  D. Increased thromboxane A_2 production[46]
III. Lipid effects
  A. Decreased high-density lipoprotein levels[89]
IV. Coagulation effects
  A. Decreased fibrinolytic activity[90]
  B. Increased blood viscosity[91]
  C. Increased fibrinogen level[91]
V. Whole vessel effects
  A. Vasoconstriction
  B. Hypertension

of this step probably represent the population of unaddicted users. How best to approach the problem of more severely addicted patients remains unsolved. It is both appropriate and desirable to indicate carefully and in detail to patients that cessation of smoking not only removes a strong negative influence but also is associated with tangible positive benefits.

In one study[45] patients with intermittent claudication who stopped smoking had significant improvement in both ankle pressure and treadmill walking when compared with continued smokers. Mean walking distance improved from 214 to 300 m. In general patients with claudication who stop smoking experience prompt improvement in walking distance that averages a doubling of the initial distance.

Patency of lower extremity arterial repairs is also related to smoking. Greenhalgh and colleagues[46] found patients with failed grafts had carboxyhemoglobin levels 2.5 times those in patients with patent grafts. Patency at 5 years in aortofemoral grafts of nonsmokers (71%) and in patients who stopped smoking (77%) were superior to continued smokers (42%) in another study.[47] Myers and associates[48] demonstrated significantly improved patency of aortofemoral grafts (90% vs 79% at 4 years) and femoropopliteal grafts (80% vs 61%) for patients who smoked fewer than five cigarettes per day. Similar findings were noted by Robicsek and coworkers[49] in patients with aortoiliac disease.

Smoking cessation results in prevention of limb loss in PAD patients. Jurgens and coworkers[37] found no patients who stopped smoking required amputation, whereas 11.4% of those who continued smoking lost their limbs. Birkenstock and coworkers[50] found that 85% of persons who stopped smoking had improvement in PAD symptoms, while only 20% of continuing smokers had improvement. This was true even in the subgroup of patients with ischemic rest pain or gangrene, in which 86% of 64 patients who stopped smoking did not require amputation, an outcome that occurred in only 10% of smokers.

Relapse after initial smoking cessation should not be regarded negatively: multiple attempts are common in the histories of successful abstinence and are a necessary part of the process, which for most who quit successfully requires from 2 to 5 *years* and includes an average of six cycles of abstinence and relapse.[51] Continuing positively expressed encouragement to stop smoking by physicians, family members, and others is identified by many ex-smokers as the most important influence leading to success. The prescription of nicotine gum or patches as an aid to ease the transition from tobacco use to abstinence is appropriate. Although the adverse effects of nicotine are well known, studies show that fewer than 5% of successful ex-smokers among those using the gum continue its use on a long-term basis.[52]

Exercise

A regular program of walking exercise results in a measurable improvement in walking distance in claudicators. Improvement from exercise ranged from an 80% increase in walking distance in one British study of 21 patients[53] to a 234% increase in a study of 148 patients from Sweden.[54] All studies have demonstrated benefit, with the greatest benefit coming from supervised programs. Gardner and Poehlman[55] found a mean increase of 179% in initial claudication distance and a mean increase of 122% in maximal walking distance in a meta-analysis of supervised programs.

Despite the beneficial effects of exercise, not all patients may be able or willing to participate in exercise training. Many patients with PAD have severe coexisting cardiac, pulmonary, arthritic, and other conditions that also limit the safety or applicability of exercise therapy. Others may simply be unwilling. In a study from Germany,[56] 34% of patients with claudication had direct contraindications to exercise treatment and 36%

were unwilling to participate, which left only 30% of 201 patients with claudication to whom a planned exercise rehabilitation program could be applied.[56]

The frequent assumption that exercise results in an improvement in the number of collateral vessels, the size of collateral vessels, or both, with a resulting increase in exercise-induced blood flow, is not supported by available data. Neither ankle blood pressure nor calf muscle blood flow improves in claudicators with improved walking tolerance after an exercise program.[53,54,57–59] The improved muscle performance caused by exercise training is partly a result of adaptive changes in muscle enzymes leading to a more efficient oxygen extraction from blood.[60] In support of this mechanism, popliteal venous blood from patients with claudication who are exercisors shows increased extraction of oxygen following regular physical training and no change in lactate levels, emphasizing that the increased muscle exercise capacity is aerobic in nature.[59] Other mechanisms may also be important. One study[61] showed improved hemorrheologic behavior of erythrocytes after regular exercise. Others have noted changes in gait to bring nonischemic muscles into greater use, improved mechanical efficiency of muscles, improved fatty acid metabolism, and increased muscle fiber : capillary ratios.[62,63]

A sedentary lifestyle is a recognized risk factor for the development of atherosclerotic disease, and most patients with claudication fit this description. Obviously, exercise programs should be individualized, but for the majority of patients a recommendation of 1 h of walking at a comfortable pace each day is well accepted. Patients are instructed to walk until claudication occurs, then rest until it subsides, then repeat the cycle for 1 h each day. There is no demonstrated benefit associated with attempting to "walk through the pain," and the level of discomfort produced by this effort is sufficient to discourage even the most dedicated patient.

Creasy and coworkers[64] randomized patients with intermittent claudication to treatment by balloon angioplasty or to exercise therapy. The initial improvement in leg circulation, as assessed by the ankle–brachial pressure index (ABI), was greater in the angioplasty group. Despite this, after 1 year of follow-up, the patients in the exercise group could walk farther, both on the treadmill in the laboratory and as assessed by questionnaire, and there was no longer a significant difference in the ankle pressure index. This study demonstrates the important benefits associated with exercise therapy and questions the presumed superiority of invasive therapy. Obviously, future studies of claudication treatment should include a control group treated by exercise.

Pharmacological Treatment

Pharmacological treatment of PAD patients includes therapy intended to prevent complications/progression of the systemic atherosclerotic process and therapy specifically to relieve symptoms/prevent progression of PAD. There is abundant evidence that all patients with symptomatic atherosclerotic disease should be treated with antiplatelet agents. The least expensive and most applicable of these is aspirin. A meta-analysis of 189 controlled studies involving prevention of cardiovascular events in more than 100,000 patients showed a highly significant 25% reduction in the risk of fatal and nonfatal myocardial infarction, stroke, and death from cardiovascular disease.[65] The specific risk of peripheral arterial surgery was reduced by 54% in subjects treated with aspirin in the Physician's Health Study.[66] Beneficial effects of aspirin therapy have been demonstrated consistently with doses ranging from 80 mg every other day to as high as 1000 mg per day. For convenience and considerations of cost, a recommendation of a single aspirin tablet taken daily suffices for most patients. Gastrointestinal symptoms, the most serious of which is bleeding, can be addressed by reducing the dosage to

80 mg every other day, although this regimen is both more expensive (paradoxically, "baby" aspirin costs more) and more difficult for patients to remember.

For patients unable to tolerate aspirin, or who remain symptomatic despite aspirin therapy, ticlopidine[67] and clopidogrel[68] are effective antiplatelet agents, each of which has incrementally greater effectiveness than aspirin in some studies. The margin of increased benefit was minimal for each, and both medications are orders of magnitude more expensive than aspirin. Ticlopidine can produce bone marrow depression, and so requires laboratory monitoring of blood counts, further increasing cost. At present, neither of these agents has sufficient advantage in effectiveness over aspirin to justify a recommendation for use as the primary antiplatelet agent in PAD patients.

Pharmacological Treatment of Claudication

Pentoxifylline is currently approved in the United States for treatment of claudication. Effects of this medication include improvement in red and white cell deformability, lowering of fibrinogen level, and decreased white cell and platelet aggregation, all of which are felt to result in improvement in the microcirculation. In a large multicenter trial performed in the United States, pentoxifylline produced a 22% improvement over placebo in initial claudication distance and a 12% improvement over placebo in maximal walking distance, both of which were statistically significant.[69] No studies have been performed to evaluate the effectiveness of pentoxifylline treatment using patient-based questionnaires. The marginal improvement in walking distance in the multicenter trials is sufficiently small that prescription of pentoxifylline is probably not justified in the absence of clear recognition of improvement by the patient. At least one study has suggested that such improvement is more likely in patients with ABI less than 0.80 and symptoms for more than 1 year.[70] In the authors' practice, benefit from pentoxifylline treatment is seen most often in patients with extremely limited walking distance (<1 block) for whom an incremental improvement produces significant functional benefit. In the overall spectrum of claudicating patients, such individuals are few. For these patients, long-term therapy with pentoxifylline is well tolerated. There are no recognized major adverse effects. Gastrointestinal side effects (nausea, vomiting, and bloating) and dizziness require discontinuance of the drug in 3% to 5% of patients.

Carnitine is a naturally occurring cofactor for skeletal muscle intermediary metabolism that is required for mitochondrial oxidation of long-chain fatty acids. Supplementation with carnitine for treatment of claudication is supported theoretically by the finding of increased levels of acylcarnitines in the skeletal muscle of PAD patients.[71] Treatment of claudicating patients with carnitine has resulted in significant benefit in walking distance.[72] Preliminary unpublished results from a blinded study conducted by Hiatt and colleagues[73] showed a 26% improvement over placebo in maximal walking time ($p = .001$). Carnitine treatment has no known side effects or toxicity. Carnitine is not currently approved as a drug treatment, but as a naturally occurring substance, it can be sold as nutritional supplement and is available in health food stores and so on (frequently at considerable cost).

Cilastozol is a phosphodiesterase inhibitor and has vasodilator and antiplatelet activity. A large blinded randomized trial has shown a dose-dependent and significant improvement in treadmill walking compared with placebo.[74] Cilostazol was recently approved for use by the U.S. Food and Drug Administration.

For each of the agents described, improvement in walking distance is significant, but small. No pharmacological agents result in cure of claudication, and for many patients statistically significant improvement in walking distance may not result. The significance of presently available agents lies in the demonstration that pharmacological therapy can improve claudication. The obvious hope is that more effective agents will follow the marginally effective current generation.

Pharmacological Treatment of Limb-Threatening Ischemia

Ischemic rest pain, ischemic ulcers, and gangrene are the end-stage manifestations of progressive lower extremity arterial obstruction. Although revascularization through surgery is nearly always possible, most patients with limb-threatening ischemia are elderly and have significant comorbidities. The attractiveness of effective pharmacological therapy is obvious.

A very large number of studies, some of which are summarized in Table 24–4 have been performed to evaluate various prostaglandins in the treatment of limb-threatening ischemia. A summary of the available information indicates that no drug treatment has been shown to result in healing of ischemic ulcers or prevention of the need for amputation. A small number of studies[28,70] have shown benefit in other parameters such as patients' perception of pain or consumption of analgesics. At present, no pharmacological agents are approved for treatment of limb-threatening ischemia in the United States, and on the basis of the information in Table 24–4, none can be recommended. As mentioned previously, each of the studies performed showed a surprisingly high rate of spontaneous improvement and ulcer healing in placebo-treated patients, emphasizing that bed rest and careful wound care constitute a reasonable approach to nonoperative management of limb-threatening ischemia in some patients,

TABLE 24–4. CONTROLLED STUDIES OF PROSTAGLANDIN THERAPY OF LIMB-THREATENING ISCHEMIA

Reference	Patients (No.)	Parameters	Drug	Result	Significance
Nizandowski et al., 1985	30	Ischemic ulcer	PGI2	Reduced size	$p < .02$
		Rest pain		No difference	NS
Negus et al., 1987	29	Ischemic ulcer	PGI2	No difference	NS
		Rest pain		No difference	NS
Eklund et al., 1982	24	Ischemic ulcer	PGE1	No difference	NS
		Rest pain		No difference	NS
Schuler et al., 1984	120	Ischemic ulcer	PGE1	No difference	NS
		Rest pain		No difference	NS
Telles et al., 1984	30	Ischemic ulcer	PGE1	No difference	NS
		Rest pain		No difference	NS
		Amputation		No difference	NS
Belch et al., 1983	28	Rest pain	PGI2	Early benefit	NS
		Anal cons		Sign improv	$p < .05$
		Ankle pressure		No difference	NS
Cronenwett et al., 1986	26	Ischemic ulcer	PGI2	No difference	NS
		Rest pain		No difference	NS
Trubestein et al., 1989	70	Ischemic ulcer	PGE1	Reduced size	$p < .05$
		Rest pain		No difference	NS
		Anal cons		Sign improv	$p < .005$
Norgren et al., 1990	103	Ischemic ulcer	Iloprost	No difference	NS

NS, not significant; Anal cons, consumption of analgesic medications; Sign improv, significant improvement; PGI2, prostacyclin; PGE1, epoprostanol.

and that improvement may be expected in as many as 25% to 40% of those so treated. This finding also illustrates the extreme importance that any newly proposed treatment for limb-threatening ischemia be evaluated by properly constituted placebo-controlled trials.

REFERENCES

1. Abbott RD, Yin Y, Reed DM, et al. Risk of stroke in male cigarette smokers. *N Engl J Med.* 1986;315:717.
2. Ad Hoc Committee on Reporting Standards, Society for Vascular Surgery, North American Chapter, International Society for Cardiovascular Surgery. Standards for reports dealing with lower extremity ischemia. *J Vasc Surg.* 1986;4:80.
3. Aronow WS, Stemmer EA, Isbell MW. Effect of carbon monoxide exposure on intermittent claudication. *Circulation.* 1974;49:415.
4. Criqui MH, Fronck A, Klauber MR, et al. The sensitivity, specificity and predictive value of traditional clinical evaluation of peripheral arterial disease: results from noninvasive testing in a defined population. *Circulation.* 1985;71:516.
5. Rutkow IM, Ernst CB. An analysis of vascular surgical manpower requirements and vascular surgical rates in the United States. *J Vasc Surg.* 1986;3:74.
6. Hertzer NR, Beven EG, Young JR, et al. Coronary artery disease in peripheral vascular patients: a classification of 1000 coronary angiograms and results of surgical management. *Ann Surg.* 1984;199:223.
7. Hertzer NR. Fatal myocardial infarction following lower extremity revascularization: two hundred and seventy-three patients followed six to eleven post-operative years. *Ann Surg.* 1981;193:492.
8. Executive Committee for the Asymptomatic Carotid Atherosclerosis Study. Endarterectomy for asymptomatic carotid artery stenosis. *JAMA.* 1995;273:1421.
9. Ahn SS, Baker JD, Walden K, Moore WS. Which asymptomatic patients should undergo routine screening carotid duplex scan? *Am J Surg.* 1991;162:180.
10. Gentile AT, Taylor LM Jr, Moneta GL, Porter JM. Prevalence of asymptomatic carotid stenosis in patients undergoing infrainguinal bypass surgery. *Arch Surg.* 1995;130:900–904.
11. Hughson WG, Munn JI, Garrod A. Intermittent claudication: prevalence and risk factors. *Br Med J.* 1978;1:1379.
12. Reid DD, Brett GZ, Hamilton PJ, et al. Cardiorespiratory disease and diabetes among middle aged male civil servants. *Lancet.* 1974;1:469.
13. Widmer LK, Greensher A, Kannel WB. Occlusion of peripheral arteries: a study of 6400 working subjects. *Circulation.* 1964;30:836.
14. Reunanen A, Takkunen H, Aromaa A. Prevalence of intermittent claudication and its effect on mortality. *Acta Med Scand.* 1982;211:249–256.
15. Boyd AM. The natural course of arteriosclerosis of the lower extremities. *Angiology.* 1960;11:10.
16. Kannel WB, Skinner JJ, Schwarz MJ, et al. Intermittent claudication: incidence in the Framingham study. *Circulation.* 1970;41:875.
17. Imparato AM, Kim GE, Davidson T, et al. Intermittent claudication: its natural course. *Surgery.* 1975;78:795.
18. Cronenwett JL, Warner KG, Zelenock GB, et al. Intermittent claudication: current results of nonoperative management. *Arch Surg.* 1984;119:430.
19. Jonason T, Ringqvist I. Factors of prognostic importance for subsequent rest pain in patients with intermittent claudication. *Acta Med Scand.* 1985;218:27.
20. Peabody CN, Kannel WB, McNamara PM. Intermittent claudication: surgical significance. *Arch Surg.* 1974;109:693.
21. Renaunen A, Takkunen H, Aromaa A. Prevalence of intermittent claudication and its effect on mortality. *Acta Med Scand.* 1972;537(Suppl):8.

22. Malone JM, Moore WS, Goldstone J. Life expectancy following aortofemoral arterial grafting. *Surgery.* 1977;81:551.

23. Veith FJ, Gupta SK, Samson RH, et al. Progress in limb salvage by reconstructive arterial surgery combined with new or improved adjunctive procedures. *Ann Surg.* 1981;194:386.

24. Edwards JM, Taylor LM Jr, Porter JM. Treatment of failed lower extremity bypass grafts with new autogenous vein bypass. *J Vasc Surg.* 1990;11:132.

25. McDermott MM, Feinglass J, Slavensky R, Pearce WH. The ankle–brachial index as a predictor of survival in patients with peripheral vascular disease. *J Gen Intern Med.* 1994;9:445–449.

26. Salmasi A-M, Nicolaides A, Al-Katoubi A, et al. Intermittent claudication as a manifestation of silent myocardial ischemia: a pilot study. *J Vasc Surg.* 1991;14:76.

27. Rivers SP, Veith FJ, Ascer E, et al. Successful conservative therapy of severe limb threatening ischemia: the value of nonsympathectomy. *Surgery.* 1986;99:759.

28. Eklund AE, Eriksson G, Olsson AG. A controlled study showing significant short term effect of prostaglandin E1 in healing of ischemic ulcers of the lower limb in man. *Prost Leuk Med.* 1982;8:265.

29. Schuler JJ, Flanigan DP, Holcroft JW, et al. Efficacy of prostaglandin E1 in the treatment of lower extremity ischemic ulcers secondary to peripheral vascular occlusive disease: results of a prospective randomized, double-blind, multicenter clinical trial. *J Vasc Surg.* 1984;1:160.

30. Belch JJF, McArdle B, Pollack JG, et al. Epoprostenol (prostacyclin) and severe arterial disease: a double-blind trial. *Lancet.* 1983;1:315.

31. Cronenwett JL, Zelenock GB, Whitehouse WM Jr, et al. Prostacyclin treatment of ischemic ulcers and rest pain in unreconstructible peripheral arterial occlusive disease. *Surgery.* 1986;100:369.

32. Lowe GDO, Dunlop DJ, Lawson DH, et al. Double-blind controlled clinical trial of ancrod for ischaemic rest pain of the leg. *Angiology.* 1982;33:46–50.

33. Norgen L, Alwark A, Angqvist KA, et al. A stable prostacyclin analog (Iloprost) in the treatment of ischaemic ulcers of the lower limb. A Scandinavian–Polish placebo-controlled randomised multicentre study. *Eur J Vasc Surg.* 1990;4:463–467.

34. Bliss B, Wilkins D, Campbell WB, et al. Treatment of limb-threatening ischaemia with intravenous Iloprost: a randomised double-blind placebo-controlled study. *Eur J Vasc Surg.* 1991;5:511–516.

35. Eastcott HHG. *Arterial Surgery,* 2nd ed. London: Pitman Medical Publishers; 1973;3.

36. Lithell H, Hedstrand H, Karlsson R. The smoking habits of men with intermittent claudication. *Acta Med Scand.* 1975;197:473.

37. Jurgens IL, Barker NW, Hines EA. Arteriosclerosis obliterans: a review of 520 cases with special reference to pathogenic and prognostic factors. *Circulation.* 1960;21:188.

38. Wynder EL. Tobacco and health: a societal challenge. *N Engl J Med.* 1979;300:894.

39. Aronow WS, Stemmer EA, Isbell MW. Effect of carbon monoxide exposure on intermittent claudication. *Circulation.* 1974;49:415.

40. Abbott RD, Yin Y, Reed DM, et al. Risk of stroke in male cigarette smokers. *N Engl J Med.* 1986;315:717.

41. Ulietstra RE, Kronmal RA, Oberman A, et al. Effect of cigarette smoking on survival of patients with angiographically documented coronary artery disease. *JAMA.* 1986;255:1023.

42. Clyne CA, Arch PJ, Carpenter D, et al. Smoking, ignorance, and peripheral vascular disease. *Arch Surg.* 1982;117:1062.

43. Kirk CJC, Lund VJ, Woolcock NE, et al. The effect of advice to stop smoking on arterial disease patients, assessed by serum thiocyanate levels. *J Cardiovasc Surg.* 1970;21:568.

44. Pollin W. The role of the addictive process as a key step in causation of all tobacco related diseases. *JAMA.* 1984;252:2874.

45. Quick CRG, Cotton LT. The measured effect of stopping smoking on intermittent claudication. *Br J Surg.* 1982;69(Suppl):524.

46. Greenhalgh RM, Laing SP, Colap V, et al. Progressing atherosclerosis following revascularization. In Bernhard VM, Towne JB, eds. *Complications in Vascular Surgery.* New York: Grune & Stratton; 1980;39.

47. Provan JL, Sojka SG, Murnaghan JJ, et al. The effect of cigarette smoking on the long term success rates of aortofemoral and femoropopliteal reconstructions. *Surg Gynecol Obstet.* 1987;165:49.

48. Myers KA, King RB, Scott DF, et al. The effect of smoking on the late patency of arterial reconstructions in the legs. *Br J Surg*. 1978;65:267.

49. Robicsek F, Daugherty HK, Mullen DC, et al. The effect of continued cigarette smoking on the patency of synthetic vascular grafts in Lericle syndrome. *J Thorac Cardiovasc Surg*. 1975;70:107.

50. Birkenstock WE, Louw JHY, Terblanche J, et al. Smoking and other factors affecting the conservative management of peripheral vascular disease. *S Afr Med J*. 1975;49:1129.

51. Stachnik T, Stoffelmayr B. Worksite smoking cessation programs: a potential for national impact. *Am J Pub Health*. 1983;73:1395.

52. Hjalmarson AIM. Effect of nicotine chewing gum in smoking cessation. *JAMA*. 1984;252:2835.

53. Clifford PC, Davies PW, Hayne JA, et al. Intermittent claudication: is a supervised exercise class worthwhile? *Br Med J*. 1980;280:1503.

54. Ekroth R, Dahllöf AG, Gundevall B, et al. Physical training of patients with intermittent claudication: indications, methods and results. *Surgery*. 1978;84:640.

55. Gardner AW, Poelhman ET. Exercise rehabilitation programs for the treatment of claudication pain. A meta-analysis. *JAMA*. 1995;274:975–980.

56. De La Haye R, Diehm C, Blume J et al. An epidemiological study of the value and limits of physical therapy/exercise therapy in Fontaine stage II arterial occlusive disease. *VASA*. 1992;38:1–40.

57. Dahllöf AG, Holm J, Sclersten T, et al. Peripheral arterial insufficiency. Effect of physical training on walking tolerance, calf blood flow and blood flow resistance. *Scand J Rehabil Med*. 1976;8:19.

58. Saltin B. Physical training in patients with intermittent claudication. In Cohen LS, Mock MB, Ringquist I, eds. *Physical Conditioning and Cardiovascular Rehabilitation*. New York: Wiley; 1981;181.

59. Sprlie D, Myhre K. Effects of physical training in intermittent claudication. *Scand J Clin Lab Invest*. 1978;38:217.

60. Bylund AC, Hammersten J, Holm J, et al. Enzyme activities in skeletal muscles from patients with peripheral arterial insufficiency. *Eur J Clin Invest*. 1976;6:425.

61. Ruell PA, Imperial ES, Bonor FJ, et al. Intermittent claudication. The effect of physical training on walking tolerance and venous lactate concentration. *Eur J Appl Physiol*. 1984;52:420.

62. Dahllöf A, Bjorntorp P, Holm J, Schersten T. Metabolic activity of skeletal muscle in patients with peripheral arterial insufficiency. Effect of physical training. *Eur J Clin Invest*. 1974;4:9–15.

63. Hiatt WR, Regensteiner JG, Wolfel EE, Carry MR, et al. Effect of exercise training on skeletal muscle histology and metabolism in peripheral arterial disease. *J Appl Phys*. 1996;81(2): 780–788.

64. Creasy TS, McMillan PJ, Fletcher EW, et al. Is percutaneous transluminal angioplasty better than exercise for claudication? Preliminary results from a prospective randomized trial. *Eur J Vasc Surg*. 1990;4:135.

65. Antiplatelet Trialists' Collaboration. Secondary prevention of vascular disease by prolonged antiplatelet treatment. *Br Med J Clin Res Ed*. 1988;296:320–331.

66. Goldhaber SZ, Manson JE, Stampfer MJ, et al. Low-dose aspirin and subsequent peripheral arterial surgery in the Physicians' Health Study. *Lancet*. 1992;340:143–145.

67. Janzon L, Bergqvist D, Boberg J, et al. Prevention of myocardial infarction and stroke in patients with intermittent claudication: effects of ticlopidine. Results from STIMS, the Swedish ticlopidine multicenter study. *J Int Med*. 1990;227:301–308.

68. CAPRIE Steering Committee. A randomized, blinded trial of clopidogrel versus aspirin in patients at risk of ischemic events (CAPRIE). *Lancet*. 1996;348:1329–1339.

69. Porter JM, Cutler BS, Lee BY, et al. Pentoxifylline efficacy in the treatment of intermittent claudication: multicenter controlled double-blind trial with objective assessment of chronic occlusive arterial disease patients. *Am Heart J*. 1982;104:66–72.

70. Lindegard F, Jelnes R, Bjorkman H, et al. Scandanavian study group: conservative drug treatment on patients with moderately severe chronic occlusive peripheral arterial disease. *Circulation*. 1989;80:1549–1556.

71. Hiatt WR, Wolfel EE, Regensteiner JG, Brass EP. Skeletal muscle carnitine metabolism in patients with unilateral peripheral arterial disease. *J Appl Physiol*. 1992;73:346–353.

72. Brevetti G, Diehm C, Lambert D. European multicenter study of Propionyl-L-carnitine in intermittent claudication: double-blind, placebo-controlled, dose titration, multicenter study. *J Am Coll Cardiol.* 1995;26:1411–1416.

73. Hiatt W. A medical approach to the management of patients with claudication. Sixty-Ninth Scientific Session, American Heart Association. New Orleans 11/96

74. Money SR, Herd JA, Isaacsohn JL, et al. Effect of cilastozol on walking distances in patients with intermittent claudication caused by peripheral vascular disease. *J Vasc Surg.* 1998; 27:267–275.

75. Murabito JM, D'Agostino RB, Silbershatz H, Wilson PWF. Intermittent claudication. A risk profile from the Framingham Heart Study. *Circulation.* 1997;96:44–49.

76. Fowkes GR, Housley E, Riemersma RA, et al. Smoking, lipids, glucose intolerance and blood pressure as risk factors for peripheral atherosclerosis compared with ischemic heart disease in the Edinburgh Artery Study. *Am J Epidemiol.* 1992;135:331–340.

77. Bowlin SJ, Medalie JH, Flocke SA, et al. Epidemiology of intermittent claudication in middle-aged men. *Am J Epidemiol.* 1994;140:418–430.

78. Cheng SWK, Ting ACW, Wong J. Lipoprotein (a) and its relationship to risk factors and severity of atherosclerotic peripheral vascular disease. *Eur J Vasc Endovasc Surg.* 1997;14:17–23.

79. Clarke R, Daly L, Robinson K, et al. Hyperhomocysteinemia: an independent risk factor for vascular disease. *N Engl J Med.* 1991;324:1149–1155.

80. Nizandowski R, Krolikowski W, Beilatowicz J, Szczeklik A. Prostacyclin for ischemic ulcers in peripheral arterial disease: a random-assignment, placebo-controlled study. *Thromb Res.* 1985;37:21.

81. Negus D, Irving JD, Friedgood A. Intra-arterial prostacyclin compared to praxilene in the management of severe lower limb ischemia: a double-blind trial. *J Cardiovasc Surg.* 1987;28:196.

82. Telles GS, Campbell WB, Wood RFM, et al. Prostaglandin E1 in severe lower limb ischemia: a double-blind controlled trial. *Br J Surg.* 1984;71:506.

83. Trubestein G, von Bary S, Breddin K, et al. Intravenous prostaglandin E1 versus pentoxifylline therapy in chronic arterial occlusive disease—a controlled randomized multicenter study. *Vasa.* 1989;28:44.

84. Norgren L, Alwmark A, Angqvist KA, et al. A stable prostacyclin analog (Iloprost) in the treatment of ischaemic ulcers of the lower limb: a Scandanavian–Polish placebo-controlled, randomized multicenter study. *Eur J Vasc Surg.* 1990;4:463.

85. Davis JW, Shelton L, Eigenberg DA, et al. Effects of tobacco and non-tobacco cigarette smoking on endothelium and platelets. *Clin Pharmacol Ther.* 1985;37:527.

86. Reinders JH, Brinkman HJM, Van Mourik JA, et al: Cigarette smoke impairs endothelial cell prostacyclin production. *Arteriosclerosis.* 1986;6:15.

87. Fielding JE: Smoking: health effects and control. *N Engl J Med.* 1985;313:555.

88. Birnstingl MA, Brinson K, Chakrabarti BK. The effect of short-term exposure to carbon monoxide on platelet stickiness. *Br J Surg.* 1971;58:837.

89. Hully SB, Cohen R, Widdowson G. Plasma high-density lipoprotein cholesterol level. Influence of risk factor intervention. *JAMA.* 1977;238:2269.

90. Hurlow RA, Strachan CJL, George AJ, et al. Thrombosis tests in smokers and non-smokers and patients with peripheral vascular disease. In Greenhalgh RM, ed. *Smoking and Arterial Disease.* London: Pitman Medical Publisher; 1981;35–45.

91. Dintenfass L. Elevation of blood viscosity, aggregation of red cells, hematocrit values and fibrinogen levels in cigarette smokers. *Med J Aust.* 1975;1:617.

92. Debacker IG, Kornitzer M, Sobolski J, Denolin H. Intermittent claudication—epidemiology and natural history. *Acta Cardiol* 1979;34:115–124.

93. Schroll M, Munck O. Estimation of peripheral arteriosclerotic disease by ankle blood pressure measurements in a population study of 60-year-old men and women. *J Chron Dis* 1981;34:261–269.

94. Fowkes FGR, Housley E, Cawood EHH, et al. Edinburgh artery study: prevalence of asymptomatic and symptomatic peripheral arterial disease in the general population. *Int J Epidemiol* 1991;20:384–392.

VII

Nonoperative Management of Vascular Problems

25

Simplified Approach to
Thrombolytic Therapy of Arterial
and Graft Occlusion

Anthony J. Comerota, MD, FACS and
Michael D. Malone, MD

INTRODUCTION

Drs. Yao and Pearce have assigned the task of simplifying the use of catheter-directed thrombolytic therapy for arterial and graft occlusion. This is most appropriate, because catheter-based thrombolytic therapy remains an important option for the treatment of this often potentially limb-threatening problem, yet there is an enormous volume of information, both supporting and condemning the use of catheter-directed thrombolysis for arterial and graft occlusion. We review selected data that may offer insight into the approach suggested, with two large prospective randomized trials comparing catheter-directed thrombolytic therapy to standard operative intervention being the central focus.[1,2] Furthermore, it is interesting to note that different conclusions are possible from analysis of the same data from the prospective trials, depending on the endpoints selected. We emphasize, however, that patient selection and clinical judgment and experience are critical to appropriate use of lytic therapy.

Because the most effective means of dissolving clot is activation of the plasminogen bound to fibrin within the matrix of the clot,[3] it is natural that current approaches to medium and large vessel thrombolysis for acute occlusion is based on catheter delivery of the plasminogen activator directly into the thrombus. The fibrin bond to the plasminogen molecule within the thrombus makes that plasminogen molecule particularly susceptible to activation by plasminogen activators. If delivered into the thrombus, the plasminogen activator is protected from neutralization by circulating plasminogen activator inhibitors. Once plasminogen is activated, plasmin can act efficiently within the thrombus, effecting lysis while being protected from neutralization by circulating plasminogen activator inhibitors. Despite the local or regional delivery, ongoing intra-thrombus infusion of lytic agents often results in systemic activation of plasminogen with breakdown of fibrinogen, clotting factors, and other plasma proteins. The degree to which this occurs depends on the dose of plasminogen activator used, the duration of infusion, and other factors.

OBJECTIVES OF TREATMENT

The primary therapeutic objective of catheter-directed thrombolysis is to dissolve the occluding thrombus. Achieving that, perfusion is usually restored and an underlying cause of the arterial or graft thrombosis can be identified, thereby allowing definitive correction of an underlying lesion. Important additional goals of thrombolytic therapy are to:

1. Convert an urgent surgical procedure into an elective procedure.
2. Gain patency of an occluded but nondiseased inflow source for subsequent bypass.
3. Lyse thrombi in the distal vasculature, thereby restoring patency to the outflow tract.
4. Convert a major vascular reconstruction into a limited, less extensive procedure.
5. Prevent arterial intimal injury from balloon catheter thrombectomy.
6. Restore patency of branch vessels inaccessible to mechanical thrombectomy.
7. Reduce the level of amputation in patients in whom complete success (limb salvage) cannot be achieved.

Although these are desirable goals, the likelihood of achieving them requires an understanding of the underlying problem, knowledge of the risks and benefits of alternative therapeutic options, and familiarity with the techniques and potential complications of each phase of intra-arterial thrombolytic therapy.

The outcome of patients treated with catheter-directed thrombolysis frequently depends on a variety of factors. The type and location of the vessel treated, the etiology and duration of occlusion, technique of lysis, and whether correction of the underlying disease was successful. The problems with lack of standard definitions and criteria for determining outcome (as evidenced by the two large prospective randomized trials) have contributed to the difficulty in developing a consensus on the indications for intra-arterial catheter-directed thrombolysis. In this chapter, we attempt to evaluate these data through the eyes of clinicians and conclude by identifying patients who are likely to benefit from catheter-directed thrombolysis as part of a strategy for revascularization of their ischemic limb.

BACKGROUND

McNichol and colleagues[4] first attempted the direct local delivery of a fibrinolytic agent for arterial thrombosis in 1963. Dotter and associates[5] extended and promoted catheter directed intra-arterial delivery of thrombolytic agents, and Katzen and van Breda[6] reported good results of low dose streptokinase infusion. However, they subsequently demonstrated that urokinase was safer and potentially more effective than streptokinase infusion.[7]

McNamara and Bomberger[8] captured the attention of vascular surgeons and interventional radiologists when they reported their good results of catheter-directed thrombolysis for patients with acute lower limb ischemia. They demonstrated that the outcome of patients with lesser degrees of ischemia was better than the outcome of patients with severe ischemia, no doubt due to multiple levels of occlusive disease in the patients with poor outcome. They also demonstrated that arterial emboli are treated more successfully than primary graft thrombosis. This is likely due to the volume of thrombus and the extent of underlying arterial disease.

Sullivan and Gardiner,[9] in their experience with catheter-directed thrombolysis for lower extremity graft occlusion, demonstrated that suprainguinal grafts are treated more successfully than infrainguinal grafts, with patency reports being 85% to 91% for the former and 59% to 68% for the latter. Interestingly, they found that the most durable patency was achieved in those with occluded autogenous grafts. However, other authors have failed to demonstrate the same degree of effectiveness of catheter-directed thrombolysis for graft failure, reporting a 1-year patency rate of only 30% to 40%.[10,11]

Because a spectrum of clinical observations have resulted from retrospective reviews and nonrandomized patient care, randomized trials were developed to answer key questions regarding thrombolytic therapy for arterial and graft occlusion.

RANDOMIZED TRIALS

The efficacy and safety of thrombolytic therapy for arterial and bypass graft occlusion have been studied in a number of well-performed prospective randomized trials. Patient selection varied somewhat and endpoint analysis has not been consistent, therefore the reader must examine these studies carefully to determine the appropriate application to individual clinical scenarios.

Berridge et al.[12] addressed the important issue of systemic thrombolysis vs. catheter-directed thrombolysis for acute arterial occlusion while investigating whether catheter-directed streptokinase (SK) was equivalent to catheter-directed tissue plasminogen activator (tPA). Results indicated that catheter-directed thrombolysis was significantly more effective than systemic thrombolysis for acute arterial thrombotic and embolic occlusion, and that catheter-directed tPA was more effective than catheter-directed SK.

Ouriel et al[13] performed a prospective randomized study to evaluate the efficacy and safety of intra-arterial catheter directed urokinase (UK) for acute limb ischemia (<7 days) compared with standard operative revascularization. One hundred fourteen patients who presented with acute limb ischemia of less than 7 days were randomized to either catheter-directed UK infusion or surgical revascularization. Patients enrolled in this study included those with embolic and thrombotic occlusion as well as native arterial and bypass graft occlusion (autogenous and prosthetic grafts). Seventy percent of the patients randomized to catheter-directed UK achieved arteriographically successful thrombolysis. An underlying lesion responsible for the arterial or graft occlusion was identified in only 37%, but each of these patients had correction of their underlying lesion by percutaneous balloon dilation or operative revision. The cumulative limb salvage was similar for the two treatment groups (82% at 12 months); however, the cumulative survival rate was significantly improved in patients randomized to thrombolysis (84% vs. 58% at 12 months, $p = .01$).

Interestingly, there was no difference in limb salvage in patients with acutely ischemic limbs; however, there was a significant reduction in mortality in patients randomized to thrombolysis, a similar observation found in the prospective blinded intraoperative UK study.[14] Although the authors attributed the high mortality in the surgical group to in-hospital cardiopulmonary complications as a consequence of the operative procedure, there may be other beneficial effects of lytic therapy that were not readily apparent.

STILE Trial

The first large prospective randomized multicenter trial evaluating catheter-directed thrombolysis vs. surgical revascularization for the ischemic lower extremity was the STILE (surgery vs. thrombolysis for the ischemic lower extremity) Trial.[1] The stated purpose was to evaluate the role of catheter-directed thrombolysis compared with routine operative revascularization in the management of the spectrum of patients with nonembolic limb ischemia. This was designed as an all-inclusive study of nonembolic limb ischemia and entered patients into the trial who had progression of ischemic symptoms within the prior 6 months. This design was a point of contention among the investigators; however, there was optimism and enthusiasm expressed by interventionists that patients with chronic limb ischemia could be treated successfully with catheter-based techniques. Randomization followed arteriographic documentation of obstruction of a native artery or bypass graft. Patients were randomized to recombinant tissue plasminogen activator (rt-PA) infusion, UK infusion, or operative revascularization. The primary endpoint was a composite clinical outcome consisting of death, amputation, ongoing or recurrent ischemia, or defined major morbidity. The trial was stopped by the data and safety monitoring committee because the pretrial boundary limits were achieved following interim analysis of the outcome of treatment of the "target vessel" (ongoing/recurrent ischemia). Overall, results indicated that lower limb ischemia was treated more effectively with operative revascularization compared with catheter-directed thrombolysis. However, when the outcome was stratified by duration of ischemia, it became apparent that acutely ischemic patients (<14 days of ischemia) had a significantly better outcome when treated with catheter-directed thrombolysis compared to patients randomized to operative revascularization. Bleeding complications occurred more often in lytic patients compared to surgical patients (6% vs. 1%, $p = .014$), and intracranial bleeding occurred in 1.2%.

Two large groups of patients stratified within in the STILE study were patients with native arterial occlusion and patients with occluded lower extremity bypass grafts. It is important to separate these two groups because the treatment outcome may be quite different. Comerota et al.[15] reviewed the results of patients with occluded lower extremity bypass grafts. It was interesting that the average duration of graft occlusion was 34 days. Catheter placement proved to be a problem, in that 39% randomized to lysis failed to have the catheter properly positioned and therefore reverted to surgical revascularization. However, following successful catheter placement, patency was restored in 84%, and in the lytic group overall, 42% had a major reduction in their planned operation. One-year results of successful lysis compared favorably with the best surgical procedure, which was new graft placement. Acutely ischemic patients (0 to 14 days) randomized to lysis showed a trend toward a lower major amputation rate at 30 days ($p = .07$) achieving significance at 1 year ($p = .026$) compared with surgical patients. However, patients with more than 14 days of ischemia showed no difference in limb salvage, but experienced a high rate of lytic failure (ongoing/recurrent ischemia) ($p < .001$). Patients with prosthetic graft occlusion had greater overall morbidity than patients with occluded autogenous grafts ($p < .02$).

Weaver et al.[16] reviewed the results obtained in the 237 STILE patients with native artery occlusion. The results indicated that 78% of the patients could have the catheter properly positioned and a lytic agent infused. This lead to a reduction in the predetermined surgical procedure in 56% of the patients. Although lysis time was shorter with rt-PA compared to UK (8 h vs. 24 h; $p < .05$), there was no difference in efficacy or safety. At 1 year, the incidence of recurrent ischemia and major amputation was higher in patients randomized to lysis. Interestingly, diabetics randomized to surgery had a 32% mortality at 1 year compared to 7.5% mortality in those randomized to catheter directed thrombolysis ($p < .05$).

TOPAS II Trial

Ouriel and colleagues[2] reported their analysis of recombinant urokinase (rUK) vs. operative revascularization as the initial treatment for acute lower extremity arterial or graft occlusion (TOPAS II). This was a randomized trial conducted at 113 centers evaluating catheter-directed intra-arterial rUK vs. operative revascularization in 544 patients with acute arterial or graft occlusion of 14 days or less. The dose of rUK was that identified by the TOPAS I trial[17] (a dose ranging trial), 4000 IU/min × 4 h, then reduced to 2000 IU/min. Interestingly, the primary endpoint for both TOPAS I and TOPAS II was "amputation-free survival."

The results of TOPAS II indicated that 68% of patients randomized to lysis achieved complete clot dissolution. Both groups had similar improvement in their ankle–brachial pressure index (ABI). Amputation-free survival rates in the rUK group was 72% at 6 months and 65% at 1 year, as compared to 75% and 70% in the surgical group, respectively. At 6 months, patients randomized to lysis underwent 315 operative procedures, compared to 551 operative procedures in the surgical group (43% reduction). However, bleeding complications occurred in 13% of the rUK group, compared to 6% in the surgical group ($p = .005$). There was a 1.6% incidence of intracranial hemorrhage.

Amputation-free survival does not seem to be an appropriate primary endpoint for a study such as this, because most patients do not die and most do not lose a limb. One might also argue that comparing "target vessel patency" in lytic patients to surgical revascularization, as was done in the STILE Trial,[1] was unlikely to demonstrate the benefit of thrombolysis because surgical results are reasonably good. With these two trials there is a large experience with catheter-directed thrombolysis from which one should be able to glean meaningful guidance as to the appropriate place of catheter-directed thrombolysis.

Despite the apparently different outcomes between the STILE and TOPAS II trials, there may be more similarities than there are differences. If the STILE data are tabulated according to the TOPAS II endpoints, one observes remarkably similar outcomes, with perhaps a trend toward better outcomes in lytic patients, especially those with acute graft occlusion (Table 25–1). There appears to be an inescapable 1% to 2% incidence of intracranial hemorrhage, with patency restored to 60% to 70% of occluded vessels. Interestingly, if the STILE investigators were to have chosen amputation-free survival as an endpoint, the trial undoubtedly would have continued to reach the target of 1000 patients, anticipating a benefit in the patients randomized with bypass graft occlusion.

TABLE 25–1. COMPARISON OF RESULTS OF TOPAS II AND STILE TRIALS USING SIMILARLY DEFINED ENDPOINTS

	TOPAS II		STILE[a]	
	Lysis	*Surgery*	*Lysis*	*Surgery*
Complete lysis patency	68%	N/A	61%	N/A
Amputation-free survival	65%	70%	81%	64%
Grafts	68%	69%	74%	52%
Arteries	61%	71%	87%	81%
Duration rUK/UK infusion (mean)	24 h	N/A	24 h	N/A
Reduction surgical procedures	43%	N/A	56%	N/A
Hemorrhage	13%	6%	6%	1%
Intracranial bleed	1.6%	0%	1.2%	0%

[a] Data from STILE Trial reformatted to endpoints defined by TOPAS II trial.

Because a "target vessel" endpoint was used, the STILE trial was stopped because of the more effective revascularization of the target vessel by surgical means.

TECHNIQUE

In patients with acute limb ischemia, planning for intra-arterial lytic therapy should begin prior to arteriography. The approach is usually from the contralateral femoral artery, threading the catheter around the aortic bifurcation. Vessels considered for thrombolysis should have an attempt at guidewire penetration of the occlusion. If a guidewire can be passed well into or through the thrombus, then successful thrombolysis is likely. If a guidewire cannot be passed through the occlusion, either atherosclerotic disease, neointimal fibroplasia, or highly organized and calcified thrombus is present that will not respond to a lytic agent; therefore, primary operative reconstruction is generally recommended. General factors predictive of outcome of catheter-directed lysis are listed in Table 25–2.

If guidewire passage is successful, the infusion catheter should be embedded well into the occluded vessel. Once catheters are appropriately positioned, either UK or rt-PA is the recommended agent. Our prior experience with SK resulted in unacceptably high bleeding complications. The initial dose of UK is usually a 500,000-unit bolus, followed by 4000 U/min until recanalization is achieved, at which point the dose can be reduced to 1000 to 2000 U/min. If rt-PA is chosen, a dose of 0.05 mg/kg per h is used for a period of up to 12 h. These generic recommendations can be modified by using higher dosages if more rapid lysis is required.

Patients are given broad-spectrum antibiotics intravenously while the catheter is in place. Routine blood studies are performed prior to and during treatment, and include a complete coagulation profile. A guiac test on a stool specimen is performed prior to treatment for documentation. All patients remain at absolute bedrest, and most are treated in the intensive care unit. Puncture sites are frequently observed, and the circulatory status of the infused extremity is monitored clinically, and ankle pressures performed when either improvement or deterioration is observed.

Periodic arteriography is performed to follow the therapeutic response and guide positioning of the catheter. The initial 2 to 4 h of infusion is generally performed in the radiology suite. Catheters are then advanced into the thrombus as required, appreciating that inappropriate catheter position increases the risk of failure.

TABLE 25–2. FACTORS PREDICTIVE OF THE SUCCESS OF CATHETER-DIRECTED INTRA-ARTERIAL THROMBOLYSIS

Factor	Likelihood of Successful Lysis	
	High	*Low*
Guidewire	Passes into clot	Cannot pass
Duration of occlusion	Short (hours or days)	Long (weeks)
Location of occlusion	Proximal	Distal
Distal vessels (by arteriogram)	Visualized	Not visualized
Distal Doppler signals	Audible	None
Relative contraindications	None/few	Some/many

TABLE 25–3. THREATENED FEMOROPOPLITEAL/TIBIAL AUTOGENOUS BYPASS: COMPARISON OF DURABILITY OF TECHNIQUES OF GRAFT REVISION

Author	Five-Year Durability	
	Balloon Dilatation	Operative Revision
Bandyk et al., 1991[30]	50% (9/18)	86% (55/64)
Perler et al., 1990[31]	22% (4/18)[a]	62% (5/19)
Cohen et al., 1986[32]	43% (3/7)	82% (18/22)

[a] Three-year durability.

If one is faced with multisegment occlusion and infusion guidewires can be advanced into the distal segment, infusion of lytic agents is performed through a coaxial system. The dose of the lytic agent is then split between the catheters, with relatively higher doses delivered to the distal occlusion.

The concurrent administration of heparin with SK has been associated with excessive hemorrhagic complication rates. The severity of bleeding complications by infusing heparin during UK administration has not been similarly observed. However, most clinicians agree that the concurrent use of heparin with all thrombolytic agents tends to increase the risk of bleeding. Heparin is used to reduce the risk of pericatheter thrombosis. If a catheter is placed into a long static arterial segment, or if the catheter traverses a high grade stenosis to reach the occluding thrombus, higher doses of heparin are given to achieve adequate anticoagulation.

The systemic effect of lytic therapy is monitored by the fibrinogen level, prothrombin time, partial thromboplastin time, and fibrin degradation products during infusion. Although bleeding can occur in any patient receiving lytic therapy, patients with significant hypofibrinogenemia appear to be at greatest risk of a serious hemorrhagic complication.[1] If the fibrinogen level drops below 100 mg/dl, we slow or stop the infusion to allow the restoration of circulating fibrinogen and clotting factors. On rare occasion, fresh-frozen plasma or cryoprecipitate can be administered to patients having a serious bleeding event.

After successful infusion, an arteriogram is performed and blood studies are repeated. The catheter is removed when the fibrinogen level returns to 100 mg/dl or more. After successful lysis, the underlying cause of the occlusion should be identified and corrected immediately by means of standard interventional techniques. If percutaneous correction is not possible, systemic anticoagulation is continued until the definitive operative procedure is completed.

The technique selected to repair the underlying lesion may have substantial impact on long-term success. In general, operative repair is more durable than percutaneous techniques, especially when dealing with infrainguinal lesions. This has been demonstrated by several studies evaluating the threatened femoropopliteal/tibial saphenous vein bypass graft (Table 25–3). Because neointimal fibroplasia is important in the etiology of autogenous graft failure, operative revision is recommended.

PATIENT SELECTION

Appropriate patient selection is critical to successful therapy. If one determines that elimination of the occluding thrombus will benefit the patient, the first step in patient selection is accomplished. We now know that long segments of the vascular tree can be obliterated by acute thrombus precipitated by severe but relatively segmental atherosclerotic disease. Also, failure of a bypass graft is often due to a segmental pathological condition, either anastomotic or within the graft, with the remainder of the graft being a potentially well-functioning conduit. This is particularly true for bypass grafts functioning for a year or more prior to thrombosis. In these clinical scenarios, the ability to eliminate the thrombus and identify and correct the segmental pathology is an important advantage of fibrinolytic therapy.

Patients diagnosed with clearcut acute embolic occlusion of large arteries that are easily accessible by a limited incision under local or regional anesthesia can be treated quickly and efficiently with standard operative embolectomy. However, patients with multivessel and distal vessel embolic occlusion may not have a favorable operative outcome, especially if associated with other critical illness or acute myocardial infarction. Intra-arterial fibrinolytic therapy should be considered as adjunctive therapy to what can be achieved operatively. However, some patients should not be offered fibrinolytic therapy, either because the risk of complications is excessively high or because the operative alternative is more efficient.

Patients with acute postoperative bypass graft thrombosis should not be treated with intra-arterial thrombolysis for several reasons. Early postoperative thrombosis usually represents a technical error or poor patient selection for the revascularization procedure. For the former problem, operative thrombectomy with concurrent correction of the technical problem is recommended. For the latter situation, recurrent thrombosis is certain after mechanical or pharmacological thrombectomy, and the limits of revascularization should be accepted without exposing the patient to needless additional risk.

Patients who have thrombosed knitted Dacron grafts treated with lytic agents have an increased risk of transgraft hemorrhage.[18] Transgraft extravasation does not appear to be a problem with grafts having an external covering or through woven Dacron or PTFE grafts. The presence of a knitted Dacron graft in a central location is a strong relative contraindication to lytic therapy.

Patients with modest ischemia who have tolerable intermittent claudication are not offered arteriography or operative intervention. This group of patients should not be offered intra-arterial lytic therapy for the same reason that bypass procedures are not considered, because the natural history of their disease is favorable. Although the likelihood of early success with any intervention in claudicants is high, finite complication and amputation rates exist, and each patient treated should be fully aware of such risks and participate in sharing the responsibility for the choice of treatment. The attitude of "Let's treat the lesion and see what happens because we have nothing to lose" should be avoided.

Patients who have acute thrombosis of a proximal artery causing significant ischemia are considered candidates for thrombolysis, assuming there are no contraindications to therapy. Acute thrombosis of a popliteal aneurysm causing profound ischemia is best treated with catheter-directed lytic therapy[19] to restore patency of the outflow vessels. This severe degree of ischemia occurs more frequently when the popliteal trifurcation is involved. Emergent operative reconstruction in these patients is associated with an excessive amputation rate.[20] Reestablishing patency of infrapopliteal vessels by the regional delivery of a fibrinolytic agent eliminates the severe ischemia, frequently opens the occluded outflow tract, and allows an elective operation. This approach increases the chance of limb salvage and successful aneurysm repair. If the patient has thrombosis of a popliteal aneurysm but the limb is not threatened, vascular reconstruction (if indicated) should be planned without prior thrombolysis.

Patients with acute occlusion of a saphenous vein bypass, either *in situ* or reversed, can have their graft salvaged by intragraft infusion by fibrinolytic agents.[9] Operative thrombectomy is generally associated with poor long-term results.[21] Thrombosed femorotibial grafts likewise carry a high operative failure rate, as does any bypass graft occlusion in which the runoff vessels are thrombosed. Thrombosis of a prosthetic bypass resulting in ischemia similar to the original indication for the bypass is treated by surgical revascularization (if indicated). However, if the patient's ischemia is more severe due to additional arterial segment thrombosis, catheter-directed lysis is recommended to restore patency to occluded native arteries. Patients who have undergone multiple previous reconstructive procedures with acute thrombosis are at high risk for an unsuccessful operative reconstruction. Numerous reasons exist for graft failure in such patients, and it is often difficult to define accurately the cause and perform appropriate correction at the time of emergency thrombectomy.

Patients who have acute embolic occlusion of vessels inaccessible to mechanical thrombectomy and patients with wound complications in whom another wound would carry significant morbidity should be considered potential candidates for intra-arterial fibrinolytic therapy.

COMPLICATIONS OF THROMBOLYTIC THERAPY

Complications encountered with catheter-directed delivery of thrombolytic agents can be categorized as complications secondary to the drug and its subsequent effects on the fibrinolytic and coagulation system and mechanical (arteriographic) complications associated with the technique (Table 25–4).

Allergic Reactions

Because bacteria are the source of SK, a foreign protein from the cell wall of the bacteria accounts for the allergic and pyretic side effects observed in up to 30% of the patients. If SK infusion is anticipated, pretreatment with 100 mg of hydrocortisone and administration of acetaminophen every 6 h reduces the allergic response. Allergic reactions are rare with UK, so pretreatment with steroids is unnecessary. Some patients have developed low-grade fevers with UK infusion that are treated with oral acetaminophen.

TABLE 25–4. COMPLICATIONS OF INTRA-ARTERIAL LYTIC THERAPY

I. Drug-Associated Complications
   A. Hemorrhage
      1. Due to lysis of hemostatic fibrin
      2. Due to the induced coagulopathy
   B. Distal emboli
   C. Allergic reaction
   D. Pyretic reaction
   E. Serum sickness (SK)
   F. Transgraft extravasation (hemorrhage)
II. Technique-Associated Complications
   A. Pericatheter thrombosis
   B. Catheter-induced arterial occlusion
   C. Toxic complications of contrast
   D. Pseudoaneurysm of puncture site
   E. Arteriogram complications

Hemorrhage

Bleeding is the most common and most feared complication of thrombolytic therapy. Bleeding usually occurs as a result of the active lytic state following dissolution of "hemostatic" thrombus, but can also be due to the induced coagulopathy (fibrinogen and clotting factor depletion) caused by the lytic agent. It is often difficult to distinguish the incidence of major bleeding complications from less serious bleeding complications in many reports. Major bleeding complications should be defined as those which cause permanent disability, prolong hospital stay, or require blood transfusion.

Patients who have major invasive procedures, especially arterial cannulation, have higher rates of bleeding complications than patients who do not, a fact that has been observed in myocardial infarction trials in which patients with arterial interventions had a 30% bleeding complication rate compared with 5% or less in patients without.[22] Intracerebral bleeding is the most dreaded of all hemorrhagic events, and its incidence is probably an inescapable 1% to 2%. Data have been gathered from several myocardial infarction trials that demonstrate that the risk of intracerebral bleeding is increased by age, hypertension, low body weight, coincident head injury, previous cerebrovascular accident, and previous warfarin anticoagulation.[22]

The mechanisms for bleeding during thrombolytic therapy can be characterized as:

1. Lysis of hemostatic thrombi
2. Consequences of clotting factor and fibrinogen depletion
3. Continued anticoagulation

Most of the bleeding during the infusion of the lytic agents was not caused by biochemical changes created by the lytic agents, but rather by the lysis of hemostatic clot. Patients treated with lytic agents who have complete vascular integrity have a smooth therapeutic course without bleeding complications.

Most bleeding occurs due to the trauma of invasive diagnostic or therapeutic procedures. By definition, invasive procedures are required for catheter-directed thrombolysis; therefore, an unavoidable minimal number of bleeding complications occur. However, if lytic therapy is anticipated prior to diagnostic arteriography, the appropriate entry site can be chosen using a single-wall puncture technique, permitting appropriate catheter or sheath placement with minimal additional trauma.

The purpose of laboratory monitoring of thrombolytic therapy is to document accurately that the thrombolytic agent chosen is producing an effective lytic state. However, whereas this is a necessary part of systemic thrombolysis, the efficacy of catheter-directed thrombolysis is evaluated clinically and angiographically and does not depend on laboratory markers of systemic fibrinolysis. In general, laboratory values do not correlate with hemorrhagic complications or efficacy of lysis.

It has been found that the importance of fibrinogen depletion as stressed early in the clinical experience with thrombolysis was probably overrated. Subsequent analyses have demonstrated that there was no correlation with bleeding complications.[23] However, the majority of these observations were made in patients treated for venous thromboembolism or acute myocardial infarction. Conversely, the clinical experience with catheter-directed thrombolysis for peripheral arterial and graft occlusion suggested that fibrinogen depletion was linked to the incidence of serious bleeding complications. A number of factors are relevant to these observations, including:

1. Patients treated for peripheral arterial or graft occlusion require arterial puncture and prolonged cannulation.
2. The duration of therapy extends far beyond that needed for myocardial infarction and may exceed that required for venous thromboembolism.

3. The fibrinogen concentration measured may detect hemostatically ineffective fibrinogen.[24]

4. Certain individuals with low fibrinogen concentrations (patients treated with thrombolytic agents and patients with hereditary afibrinogenemias) do not uniformly have hemorrhagic complications.[25]

5. The fibrinogen associated with platelets may be as important hemostatically ascirculating fibrinogen.[26]

Transgraft Extravasation

Extravasation of contrast material and blood has been reported in patients treated with SK or UK who have prostheses in place.[27,28] Extravasation has been observed most often through knitted Dacron grafts. The larger mesh of the knitted graft is the likely explanation for this observation. Plasmin lyses the fibrin seal of the graft, which opens the interstices and allows subsequent extravastion of dye and blood. Reports of extravastion from grafts in place for more than a year indicate that the fibrin meshwork is continually susceptible to lysis despite a long graft inplant time. Therefore, patients with knitted prostheses have a major added hemorrhagic potential when treated with lytic agents. In our opinion, these patients may be considered to have a relative contraindication to thrombolytic therapy. In the event of a knitted prostheses in a central location (chest or abdomen), if hemorrhage occurs it can be life-threatening; therefore, alternative therapy is suggested. Because many patients with aortic aneurysmal and occlusive disease subsequently suffer myocardial infarction and because high-dose fibrinolytic therapy can benefit many patients with myocardial infarction, we suggest that knitted Dacron grafts not be used in the chest or abdomen.

Distal Emboli

Embolic complications distal to the occluded artery or graft can occur during intra-arterial thrombolytic therapy that is usually the result of either partial lysis of thrombus, with fragments carried distally during reperfusion; or, less frequently, a mechanical complication due to catheter manipulation or volume of infusate.

In our experience, distal embolic occlusion is observed infrequently during treatment of thrombosed native arteries or saphenous vein grafts. It has been observed occasionally during treatment of acute arterial emboli and more frequently during treatment of thrombosed PTFE grafts with patent runoff vessels.

Appropriate treatment of distal emboli that occur during catheter-directed thrombolysis is catheter advancement and continued infusion, perhaps at a higher dose. Whereas this tends to lyse distal emboli, occasionally occlusions of the smaller arteries are resistant to lysis. If lysis does not occur in the face of progressive ischemia, the risk of irreversible ischemic damage escalates rapidly, and clinical judgment as to the appropriate treatment can be difficult.

Technical Complications

Technique-related complications are those associated with arteriography and catheter placement. Intimal dissection, thrombosis, allergic and toxic reactions to contrast agents, and femoral neuropathy have been reported.

Whenever the catheter passes through an existing stenosis to treat an occlusion, the risk of pericatheter thrombosis increases and concurrent anticoagulation should be considered. Repeat arteriography is accompanied by an increased contrast dye load and thereby escalates the risk of renal impairment.

CURRENT CLINICAL APPLICATIONS

All who have participated in randomized trials such as the trials previously reviewed in this chapter appreciate that patients can meet entry criteria and be randomized, yet not represent the typical patient an experienced clinician would choose to treat with catheter-directed lysis. The characteristics of patients likely to benefit from catheter-directed thrombolysis are summarized in Table 25–5. Patients presenting with acute limb ischemia due to thrombosed lower extremity bypass grafts are treated preferentially with catheter-directed thrombolysis. This is especially true if the graft has been functional for an extended period of time after insertion. Once a guidewire and a catheter are positioned appropriately, one can anticipate a high likelihood of success. Key to long-term benefit is the identification and correction of an underlying lesion that may lead to graft failure.

Acute embolic occlusion, especially if multiple vessels are involved, is treated appropriately with catheter-directed thrombolysis. It has been our experience that embolic occlusions lyse relatively rapidly. Acute native artery thrombosis can be treated successfully if a guidewire can be advanced through the occluded segment and if a catheter can be positioned appropriately (Fig. 25–1). However, one must use considerable clinical judgment, because long segments of diseased vessels will ultimately require surgical revascularization. Therefore, it may not be prudent to subject the patient to prolonged lytic infusions if the final operation cannot be avoided.

Intraoperative intra-arterial infusions of UK and tPA offers useful adjunctive lysis to mechanical thromboembolectomy. Although it was not the subject of this review, intraoperative intra-arterial lytic infusion can be used safely to improve the chance of success following balloon catheter thromboembolectomy.[14,29] We now routinely infuse lytic agents in the distal circulation of all patients when thrombus is removed. It has been shown that complete mechanical removal is the exception rather than the rule, and residual distal thrombotic material can undergo accelerated lysis with intraoperative intra-arterial infusions.

In summary, catheter-directed thrombolysis and intraoperative intra-arterial thrombolysis are important adjuncts in the care of patients with acute arterial and bypass graft occlusion. It is important that intra-arterial thrombolysis not be thought of as a competitor to operative revascularization, but rather as a part of an overall treatment strategy in properly selected patients. This enables the responsible physician to offer the best of what is available for these patients.

TABLE 25–5. CHARACTERISTICS OF PATIENTS LIKELY TO BENEFIT FROM CATHETER-DIRECTED THROMBOLYSIS

1. Acute occlusion of saphenous vein bypass grafts, especially grafts that have functioned well for 1 or more years.

2. Acute thrombosis of prosthetic bypass graft, with more severe ischemia than present at time of initial bypass (additional arterial segment thrombosis).

3. Acute embolic or thrombotic occlusion causing critical ischemia in vessels inaccessible to mechanical thromboembolectomy.

4. Acute embolic or thrombotic occlusion causing critical ischemia in poor-risk surgical patients.

5. Acute thrombosis of popliteal aneurysms causing critical limb ischemia due to occlusion of tibial and peroneal arteries.

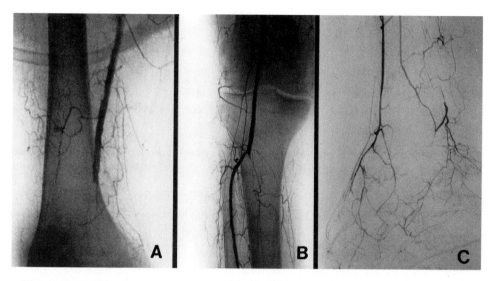

Figure 25–1. (A) Arteriogram of a diabetic patient with an acutely ischemic foot who suffered an acute myocardial infarction 4 days earlier. Arteriography demonstrates occlusion of the popliteal artery and all runoff vessels. **(B)** Following catheter-directed urokinase (UK), the popliteal artery and anterior tibial artery were opened. A lesion of the midpopliteal artery was thought to be the culprit lesion and responded well to balloon dilatation. **(C)** Foot film showing perfusion at the ankle and foot level.

REFERENCES

1. The STILE Investigators. Results of a prospective randomized trial evaluating surgery versus thrombolysis for ischemia of the lower extremity. The STILE Trial. *Ann Surg.* 1994;220: 251–268.
2. Ouriel K, Veith FJ, Sasahara AA, et al. A comparison of recombinant urokinase with vascular surgery as initial treatment for acute arterial occlusion of the legs. *N Engl J Med.* 1998;338:1105–1111.
3. Alkjaersig N, Fletcher AP, Sherry S. The mechanism of clot dissolution by plasmin. *J Clin Invest.* 1959;38:1086.
4. McNichol GP, Reid W, Bain WH, Douglas AS. Treatment of peripheral arterial occlusion of peripheral arterial occlusion by streptokinase perfusion. *Br Med J.* 1963;1:1508.
5. Dotter CT, Rosch J, Seamen AJ. Selective clot lysis with low dose streptokinase. *Radiology.* 1974;111:31.
6. Katzen BT, van Breda A. Low dose streptokinase in the treatment of arterial occlusions. *Am J Radiol.* 1986;36:1172.
7. van Breda A, Katzen BT, Deutsch AF. Urokinase vs. streptokinase in local thrombolysis. *Radiology.* 1987;176:109.
8. McNamara TO, Bomberger RA. Factors affecting initial and 6 month patency rates after intraarterial thrombolysis with high dose urokinase. *Am J Surg.* 1986;152:709.
9. Sullivan KL, Gardiner GA Jr, Kandarpa K, et al. Efficacy of thrombolysis in infrainguinal bypass grafts. *Circulation.* 1991;83(Suppl I):1–99.
10. Belkin M, Donaldson MC, Wittemore AD, et al. Observations on the use of thrombolytic agents for thrombotic occlusion of infrainguinal vein grafts. *J Vasc Surg.* 1990;11:289.
11. Sicard G, Schier JJ, Totty WG, et al. Thrombolytic therapy for acute arterial occlusion. *J Vasc Surg.* 1985;2:65.
12. Berridge DC, al Kutoubi A, Mansfield AU, et al. Thrombolysis in arterial graft thrombosis. *Eur J Vasc Endovasc Surg.* 1995;9:129–132.

13. Ouriel K, Shortell CK, DeWeese JA, et al. A comparison of thrombolytic therapy with operative revascularization in the treatment of acute peripheral arterial ischemia. *J Vasc Surg.* 1994;19:1021–1030.

14. Comerota AJ, Rao AK, Throm RC, et al. A prospective randomized, blinded and placebo controlled trial of intraoperative urokinase infusion during lower extremity revascularization: regional and systemic effects. *Ann Surg.* 1993;218:534.

15. Comerota AJ, Weaver FA, Hoskins JD, et al. Results of a prospective, randomized trial of surgery versus thrombolysis for occluded lower extremity bypass grafts. *Am J Surg.* 1996;172:102–112.

16. Weaver FA, Comerota AJ, Youngblood M, et al. Surgical revascularization versus thrombolysis for nonembolic lower extremity native artery occlusions: results of a prospective randomized trial. *J Vasc Surg.* 1996;24:513–523.

17. Ouriel K, Veith F, Sasahara A. Thrombolysis or peripheral arterial surgery: phase I results. *J Vasc Surg.* 1996;23:64–75.

18. Comerota AJ, White, JV. Overview of catheter directed thrombolytic therapy for arterial and graft occlusion. In Comerota AJ, ed. *Thrombolytic Therapy for Peripheral Vascular Disease.* Philadelphia: JP Lippincott Co.; 1995;225–252.

19. Taylor LM, Porter JM, Baur GM. Intraarterial streptokinase infusion for acute popliteal and tibial artery occlusion. *Am J Surg.* 1984;147:583.

20. Bouhoustos J, Martin P: Popliteal aneurysm: a review of 116 cases. *Br J Surg.* 1974;61:469.

21. Green RM, Ouriel K, Ricotta JJ, DeWeese JA. Revision of failed infrainguinal bypass grafts: principles and management. *Surgery.* 1986;100:646.

22. deBono DP, More RS. Prevention and management of bleeding complications after thrombolysis. *Int J Cardiol.* 1993;38:1.

23. Marder VJ. The use of thrombolytic agents: choice of patient, drug administration, laboratory monitoring. *Ann Intern Med.* 1973;90:802.

24. Ranjadayalan K, Stevenson R, Marchant B, et al. Streptokinase induced defibrination assessed by thrombin time: effects on residual coronary stenosis and left ventricular ejection fraction. *Br Heart J.* 1992;68:171.

25. Sharp RA, Forbes CD. Congenital coagulation disorders. In: Ludlam CA, ed. *Clinical Haemotology.* Edinburgh: Churchill Livingstone; 1990;351.

26. Coller BS. Platelets and thrombolytic therapy. *N Engl J Med.* 1990;322:33.

27. Hargrove WC, Barker CF, Berkowitz HD, et al. Treatment of acute peripheral arterial and graft thromboses with low dose streptokinase. *Surgery.* 1982;92:981.

28. Rabe FE, Becker GJ, Richmond BD, et al. Contrast extravasation through Dacron grafts: a sequela of low dose streptokinase therapy. *Am J Radiol.* 1982;138:917.

29. Comerota AJ, Rao AK. Intraoperative intraarterial thrombolytic therapy. In: Comerota AJ, ed. *Thrombolytic Therapy for Peripheral Vascular Disease.* Philadelphia: JB Lippincott Co.; 1995;313–328.

30. Bandyk DF, Bergamini TM, Towne JB, et al. Duration of vein graft revisions: the outcome of secondary procedures. *J Vasc Surg.* 1991;61:159–165.

31. Perler BA, Osterman FA, Mitchell SE, et al. Balloon dilation versus surgical revision of infra-inguinal autogenous vein graft stenoses: long term follow-up. *J Cardiovasc Surg.* 1990;31(5):656–660.

32. Cohen FR, Mannick JA, Couch NP, et al. Recognition and management of impending vein graft failure. *Arch Surg.* 1986;121:758.

26

The Management of Mesenteric Venous Thrombosis

Michael C. Dalsing, MD

INTRODUCTION

The management of acute mesenteric venous thrombosis (MVT) was entirely surgical prior to 1985. Without surgical intervention, only 8% of patients survived.[1] Proper operative intervention involving bowel resection could salvage approximately 65% of patients and the addition of anticoagulation could improve the patient's chances by approximately 12%.[1] However, animal experimentation, clinical observation, and operative findings all suggested that this disease should present as a spectrum of severity from the asymptomatic state to a condition of complete bowel infarction. The problem, of course, was the imprecise presentation and lack of diagnostic tools that could confirm the diagnosis prior to clinical deterioration. The advent of noninvasive, diagnostic imaging that is readily available and accurate has dramatically changed our approach to the management of these patients.

INCIDENCE

The incidence of MVT as a cause of acute mesenteric ischemia has varied historically based first on the realization that it existed and then the ability to accurately make the diagnosis. The first operative description of this type of bowel infarction was provided by Elliott in 1895.[2] This observation lay in relative obscurity until Warren and Eberhard described MVT as a distinct clinical entity in 1935.[3] With its rediscovery, MVT was increasingly considered the cause of bowel ischemia over the next 25 years. Thirty to 50% of mesenteric infarction with a known cause was attributed to MVT during this period.[4] However, with the discovery in the late 1950s that mesenteric ischemia may be due to a nonocclusive generalized low-flow phenomena, the diagnosis of MVT as a cause of bowel ischemia declined. It was reported as the etiologic factor of mesenteric infarction in 4% to 13% of cases in series from 1960 to 1980.[5,6] The introduction of noninvasive diagnostic imaging that allowed detailed evaluation of the abdominal cavity appears to have generated a resurgence of this diagnosis especially in patients who might otherwise have never been discovered. A review from the Mayo Clinic reports a 17.9% rate of MVT as the cause of acute mesenteric ischemia.[7] In this study, 37 patients were discovered in a 10-year period after 1984, whereas only 16 cases were observed from 1972 to 1983.

Even though MVT is being rediscovered because of improved diagnostic procedures and physician awareness, it is still an uncommon surgical problem. This diagnosis is reported to account for only 0.002% to 0.06% of all emergency surgical admissions to acute care hospitals.[5,6]

EXPERIMENTAL STUDIES AND PATHOPHYSIOLOGY

The majority of experimental work on MVT and the bowel ischemia it imparts was performed in the dog model. These experimental findings provide some useful insight into what is observed clinically.

Donaldson and Stout[8] ligated the main venous radicals together with bowel wall collaterals draining venous blood from 8 to 25 cm of ileum. They observed the soggy edematous bowel wall seen clinically in acute MVT. The bowel demonstrated active peristalsis when stimulated, suggesting that bowel movements could still occur in this condition. The arterial system routinely remained patent. Using this model, the majority of animals survived. Progression of the disease from an early swollen bowel to a state of local adhesions with normal appearing bowel was observed by delayed sacrifice. This study suggested that a moderate length of bowel could experience mesenteric venous occlusion reflected as significant edema of the bowel but that the process could eventually resolve with few ill effects.

Laufman[9] observed total occlusion of the superior mesenteric vein (SMV) in 20 necropsies without intestinal damage, an observation that spurred his interest to study a dog model of slow mesenteric venous occlusion. A loose cellophane wrapping of the SMV in the dog slowly narrowed and could eventually occlude the vein. No intestinal lesion resulted, and venography demonstrated the remarkable collateral network that had developed to alleviate the venous hypertension.[9] This suggested that MVT of major veins could occur without bowel infarction if appropriate collateralization developed.

In a follow-up investigation by Laufman and Method,[10] acute ligation of the SMV clearly demonstrated tremendous swelling of the bowel and mesentery with the formation of a bloodstained peritoneal transudate. Arterial spasm produced as a response to the acute venous hypertension was not always relieved with the release of venous occlusion, resulting in continued bowel ischemia.[10] The animals appeared to die from shock generally within 3 h. This study suggested that arterial vasospasm may contribute to bowel ischemia but that death appeared to be a shock phenomena.

Polk, Friedenberg, and colleagues in the mid-1960s reported a series of experiments to study MVT. Simple ligation of the SMV was compatible with survival but did result in significant bowel changes and transudates as noted in previous studies.[11] Measurable fluid losses exceeding 100 ml/kg in the first hour (equivalent to 10 L in a 70 kg man) were amenable to correction with proper fluid replacement. Leukocytosis was present early in the disease process but would normalize over several weeks. Although the mesenteric venous pressure was extremely high immediately after ligation (1200 mm Hg), patients who survived demonstrated a rapid decline in intravenous pressure within 5 min. Peritoneal fluid was present but was not toxic to mice, and therefore was likely sterile. It would appear that the treatment of clinical MVT must consider tremendous fluid shifts likely be manifest as shock whereas infection in the early stages without frank bowel infarction may be of less concern. Appropriate treatment of early shock can result in long-term survival.

The addition of intravenous thrombin injection caudal to the SMV ligature resulted in clotting well into the peripheral veins and resulted in death within 1 to 4 h.[12] The volume loss in these animals was more severe and showed less response to deficit correction than simple ligation of the SMV. It appeared that thrombosis of the small venules that drain the bowel directly might prevent collateral networks from developing, resulting in bowel loss, whereas more central occlusions may be ultimately tolerable.

If the body is given time to adapt by recruiting collaterals, the bowel can survive. The anticoagulant heparin might provide the critical time required for this process to occur by preventing continued or more extensive thrombosis. Laufman and colleagues[13] demonstrated sludge formation in small veins within 10 to 30 min of SMV occlusion. Thrombus formation began within 30 min but could be prevented by anticoagulants. Nelson and Kremen[14] clamped the SMV and observed bowel engorgement, bloody peritoneal fluid accumulation, shock, and death within 4 h. Preoperative heparinization allowed SMV clamping for as long as 6 h without significant bowel damage. Going one step further, the SMV was ligated in a heparinized group of animals and only two of the eight dogs died. Several weeks later, two animals were sacrificed and the intestine appeared normal.[14] The SMV remained occluded. Polk,[12] using a very stringent model of MVT, could demonstrate no benefit to heparin use. This discrepancy is easily explained by the overwhelming stimulus to thrombosis initiated by intravascular thrombin injection.

Superior mesenteric artery (SMA) angiography with venous phase was diagnostic for this disease showing (1) reflux of dye into the aorta, (2) spasm of the SMA and branches often more obvious with disease progression, (3) difficulty in opacifying peripheral arterial branches, (4) prolongation of the arterial phase of injection, (5) intense opacification of the thickened bowel wall (blushing), (6) occasional intraluminal contrast, and (7) failure to opacify the mesenteric venous and portal systems.[15] Obviously, angiography could provide an accurate diagnostic tool readily available to the discerning clinician.

Venous thrombectomy is a surgical intervention investigated experimentally. Thrombectomy could be lifesaving if performed within 2 h of thrombosis.[12] It may be a viable treatment option but one that is unlikely to be useful clinically if it must be performed in a time frame this short.

Experimental studies have provided useful insight into the extreme fluid shifts that occur in this disease, the presence of early stage leukocytosis, the usefulness of fluid resuscitation and heparin, and the diagnostic possibilities of abdominal paracentesis (bloody transudate) and angiography. It would appear from these studies as well as from clinical observation that the location of the initial thrombus may vary with the cause and can dramatically influence resulting bowel loss. The thrombus resulting from low-flow states (e.g., portal hypertension, congestive heart failure) as well as from a local process (e.g., pancreatitis, splenectomy, sclerotherapy) probably begins in the central veins and then progresses more distally. Thrombus resulting from hypercoagulable states and local infections probably begins in the peripheral venous system. In either case, neither would necessarily cause bowel infarction unless all collateral pathways were eliminated, which generally means that the vasae rectae and the peripheral arcades are occluded.[3,16] The rich collateral network decompressing the inferior mesenteric vein (IMV) may well explain the lack of reported bowel infarction resulting from this single event.[16-18] When the collateral circulation becomes inadequate, the progression in bowel and mesenteric swelling, thickening, serous drainage, and eventually infarction with or without arterial vasoconstriction occurs.

ANATOMY

In the mucosal membrane, blood from surface capillaries is collected by venules that then enter mucosal veins. After penetrating the muscularis mucosa, these veins drain into large submucosal veins. The blood in these veins join venae rectae that exit the bowel wall and arborize to form venous arcades. A number of main tributaries then join together to form the SMV (Fig. 26–1).[19] These named tributaries are merely identified collections of venous arcades that connect freely within the mesenteric folds. The jejunal and ileal veins join to the left of the SMV and are named after their respective arteries. The ileocolic vein is formed by the union of the cecal veins (anterioposterior), the appendicular vein, the last ileal vein, and a colic vein. It joins the SMV to the right. The right colic vein lies in the retroperitoneum and crosses over the duodenum to meet the SMV. It drains the right colon from several venous arcades and also joins the marginal vein. The middle colic vein connects with the right colic (right branch) and with the left colic vein (left branch), a tributary of the IMV, to join the SMV directly or as a component of the gastrocolic trunk. The right gastroepiploic vein drains the

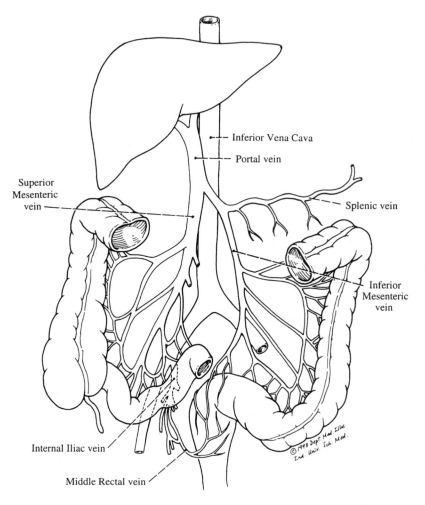

Figure 26–1. The mesenteric venous system with some indication of the collateral network available for decompression both within the mesenteric system and into the systemic circulation.

greater omentum and the distal body and antrum of the stomach. It is connected directly to the left gastroepiploc vein, which drains the spleen and part of the stomach. Together with the middle colic and anterior superior pancreaticoduodenal vein, it forms the gastrocolic trunk of the SMV or enters it directly. The pancreaticoduodenal vein (inferior and superior each with an anterior and posterior division) drains the pancreas and duodenum. The posterior and anterior inferior pancreaticoduodenal veins join the first jejunal veins, whereas the posterior superior pancreaticoduodenal enters the portal vein.

The IMV (see Fig. 26–1) begins as the superior rectal (hemorrhoidal) vein, which originates from the rectal plexus and freely forms anastomoses to the middle and inferior rectal veins.[19] It rises in the retroperitoneal to join the sigmoid and left colic veins. The left colic is joined to the middle colic vein via the marginal vein, which also extends to the sigmoid vein.

These mesenteric veins communicate with the splenic and portal venous system and with the systemic venous system. The connections with the portosplenic system is obvious from the anatomy already mentioned. The potential systemic anastomoses are basically five in number: (1) inferior gastroepiploc to short gastrics and then into the systemic system via intercostals, the azygus, and esophageal veins; (2) rectals to the systemic hypogastric venous system; (3) the umbilical vein; (4) wherever the abdominal organs meet the retroperitoneum or anterior abdominal wall (intercostals, lumbars, vein of Retzius, any adhesions or scars); and (5) connections with the left renal vein via splenic, gastric, adrenal, and so on.[19] These interconnections clearly provide a tremendous collateral network for decompression of major venous occlusions. Certainly, if vasae rectae or intraenteric veins of sufficient length become involved, there are less potential collaterals for venous decompression. However, even in these cases, local adhesions, scars, and the submucosal veins may provide a channel of egress.

ETIOLOGIC AND ASSOCIATED CONDITIONS

Primary MTV is considered the diagnosis when the patient lacks a history of predisposing conditions. A common diagnosis in early series (approximately 50% or more),[3,4] it is becoming apparent that the etiology may have simply been elusive and probably represents an underdiagnosis of a hypercoagulable state. Even in older series, a prior history of some type of deep or superficial thrombophlebitis was commonly reported.[1,3] Similar findings are noted in other series.[20,21] In addition, hypercoagulable conditions are being discovered more accurately due to improved testing and now accounts for 40% to 50% of MVT cases, verses 5% in older series.[3,7,20]

Secondary MVT is considered present when there is an ongoing pathologic process that predisposes the patient to this malady (Table 26–1).

Intraperitoneal inflammation or infection has long been associated with the onset of MVT. Peritonitis, diverticulitis, appendicitis, pelvic or intraabdominal abscesses have all been associated with MVT.[1,3,4,21] Inflammatory bowel disease has been implicated.[3,22] The inflammatory process or bacterial invasion may cause local thrombosis, which progresses more centrally, eventually resulting in the full manifestation of the disease.

Postoperative trauma may instigate the clotting cascade. The most obvious association is following splenectomy, in which the splenic vein may thromboses and the thrombus then propagate centrally.[3] Pelvic operations, abortions, deliveries, or other abdominal procedures (appendectomy, cholecystectomy, etc.) have also been associated with this process.[3,4,7,21] Blunt abdominal trauma may predispose to its onset.[1,3]

TABLE 26–1. CONDITIONS ASSOCIATED WITH AND POSSIBLE ETIOLOGIC CAUSES OF MESENTERIC VENOUS THROMBOSIS

Primary— ↓
Secondary
  Inflammation
    Peritonitis (any cause)
    Localized abscess
      Pelvic or abdominal
    Inflammatory bowel disease
  Postoperative trauma
    Splenectomy
    Other (abdominal/pelvic)
  Blunt abdominal trauma
  Portal hypertension
    Cirrhosis/hepatitis
    Sclerotherapy
  Hypercoagulable states
    Neoplasms
    Oral contraceptives
    Pregnancy
    Hematologic— ↑
      Polycythemia vera
      Thrombocytosis
      Antithrombin III deficiency
      Protein C or S deficiency
      Others
  Pancreatitis
  Others:
    Decompression sickness
    Cardiac disease

↑, decreasing incidence; ↓, increasing incidence.

Low flow within the mesenteric venous system can result from conditions such as portal hypertension (hepatitis, cirrhosis) or congestive heart failure.[1] The former was one of the first disorders clearly associated with MVT[3,5] and is still commonly noted.[7,20,22] Interestingly, treatment of a complication of portal hypertension (esophageal variceal bleeding) with sclerotherapy has resulted in MVT.[23]

Pancreatitis may cause a nonseptic inflammatory reaction within the venous system, resulting in local thrombosis.[22,24] Dehydration may be a factor. Decompression sickness and MVT have been linked and may be due to venous endothelial damage and eventual thrombosis.[1]

Hypercoagulable states resulting in MVT are numerous and becoming more evident as contributing factors. Solid organ neoplasms (stomach, pancreas, and other malignant tumors or lesions) can predispose to MVT.[1,3,7,20] Oral contraceptives are still a problem in some cases,[1,8,20,22] and pregnancy itself has been implicated.[25] Hematologic diseases are the fastest growing category due to the explosion in the discovery of prothrombotic states. Such blood dyscrasias include polycythemia vera, antithrombin III deficiencies, hyperfibrinogenemia, protein C deficiencies, protein S deficiencies, thrombocytosis, and factor IX deficiencies, to mention just a partial listing.[1,3,7,20,22]

CLINICAL PRESENTATION AND DIAGNOSIS

MVT can present to the clinician at any point along the pathophysiologic spectrum of the disease. The disease need not advance through an entire course in any given patient.

As a result, the patient can present with an acute catastrophic event or with vague signs and symptoms that may or may not lead to an acute abdomen, or with signs and symptoms of chronic MVT. The first two presentations are intimately connected and are considered as acute/subacute MVT for this review.

ACUTE/SUBACUTE MESENTERIC VENOUS THROMBOSIS

Signs and Symptoms (History and Physical)

MVT can present as an acute abdomen or as a set of vague signs and symptoms with few helpful diagnostic clues. To emphasize this fact, the diagnosis was generally made only during exploratory laparotomy or autopsy prior to accurate diagnostic imaging.[1,3,17] Abdominal pain is the presenting symptom in nearly all cases (75% to 100%),[7,18,20–22] but it is nonspecific in duration and location. Most patients have a history of intermittent and generally tolerable abdominal pain before seeking medical attention, the length of symptoms prior to hospitalization being greater than 24 h in 90% to 100% of patients.[7,21] The average length of abdominal symptoms was 17 days in one series,[22] and ranged from 2 days to 6 weeks in another.[21] Symptoms may be present for longer than 1 month but this extended duration may represent a more subacute disease process.[7] The location within the abdomen may be diffuse or localized to the segment of bowel involved.[7,22] The character of the pain is often colicky in nature, possibly due to the continued ability of the bowel to peristalsis.[1] About half the patients continue to eat.[7,20] Nausea with or without vomiting occurs in about 40% of patients.[7,20] Whereas other series have noted a higher percentage (>50%) of this complaint,[18,21] diarrhea (15% to 43%)[7,18,20,26] and more rarely constipation (10% to 23%)[7,18,26] may be described. Hematemesis or hematochezia have a varied presentation in the reported literature but may be seen in 6% to 35% of cases.[7,18,20,22,26] This nondescript presentation is dramatically interrupted by advancement of the disease to the point of bowel infarction represented clinically as peritoneal irritation. Advancement to this stage was quite common in older series,[3,17,18] and may still occur in approximately one-third of patients because of delayed patient presentation or physician-based delays.[7,20,22] The delay in diagnosis after patient presentation remains 2 to 3 days.[7,18,21]

The signs of MVT are no less vague until abdominal catastrophe intervenes. A temperature of greater than 38°C was noted in 25% to 47% of cases in some series[7,26] but were hardly mentioned in others.[20–22] Signs of volume depletion (hypotension, tachycardia) are rarely described until the onset of overt sepsis.[7,26] Although abdominal distension may be present in 50% to 80% of cases, bowel sounds are generally present, if somewhat diminished.[3,7,24,26] Abdominal tenderness is observed,[26] but guarding and rebound indicative of peritonitis is noted only in later stages of the disease. Hemocult positive stools are reported in 30% to 70% of patients.[7,20,22,26] As a rule, patients with MVT appear more ill than the physical examination would suggest.[17,22,26]

Laboratory Data

Laboratory studies suggestive of bowel ischemia in animal studies have not been helpful in the clinical diagnosis of MVT. Serum phosphorus, amylase, and creatinine kinase levels are occasionally elevated.[7,22] Leukocytosis with a left shift is a common finding, but the average white blood cell count is only 12,000 to 14,000.[7,22,26] Significant hemo-concentration is seldom noted in early to intermediate stages of the disease. A lactic acidosis is associated with bowel infarction, and is not a helpful clue to early diagnosis.[7] Abdominal paracentesis can demonstrate the serosanguinous transudate of MVT,[17] but is generally not a mentioned diagnostic study in more recent series, possibly due to the infrequent occurrence of ascites in these patients and the availability of newer diagnostic studies.[7,20–22,26] No single study or constellation of laboratory studies can confirm or exclude the diagnosis of MVT at the present time.

Radiologic Diagnosis

Patients with abdominal pain generally obtain a kidney, ureter, and bladder (KUB) and an upright abdominal roentgenogram at the time of initial evaluation. These studies usually demonstrate a nonspecific ileus pattern in patients with MVT (Fig. 26–2).[7,20,21] The typical picture suggestive of intestinal ischemia is rarely seen.[21] The addition of barium (upper or lower series) can more clearly demonstrate the separation of bowel loops due to mesenteric thickening, the swollen bowel wall itself with luminal narrowing, the loss of valvulae conniventes due to congestion, and focal hemorrhage seen as pseudotumors ("thumbprints"). When obtained, however, such studies often fail to provide a clear diagnosis.[20]

Selective mesenteric angiography shown early by animal experimentation to be specific and sensitive for the diagnosis of MVT has found clinical confirmation.[7,20–22] The invasiveness of this diagnostic tool is both an advantage and disadvantage, the

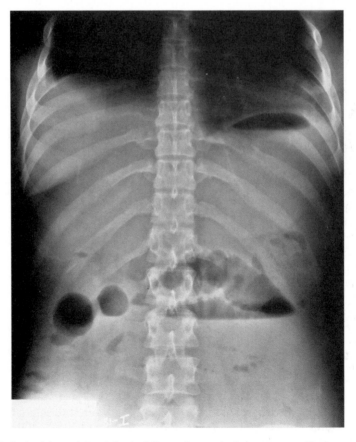

Figure 26–2. A plain upright abdominal X-ray demonstrating a nonspecific gas pattern in a patient with mesenteric venous thrombosis (also shown in Fig. 26–6).

potential advantage being an access for therapeutic intervention in select cases.[27] The diagnosis is made just as Friedenberg and coworkers[15] described in the canine with the possible addition of clear documentation of a thrombus in the SMV with partial or complete occlusion. The sensitivity of this technique approaches 100%,[7,20,22] but is less frequently obtained as noninvasive techniques emerge.

Conventional ultrasonography demonstrates SMV thrombosis or cavernous transformation in approximately 50% of cases studied.[7,18,20,22] The duplex scan adds spectral analysis to improve diagnostic accuracy. Complete lack of blood flow in the SMV or flow suggestive of partial thrombosis of the vein increases diagnostic sensitivity to approximately 90% in some series (Fig. 26–3).[18,22] Both techniques can be hindered by the timing of the study in relation to clot extension, visual clarity (bowel gas, ascites), and the habitus of the patient. Although useful as a quick screening method if positive, lack of proper visualization mandates another approach.

Contrast-enhanced abdominal computed tomography (c-CT) is surfacing as the best noninvasive method with which to make the diagnosis of acute/subacute MVT. A scan is positive if thrombus is present in the vein (Fig. 26–4) and is demonstrated by vein enlargement and a central area of low attenuation (representing intraluminal thrombus) with or without a surrounding rim of high density (Fig. 26–5).[28,29] Using this definition, the correct diagnosis was made in more than 90% of patients studied.[20,22] Adding the presence of abnormal bowel wall thickening (Fig. 26–6), pneumatosis, or dilated collateral vessels in a thickened mesentery, the overall sensitivity becomes

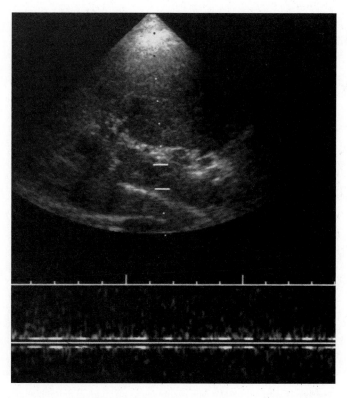

Figure 26–3. A duplex scan illustrating the absence of flow in the superior mesenteric vein (SMV). There is loss of the normal Doppler waveform.

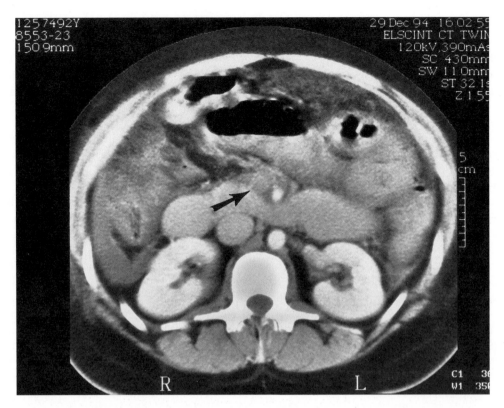

Figure 26–4. Thrombus within the SMV (*arrow*), which lies adjacent to the superior mesenteric artery, as evident in this c-CT scan.

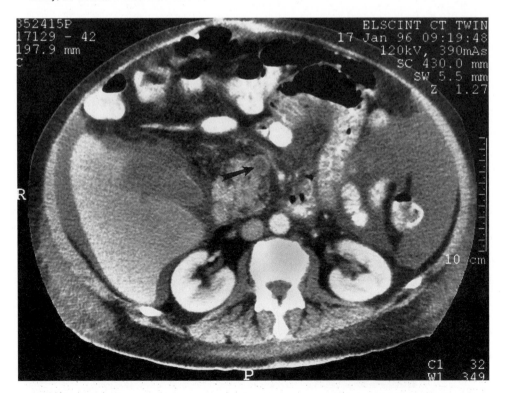

Figure 26–5. Thrombus within the SMV with an obvious surrounding rim of high density (*arrow*) that may represent a subacute stage of the disease with beginning collateral flow and recanalization of the SMV. The illustration is a c-CT scan.

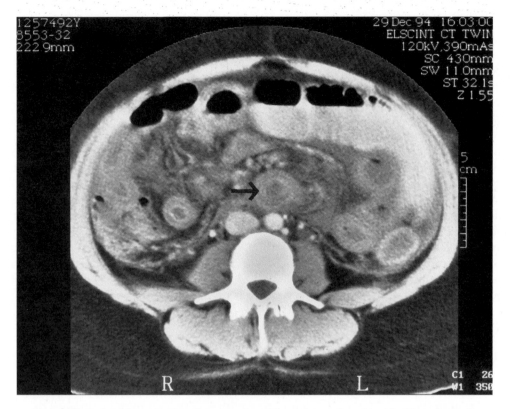

Figure 26–6. A thickened, edematous bowel wall (*arrow*) is quite evident in this patient with mesenteric venous thrombosis as demonstrated by c-CT scan.

essentially 100%.[7] These later findings may be found in other types of bowel infarction, however, and may not be specific for MVT. Nevertheless, even when using quite strict criteria, this study can confirm the diagnosis of MVT in most cases and provides an array of other information that can lead to a correct diagnosis in many of the remaining cases.

Magnetic resonance imaging (MRI) can demonstrate the venous thrombus,[30] but has not been used extensively to study patients suspected of having MVT. Its major advantage appears to be freedom from the need to use ionizing radiation, whereas its major disadvantage may be the cost of the procedure.

The ability to label agents with radioisotopes destined to localize in ischemic bowel has been investigated. Prolongation of the scintiangiographic mesenteric blush may suggest MVT.[31] These studies do not provide the information given by c-CT scanning as a screening method, nor the accuracy of SMA angiography as a confirmatory study, and therefore are rarely selected to evaluate patients with MVT.

Other Diagnostic Methods

Endoscopy may be used to study MVT patients but often does not visualize the bowel segment most likely affected in the disease—the small bowel. The presence of varices may suggest the diagnosis, but confirmatory studies are required.[20] The resurgence of laparoscopy as a diagnostic and therapeutic modality has found its proponents for the diagnosis of MVT.[32] The need for intraperitoneal insufflation with resulting increased intraperitoneal pressures may be harmful to bowel with precarious blood flow.[26] It is invasive for the very ill patient, and may not be diagnostic in very early localized cases because only the serosa of the bowel is visualized.

Laparotomy is the ultimate diagnostic and, in addition, therapeutic modality. Prior to angiography, it was the only method useful for confirming one's clinical suspicion. With the advent of treatments aimed at halting or reversing further clotting to prevent bowel infarction, a diagnostic schema aimed at early diagnosis and prevention to obviate the need for laparotomy has become the goal. Sometimes this is not always possible, and the surgical hallmarks of MVT must be recognized.[1,3,17,26] The afflicted bowel is blue-black, purple, or dark red in color, with a markedly thickened edematous wall and a bloody transudate present in the peritoneal cavity. The mesentery is similarly edematous, hemorrhagic, and discolored. When the mesentery is cut to resect the involved bowel, arterial pulsations are present, whereas the cut veins may extrude thrombi. The venous clotting may extend into mesentery, supplying normal-appearing bowel indicative of a gradual transition between normal and infarcted intestine. Involvement of the colon is infrequent. Only 6 of 99 autopsy cases[16] and 2 of 74 clinical cases[17,18] report thrombosis of the IMV. However, if it is involved, the gross findings are similar to those noted in the small bowel.

CURRENT DIAGNOSTIC ALGORITHM

Our current diagnostic algorithm in patients with suspected MVT depends on clinical presentation (Fig. 26–7). Patients presenting with severe abdominal pain with or without bowel emptying, leukocytosis, and with or without peritoneal irritation are initially evaluated to rule out other causes of severe abdominal irritation (example: bowel perforation) that could be seen easily on plain abdominal films. Selective mesenteric

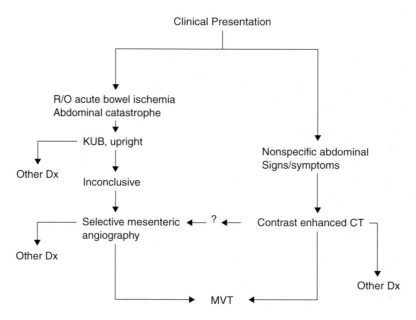

Figure 26–7. A diagnostic algorithm for patients with suspected acute/subacute MVT.

angiography can confirm or eliminate bowel ischemia (arterial, low flow, or venous) as a cause of the patient's symptoms, a critical determination because time is of the essence in the effective treatment of these patients. A c-CT scan may be recommended subsequent to a negative angiogram, but at that point, the patient is in a new diagnostic category. Those patients presenting with less acute, nonspecific abdominal complaints are studied first with a c-CT scan. This study confirms the diagnosis of MVT and allows some indication of the extent of bowel involvement. Selective mesenteric angiography may be indicated in follow-up to investigate arterial or low flow disease, or as a therapeutic maneuver, but is generally not required for confirmation of the diagnosis of MVT except in very unusual cases.

CHRONIC MESENTERIC VENOUS THROMBOSIS

Patients present with signs and symptoms resulting from chronic mesenteric venous hypertension, the sequelae of bowel ischemia, or are asymptomatic. Gastrointestinal bleeding from intestinal varices has been reported.[33] If the portal or splenic vein is involved, the physical findings of portal hypertension are seen, such as splenomegaly (localized pain or hypersplenism) and esophageal varices with or without bleeding episodes.[28] A chronic intestinal stricture presenting as obstruction can be the presenting problem.[34]

The diagnosis can be made serendipitously by c-CT scan or ultrasonography while evaluating a patient for another problem. Alternatively, the workup is directed to the evaluation of gastrointestinal bleeding or bowel obstruction. Endoscopy confirms the presence of varices. A c-CT scan or ultrasonography demonstrates the absence of major venous flow, recanalization, and collateral blood flow. Selective mesenteric angiography with venous phase is the most appropriate test to demonstrate venous anatomy if one is contemplating a surgical decompressive shunt (Fig. 26–8).

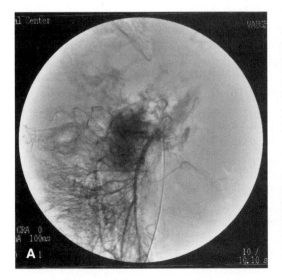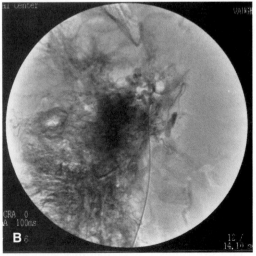

Figure 26–8. (**A**) A selected SMA angiogram demonstrating plethoric arterial perfusion but, (**B**) no reconstitution of a major SMV available for potential shunt procedure.

TREATMENT

Acute and Subacute MVT

The treatment of patients afflicted with MVT is determined initially by the presence or absence of peritoneal signs (Fig. 26–9). Proper resuscitation with aggressive hydration and broad-spectrum antibiotic coverage is determined by the patient's presenting physical condition.[1,17] If peritoneal signs are present indicative of bowel infarction, laparotomy with the intent to resect dead bowel is proper care.[7,18,20,22,26] The extent of bowel resection is always a concern, especially with increasing lengths of affected bowel. Prior to the availability of heparin, the goal was resection to include apparently normal bowel and mesentery such that all venous thrombi were encompassed.[1,17] This would decrease the likelihood of recurrent thrombosis from retained foci of venous clot. Presently, the use of heparin and second-look operations have allowed a more conservative approach. Although the Doppler has been used by some to determine the length of required resection,[1] the continued presence of arterial flow may make a proper interpretation difficult. Clinical evaluation in localized disease, or the use of flourescein and a Wood's lamp in cases of extensive lengths of bowel ischemia, appears more applicable.[7,26] Second-look operations are generally recommended only if bowel of questionable viability is left *in situ.*[7] Immediate heparin anticoagulation is recommended to prevent recurrent or progressive thrombosis.[7,22,26] In our own series, recurrent thrombosis occurred in two of three patients not treated with postoperative anticoagulation, whereas no patients treated with heparin had a recurrent event.[22] A clinical review of 173 patients demonstrated that postoperative heparin decreased the recurrence rate from 26% to 14% and the mortality rate from 59% to 22% during an era when surgery was the only therapeutic option.[1]

The situation in which limited bowel is infarcted requires resection of dead bowel and anticoagulation therapy. In those cases in which the entire or majority of the jejunoileum is necrotic, the clinical situation and patient desires influence the decision to simply close or to resect and accept the short bowel syndrome.

Cases involving lengthy or patchy areas of bowel ischemia not yet clearly infarcted requires a more varied armamentarium of therapeutic maneuvers. The goal is to salvage as much bowel as is possible for patient survival and for normal bowel function. If the major veins, SMV, and/or portal vein are involved, venous thrombectomy is an option.[7,18] In one series, this approach decreased patient mortality and also decreased the incidence of recurrence but neither on a statistical basis.[18] The use of heparin is routine, and second-look operations are planned if questionable bowel is left behind. In one series, recombinant tissue plasminogen activator was infused for 2 or 3 days via a 16 French intravenous catheter positioned in a jejunal mesenteric vein.[18] The catheter was simply pulled after completion of the infusion. Their patients required multiple operations for diffuse bleeding but not from the area where the catheter had been inserted. No patient died or experienced recurrent thrombosis. If the major veins are open or recanalized, then a second-look operation after 12 to 18 h of SMA angiography-directed papaverine infusion may relieve arterial spasm, while heparin therapy prevents further venous thrombosis.[26] Alternatively, SMA angiography-directed thrombolysis may be an option with a similar plan for reexploration to remove any frankly necrotic bowel at that time.[27]

If the patient has no peritoneal signs, prompt anticoagulation with heparin generally preserves bowel viability and allows clinical resolution of the patient's symptoms.[7,20,22] In fact, c-CT or sonography follow-up studies demonstrated recanalization of the thrombosed vein within 7 days to 4 weeks, and at 1 year, the veins were still

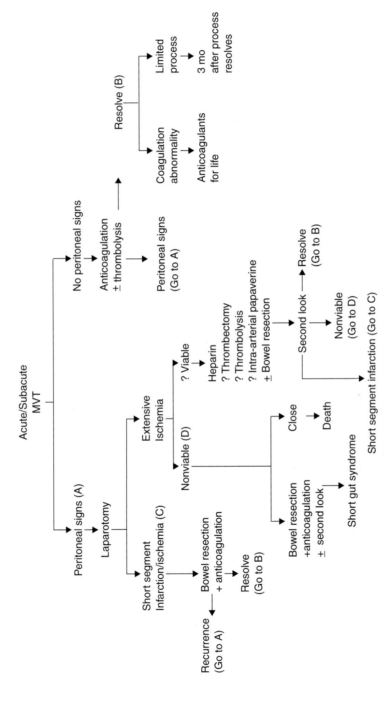

Figure 26–9. The management algorithm for patients with subacute/acute MVT.

patent.[29] The Mayo group found anticoagulation in patients without signs of bowel infarction to be as effective as bowel resection with adjuvant anticoagulation in patients requiring this approach with a respective 83.3% and 86.9% 30-day survival.[7] It may be that those patients presenting with a long (>4 week) history of abdominal complaints (possibly defining a group of patients with a subacute process) may fair even better with anticoagulation alone.[7] In our own series, no patient free of peritoneal signs and treated with anticoagulation progressed to the point of bowel infarction.[22] Conversely, patients treated with observation alone did very poorly, having only a 29.2% 30-day survival.[7] If the patient does progress to the point of bowel infarction as suggested by the onset of peritoneal signs, the approach to treatment must be changed appropriately.

Prevention of recurrence is the ultimate goal of long-term anticoagulation. The majority of recurrent thrombosis occurs within 40 days of bowel resection, suggesting that this may be a critical period of high risk.[7,17] Naitove and Weismann[17] recommend 7 to 10 days of heparin therapy followed by 10 weeks of warfarin therapy. This may certainly be a reasonable approach, an approach much like that suggested for any deep venous thrombosis. It apparently is successful treatment for patients with a temporary disease process.[22,24] Patients proved to have a hypercoagulable state, however, should be treated for life.[20,22] This suggestion must be tempered by the clinical situation because in some cases (e.g., varices) anticoagulation may pose a high risk for bleeding.[7]

Chronic MVT

The treatment of chronic MVT is the treatment of patients with bleeding varices or bowel obstruction. The latter requires nasogastric decompression and, generally, bowel resection for the ischemic stricture that has developed.[34] The management of bleeding esophageal or mesenteric varices may be quite challenging. The use of sclerotherapy, mechanical compression, various shunt procedures, and even devascularization procedures have been discussed widely, and details of these options for esophageal bleeding are beyond the scope of this review. Mesenteric varices result in lower gastrointestinal bleeding. Often the site of bleeding is not found and medical management with blood transfusions with or without intra-arterial vasopressin may be sufficient therapy.[33] If the sight of bleeding is found, resection is an option. Variceal decompression via a shunt is often not a viable option because no major SMV is patent (see Fig. 26–8), but should be considered if the anatomy is conducive.[33]

RESULTS

Survival in patients afflicted with acute/subacute MVT is related directly to early diagnosis and treatment. The natural history of MVT treated without operation or anticoagulant therapy is a survival of 5% to 15%.[1,3,7] The addition of operative resection results in a survival of 65%,[1,3] whereas the addition of heparin improves the survival by approximately 12% to 77%.[1] With early diagnosis and aggressive treatment as outlined in Figs. 26–7 and 26–9, the overall mortality is 12% to 14% and is generally due to an associated morbid condition.[20,22] If the diagnosis is made when anticoagulation alone is deemed the appropriate treatment, survival is excellent.[7,20,22]

Associated morbidity is related to the need for operation and the amount of bowel resected. Boley and associates[26] state that the length of bowel resected is often less than that required with arterial infarction and averaged 151 cm in their series. The Mayo series reports the short bowel syndrome in 22.6% of their patients treated for acute MVT.[7] A plethora of other complications also occurred in their patients, including pulmonary embolus, wound infection, sepsis, and so on, for an overall 55% of patients with an in-hospital complication.[7] Even so, for patients treated aggressively, the 30-day mortality was only 15%.[7]

The majority of deaths after 30 days are due to comorbid conditions (cirrhosis, cancer, etc.).[7,20,22] In our series, none of the five patients diagnosed with MVT prior to bowel infarction and treated with anticoagulation had further disease or any sequelae of MVT within an average follow-up of 18 months (range 1 to 32 months).[22] None of our surviving 13 patients have demonstrated signs of chronic venous hypertension, such as bleeding or ascites.[22] What percentage of these patients will progress to a state of symptomatic chronic MVT is not known but is probably small. In my own experience, I have been asked to see only a handful of patients with symptomatic bleeding who had an absent SMV on SMA angiography and then only in combination with portal thrombosis. We are still following a number of the patients from our original article and have not seen any with a chronic sequelae of MVT to my knowledge. Obviously, there are patients who advance to a chronic and symptomatic state,[28,33,34] but the deficency of reported cases in the literature would suggest that this number is small.

SUMMARY

MVT may account for approximately 15% of acute mesenteric ischemia. Some etiologic factor that promotes a hypercoagulable state is usually present. The venous thrombus may begin in the peripheral mesenteric veins or centrally, but rarely causes frank bowel infarction until the vasae rectae or intraenteric veins have occluded or collateral flow has been eliminated. Vague abdominal complaints may suggest bowel wall swelling and may progress to peritoneal signs suggestive of bowel infarction. The nonspecific nature of the signs and symptoms of MVT often delays proper diagnosis, and therefore a high-index of suspicion must exist if timely diagnosis is to be realized. An abdominal c-CT scan appears to provide optimal diagnostic information. Treatment is based on the patient's clinical presentation. Peritoneal signs mandate an abdominal exploration, whereas more vague complaints may be managed by adequate anticoagulation. With aggressive diagnostics and appropriate treatment, an overall survival following acute/subacute MVT should approach 85%.

REFERENCES

1. Abdu RA, Zakhour BJ, Dallis DJ. Mesenteric venous thrombosis—1911 to 1984. *Surgery.* 1987;101:383–388.
2. Elliot JW. The operative relief of gangrene of intestine due to occlusion of the mesenteric vessels. *Ann Surg.* 1895;21:9–23.
3. Warren S, Eberhard TP. Mesenteric venous thrombosis. *Surg Gynecol Obstet.* 1935;61:102–121.
4. Jenson CB, Smith, GA. A clinical study of 51 cases of mesenteric infarction. *Surgery.* 1956;40:930–937.
5. Ottinger LW, Austen WG. A study of 136 patients with mesenteric infarction. *Surg Gynecol Obstet.* 1967;124:251–261.
6. Hansen HJB, Christoffersen JR. Occlusive mesenteric infarction: a retrospective study of 83 cases. *Acta Chir Scand.* 1976;472(Suppl):103–108.
7. Rhee RY, Gloviczki P, Mendonca CT, et al. Mesenteric venous thrombosis: still a lethal disease in the 1990s. *J Vasc Surg.* 1994;20:688–697.
8. Donaldson JK, Stout BF. Mesenteric thrombosis. *Am J Surg.* 1935;29:208–217.

9. Laufman H. Gradual occlusion of the mesenteric vessels: experimental study. *Surgery.* 1943;13:406–410.

10. Laufman H, Method H. The role of vascular spasm in recovery of strangulated intestine. *Surg Gynecol Obstet.* 1947;85:675–686.

11. Polk HC Jr. Studies in experimental mesenteric venous occlusion. Part 1. The experimental system and its parameters. *Am J Surg.* 1964;108:693–698.

12. Polk HC Jr. Experimental mesenteric venous occlusion. III. Diagnosis and treatment of induced mesenteric venous thrombosis. *Ann Surg.* 1966;163:432–444.

13. Laufman H, Martin WB, Tanturi C. Effect of heparin and dicoumarol on sludge formation. *Science.* 1948;108:283–284.

14. Nelson LE, Kremen AJ. Experimental occlusion of the superior mesenteric vessels with special reference to the role of intravascular thrombosis and its prevention by heparin. *Surgery.* 1950;28:819–826.

15. Friedenberg MJ, Polk HC Jr, McAlister WH, Shochat SJ. Superior mesenteric arteriography in experimental mesenteric venous thrombosis. *Radiology.* 1965;85:38–45.

16. Johnson CC, Baggenstoss AH. Mesenteric venous occlusion. Study of 99 cases of occlusion of veins. *Mayo Clin Proc.* 1949;24:628–636.

17. Naitove A, Weismann RE. Primary mesenteric venous thrombosis. *Ann Surg.* 1965;161: 516–523.

18. Klempnauer J, Grothues F, Bektas H, Pichlmayr R. Results of portal thrombectomy and splanchnic thrombolysis for the surgical management of acute mesentericoportal thrombosis. *Br J Surg.* 1997;84(1):129–132.

19. Abdominal Aorta and Branches (and) Veins of the Abdomen and Pelvis. In: Uflacker R, ed, *Atlas of Vascular Anatomy.* Baltimore: Williams & Wilkins, 1997:530–534, 640–644.

20. Harward TR, Green D, Bergan JJ, Rizzo RJ, et al. Mesenteric venous thrombosis. *J Vasc Surg.* 1989;9:328–333.

21. Clavien PA, Durig M, Harder F. Venous mesenteric infarction: a particular entity. *Br J Surg.* 1988;75:252–255

22. Grieshop RJ, Dalsing MC, Cikrit DF, et al. Acute mesenteric venous thrombosis: revisited in a time of diagnostic clarity. *Am Surg.* 1991;57:573–578.

23. Ofek B, Shemesh D, Abramowitz HB. Mesenteric vein thrombosis after injection sclerotherapy for oesophageal varices. Case report. *Eur J Surg.* 1992;158:195–196.

24. Krummen DM, Cannova J, Schreiber H. Conservative management strategy for pancreatitis-associated mesenteric venous thrombosis. *Am Surg.* 1996;62:432–435.

25. Engelhardt TC, Kerstein MD. Pregnancy and mesenteric venous thrombosis. *Southern Med J.* 1989;82:1441–1443.

26. Boley SJ, Kaleya RN, Brandt LJ. Mesenteric venous thrombosis. In: Boley SJ, Brandt LJ, eds. *The Surgical Clinics of North America.* Philadelphia: WB Saunders; 1992;72:183–201.

27. Poplausky MR, Kaufman JA, Geller SC, Waltman AC. Mesenteric venous thrombosis treated with urokinase via the superior mesenteric artery. *Gastroenterology.* 1996;110:1633–1635.

28. Vogelzang RL, Gore RM, Anschuetz SL, Blei AT. Thrombosis of the splanchnic veins: CT diagnosis. *Am J Radiol.* 1988;150:93–96.

29. Rahmouni A, Mathieu D, Golli M, et al. Value of CT and sonography in the conservative management of acute splenoportal and superior mesenteric venous thrombosis. *Gastrointest Radiol.* 1992;17:135–140.

30. Gehl HB, Bohndorf K, Klose KC, Gunther RW. Two-dimensional MR angiography in the evaluation of abdominal veins with gradient refocused sequences. *J Comp Assist Tom.* 1990;14:619–624.

31. Smith RW, Selby JB. Scintiangiographic diagnosis of acute mesenteric venous thrombosis. *Am J Radiol.* 1979;132:67–69.

32. Serreyn RF, Schoofs PR, Baetens PR, Vandekerckhove D. Laparoscopic diagnosis of mesenteric venous thrombosis. *Endoscopy.* 1986;18:249–250.

33. Soper NJ, Rikkers LF, Miller FJ. Gastrointestinal hemorrhage associated with chronic mesenteric venous occlusion. *Gastroenterology.* 1985;88:1964–1967.

34. Eugiene C, Valla D, Wesenfelder L, et al. Small intestinal stricture complicating superior mesenteric vein thrombosis. A study of three cases. *Gut.* 1995;37:292–295.

27

Nonoperative Treatment of
Femoral Pseudoaneurysms

Steven S. Kang, MD and Nicos Labropoulos, PhD

The standard mode of treatment of postcatheterization femoral pseudoaneurysms has been surgical repair. Although surgical repair is very effective, it is expensive and there is significant morbidity in this high-risk population, with mortality rates of up to 8%.[1] Some centers advocate surgery as the initial treatment of many pseudoaneurysms.[2] However, there has been an increasing trend toward nonoperative treatment for most pseudoaneurysms. This has been spurred partly by the large increase in numbers of pseudoaneurysms encountered as more diagnostic and interventional catheterization procedures are being performed. The development and improvement of duplex ultrasonography have also played a role because a fast, noninvasive, and inexpensive method of diagnosis and follow-up became available and allowed demonstration that the natural history of untreated pseudoaneurysms is more benign than previously thought. This chapter reviews the different nonoperative treatment options for pseudoaneurysms. They include observation, ultrasound-guided compression, various catheter-based techniques, and the newest procedure, ultrasound-guided thrombin injection.

NATURAL HISTORY

The potential complications of untreated pseudoaneurysms are well known. Rupture is the most dramatic and life-threatening. Compression of surrounding tissues can cause pain, neuropathy, venous thrombosis, and necrosis of the overlying skin. Thrombosis or embolization of the feeding artery may occur. Infection of these pseudoaneurysms is uncommon. The natural history of postcatheterization femoral pseudoaneurysms has been described only recently.

The first reports of the spontaneous thrombosis of postcatheterization femoral pseudoaneurysms appeared in 1989. Habscheid and Landehr[3] identified 16 pseudoaneurysms that ranged from 1.5 to 4 cm in diameter by duplex ultrasound. Eight were repaired surgically but the other eight were found to thrombose spontaneously on follow-up. Sacks et al[4] used duplex ultrasound to diagnose seven pseudoaneurysms after femoral catheterization. Whereas six underwent surgical repair, one was observed and follow-up duplex scan 6 weeks later showed complete thrombosis.

In 1990, Kotval et al.[5] reported on three patients diagnosed with pseudoaneurysms who did not have early surgical repair because of clinical instability. One was followed closely with multiple duplex examinations and was seen to have progressive centripetal formation of thrombus with eventual complete thrombosis at 38 days. The other two were found to be thrombosed when imaged 9 days and 9 weeks later. In 1991, Kresowik et al.[6] described the natural history of seven pseudoaneurysms that occurred after percutaneous transluminal coronary angioplasty. The cavity size ranged from 1.3 to 3.5 cm. These pseudoaneurysms were followed by weekly duplex scans and all thrombosed by 4 weeks. The authors suggested that early surgical treatment was usually not necessary and recommended it for those aneurysms that were symptomatic, expanding, or associated with large hematomas. Later that year, Johns et al.[7] published their series of five pseudoaneurysms between 2 to 4 cm in diameter followed with serial duplex scans. All thrombosed between 7 and 42 days, but one patient had surgical drainage of a persistent hematoma.

In 1992, Paulson et al.[8] reviewed 24 pseudoaneurysms that were studied with serial duplex scans. Fourteen of these pseudoaneurysms underwent spontaneous thrombosis and 10 were repaired surgically. The reasons for surgical repair were not stated. The group that underwent spontaneous thrombosis was found to have had a smaller volume (1.8 ml ± 3.3 ml) than the group that had surgical repair (4.4 ml ± 3.2 ml). Volume was calculated as length × width × depth × 0.52. The authors concluded that smaller pseudoaneurysms were more likely to thrombose than larger ones, but this was a retrospective study with a potential for selection bias.

In a 1993 report, Kent et al.[9] prospectively followed 16 femoral pseudoaneurysms and 6 arteriovenous (AV) fistulas with repeat duplex scans at 48 h and weekly thereafter. They excluded 8 other pseudoaneurysms that were expanding rapidly or had progressive hemorrhage, which were surgically repaired. Nine pseudoaneurysms thrombosed spontaneously at an average of 22 days (range 3 to 34 days) and 7 required surgical repair for expansion greater 100%, severe pain, or femoral neuralgia. Pseudoaneurysms that were less than 6 ml in volume (calculated as the product of length, width, and depth), or about 1.8 cm in diameter, were more likely to thrombose, but 2 of 9 such aneurysms required repair and 2 of 7 larger aneurysms thrombosed. None of the patients with spontaneous thrombosis were receiving anticoagulants at the time. The authors recommended repair for patients on anticoagulation, and discharge and follow-up for patients with aneurysms smaller than 6 ml.

Several other reports followed, mostly as the subset of pseudoaneurysms that thrombosed while awaiting ultrasound-guided compression. For this reason, many authors advocate observation for small pseudoaneurysms in patients not requiring long-term anticoagulation.[2,10,11] One publication identified one additional pseudoaneurysm characteristic may help predict spontaneous thrombosis. Samuels et al.[12] monitored 11 pseudoaneurysms after measuring their volume and the length and width of the necks. All pseudoaneurysms underwent spontaneous thrombosis, but those aneurysms with necks 0.9 cm or longer thrombosed at an average of 9.8 days, compared with aneurysms with necks shorter than 0.9 cm, which took an average of 52 days. Therefore, another selection criterion for observation may be neck length.

ULTRASOUND-GUIDED COMPRESSION

In 1989, Wery et al.[13] reported their successful treatment of three femoral pseudoaneurysms by simple manual percutaneous compression of the puncture site. In 1991,

Fellmeth et al.[14] described the method of ultrasound-guided treatment of postcatheterization femoral pseudoaneurysms and AV fistulas. The technique of simple manual compression was improved by their use of the ultrasound transducer both to apply compression and to monitor the effectiveness of the compression. Their description of ultrasound-guided compression repair (UGCR) is as follows. The transducer is positioned directly over the center of the track or neck of the pseudoaneurysm or AV fistula. Straight downward pressure is applied with the transducer until flow through the track is arrested. Pressure is maintained for 10 to 20 min and then slowly released. If flow is still present, compression is immediately resumed. This cycle is repeated until the flow in the pseudoaneurysm or fistula is eliminated.

They identified 35 pseudoaneurysms and 4 AV fistulas. Four pseudoaneurysms thrombosed on their own after anticoagulation was stopped before UGCR could be attempted. Two pseudoaneurysms were repaired surgically because of overlying skin ischemia in 1 and drainage of purulent material after 10 min of compression in another. UGCR was attempted in the remaining 33 patients and was not technically possible in 4. The track could not be localized and compressed in 1 fistula because of a large hematoma, another fistula had no track, one pseudoaneurysm track could only be compressed by extreme pressure that also occluded the artery, and compression of one pseudoaneurysm caused pain severe enough to induce chest pain. Twenty-six of the remaining 27 pseudoaneurysms and 1 of the 2 fistulas were successfully treated with UGCR 1 to 16 days after catheter removal. Five patients required intravenous sedation and 1 had general anesthesia. In 5 of 9 anticoagulated patients, UGCR was initially not successful, and repeated attempts after stopping anticoagulation were successful in 4 of the 5.

Unsuccessful treatment of three older pseudoaneurysms was not included in those previously mentioned but described separately. A pseudoaneurysm with an associated AV fistula detected 3 months after removal of a catheter was treated with 50 min of compression that also compressed the femoral artery. Shortly after successful thrombosis of the pseudoaneurysm but not the fistula, the patient had leg ischemia due to a thrombus in the distal superficial femoral artery. This was lysed with urokinase and the fistula surgically repaired. Two other pseudoaneurysms, discovered 10 and 8 weeks after catheterization, could not be compressed without also collapsing the femoral artery, and UGCR was aborted.

Since the introduction of UGCR, dozens of reports have been published verifying the efficacy and overall safety of this procedure.[15-20] The typical success rate is between 60% and 90%. Besides the complication of arterial thrombosis described previously, there have been only a few published complications, including rupture during compression, rupture after successful compression, thrombosis of the femoral vein from the compression, skin necrosis caused by prolonged pressure on the skin, and vasovagal reactions. Therefore, UGCR is a good alternative to surgical repair and most centers have made it the initial treatment method.

There are several disadvantages to the procedure. In most hands, the results are poorer for patients on anticoagulants.[15,17,18,21] The recurrence rate is about 4% to 11%,[18,19,22] and as high as 20% for anticoagulated patients.[16] Up to 10% of patients cannot be treated with UGCR because they have pseudoaneurysms that are not compressible or cannot be compressed without also collapsing the underlying artery.[14,18,19] For most patients, the compression is painful, and intravenous sedation or analgesia is often necessary. Some patients have required epidural or general anaesthesia to allow compression.[18,23] Applying compression is very uncomfortable for the operator as well, motivating the use of ultrasound-positioned mechanical compression devices such as the C-clamp[24] or Femostop[25] as a substitute for manual transducer compression. It is also time-consuming and can cause significant delays in a busy vascular laboratory.

CATHETER-BASED TECHNIQUES

There have been isolated case reports and small series of femoral pseudoaneurysms treated with various catheter-based techniques. Saito et al.[26] have described the use of an embolization spring coil. A catheter was inserted over a guidewire into the left femoral artery and manoeuvered into the neck of a right femoral pseudoaneurysm. The embolization coil was then deployed within the neck, successfully occluding it with subsequent thrombosis of the pseudoaneurysm.

Jain et al.[27] attempted a similar procedure that required modification. Initial treatment of a 3-cm femoral pseudoaneurysm with UGCR failed. There was no change in the pseudoaneurysm after observation for 1 month. Attempts to catheterize the neck of the pseudoaneurysm from the contralateral femoral artery were unsuccessful. Subsequently, a balloon catheter was inflated across the neck of the pseudoaneurysm and a catheter was placed percutaneously directly into the aneurysm. Through this catheter, seven embolization coils were loaded into the aneurysm cavity with successful thrombosis.

Pan et al.[28] described coil insertion in six patients with pseudoaneurysms that failed compression therapy. Four patients had contrast injected through a catheter placed in the involved femoral artery from the contralateral femoral artery and through a needle directly punctured into the pseudoaneurysm. This allowed delineation of the anatomy. A guidewire was passed through the needle in the pseudoaneurysm through the neck and into the feeding artery. The catheter from the contralateral side was then fed over this guidewire into the neck of the pseudoaneurysm and embolization coils were deployed. In three patients, the coils were placed into the neck with successful occlusion of the neck. In one patient, the coil entered the pseudoaneurysm and flow persisted. However, 5 min of manual compression caused pseudoaneurysm thrombosis. This led to treatment of two other patients with temporary wire insertion directly into the pseudoaneurysm. Under fluoroscopic guidance, 15 to 20 cm of a standard 0.035 inch guidewire was introduced directly into the pseudoaneurysm and kept in place for up to 6 h. This caused thrombosis of the pseudoaneurysm and the guidewire was subsequently removed.

Parodi[29] has treated several traumatic pseudoaneurysms with stent-grafts, including an infected postcatheterization common femoral artery pseudoaneurysm. Specific details were not given except that retrograde access through the superficial femoral artery was used to deploy a Palmaz stent covered with autologous vein. After occlusion of the pseudoaneurysm, the remaining abscess cavity was drained and debrided.

Although the techniques mentioned are technically feasible, they seem to offer little advantage over surgical repair if indeed simpler nonoperative techniques are unsuccessful or contraindicated. However, for pseudoaneurysms arising from other, less easily accessible arteries, there may be a role.

ULTRASOUND-GUIDED THROMBIN INJECTION

Because of the shortcomings of UGCR, in 1996 we began to evaluate a new method of treating pseudoaneurysms by ultrasound-guided thrombin injection.[30] The technique has been modified a bit since the beginning and is as follows. The ultrasound transducer is centered over the pseudoaneurysm. Topical thrombin at a concentration of 1000 U/ml is placed into a small syringe and a 22G spinal needle is attached. The needle is inserted at an angle into the pseudoaneurysm along the same plane as the transducer (Fig. 27–1). A needle biopsy guide that is attached to the transducer can be used in most circumstances and can eliminate the guesswork in determining the angle that the needle must take. There is a function in the ATL machine (Advanced Technology Laboratories, Bethell, Washington) we use and in others that shows the path that the needle will take within the biopsy guide. A cursor can measure the distance from the top of the biopsy guide to any point along the path. Ultrasound imaging without color Doppler is used to confirm that the needle tip is near the center of the pseudoaneurysm (Fig. 27–2). Visualization of the needle tip appears to be enhanced by the small amount of thrombus that forms on the needle bevel as it enters the pseudoaneurysm. Special needles that are etched near the tip are available that seem to improve ultrasound visualization. With color-flow back on, about 0.5 ml of thrombin solution is slowly injected into the pseudoaneurysm. Within seconds, thrombus forms within the pseudo-aneurysm and the color-flow signals fade out. When there is incomplete thrombosis, the needle is redirected into the remaining flow cavity and more thrombin is injected.

So far we have had great success with this procedure. Of the first 40 femoral pseudoaneurysms, 12 of which were in anticoagulated patients, all but 1 were success-fully treated. The one failure, which was the second patient in our series, might have been successful had we injected a second time but the protocol at the time allowed only one injection. There were no changes in distal pulses and ankle–brachial indices. The procedure was not painful and no patient required any analgesia or sedation. We allow patients to get out of bed immediately after treatment and outpatients are sent

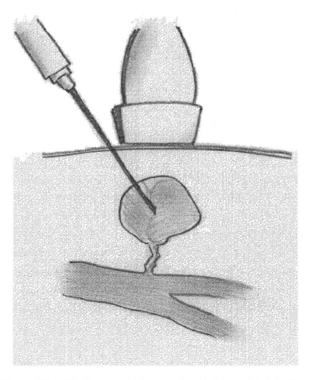

Figure 27–1. Technique of ultrasound-guided thrombin injection.

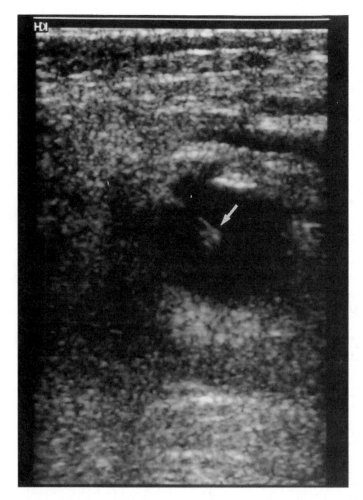

Figure 27–2. Duplex ultrasound of femoral pseudoaneurysm. The tip of the needle is seen in the center of the pseudoaneurysm (*arrow*).

home soon after the procedure. One patient had an early recurrence that was successfully and permanently treated by repeat thrombin injection. There have been no late recurrences.

There were no complication in this series but we did have a complication with thrombin injection of a brachial artery pseudoaneurysm. After one injection of thrombin, most of the pseudoaneurysm was thrombosed but there was a persistent neck. The needle tip was positioned within this neck and less than 0.2 ml of thrombin was injected with successful thrombosis. However, a few minutes later, the patient had hand ischemia and ultrasound showed thrombus in the distal brachial artery. On review of the videotape, it appeared that some of the thrombin solution was injected directly into the artery. The patient was already on a heparin infusion and an additional 5000 U was bolused. A few minutes later, while waiting for an operating room, the patient's hand ischemia resolved. Ultrasound showed partial lysis of the thrombus, and 3 days later it had completely disappeared. The pseudoaneurysm remained thrombosed. Based on this experience, we no longer inject persistent necks, and five have been observed with spontaneous thrombosis in four and a recurrence the following day in one.

The potential complication of intrarterial thrombosis has not been seen when the injection is within the pseudoaneurysm cavity itself. The high concentration of thrombin results in almost immediate conversion of the solution into a solid (thrombus) when it mixes with relatively stagnant blood. Because the neck of the pseudoaneurysm is always narrower than the aneurysm cavity, the thrombus cannot enter the artery. As long as the volume of the thrombin injected does not approach or exceed the volume of the pseudoaneurysm, which may result in forcing some of the solution out of the cavity, the risk of native artery thrombosis should be small.

The use of thrombin for treating aneurysms has been reported by others. Rogoff and Stock[31] injected thrombin percutaneously into a previously excluded but still patent common iliac artery aneurysm. Cope and Zeit[32] injected thrombin percutaneously into a ruptured anastomotic femoral pseudoaneurysm for temporary control before the patient was taken to surgery. They also treated a common iliac pseudoaneurysm, a peroneal artery pseudoaneurysm after trauma, and a hepatic artery aneurysm. Walker et al.[33] injected thrombin through a catheter from the contralateral side into a profunda pseudoaneurysm that had developed after treatment of a femoral neck fracture. All of the procedures mentioned required fluoroscopy for localizing the aneurysms and for determining successful thrombosis. Liau et al.[34] described successful thrombin injection of five femoral pseudoaneurysms using a technique very similar to ours. Instead of direct injection of thrombin through a needle, a catheter was placed percutaneously into the pseudoaneurysm. Because this catheter was not visible on ultrasound, its location within the pseudoaneurysm was confirmed by injection of saline containing microair bubbles before thrombin was injected.

CONCLUSIONS

Since the late 1980s, there have been significant advances in the knowledge of the natural history of femoral pseudoaneurysms and the ability to diagnose and treat them. Many treatment options are available and there are advocates of each. Currently, the majority perform ultrasound-guided compression repair as the initial therapy for these pseudoaneurysms. Ultrasound-guided thrombin injection seems to be extremely efficacious and cost-effective. More experience is needed to determine if it is the best option.

REFERENCES

1. Messina LM, Brothers TE, Wakefield TW, Zelenock GB, et al. Clinical characteristics and surgical management of vascular complications in patients undergoing cardiac catheterization: interventional versus diagnostic procedures. *J Vasc Surg.* 1991;13:593–600.
2. Toursarkissian B, Allen BT, Petrinec D, Thompson RW, et al. Spontaneous closure of selected iatrogenic pseudoaneurysms and arteriovenous fistulae. *J Vasc Surg.* 1997;25:803–808.
3. Habscheid W, Landwehr P. [Aneurysma spurium of the femoral artery following heart catheterization: a prospective ultrasound study]. [German]. *Zeitschrift fur Kardiologie.* 1989;78:573–577.
4. Sacks D, Robinson ML, Perlmutter GS. Femoral arterial injury following catheterization. Duplex evaluation. *J Ultrasound Med.* 1989;8:241–246.
5. Kotval PS, Khoury A, Shah PM, Babu SC. Doppler sonographic demonstration of the progressive spontaneous thrombosis of pseudoaneurysms. *J Ultrasound Med.* 1990;9:185–190.
6. Kresowik TF, Khoury MD, Miller BV, Winniford MD, et al. A prospective study of the incidence and natural history of femoral vascular complications after percutaneous transluminal coronary angioplasty. *J Vasc Surg.* 1991;13:328–333.

7. Johns JP, Pupa LE Jr, Bailey SR. Spontaneous thrombosis of iatrogenic femoral artery pseudo-aneurysms: documentation with color Doppler and two-dimensional ultrasonography. *J Vasc Surg.* 1991;14:24–29.

8. Paulson EK, Hertzberg BS, Paine SS, Carroll BA. Femoral artery pseudoaneurysms: value of color Doppler sonography in predicting which ones will thrombose without treatment. *Am J Roentgenol.* 1992;159:1077–1081.

9. Kent KC, McArdle CR, Kennedy B, Baim DS, et al. A prospective study of the clinical outcome of femoral pseudoaneurysms and arteriovenous fistulas induced by arterial puncture. *J Vasc Surg.* 1993;17:125–131.

10. Rivers SP, Lee ES, Lyon RT, Monrad S, et al. Successful conservative management of iatrogenic femoral arterial trauma. *Ann Vasc Surg.* 1992;6:45–49.

11. Kronzon I. Diagnosis and treatment of iatrogenic femoral artery pseudoaneurysm: a review. *J Am Soc Echocardiog.* 1997;10:236–245.

12. Samuels D, Orron DE, Kessler A, Weiss J, et al. Femoral artery pseudoaneurysm: Doppler sonographic features predictive for spontaneous thrombosis. *J Clin Ultrasound.* 1997;25:497–500.

13. Wery D, Delcour C, Jacquemin C, Richoz B, et al. [Iatrogenic femoral pseudoaneurysm. Analysis of the causes, diagnosis and treatment. Study of 12,248 arterial catheterizations]. [French]. *Journal de Radiologie.* 1989;70:609–611.

14. Fellmeth BD, Roberts AC, Bookstein JJ, Freischlag JA, et al. Postangiographic femoral artery injuries: nonsurgical repair with US-guided compression. *Radiology.* 1991;178:671–675.

15. Feld R, Patton GM, Carabasi RA, Alexander A, et al. Treatment of iatrogenic femoral artery injuries with ultrasound-guided compression. *J Vasc Surg.* 1992;16:832–840.

16. Cox GS, Young JR, Gray BR, Grubb MW, et al. Ultrasound-guided compression repair of postcatheterization pseudoaneurysms: results of treatment in one hundred cases. *J Vasc Surg.* 1994;19:683–686.

17. Schaub F, Theiss W, Heinz M, Zagel M, et al. New aspects in ultrasound-guided compression repair of postcatheterization femoral artery injuries. *Circulation.* 1994;90:1861–1865.

18. Coley BD, Roberts AC, Fellmeth BD, Valji K, et al. Postangiographic femoral artery pseudo-aneurysms: further experience with US-guided compression repair. *Radiology.* 1995;194:307–311.

19. Hood DB, Mattos MA, Douglas MG, Barkmeier LD, et al. Determinants of success of color-flow duplex-guided compression repair of femoral pseudoaneurysms. *Surgery.* 1996;120:585–588.

20. Kazmers A, Meeker C, Nofz K, Kline R, et al. Nonoperative therapy for postcatheterization femoral artery pseudoaneurysms. *Am Surg.* 1997;63:199–204.

21. Hodgett DA, Kang SS, Baker WH. Ultrasound-guided compression repair of catheter-related femoral artery pseudoaneurysms is impaired by anticoagulation. *Vasc Surg.* 1997;31:639–644.

22. Hajarizadeh H, LaRosa CR, Cardullo P, Rohrer MJ, et al. Ultrasound-guided compression of iatrogenic femoral pseudoaneurysm failure, recurrence, and long-term results. *J Vasc Surg.* 1995;22:425–430.

23. Khoury M, Batra S, Berg R, Rama K. Duplex-guided compression of iatrogenic femoral artery pseudoaneurysms. *Am Surg.* 1994;60:234–236.

24. Fellmeth BD, Buckner NK, Ferreira JA, Rooker KT, et al. Postcatheterization femoral artery injuries: repair with color flow US guidance and C-clamp assistance. *Radiology.* 1992;182:570–572.

25. Trertola SO, Savader SJ, Prescott CA, Osterman FA Jr. US-guided pseudoaneurysm repair with a compression device. *Radiology.* 1993;189:285–286.

26. Saito S, Arai H, Kim K, Aoki N, et al. Percutaneous transfemoral spring coil embolization of a pseudoaneurysm of the femoral artery. *Catheter Cardiovasc Diagn.* 1992;26:229–231.

27. Jain SP, Roubin GS, Iyer SS, Saddekni S, et al. Closure of an iatrogenic femoral artery pseudoaneurysm by transcutaneous coil embolization. *Catheter Cardiovasc Diagn.* 1996;39:317–319.

28. Pan M, Medina A, Suarez de Lezo J, Romero M, et al. Obliteration of femoral pseudoaneurysm complicating coronary intervention by direct puncture and permanent or removable coil insertion. *Am J Cardiol.* 1997;80:786–788.

29. Parodi JC. Endovascular repair of abdominal aortic aneurysms and other arterial lesions. *J Vasc Surg.* 1995;21:549–555.
30. Kang SS, Labropoulos N, Mansour MA, Baker WH. Percutaneous ultrasound guided thrombin injection: a new method for treating postcatheterization femoral pseudoaneurysms. *J Vasc Surg.* 1998;27:1032–1038.
31. Rogoff PA, Stock JR. Percutaneous transabdominal embolization of an iliac artery aneurysm. *Am J Roentgenol.* 1994;145:1258–1260.
32. Cope C, Zeit R. Coagulation of aneurysms by direct percutaneous thrombin injection. *Am J Roentgenol.* 1994;147:383–387.
33. Walker TG, Geller SC, Brewster DC. Transcatheter occlusion of a profunda femoral artery pseudoaneurysm using thrombin. *Am J Roentgenol.* 1994;149:185–186.
34. Liau CS, Ho FM, Chen MF, Lee YT. Treatment of iatrogenic femoral artery pseudoaneurysm with percutaneous thrombin injection. *J Vasc Surg.* 1997;26:18–23.

28

Deep Venous Thrombosis

Catheter-Directed Thrombolytic Therapy

Robert L. Vogelzang, MD and Mark W. Mewissen, MD

Acute deep venous thrombosis (DVT) is a common condition with considerable public health implications due to the long-term morbidity and utilization of health care resources that a major episode of DVT can cause. Acute morbidity and complications associated with this disorder include pulmonary embolism and (very rarely) the development of venous gangrene, but chronic morbidity is as large or larger an issue because one-half to two-thirds of patients with proximal (iliofemoral) DVT develop the post-thrombotic (postphlebitic) syndrome. Problems related to development of this syndrome have been well established and described: venous claudication, venous ulceration, permanent valvular insufficiency, and chronic leg edema occur in a high of percentage of those patients.[1,2]

Deep venous thrombosis has been treated principally by anticoagulation: heparin (or the newer heparinoids) early and longer term warfarin therapy. Thrombolytic agents, although available for many years, have been little used for DVT in the United States, despite studies that have shown their superiority over heparin.[3–5] Several of these major well-controlled trials showed a significant advantage of systemic thrombolysis over heparin, with complete thrombolysis rates as high as 10 times greater than patients treated with heparin only. These treatment regimens, however, did not achieve adequate venous patency rates due to insignificant or ineffective delivery of drug to occluded segments. Additional concerns about other major complications of thrombolytic therapy, such as intracranial bleeding, also continue to limit its use. A third treatment option, surgical thrombectomy, has fallen into relative disfavor in the United States due to relatively poor results and is now rarely used.[6]

RATIONALE FOR CATHETER-DIRECTED THROMBOLYSIS OF DEEP VENOUS THROMBOSIS

Catheter-directed thrombolysis has now been a mainstay in the treatment of peripheral arterial occlusive disease since the late 1980s. In peripheral arterial disease, the rationale for thrombolysis is to deliver a concentrated plasminogen activator directly into the thrombus and thereby improve the rate of thrombolysis and permit vascular access for stent placement or angioplasty, or to allow surgical correction of vascular lesions.[7,8] Because these plasminogen activators (principally urokinase) can be delivered directly into the thrombus, treatment duration can be reduced and complete lysis rates improved while major bleeding and other complications associated with systemic therapy can be lessened. The concept for venous thrombolysis was essentially identical. In 1994, Dake and Semba at Stanford University published a landmark study of 21 patients with iliofemoral DVT who were treated with catheter-directed therapy. They achieved a very encouraging 72% complete lysis rate; their work clearly suggested the need to examine this treatment option on a wider scale.[9]

At the same time, other workers throughout the United States and Europe were performing their own institutional evaluations of the efficacy of thrombolysis of the deep veins. As is always true in initial efforts, a variety of infusional and catheterization techniques were used.[10,11] Angioplasty and stents were part of the treatment regimen but were not uniformly applied, nor were treatment criteria widely developed or understood.

THE VENOUS REGISTRY

In order to validate the initial positive results obtained from the work at Stanford and other centers, a multi-institutional registry was established in January 1995 for the purpose of collecting and evaluating data on catheter-directed thrombolysis of symptomatic deep venous thrombosis.[12] Ultimately, 73 medical centers participated and over a 2-year period that terminated in December 1996, and 481 patients were enrolled. Complete data sets including a set of pre- and postlysis venograms and duplex follow-up of at least 10 days was available in 287 patients (61%). A full report will be published shortly, but this chapter discusses the basic results and summarizes the major lessons learned that have proved to be significant.

Overall Results of the Venous Registry

As indicated previously, 287 out of 473 patients had complete data sets available for evaluation (61%). A total of 312 urokinase infusions were used to treat 303 limbs in these 287 patients. Forty-eight percent were men and 52% were women. Sixty-six percent had acute symptoms, 16% had chronic symptoms, and the other 19% had acute changes of pain or edema in a chronically symptomatic limb. Iliofemoral DVT was seen in 71% of patients with about one-fifth (21%) of iliofemoral DVT extending into the inferior vena cava. There was isolated femoropopliteal DVT in 25%, isolated iliac DVT in 3%, and isolated IVC thrombosis in 1%. An average of 6.77 million units of urokinase was infused directly in the thrombus over an average of 48 h using standard coaxial infusion techniques.

The overall rate of lysis in limbs was calculated, which resulted in a percentage of thrombolysis achieved. This *thrombolytic percentage* was then used to assign patients into three groups for analysis: Grade 1: less than 50% lysis; grade 2: greater than 50% lysis; and grade 3: 100% or complete lysis. Based on these scores, complete lysis (grade 3) was achieved in 31% of limbs, grade 2 or greater than 50% of lysis in 52%, and less than 50% lysis (grade 1) in 17% (Fig. 28–1). Therefore, the combined incidence of significant lysis (grade 2 or 3 lysis) was 83%. As might be expected, the prevalence of complete lysis was significantly greater for patients with chronic symptoms versus patients with acute symptoms (34% vs 19%) and for patients with a history of DVT

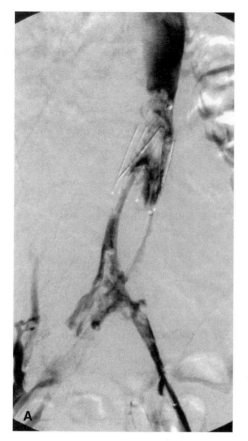
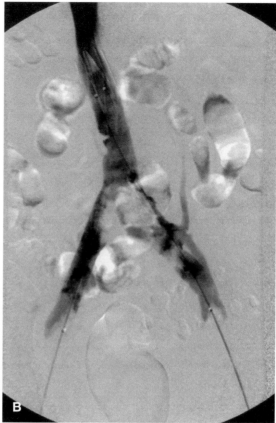

Figure 28–1. Complete lysis (grade 3) of massive iliocaval thrombosis. (**A**) Prethrombolysis cavagram demonstrating extensive thrombus. Forty-eight hours after initiation of bilateral thrombolytic therapy (**B**), there is considerable resolution and increased flow. After 72 h of lytic therapy (**C**), there is complete resolution of iliocaval thrombus. This injection was from the right side. The left iliac vein was also widely patent.

(36% complete lysis for those without a prior history vs 21% for those with a prior history of DVT).

The primary patency of all treated limbs was 65% and 60% at 6 and 12 months, respectively. As might be expected, the degree of thrombolysis achieved was a major predictor of long-term patency irrespective of thrombus location. At 12 months, 79% of limbs with complete or grade 3 thrombolysis were patent, compared with only 32% of limbs with less than 50%, or grade 1 thrombolysis. This difference was statistically significant. As indicated earlier, the patency was also improved with the use of stents in the iliac vein; at 1 year, 70% of stents remained patent, compared to 53% without stent placement.

Finally, major complications were noted in 54 of 473 patients, or 11.5%. Thirty-nine percent of the complications occurred at the venous insertion site and 13% of patients had retroperitoneal hematoma. Twenty-eight percent of bleeding complications involved musculoskeletal, GI, or GU systems, and in another 20% the source of bleeding was not reported. Minor bleeding occurred at 16%. Intracranial hemorrhage occurred in two patients: one fatal intracranial hemorrhage and one with a subdural hematoma. Thus the overall incidence of major neurological complications was 0.4%. Pulmonary

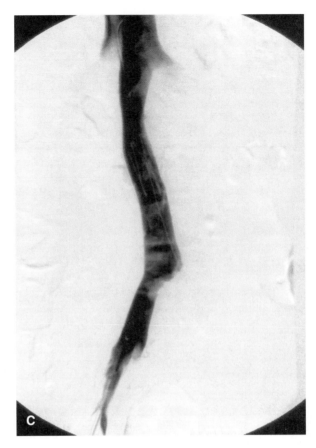

Figure 28–1. (*Continued*)

embolism occurred in six patients (1.3 percent), and there was one patient who had a fatal pulmonary embolism 16 h after initiation of urokinase. The overall mortality rate in this group was 0.4%, or two patients.

Some of the major technical and clinical issues that were raised as this therapy was initiated are now either answered or much better understood. Next, we highlight how the experience gained to date has clarified three of the most pressing of these problems: venous access, the use of stents and angioplasty and the rate of pulmonary embolism, and the need for IVC filters during treatment.

VENOUS ACCESS SITE FOR THROMBOLYSIS

In the Venous Registry and in the early experience, venous access was variable. Investigators initially used the jugular (21%), femoral (28%), and tibial (12%) venous access, but as experience accumulated, it become clear that the popliteal approach was clearly the superior access method of choice for a number of reasons, the principal of which was the fact that catheterization of the venous valves in the femoropopliteal segment was easier and less traumatic. Attempts to cross these valves in thrombosed venous segments from a retrograde approach frequently met with limited success, and concern was raised about the possibility of damaging the venous valves during catheterization.

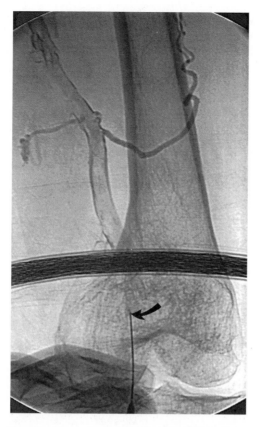

Figure 28–2. Popliteal venous access. Typical location of popliteal vein entry with needle (*arrow*) entering thrombosed popliteal vein.

The use of the popliteal puncture under ultrasound guidance (Fig. 28–2) greatly simplified catheter and guidewire exchanges and allowed patients to be moved and transported with much greater comfort and ease. Popliteal access also permitted complete lysis of femoral venous segments, a difficult if not impossible task via common femoral venous catheterization. In addition, compression of the femoral venous puncture site after termination of successful thrombolytic therapy often caused rethrombosis of a segment. We and most other investigators found the popliteal vein to be simple to puncture under ultrasound guidance, and now consider it to be the principal access route of choice.

ADJUNCTIVE USE OF STENTS AND ANGIOPLASTY

Fairly early in the course of this therapy, it became apparent to most investigators that even successful lysis frequently left residual underlying chronic venous lesions that were responsible for substantial stagnation of venous flow as evidenced by sluggish washout of contrast on follow-up venography. Early anecdotal experience also indicated that failure to treat these hemodynamically significant lesions with either angioplasty or stents led to rapid rethrombosis of the freshly treated and damaged venous endothelium. Aggressive use of angioplasty was found to be extremely helpful by promoting flow and breaking venous webs, bands, and stenoses that impaired flow, but after maximal lytic effect had been achieved, venous stents were the mainstay of therapy to treat underlying chronic venous lesions or venous compressions (Figs. 28–3 and 28–4). In the Venous Registry, adjunctive stents were placed to maintain venous patency in 33% of limbs treated and more stents were placed on the left (71% vs. 29%). This interesting observation leads us to the tentative conclusion in many cases that acute venous thrombosis on the left is caused by some form of extrinsic compression by the right common iliac artery. Overall, adjunctive metallic stent procedures were necessary to treat persistent lesions in 105 limbs (33%): 99 in the iliac segments, 5 in the femoral popliteal vein, and 1 in the inferior vena cava. Stents also improved long-term patency in limbs; 74% of stented limbs remained patient whereas 53% without stent placement remained patent. The results in femoropopliteal stents was very poor, with 4 of 5 stents occluding within a mean of 42 days, and the last stent remaining patent at 2 months but lost to follow-up thereafter. These dismal results lead us to no longer recommend stent placement below the inguinal ligament.

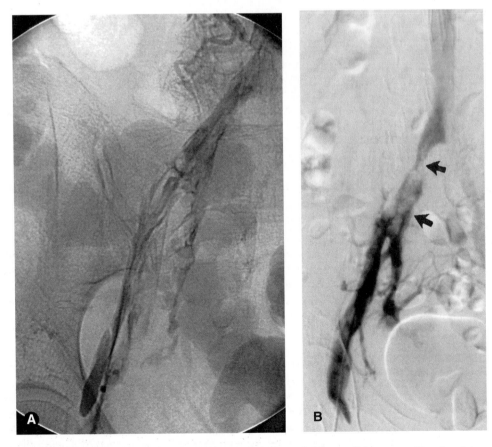

Figure 28–3. Use of stents to eliminate residual lesions. A 66-year-old woman with extensive iliocaval thrombosis. Pretreatment venogram (**A**) shows extensive thrombus. After 44 h of lytic therapy and angioplasty (**B**), a persistent common right iliac vein narrowing is seen (*arrows*). After placement of a 14-mm diameter Wallstent (**C**) there is excellent flow with full restoration of venous patency.

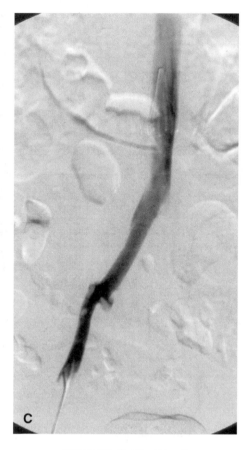

Figure 28–3. (*Continued*)

FREQUENCY OF PULMONARY EMBOLISM AND THE NEED FOR FILTERS DURING CATHETER-DIRECTED THERAPY

A major initial concern of investigators was whether massive pulmonary embolism would occur during therapy of extensive caval, iliac, or femoral venous thrombosis. Although some caval filters were implanted in the early experience, one surprising result in this group of patients was the low incidence of pulmonary embolism. Although the true incidence of pulmonary embolism is unknown, only 6, or 1.3%, had symptomatic embolism. There was one fatal pulmonary embolism, as noted previously. We are also aware anecdotally of other episodes of pulmonary embolism during this therapy, and while we currently do not recommend the placement of a permanent vena cava filter in all patients, the availability of temporary filters may simplify decision making on this important and somewhat controversial point. More clearly needs to be learned, but it would appear that thrombolytic therapy does not cause as much symptomatic pulmonary embolism as originally assumed.

OVERVIEW AND CONCLUSIONS

Catheter-directed therapy for DVT is clearly still in its infancy. The Venous Registry data provides important preliminary information on the efficacy of this significant new

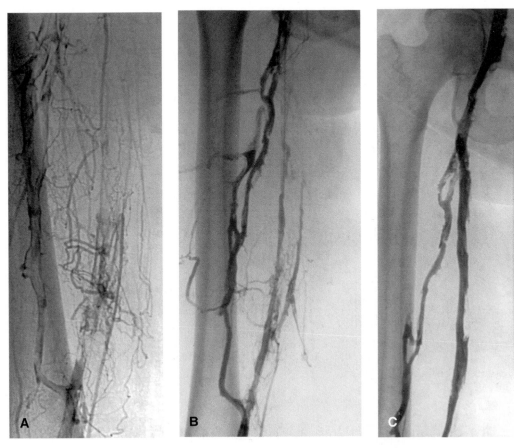

Figure 28–4. Femoropopliteal venous thrombolysis with angioplasty. Femoropopliteal venogram pretreatment of a 53-year old woman with venous gangrene of the lower extremities (**A**). After 40 h of thrombolytic therapy (**B**), there is persistent narrowing of the femoral popliteal vein. Following angioplasty of the femoral vein, there is residual disease but improved flow (**C**). The patient's phlegmasia resolved, and tissue loss was limited to the forefoot.

technique, but many issues remain unresolved. Because the Registry was not a controlled trial, a wide variety of patients with varied and diverse symptom duration, thrombus location, history of deep venous thrombosis, and even thrombolytic technique were enrolled. For this group, the complete lysis rate was only 31%; however, this only underscores the need for further analysis of specific subgroups of patients to determine optimal patient selection. In addition, it should be recognized that other devices and techniques will undoubtedly emerge that should further improve our results. For example, the new generation of mechanical catheter-based thrombectomy devices may well improve the efficiency of clot removal and shorten the time of therapy that in current experiences averages several days of infusion.

Nevertheless, the conclusions of the preliminary experience as reported by the Venous Registry are, we believe, fairly powerful ones. Catheter-directed therapy of DVT is a method of treatment that will undoubtedly gain in acceptance as we learn more but even at this early phase, it is clear that the treatment has a very important potential for preventing or significantly modifying the problems of chronic insufficiency and preventing postthrombotic syndrome.

REFERENCES

1. O'Donnell TF, Browse WL, Burnand KE, Thomas ML. Socioeconomic effects of an iliofemoral deep venous thrombosis. *J Surg Res.* 1977;22:483–488.
2. Akesson H, Brudin L, Dahlstrom JD, et al. Venous function assessed during a five year period after acute iliofemoral venous thrombosis treated with anticoagulation. *Eur J Vasc Surg.* 1990;4:43–48.
3. Kakkara VV, Sagar S, Lewis M. Treatment of deep vein thrombosis with intermittent streptokinase and plasminogen infusion. *Lancet.* 1995;2:674–676.
4. Elliott MS, Immelsman EJ, Jeffrey L, et al. A comparative randomized trial of heparin versus streptokinase in the treatment of acute proximal venous thrombosis: an interim report of a prospective trial. *Br J Surg.* 1979;66:838–843.
5. Amesen H, Hoiseth A, Ly B. Streptokinase or heparin in the treatment of deep vein thrombosis: follow-up results of a prospective study. *Acta Med Scand.* 1982;211:65–68.
6. Plate G, Einarsson E, Ohlin P, et al. Thrombectomy and temporary arterio-venous fistula in acute iliofemoral venous thrombosis. *J Vasc Surg.* 1990;12:467–475.
7. Ouriel K, Shortell CK, De Weese JA, et al. A comparison of thrombolytic therapy with operative revascularization in the initial treatment of acute peripheral arterial ischemia. *J Vasc Surg.* 1994;19:1021–1030.
8. The STILE Investigators. Results of a prospective randomized trial evaluating surgery venous thrombolysis for ischemia of the lower extremity: the STILE trial. *Ann Surg.* 1994;220:251–268.
9. Coons WW, Willis PW, Keller JB. Venous thromboembolism and other venous disease in the Tecumseh Community Health Study. *Circulation.* 1973;48:839–846.
10. Comerota A, Aldridge SC. Thrombolytic therapy for deep venous thrombosis: a clinical review. *Can J Surg.* 1993;36:359–364.
11. Kandarpa K. Technical determinant of success in catheter-directed thrombolysis for peripheral arterial occlusions. *J Vasc Interv Radiol.* 1995;18:367–372.
12. Mewissen MW, Haughton SH. *Catheter-Directed Thrombolysis for Lower Extremity Deep Vein Thrombosis. A Clinical Approach to Vascular Intervention.* New York: Thieme Publishers; 1998.

VIII

Trauma and Emergency Surgery

29

A New Strategy in the
Resuscitation of Trauma Patients

Kenneth L. Mattox, MD

INTRODUCTION

Surgeons, especially vascular, trauma, and critical care surgeons caring for patients with acute blood loss that is often secondary to interruption in vascular wall integrity, are faced with a long series of evaluative and treatment decisions, including those relating to resuscitation, a delicate but complex interaction among a body's natural compensations, control of vascular integrity (both loss of wall substance and chemical and neurological changes), and restoration of physiology toward what is considered to be normal. Approaches to these objectives have continued to evolve over the past 300 years due to better understanding of physiology, including cell and subcellular biology. As technical advances are introduced, such as emergency medical services (EMS); surgical critical care units (ICUs); new devices, drugs, and fluids (hypertonic saline, Ringer's lactate, etc.); new diagnostics [computed tomography (CT) scanning, laparoscopy, ultrasound, etc.]; and a more aggressive approach to initial (EMS and emergency room) reversal of blood pressure by new drugs, devices, and fluids, it is logical that syndromes never before described would emerge as patients with these complications never lived long enough in the past to develop them. Many of the resuscitation and surgical critical care problems are secondary to our advancing technology.

Paradigm shifts evolve with observation, description, explanations, hypotheses, evaluation of the description (research), analysis of results, publication of analysis, and societal reaction. If at any point in this continuum the observation, description, hypothesis, analysis, publication, or reaction is incorrect or flawed, the final conclusions must also be questioned. Some such faulted conclusions include: the sun revolves around the Earth, the Earth is flat, circumcision prevents penile cancer, and wrinkle-removing creams work. In the field of resuscitation following traumatic or hypovolemic shock, much of the thought processes were governed by controlled hemorrhage animal models or testimonials, rather than Class I or Class II evidence-based outcomes. Consequentially, the resulting conclusions had to be questioned.

NEED FOR RESUSCITATION

Resuscitation is a term that encompasses many concepts and doctrines. Resuscitation doctrines range from attempting to return all body functions to "normal" prior to operation to "packaging" a patient for transfer. Resuscitation is performed by various health care personnel in a variety of locations, including prehospital by first responders or EMS personnel, the emergency center by emergency room physicians and surgeons, the radiology suite using interventional radiologic techniques, the operating room by surgeons, and the ICU by a variety of personnel. In patients with an acute vascular or trauma abnormality, resuscitation is required to prevent further loss of tissue perfusion, including renal and cerebral function. With advances in alerting (calls to 911), care during transport (emergency medical services), trauma system development (trauma centers), and emergency medicine, patients who might not have previously reached a surgeon alive are presenting with hypotension, acidosis, hypothermia, and acute blood loss. These patients require rapid evaluation and treatment. Any resuscitation is part of an integrated continuum of care that may include surgical intervention (sometimes nonoperative surgical judgment and care). The process and the end points of this resuscitation are currently undergoing reevaluation and changes.

NATURAL HISTORY OF PATIENTS WITH HEMORRHAGIC/TRAUMATIC SHOCK

Following injury, hemorrhagic or traumatic "shock" is seen in less than 10% of the injured population. One-third (33%) of patients in hemorrhagic or traumatic shock have minor injury. The etiology of shock, usually indicated by hypotension (blood pressure of less than 90/-), is due to conditions such as pneumothorax, effects of imbibed alcohol or drugs, distended stomach, and other "benign" causes. One-third (33%) of hypotensive trauma patients have a nonsurvivable injury, regardless of the timing and extent of treatment. An irreversible injury is not always apparent on initial evaluation; therefore, this subgroup of patients tends to consume considerable time, expense, and manpower. One-third (33%) of patients who are hypotensive following hemorrhage or trauma have injuries that require control or repair. In these patients, hemodynamic compensation is prompted by a long list of neurological, endocrine, metabolic, and biochemical stimuli that have been described for decades and have resulted in the term *reversible* shock. Since the late 1940s, a number of "shock" treatments have been aimed at attempting to duplicate these intrinsic compensations. The use of vasopressors, attempting to elevate blood pressure; aggressive administration with large volumes of crystalloid fluids; administration of steroids; application of antishock garments; and many other treatments have been attempted with variable outcomes.

HISTORICAL APPROACH TO RESUSCITATION

During the early part of the 20th century, limited crystalloid resuscitation in trauma patients was the rule. Following a series of "controlled hemorrhage shock model" experiments, the recommendations for replacement with 3 ml of crystalloid for each

1 ml of estimated blood volume loss became a "standard" approach for operative management of patients with hemorrhage during the late 1950s and early 1960s. This was a time when the specialty of emergency medicine and EMS did not functionally exist. The "3:1 rule" became a standard policy without prospective, randomized, controlled, human evaluations. During the late 1960s and early 1970s, when emergency medicine became a discipline and prehospital EMS began to extend resuscitation, it was logical to "start IVs" in the ambulance and attempt aggressive resuscitation, often initiated prior to a surgeon's presence and without physician supervision. Protocols were developed that included devices capable of "rapid fluid infusion" in the ambulance, emergency center, operating room, and ICU. Even the Advanced Trauma Life Support Course (ATLS) of the American College of Surgeon's Committee on Trauma initially recommended two "large bore" intravenous sites to rapidly infuse crystalloid fluids at the "3:1" rate.[1-3] Often, fluids were administered at even greater volumes. For patients with chest injury, especially blunt chest trauma and pulmonary contusion, this aggressive volume resuscitation often resulted in pulmonary insufficiency and systemic inflammatory response syndromes (SIRS) with its pulmonary manifestation [adult respiratory distress syndrome (ARDS)].[4-7] The goal of field and emergency center resuscitation was often elevation of the blood pressure to normal or supernormal levels, rather to an appropriate life-sustaining level.

ANOMALIES

Other clinical conditions exist with physiological changes similar to those seen in trauma patients with hypovolemia and hypotension. Ironically, different practice approaches exist for many of these conditions in opposition to conditions for trauma. When a hypotensive patient is diagnosed or presumed to have a leaking abdominal aortic aneurysm, *no* efforts are made to elevate the blood pressure or to dilute the coagulation factors until operative proximal control has been achieved.[8] Blood pressure is deliberately reduced in patients with a dissecting aneurysm of the descending thoracic aorta, often in lieu of operative management.[9] Many internists request that a patient with a bleeding duodenal ulcer be kept hypotensive, without aggressive fluid/blood replacement, for fear that replacement will cause the patient to bleed more. Fluid restriction has resulted in a marked reduction in the mortality and morbidity in flail chest. A patient with a vascular penetration from trauma is very similar to this scenario. A question must be asked, "Why one therapy for one form of hemorrhagic shock and a completely opposite therapy for another presentation of hemorrhagic shock?" This question was not raised until the early 1990s.

RESEARCH AND CLINICAL DISCOVERY

During the 1980s, several forms of laboratory, theoretical, and clinical research raised serious questions about the aggressive fluid resuscitation concept that had been a major part of hypovolemic hypotensive resuscitation philosophy for more than 35 years. The rhetorical question regarding aneurysm versus trauma hypotension began to be asked. Uncontrolled hemorrhagic shock models revealed that aggressive volume resuscitation was detrimental and caused an increase in mortality.[10-19] Computerized modeling indicated that prehospital administration of crystalloid fluid to shock patients was not

TABLE 29–1. MORTALITY RATES AND PREOPERATIVE FLUID VOLUMES AMONG TRAUMA PATIENTS

Volume (ml)	No. of Patients	Mortality Rate (%)
0–500	55	9.1
501–1000	162	11.7
1001–1500	117	17.9
>1500	64	20.3

beneficial for up to 40 min.[20] Several EMS reports raised serious questions as to the value of crystalloid fluids given to trauma patients in an ambulance. A classic evaluation of antishock garments [medical anti-shock trousers (MAST)] revealed that this device was not beneficial and did produce significant new problems.[21-24] A pilot and then a multicenter study of hypertonic saline were prematurely terminated when a number of problems were encountered.[25,26] In these studies, the volume of resuscitative fluid administered in the ambulance, emergency center, and preoperatively in the operating room were known. In equally matched patients for time and injury, increasing volumes of resuscitative crystalloid fluid had a linear relationship to an increasing mortality (Table 29–1).

Based on the historical anomalies, the uncontrolled hemorrhage animal models, the computer modeling, and the retrospective observations, the surgeons at Ben Taub General Hospital affiliated with Baylor College of Medicine in Houston, Texas, conducted what is now heralded as a landmark study.[27] This prospective randomized study compared standard preoperative resuscitative crystalloid resuscitation in post-traumatic hypotension to fluid restriction until the time of surgery, even if delayed for more than 20 h (Table 29–2). At no time on the survival curve was there any survival advantage to immediate (and traditional) crystalloid resuscitation (Fig. 29–1). Postoperatively, the rate of complications in the aggressive immediate fluid

TABLE 29–2. COMPARISON OF BLOOD PRESSURE AND LABORATORY FINDINGS IN THE EMERGENCY CENTER IN PATIENTS WITH IMMEDIATE VERSUS DELAYED CRYSTALLOID RESUSCITATION FOLLOWING PENETRATING INJURY TO THE TORSO AND INITIAL HYPOTENSION

Blood Pressure and Laboratory Findings	Immediate Resuscitation Group ($n = 309$)	Delayed Resuscitation Group ($n = 289$)	p Value
Blood pressure (mm Hg)	79 ± 46	72 ± 43	.016
Hemoglobin (mg/dL)	11.2 ± 2.6	12.9 ± 2.2	.0001
Platelet count	274 ± 84	297 ± 88	.0037
Prothombin time (s)	14.1 ± 16	11.4 ± 1.8	.0001
Partial thrombin time (s)	31.8 ± 9.3	27.5 ± 1.2	.007
Systemic arterial pH	7.29 ± 0.17	7.28 ± 0.15	NS

NS, nonsignificant.

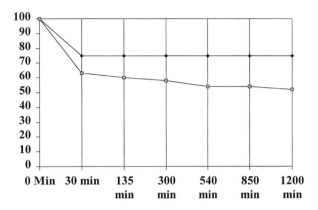

Figure 29–1. Survival curves for immediate (solid squares) versus delayed (open squares) resuscitation groups.

resuscitation was greater than in patients with restriction of fluid administration until time of the operation (Table 29–3).

The complications seen more commonly in the aggressive fluid resuscitation group were renal failure, abdominal compartment syndrome, and ARDS. The length of hospital stay was shorter in the delayed resuscitation group.

Additional information was gleaned from the large database, some of which was not published in the original article. All hypotensive patients with minor injuries not requiring surgery survived regardless of treatment or time to treatment. All hypotensive patients with initial vital signs and trauma scores with predictably nonsurvivable injuries died, regardless of the treatment group. The initial clotting factors and platelet counts (drawn on arrival in the emergency department) in the aggressive fluid resuscitation group were statistically abnormal compared to the

TABLE 29–3. POSTOPERATIVE COMPLICATIONS IN PATIENTS WITH HYPOTENSION FOLLOWING PENETRATING TRAUMA AND RANDOMIZED TO IMMEDIATE AND DELAYED FLUID RESUSCITATION GROUPS AND PATIENTS WHO SURVIVED TO REACH THE SURGICAL INTENSIVE CARE UNIT

Complication	Immediate Resuscitation Group ($n = 309$)	Delayed Resuscitation Group ($n = 289$)	p Value
ARDS	8	3	.108
Sepsis syndrome	12	11	.741
Acute renal failure (requiring dialysis)	8	3	.108
Coagulopathy	24	19	.335
Wound infection	29	24	.361
Pneumonia	28	22	.282
Total	109	82	.003

ARDS, adult respiratory distress syndrome.

TABLE 29–4. PATIENTS IN DELAYED AND IMMEDIATE FLUID RESUSCITATION GROUPS WHO AWAITED SURGERY AND THE TIMES THEY WAITED IN EMERGENCY CENTER OR PREOPERATIVE HOLDING AREA FOR AN OPERATING ROOM

Resuscitation Group	Time (min)						
	0–20	*21–40*	*41–60*	*61–80*	*81–100*	*101–120*	*>120*
Delayed (%)	44	31	14	5	2	2	2
Immediate (%)	36	31	14	6	4	2	7

delayed resuscitation group, demonstrating an acquired coagulopathy with less than 1000 ml of crystalloid prior to arrival in the emergency center. Within each group were patients who waited for more than 80 min for an operation, most often due to logistic reasons. Some patients waited for an operating site for more than 22 h (Tables 29–4 and 29–5). Among patients who received continuing fluid resuscitation, including blood, and who waited more than 80 min for an operation, there was a 13% mortality. Among an equally matched group who received no fluid resuscitation while awaiting surgery, there was *no mortality*, suggesting that the continuing hypotension and absence of hemodilution was protective. Ironically, whether by compensation or by therapy, by the time the patients arrived in the operating room, both groups had comparable averaged blood pressure readings.

These data suggest several conclusions:

- Aggressive fluid resuscitation prior to operation in patients who were hypotensive from penetrating trauma has no survival advantage when compared to fluid resuscitation delayed until the time of operation.
- Minimal fluid administration results in a dilutional coagulopathy.
- The complication rate is greater for patients receiving aggressive fluid resuscitation.
- For patients whose operation is delayed, continuing fluid resuscitation appears to increase bleeding and the mortality rate.
- Blood pressure is not an ideal monitor of adequacy of resuscitation, and may actually be misleading.
- Moderate hypotension in patients with penetrating trauma appears actually to be protective.

TABLE 29–5. MORTALITY PERCENTAGES AMONG PATIENTS WITH IMMEDIATE AND DELAYED FLUID RESUSCITATION BY THE TIME EACH AWAITED AN OPERATING ROOM FOR AN OPERATION

Resuscitation Group	Time (min)						
	1–20	*21–40*	*41–60*	*61–80*	*81–100*	*101–120*	*>120*
Delayed (%)	34	12	4	30	0	0	0
Immediate (%)	48	30	30	21	8	0	5

HYPOVOLEMIC AND/OR MODERATE RESUSCITATION

Aggressive resuscitation (>80 ml/kg/h) is excessive and leads to complications in both experimental animals and hypotensive hypovolemic patients. No preoperative resuscitation in such patients carries the risk of inadequate tissue perfusion, particularly to the brain. The range and limits of moderate fluid resuscitation is currently being defined, debated, and researched. The 3:1 rule is also being reconsidered in view of more recent clinical data. In the 1998 edition of the American College of Surgeon's Committee on Trauma's course on Advanced Trauma Life Support (ATLS), attempts to elevate the blood pressure and volume resuscitation is deemphasized in favor of the more important concept of stop the bleeding and then fluid resuscitate. An individual surgeon's interpretation of "moderate" resuscitation is based on past experience. As in the patient with a leaking abdominal aortic aneurysm, keeping the patient hypotensive, maintaining critical tissue perfusion, and attempting to prevent coagulopathy are noble goals. Teleologically, hypotension is undoubtedly a protective compensation.[28] Attempts simply to raise the blood pressure to normal or even supernormal often is counterproductive. Normal urine output and cerebral activity are perhaps as satisfactory clinical monitors as exist. The surgeon is well served to continue to maintain essential but hypotensive fluid volumes prior to operative control. Blood pressure as a single and guiding monitor has become as much an enemy as a friend in patients with hypovolemic hypotension.

END POINTS OF RESUSCITATION

Surgeons have long sought techniques to determine when resuscitation has been successful. Similarly, surgeons have looked for markers that reflect an irreversible state, determined by clinical, laboratory, or other monitoring techniques. In the past, blood pressure, pulse, respiration, capillary refill, respiratory effort, and the Glasgow Coma Scale were the physiological measures that made up the trauma score. Although its greatest value is not as a predictor of outcome, the trauma score is often used both as a triage instrument and as a method of estimating survival. Some generalizations have been developed at the Ben Taub General Hospital Comprehensive Resuscitation Center to aid the surgeon in making a decision.

- An unintubated patient presenting with posttraumatic cardiac arrest and requiring external cardiac massage for more than 4 min prehospital virtually never survives.[29]
- An intubated posttraumatic patient presenting with more than 10 min of prehospital cardiopulmonary resuscitation (CPR) virtually never survives.
- In most instances, an initial arterial blood gas with pH of less than 6.8 is associated with death.
- An initial arterial blood gas with a base deficit of greater than −30 is associated with an extremely high mortality.
- With increasing need for banked blood replacement in excess of 12 to 15 units, the mortality rate is greater than 50%, and with each additional unit of blood, the mortality rate increases logarithmically.
- Several research technologies are being evaluated in trauma patients, such as oxygen consumption, gastric tonometry, and near-infrared spectroscopy, none of which are presently available for widespread aid in determining end points of resuscitation.

SPECIFIC RECOMMENDATIONS

Based on long experience, more recent trauma research, continuing evaluation of resuscitation approaches, and review of more recent literature, some specific recommendations are in order regarding hypotensive trauma patients. Some of these recommendations are becoming firmly established as one standard of practice in the literature, in the ATLS course, and in many trauma centers. Other recommendations are based on the author's observations and bias and are supported by years of trauma treatment at one of the busiest trauma centers in the world. These are submitted for the consideration of all who read this chapter as a practical approach for specific conditions.

Time

Widely cited, the "golden hour" has been a marketing tool for trauma for decades, and no studies have demonstrated its existence. The concept of expeditious evaluation and treatment is universally accepted, but ironically, the average time from injury to operation remains greater than 2.5 h in most trauma centers around the world. Many of our treatment modalities, such as prehospital helicopter use in an urban setting, may actually *increase* the time interval from wounding to arrival at a trauma center.[30,31] One study even suggests that in an urban area where the ambulance attendants spend a great deal of time stabilizing a trauma patient at the scene, the mortality rate is higher when transported by an advance life support vehicle than when transported in the van or car of a friend.[32]

Resuscitative Fluid

Types
Many varieties of fluids are available around the world for use by ambulance attendants, emergency center personnel, surgeons, anesthesiologists, and intensivists. Tremendous individual preferences and biases exist relating to colloid, balanced salt solutions, hypertonic saline (with and without dextran), "artificial" blood, and many many others. Many of these solutions actually dilute the clotting factors, activate cytokines, and expand the intravascular volume for only a short period of time.[33] In the United States, balanced salt solutions such as Ringer's lactate or acetate were the most widely used resuscitative fluids, prior to the availability of banked blood.

Volumes
The volume of resuscitative fluid to be administered to a hypotensive hypovolemic patient is currently under great discussion. Almost all investigators acknowledge that aggressive volume replenishment (>80 ml/kg/h) is detrimental. Other researchers recommend 20 ml/kg/h. Still other investigators recommend extremely judicious low volume administration to keep the oxygen consumption at an optimal level. In such instances the blood pressure is usually *not* at normal levels. This author sides with the latter recommendations.

Damage Control

Integral to new approaches to resuscitation is the concept of damage control.[34] Trauma damage control concepts have been developed for most body cavities and organ injuries, but it is in the abdomen that damage control tactics have received the greatest potential for resuscitative contributions and are as follows:

- Decision for a staged approach to control abdominal injuries should be made shortly after incision is made, if not before, and is based on physiological and clinical findings.[35]
- Control of ongoing hemorrhage and gross enteric spillage is the major initial objective.
- Secondary complications such as abdominal infections and abdominal compartment syndrome must be considered and perhaps avoided by the use of early second-look operations and preemptive use of a temporary "Bogota Bag" (plastic bag) bridging of an abdominal wall defect.[36]
- Temporary intravascular stenting, fasciotomies, balloon tamponade, and perihepatic packing are all forms of damage control.

Sites of Vascular Access for Fluid Resuscitation

- Subclavian, internal jugular, dorsum of hand, and forearm cephalic vein sites are preferred.
- Paramedics and nurses are discouraged from *ever* using the veins at the anticubital fossa.
- Catheters into the common femoral vein are discouraged.
- If the patient is *in extremis,* a cutdown into the greater saphenous vein at the groin is preferred. A venous extension tubing is used as the 4 to 6 French cannula of choice.
- In patients with potential injury to the thoracic outlet, at least one large venous portal is placed in the lower extremity.

Prehospital EMS

- "Load-and-go" philosophy.
- Attempt to obtain a venous portal during transport.
- Maintain volume administered in this venous portal to keep open only.
- Intubate trachea, if deemed necessary, by the paramedic using on-line or protocol medical control.
- Do not stop at the closest facility for stabilization, but go initially to the closest appropriate facility, as determined by regional trauma guidelines.
- Do *not* administer vasopressors either endotracheally or intravenously for the purpose of elevating the blood pressure in either adults or children.
- Needles and cannula should *not* be placed into the anticubital fossa.

Children

For the purposes of this chapter, *children* are defined as persons age 14 years or younger who are also physiologically prepubertal.

- Establish an intravenous (*not interosseous*) site in the resuscitation area of the trauma center.
- Assure that trauma surgeons, general surgeons, or pediatric surgeons are the patient's primary physician and responsible for decision making and treatment options.
- Administer *limited* fluids until the extent of injuries is known.
- Use central nervous system (CNS) status and possibly urinary output as end points to adequacy of organ perfusion.

- Consider substituting very limited colloids as the resuscitation fluid instead of crystalloids.
- Do *not* use any rapid infusor devices.
- Admit the patient to the operating room or monitored area under the direction of the trauma service with the surgeon having *sole* responsibility for managing the care of the patients.

Adults

For the purposes of this section, an *adult* is defined as a person between the ages of 14 years and 55 years who is postpubertal.

- Restrict intravenous fluid volumes in the prehospital phase to either *no* access or access with keep open only rate.
- For penetrating trauma, limit crystalloid fluid administration to keep open or volumes required to administer antibiotics and so on until a skin incision is made.
- For blunt trauma (pelvic fractures), should volume expansion be required prior to operation, pelvic fixitor, or angiographic control of hemorrhage, judicious use of crystalloid fluid or blood.
- Systemic blood pressure is kept less than 100/- mm Hg.
- Venous pressure (especially in the abdomen) is kept less than 10 cm H_2O.
- For blunt trauma to the chest, crystalloid resuscitation is limited to 800 ml every 24 h. Should volume expansion be required, colloid, including blood, is used.
- Blood pressure is kept below 120/- and preferably below 110/- mm Hg, in order to not "blow out" soft forming clots.
- Should the patient become somnolent, he or she is given priority operating room status among patients awaiting surgery.

Elderly Adults

For the purposes of this section, *elderly adults* are defined as persons who are older than 55 years.

- Recognize that the margin of safety for aggressive, moderate, and limited fluid resuscitation is narrower in this group of patients.
- Keep the systemic blood pressure greater than 80/- and less than 130/- mm Hg.
- If the systemic blood pressure is greater than 100/- mm Hg, consider administering beta blockage in the emergency center in order to alter the Dp/Dt (delta pressure/delta time) in the arterial tree.
- Limit crystalloid fluid resuscitation in the resuscitation area to less than 500 ml every 24 h. Should volume expansion be required, blood products or the judicious use of colloids is recommended.
- Consider use of vasopressors or intra-aortic balloon pump (IABP), if indicated.
- Under *no* circumstance use a rapid infusor of any type.
- Keep the venous pressure less than 15 cm H_2O.
- Strongly consider early movement to the surgical ICU and insert a pulmonary artery catheter for monitoring purposes.

Patients with Head Trauma

- Recognize that cerebral perfusion is mandatory for functional survival.
- Assure moderate fluid resuscitation.
- Assure that aggressive and excessive fluid resuscitation, contributing to fluid administration related intracranial compartment syndrome, does not occur.

- Involve the neurosurgeons to consider the most appropriate form of monitoring.
- Assure that the cerebral perfusion pressure is optimized depending on the monitoring techniques available to the trauma team.
- If blood pressure is the only monitoring available, assure that the systemic blood pressure is optimally between 90/- and 110/- mm Hg, and does not go below 70/- mm Hg.

A landmark experimental study regarding the value of moderate to aggressive fluid resuscitation in patients with head injury and posttraumatic hypovolemic hypotension has been reported.[37] This study, like the Houston study addressing aggressive fluid resuscitation in victims of penetrating truncal trauma, supports a concept of limited fluid resuscitation over aggressive fluid resuscitation, even in patients with head injury. This one study will require additional experimental and clinical studies before this approach becomes standard for head injury patients with hypotension.

Patients in Extremis and Undetectable Blood Pressures

- Determine the ultimate viability and resuscitatability rapidly.
- Proceed directly to the operating room (if one is available).
- Perform operation in the resuscitation area of the trauma center, by surgical personnel, if indicated, in order to stop internal hemorrhage and to aid in resuscitation.
- Immediately begin fluid resuscitation in the form of packed red cells and crystalloid fluid concomitant with internal control of hemorrhage.

Patients with Spinal Cord Trauma

- Assess neurological status early.
- Determine whether any spinal cord injury is complete or incomplete.
- Use vasopressors early if there is evidence of "spinal shock."
- Administer fluid volume replacement greater than the "normal" hypotensive patient described earlier if needed due to peripheral vasodilatation.
- Consider placement of a pulmonary artery catheter to calculate the peripheral vascular resistance.

Patients with Pelvic Fractures

- Assess the volume of blood loss in the pelvis early.
- Consider the application of a pelvic fixitor early if ongoing pelvic bleeding is probable, although this modality is now being debated as to its real efficacy.
- Maintain the systolic pressure at no greater than 100 mm Hg
- Maintain the venous pressure [especially in the inferior vena cava (IVC)] at less than 10 cm H_2O.
- Limit administration of crystalloid fluids and limit the first 24-h crystalloid fluid volume to less than 800 ml if possible, and a maximum 24-h crystalloid fluid volume of 2000 ml, unless an operation is required for nonpelvic bleeding.

Patients with Blunt Chest Trauma and a Potential for Pulmonary Contusion

- Limit crystalloid fluid administration to 800 ml every 24 h, if possible.
- Should volume expansion be required, colloids, especially blood, is used.
- Always avoid the use of albumin.

Patients with Trauma, Hypotension, and Known Cirrhosis

- Recognize that advanced cirrhosis and *any* trauma often result in an "undesirable" outcome.
- Limit use of crystalloid fluid even more severely than in other trauma patients.
- When crystalloid solutions are required, use Ringer's acetate rather than Ringer's lactate.
- Use blood and blood products early should intravascular expansion be required.
- Use autotransfusion whenever possible.
- Consult a hematologist or pathologist with special interest in coagulation early.
- Accept a lower blood pressure than in other trauma patients.
- Keep a close eye on the anesthesiologist and other members of the trauma team to assure that excessive fluids are not given, resulting in further dilution of clotting factors and platelets. Communicate with the anesthesiology personnel prior to the operation regarding limited administration of crystalloid fluid.

Patients with a "Stable" Blood Pressure Between 70/- and 90/- mm Hg and Awaiting an Operative Site

- Admit the patient to the hospital and move from the emergency center as soon as possible.
- Continue to limit the crystalloid fluid volume resuscitation.
- Educate the nurses, house staff, and anesthesiologist as to the nonnecessity to add volume aggressively.
- Move the patient to the operating room or a monitored preoperative holding area as soon as possible.
- Watch the patient for any change and need for new prioritization.

Patients with Hypovolemia and Any Blood Pressure and in Whom the CNS Status Is Deteriorating Secondary to the Hypovolemia

- Move rapidly to the operating room to control ongoing hemorrhage.
- At induction of anesthesia, give a bolus of 500 ml crystalloid fluids as the skin incision is made.
- Do not elevate the blood pressure with excessively aggressive crystalloid administration in lieu of operative control of hemorrhage.

Patients with Signs of Continuing or Accelerated Internal Hemorrhage

- As soon as possible, move to the operating room for control of hemorrhage.
- *Stop the bleeding.*
- Do *not* be tempted to aggressively administer fluids in lieu of operative control of hemorrhage.

At Induction of Anesthesia

- Watch the anesthesiologist or CRNA closely to prevent premature or unnecessary elevation of blood pressure with aggressive and excessive crystalloid fluid administration or vasopressor use, to make the anesthesiology record look good. Communicate with the anesthesiology personnel prior to the operation regarding the use of any vasoactive medication that might be used.

- Limited crystalloid fluids administration.
- Early controlled intubation and ventilation.

During the Operation

- Watch the anesthesiologist or CRNA closely to prevent the premature or unnecessary elevation of blood pressure with aggressive and excessive crystalloid fluids administration or vasopressor use, merely to make the anesthesiology record look good.
- Volume replacement is based on calculated volume losses.
- Frequent dialog is essential between all members of the operative team concerning the type and volumes of fluid administration.

In the ICU

- Maintenance fluids (both volume and type) are determined by analysis of the intake and output and daily electrolyte determinations.
- Resuscitative fluids and consideration for supernormal volume administration is extremely rarely indicated, and when aggressively administered, the iatrogenic complications of abdominal compartment syndrome, respiratory insufficiency, and excessive weight gain are considerable.
- When trauma patients are unstable and apparently require repeated volume challenges postoperatively, a pulmonary artery catheter is inserted and fluid management is determined by using all monitoring devices available.

SUMMARY

Resuscitation concepts are currently in the midst of a paradigm shift. Resuscitation is now focusing on outcomes analysis rather than immediate and misleading single physiological parameters, such as an elevation of the blood pressure. Especially in the urban setting, a review of prehospital transportation, including both ground and air ambulances, is in order. Aggressive fluid resuscitation with balanced salt solutions prior to operative control of ongoing bleeding is very often counterproductive. The operation is a major part of resuscitation, not a sequel. Damage control is integral to adequate surgical resuscitation, which may require repeated staged operation.

REFERENCES

1. American College of Surgeons, Committee on Trauma. Chapter 3: Shock. In: *Advanced Trauma Life Support Program for Physicians, Instructor's Manual,* Chicago: American College of Surgeons; 1993;75–110.
2. Caroline NL. *Emergency Care in the Streets,* 2nd ed. Boston: Little, Brown and Co.; 1983; 57–99.
3. Fowler RL. Chapter 5: Shock. *Basic Trauma Life Support Advanced Prehospital Care,* 2nd ed. Campbell IE, ed. Alabama Chapter, American College of Emergency Physicians, Englewood Cliffs, NJ; Brady Pub.; 1988;107–119.
4. Teschan PE, Post RS, Smith LH, et al. Post traumatic renal insufficiency in military casualties. *Am Intern Med.* 1955;15:172–186.

5. Collins IA, James PM, Bredenberg CE, et al. The relationship between transfusion and hypoxemia in combat casualties. *Ann Surg.* 1978;188:513–520.
6. Collins JA. The causes of progressive pulmonary insufficiency in surgical patients. *J Surg Res.* 1969;9:685–704.
7. McNamara JJ, Molot MD, Stremple IF. Screen filtration pressure in combat casualties. *Ann Surg.* 1970;172:334.
8. Crawford ES. Ruptured abdominal aortic aneurysm. *J Vasc Surg* 1991;13:348–350.
9. Wheat MW, Shumaker HB. Dissecting aneurysm: problems of management. *Chest.* 1976;70:650.
10. Kowalenko T, Stern S, Wang X, Dronen S. Improved outcome with "hypotensive" resuscitation of uncontrolled hemorrhagic shock in a swine model. *J Trauma.* 1991;31:1032.
11. Miles G, Koucky CI, Zacheis GM. Experimental uncontrolled arterial hemorrhage. *Surgery.* 1966;60:434–442.
12. Stern SA, Dronen SC, Birrer P, Wang X. Effect of blood pressure on hemorrhage volume and survival in a near-fatal uncontrolled hemorrhage model. *Ann Emerg Med.* 1991;20:480.
13. Gross D, Landau EH, Assalla A, Drausz MM. Is hypertonic saline resuscitation safe in "uncontrolled" hemorrhagic shock? *J Trauma.* 1988;28:751–756.
14. Bickell WN, Bruttig SP, Millnamow GA, O'Benar I, et al. The detrimental effects of intravenous crystalloid after aortotomy in swine. *Surgery.* 1991;110:629–636.
15. Ehrlich FE, Kramer SG, Watkins E. An experimental shock model simulating clinical hemorrhagic shock. *Surg Gynec Obstet.* 1969;129:1173–1180.
16. Gross D, Landau EN, Klin B, et al. Quantitative measurements of bleeding following hypertonic saline therapy in "uncontrolled" hemorrhagic shock. *J Trauma.* 1989;29:79–83.
17. Gross D, Landau EN, Klin B, Krausz MM. Treatment of uncontrolled hemorrhagic shock with hypertonic saline solution. *Surg Gynec Obstet.* 1990;170:106–112.
18. Harris BH, Shaftan GW, Chiu CJ, Limson A. The treatment of massive venous hemorrhage: an experimental re-appraisal. *J Surg.* 1967;61:891.
19. Bickell WN, Bruttig SP, Wade CE. Hemodynamic response to abdominal aortotomy in the anesthetized swine. *Circ Shock.* 1989;28:23–32.
20. Lewis FL. Prehospital intravenous fluid therapy: physiologic computer modeling. *J Trauma.* 1986;26:804–811.
21. Mattox KL, Bickell WH, Pepe PE, et al. Prospective evaluation of MAST in 911 patients with post-traumatic hypotension—the final report. *J Trauma.* 1989;29:1104–1112.
22. Cogbill TH, Moore FE, Millikan IS, et al. Pulmonary function after military antishock trouser inflation. *Surg Forum.* 1981;32:302.
23. Cayten CG, Berendt PM, Byrne DW, Murphy JG, et al. A study of pneumatic antishock garments in severely hypotensive trauma patients. *J Trauma.* 1993;34:728–735.
24. Cooper A, Barlow B, DiScala C, String O. Efficacy of MAST use in children who present in hypotensive shock. *J Trauma.* 1992;33:151.
25. Laudau EM, Gross D, Assalia A. Treatment of uncontrolled hemorrhagic shock by hypertonic saline and external counter pressure. *Ann Emer Med.* 1989;18:1039–1043.
26. Mattox KL, Maningas PA, Moore EB, et al. Prehospital hypertonic saline/dextran infusion for post-traumatic hypotension: the USA multicenter trial. *Ann Surg.* 1991;213:482–491.
27. Bickell WH, Wall MJ, Pepe PE, et al. A comparison of immediate versus delayed fluid resuscitation for hypotensive patients with penetrating torso trauma. *N Engl J Med.* 1994;331:1105–1109.
28. Butler FK, Hagmann J, Butler EG. Tactical combat casualty care in special operations. *Mil. Med.* 1996;161(Suppl):3–16.
29. Durham A, Richardson RJ, Wall MJ, et al. Emergency center thoracotomy: impact of prehospital resuscitation. *J Trauma.* 1992;32:775–779.
30. Schiller WR, Knox R, Zinnecker H, et al. Effect of helicopter transport of trauma victims on survival in an urban trauma center. *J Trauma.* 1988;28:1127–1134.
31. Cocanour CS, Fischer RP, Ursic CM. Are scene flights for penetrating trauma justified? *J Trauma.* 1997;43:83–87.
32. Demetriades D, Chan L, Cornwell E, et al. Paramedic vs private transportation of trauma patients. *Arch Surg.* 1996;131:133–138.

33. Rhee P, Burris D, Kaufmann C, et al. Lactated Ringer's solution resuscitation causes neutrophil activation after hemorrhagic shock. *J Trauma.* 1998;44:313–319.
34. Hirshberg A, Walden R. Damage control for abdominal trauma. *SCNA.* 1997;77(4):813–820.
35. Hirshberg A, Stein M, Adar R. Reoperation: planned and unplanned. *SCNA.* 1997;77(4): 897–908.
36. Ivatury RR, Diebel L, Porter JM, et al. Intra-abdominal hypertension and the abdominal compartment syndrome. *SCNA.* 1997;77(4):783–800.
37. Bourguignom PR, Shackford SR, Shiffer C, et al. Delayed fluid resuscitation of head injury and uncontrolled hemorrhagic shock. *Arch Surg.* 1998;133:390–398.

30

Carotid Trauma

When to Operate

David V. Feliciano, MD

INTRODUCTION

Injuries to extracranial cervical carotid arteries are most commonly caused by penetrating wounds in the anterior triangle of the neck and account for approximately 3% to 5% of arterial injuries in urban centers.[1,2] With the increased use of shoulder-harness restraint devices in motor vehicle crashes, blunt injuries to the carotid arteries are being detected much more frequently, also. For example, the incidence of blunt carotid injury was 0.67% after motor vehicle crashes in one recent review and 0.75% in admissions after blunt trauma in another.[3,4] Finally, on rare occasions, a mycotic aneurysm of the carotid artery may result from misplaced injection of illicit drugs into the carotid sheath.[5]

DIAGNOSTIC EVALUATION

Hard Signs

Any discussion of the diagnostic evaluation of possible injuries to the cervical carotid arteries must review the different classification systems. Monson et al.[6] from Cook County Hospital first described the division of the cervical region into three zones in 1969. These included zone I (below the sternal notch), zone II (midcervical region between the sternal notch and the angle of the mandible), and zone III (above the angle of the mandible and below the base of the skull). This classification remains the easiest to remember and use, but is often confused with that described by Roon and Christensen[7] from San Francisco General Hospital in 1979. In this classification, the description of the "low" zone (I) is below the inferior border of the cricoid cartilage. The "middle" zone (II) then became the area between the inferior border of the cricoid cartilage and the angle of the mandible, whereas the definition of the "high" zone (III) remained the same.

Much as with the diagnosis of arterial injuries in other locations, a patient with an injury to the carotid artery presents with either "hard" or "soft" symptoms or signs. Examples of "hard" symptoms or signs of an injury to the cervical carotid artery include the following: (1) pulsatile hemorrhage through the penetrating wound or into the oropharynx; (2) a stable or expanding hematoma with deviation of the trachea or elevation of the floor of the mouth, causing compromise of the airway (Fig. 30–1); (3) a palpable thrill/audible bruit over a carotid–jugular arteriovenous fistula; or (4) loss of the palpable carotid pulse with or without associated neurological symptoms.

In patients with the symptoms or signs listed, immediate cervical exploration obviously is indicated for those with pulsatile hemorrhage, an expanding hematoma, or loss of carotid pulse with an associated neurological deficit. When a stable hematoma, unclear level of a carotid–jugular arteriovenous fistula (Fig. 30–2), or loss of the carotid pulse in a patient without a neurological deficit is present, further diagnostic evaluation is indicated. Either arch aortography with selective carotid arteriograms or duplex ultrasonography with color-flow imaging may be used, depending on local availability and expertise, and is the determining factor in whether operation is necessary in the patient with a stable hematoma or asymptomatic occlusion.[8] Potential diagnoses that may result from these studies and the proposed management include the following:

1. Intramural hematoma or intimal defect with intact distal flow (Fig. 30–3)—
   Options for management include operation; endovascular stenting; or observation with repeat diagnostic evaluation in 1 to 2 weeks. Operation would rarely be chosen in the modern era, whereas endovascular stenting would commonly be performed if the lesion is in the internal carotid artery.

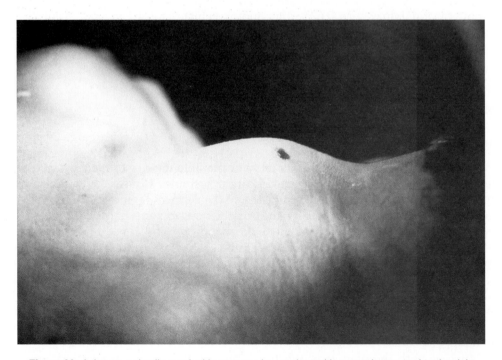

Figure 30–1. Large, pulsatile cervical hematoma in a patient with a gunshot wound to the right common carotid artery. (*From Brown MF, Graham, JM, Feliciano DV, et al. Carotid artery injuries. Am J Surg. 1982;144:748–753. Used by permission*).

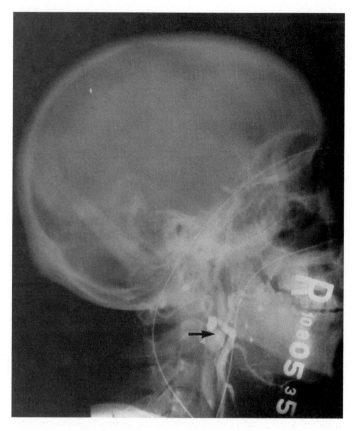

Figure 30–2. Lateral view of a right internal carotid artery–internal jugular vein fistula from gunshot wound to the right side of the face. (*From Feliciano DV. In: Maull KI, Cleveland HC, Feliciano DV, Rice CL, Trunkey DD, eds.* Advances in Trauma and Critical Care, *Vol. 9. St. Louis: Mosby; 1994;319–345. Used by permission*).

2. Pseudoaneurysm (acute pulsatile hematoma)—Options for management include operation; endovascular stenting; or, if a small-sized lesion is present, observation with repeat diagnostic evaluation in 1 to 2 weeks. Large pseudoaneurysms should undergo immediate operation or endovascular stenting depending on local expertise and the level of the injury (Fig. 30–4). For example, a medium-to-large pseudoaneurysm near the base of the skull is best treated with endovascular stenting to avoid the extensive dissection and vertical ramus osteotomy of the mandible necessary for exposure.[9]

3. Occlusion—The asymptomatic patient with an isolated occlusion of the internal carotid artery (Fig. 30–5) is currently treated with heparinization.[3,4,10] In the review by Fabian et al.,[3] this was performed to "1) minimize clot formation at the site of intimal injury; 2) decrease further propagation of clot which has formed allowing the internal fibrinolytic system to dissolve the clot; and, 3) prevent embolization of clot from the sac of the aneurysm."

Soft Signs

Examples of "soft" symptoms or signs of an injury to the cervical carotid artery include the following: (1) history of arterial bleeding from the wound in the prehospital period;

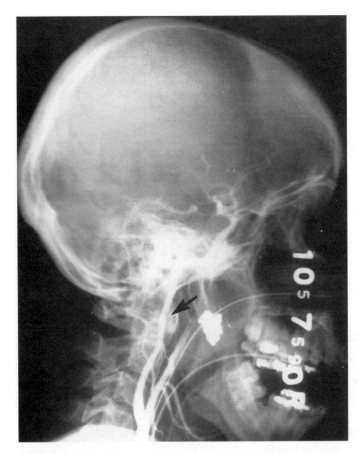

Figure 30–3. Intimal defect in right internal carotid artery in zone III caused by a gunshot wound. (*From Feliciano DV. In: Maull KI, Cleveland HC, Feliciano DV, Rice CL, Trunkey DD, eds.* Advances in Trauma and Critical Care, *Vol. 9. St. Louis: Mosby; 1994;319–345. Used by permission*).

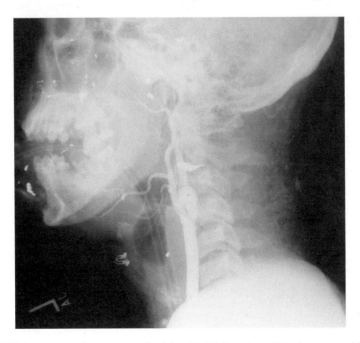

Figure 30–4. Large pseudoaneurysm at origin of left internal carotid artery caused by a gunshot wound.

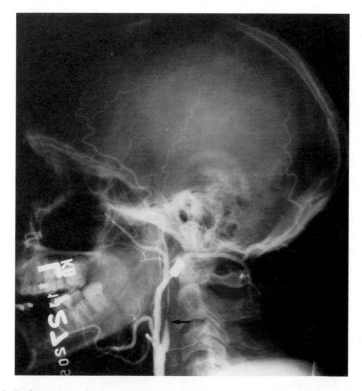

Figure 30–5. Occlusion of the left internal carotid artery caused by a gunshot wound in an asymptomatic patient. (*From Feliciano DV. In: Maull KI, Cleveland HC, Feliciano DV, Rice CL, Trunkey DD, eds.* Advances in Trauma and Critical Care. *Vol. 9. St. Louis: Mosby; 1994;319–345. Used by permission*).

(2) proximity of track of stab or missile wound to the carotid sheath; (3) small nonpulsatile hematoma in the anterior triangle of the neck; and (4) neurological deficit (altered mental status, focal neurological deficit, or Horner's syndrome).

Although there is some enthusiasm for observation only in asymptomatic patients without physical findings after sustaining penetrating stab wounds in zone II (proximity wound),[11-13] further diagnostic evaluation with a selective carotid arteriogram or duplex ultrasound is indicated when a gunshot wound has occurred or when any of the other "soft" symptoms or signs are present.[10]

Much as in patients with "hard" symptoms or signs, the decision to intervene or operate is based on these further diagnostic studies.

OPERATIVE TECHNIQUES

Management of the Airway

In the patient with exsanguinating hemorrhage into the airway, manual compression of the common carotid artery at the base of the neck or directly over the penetrating wound may temporarily control bleeding. A rapid orotracheal intubation is then performed. If intraoral hemorrhage can be controlled only by direct application of a finger, balloon catheter, or gauze pack, then a cricothyroidotomy is performed.

Patients presenting with pulsatile hematomas in the neck often develop marked deviation of the trachea and elevation of the floor of the mouth that may precipitate sudden asphyxiation.[10] Therefore, such a patient is moved rapidly to the operating room, where orotracheal intubation, nasotracheal intubation, or cricothyroidotomy is performed. In the patient who still has an airway, controlled fiberoptic bronchoscopy with nasotracheal intubation under appropriate sedation is an ideal choice. Impending asphyxiation is managed with orotracheal intubation by an experienced anesthesiologist using paralytic agents. Should this technique be unsuccessful, a rapid cricothyroidotomy is performed despite the risk of contamination to the subsequent arterial repair.

Control of Hemorrhage

An oblique cervical incision along the anterior border of the sternocleidomastoid muscle is still the ideal incision for exposure of unilateral injuries to the cervical carotid artery. With possible bilateral injuries in the carotid sheaths, a high transverse anterior cervical incision with bilateral extensions along the anterior borders of the sternocleidomastoid muscles may be considered, but is rarely performed.

Although proximal arterial control may be somewhat difficult for cervical carotid wounds in low zone II or in zone I, an experienced surgeon can usually elevate the

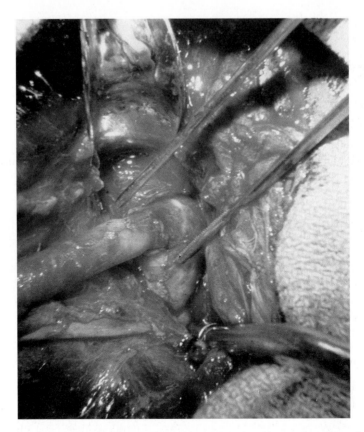

Figure 30–6. End-to-end anastomosis of the right common carotid artery just above the bifurcation of the innominate artery was performed through a cervical incision in a patient with a shotgun wound of the anterior neck. (*From Feliciano DV. In: Maull KI, Cleveland HC, Feliciano DV, Rice CL, Trunkey DD, eds.* Advances in Trauma and Critical Care, *Vol. 9. 1994;319–345. Used by permission*).

proximal common carotid artery into the cervical incision using traction (Fig. 30–6). If proximal arterial control cannot be attained through the oblique cervical incision, manual or pack compression is applied to the site of hemorrhage as a median sternotomy is performed.

Hemorrhage from the distal internal carotid artery in zone III at the base of the skull cannot always be controlled by external manual compression or even by clamping of the common carotid artery at the base of the neck. On occasion, the passage of a #3–#8 Fogarty or 5-ml Foley balloon catheter directly into the penetrating wound at the base of the skull and sequential inflation may eventually result in control of hemorrhage by direct compression (Fig. 30–7).[14] An alternate approach is to make a common carotid arteriotomy and pass the balloon catheter into the distal internal carotid artery with sequential inflation until hemorrhage is controlled. A decision must then be reached on whether surgical repair or reconstruction is possible using the vertical ramus mandibulotomy approach for formal exploration. With an injury just outside the skull, continued balloon compression for 48 h without surgical repair is appropriate in the patient who was neurologically intact on arrival in the emergency center. Deflation of the balloon and removal at 48 h is then performed. Another option would be transfer of the patient to the arteriography suite for stenting or internal balloon occlusion of the distal internal carotid artery if external balloon compression only has been applied.[15]

Arterial Repair

Because of the elasticity of the carotid artery in young trauma patients, puncture wounds or wall defects are easily repaired by wedge excision and transverse arteriorrhaphy with interrupted 6-0 polypropylene sutures. On occasion, wall defects near the carotid

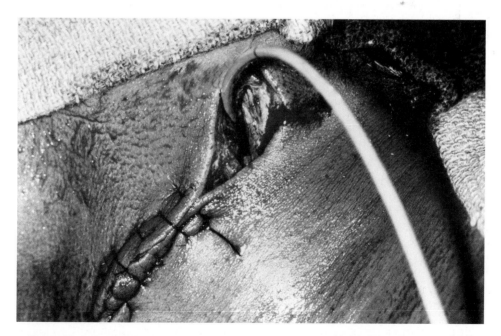

Figure 30–7. A #8 Fogarty balloon catheter was inserted in a high left cervical stab wound to control exsanguinating hemorrhage from the base of the skull. Deflation of the balloon and removal of the catheter were performed on the fourth day after insertion.

bifurcation are best repaired with vein or polytetrafluoroethylene (PTFE) patch arterio-plasty using a continuous 6-0 polypropylene suture.

Major segmental defects in the common carotid artery are repaired with segmental resection and a saphenous vein or polytetrafluoroethylene (PTFE) interposition graft.[16] Although much has been written about transposition of the external carotid artery to replace an injury to the proximal internal carotid artery, this author is aware of only one patient treated in this manner at the major trauma centers in which he has worked. Interposition grafting in the internal carotid artery is best accomplished using a reversed saphenous vein graft based on improved patency as compared to PTFE grafts in this location.[17]

CONTROVERSIES

Carotid Artery Injury with Associated Stroke or Coma

Controversy regarding the management of a patient with an injury to the carotid artery and an associated stroke or coma on admission to the emergency center is now nearly 80 years old.[18] Based on older reports from Cohen et al.[19] and Bradley,[20] it was suggested that ligation of the injured carotid artery might be appropriate in some patients with preoperative neurological deficits. The subsequent comprehensive review by Liekweg and Greenfield[21] in 1978 is still one of the most helpful articles in understanding this controversial area. In 40 patients with a neurological deficit short of coma, 34 underwent revascularization with 85% having a favorable outcome. Six patients with similar preoperative deficits underwent ligation of the carotid artery, and only 50% had a favorable outcome ($p < .05$). In the review by Brown et al.,[22] 19 patients with neurological deficits short of coma underwent revascularization, and 14 had no deficit or a decreased deficit at hospital discharge. Three patients with neurological deficits underwent ligation, and two died. A review by Ramadan et al.[23] using patients in the North Carolina Trauma Registry emphasized that "operative repair offers the best chances for recovery in all categories of patients regardless of injury mechanism" (p. 46).

When reviewing patients with preoperative coma, Liekweg and Greenfield[21] described 15 patients undergoing revascularization and 8 patients with ligation. Only 4 (27%) and 2 (25%) patients, respectively, had a favorable outcome. Brown et al.[22] noted partial or complete clearing of coma in 6 of 9 (67%) patients undergoing revascularization. In contrast, 5 of 7 (71%) patients with coma and treatment by ligation died.

In summary, all patients with neurological deficits short of coma resulting from penetrating wounds to the carotid arteries should be treated with immediate revascularization. Comatose patients should undergo immediate reconstruction as well, particularly if hypotension has distorted the preoperative neurological examination.[10] Improvement or clearing of the preoperative coma has occurred in 27% to 66% of patients, especially if the Glasgow Coma Scale score is greater than 9.[10,24]

Exposure of Injuries in Zone III

In emergency situations, the following operative approaches have been recommended: (1) subluxation of the temporomandibular joint by wiring around the mandible and across the nose;[25] (2) subluxation of the temporomandibular joint by diagonal interdental wiring;[26] (3) a variety of mandibular osteotomy approaches including the "stepladder" described by Dichtel et al.;[27] and (4) the vertical ramus osteotomy approach described by Larsen and Smead.[9]

The choice of approach is based on local availability and expertise, but the vertical ramus osteotomy has particular appeal in terms of simplicity, excellence of exposure, and minimal morbidity.

Blunt Injury to the Carotid Artery

Two reviews have summarized the current aggressive diagnostic approach to potential blunt carotid injuries as well as the importance of instituting heparinization.[3,4] In the review by Fabian et al.[3] of 67 patients with blunt carotid injuries, 43% (29) were diagnosed after the onset of new neurological symptoms, 34% (23) by incompatible neurological and CT findings, and 23% (15) by physical examination. Using logistic regression analysis, heparinization was found to be associated independently with improvements in survival and neurological outcome.

The review of 32 patients with blunt carotid injury at the Denver Health Medical Center by Biffl et al.[4] also emphasized the importance of aggressive diagnostic screening and heparinization. Of interest was the stenting of the injured internal carotid artery performed in 11 of the 21 patients undergoing anticoagulation.

REFERENCES

1. Feliciano DV, Bitondo CG, Mattox KL, et al. Civilian trauma in the 1980s. A 1-year experience with 456 vascular and cardiac injuries. *Ann Surg.* 1984;199:717–724.
2. Mattox KL, Feliciano DV, Burch J, Beall AC Jr, et al. Five thousand seven hundred sixty cardiovascular injuries in 4459 patients. Epidemiologic evolution 1958 to 1987. *Ann Surg.* 1989;209:698–707.
3. Fabian TC, Paton JH Jr, Croce MA, Minard G, et al. Blunt carotid injury. Importance of early diagnosis and anticoagulant therapy. *Ann Surg.* 1996;223:513–525.
4. Biffl WL, Moore EE Jr, Ryu RK, Coldwell DM, et al. The unrecognized epidemic of blunt carotid arterial injuries: aggressive surveillance reduces morbidity. *Ann Surg.* 1998. [In press]
5. Ledgerwood AM, Lucas CE. Mycotic aneurysm of the carotid artery. *Arch Surg.* 1974; 109:496–498.
6. Monson DO, Saletta JD, Freeark RJ. Carotid vertebral trauma. *J Trauma.* 1969;9:987–999.
7. Roon AJ, Christensen N. Evaluation and treatment of penetrating cervical injuries. *J Trauma.* 1979;19:391–397.
8. Demetriades D, Theodorou D, Cornwell E III, et al. Penetrating injuries of the neck in patients in stable condition. Physical examination, angiography, or color flow Doppler imaging. *Arch Surg.* 1995;130:971–975.
9. Larsen PE, Smead WL. Vertical ramus osteotomy for improved exposure of the distal internal carotid artery: a new technique. *J Vasc Surg.* 1992;15:226–231.
10. Feliciano DV. A new look at penetrating carotid artery injuries. In: Maull KI, Cleveland HC, Feliciano DV, Rice CL, Trunkey DD, eds. *Advances in Trauma and Critical Care*, Vol. 9. St. Louis: Mosby; 1994:319–345.
11. Wood J, Fabian TC, Mangiante EC. Penetrating neck injuries: recommendations for selective management. *J Trauma.* 1989;29:602–605.
12. Noyes LD, McSwain NE Jr, Markowitz IP. Panendoscopy with arteriography versus mandatory exploration of penetrating wounds of the neck. *Ann Surg.* 1986;204:21–31.
13. Ngakane H, Muckart DJJ, Luvuno FM. Penetrating visceral injuries of the neck: results of a conservative management policy. *Br J Surg.* 1990;77:908–910.
14. Feliciano DV, Burch JM, Mattox KL, Bitondo CG, et al. Balloon catheter tamponade in cardiovascular wounds. *Am J Surg.* 1990;160:583–587.
15. Liebman KM, Rosenwasser RH, Heinel LA. Endovascular management of aneurysm and carotid–cavernous fistulae from gunshot wounds to the skull base and oropharynx. *J Cranio-Maxillofacial Trauma.* 1996;2:10–16.

16. Feliciano DV, Mattox KL, Graham JM, Bitondo CG. Five-year experience with PTFE grafts in vascular wounds. *J Trauma.* 1985;25:71–82.

17. Becquemin JP, Cavillon A, Brunel M, Desgranges P, et al. Polytetrafluoroethylene grafts for carotid repair. *Cardiovasc Surg.* 1996;4:740–745.

18. Makins GH. *Gunshot Injuries to the Blood Vessels.* Bristol, England: John Wright & Sons; 1919.

19. Cohen A, Brief D, Mathewson C Jr. Carotid artery injuries. An analysis of eighty-five cases. *Am J Surg.* 1970;120:210–214.

20. Bradley EL III. Management of penetrating carotid injuries: an alternative approach. *J Trauma.* 1973;13:248–253.

21. Liekweg WG Jr, Greenfield LJ. Management of penetrating carotid arterial injury. *Ann Surg.* 1978;188:587–592.

22. Brown MF, Graham JM, Feliciano DV, Mattox KL, et al. Carotid artery injuries. *Am J Surg.* 1982;144:748–753.

23. Ramadan F, Rutledge R, Oller D, Howell P, et al. Carotid artery trauma: a review of contemporary trauma center experiences. *J Vasc Surg.* 1995;21:46–56.

24. Teehan EP, Padberg FT Jr, Thompson PN, et al. Carotid arterial trauma: assessment with the Glasgow Coma Scale (GCS) as a guide to surgical management. *Cardiovasc Surg.* 1997;5:196–200.

25. Fisher DF Jr, Clagett GP, Parker JI, et al. Mandibular subluxation for high carotid exposure. *J Vasc Surg.* 1984;1:727–733.

26. Dossa C, Shepard AD, Wolford DG, Reddy DJ, et al. Distal internal carotid exposure: a simplified technique for temporary mandibular subluxation. *J Vasc Surg.* 1990;12:319–325.

27. Dichtel WJ, Miller RH, Woodson GE, Feliciano DV, et al. Lateral mandibulotomy: a technique of exposure for penetrating injuries of the internal carotid artery at the base of the skull. *Laryngoscope.* 1984;94:1140–1144.

31

Noninvasive Tests in the Diagnosis of Vascular Trauma

Kaj Johansen, MD, PhD

INTRODUCTION

The diagnosis of vascular trauma has particular immediacy. Unlike chronic arterial and venous disease, limb- or even life-threatening acute ischemia or hemorrhage is an ever-present threat in trauma victims. Historically, the diagnosis of vascular trauma has been made by physical examination followed by contrast arteriography. However, the validation of a series of lesser or noninvasive diagnostic modalities first utilized in the evaluation of chronic arterial and venous disease resulted in a reassessment of the optimal vascular diagnostic approach to the trauma patient who may harbor a vascular injury.

HISTORICAL BACKGROUND

Classically, accurate preoperative diagnosis of vascular injury most commonly was made in the setting of extremity or neck trauma: Truncal vascular trauma has been more commonly diagnosed only at laparotomy for bleeding or hypotension. In the limbs, loss of arterial pulsation, presence of bruits or thrills, or evidence for significant external or internal bleeding are generally readily identifiable. Although the diagnosis of overt hemorrhage or ischemia is thus usually confirmed easily, the diagnosis of an occult vascular injury has been far more difficult. A history and physical examination seeking evidence for neurological dysfunction, stable hematomas, a history of bleeding or ischemia, proximity of wound to limb arteries, or other such "soft" findings had been thought to be accurate in ruling in or out an underlying vascular injury. However, the sensitivity and specificity of the physical examination are not optimal: false positives may occur in the context of relatively benign and self-limited conditions like arterial spasm, whereas (much more worrisome) false negatives may occur in the presence of lesions such as intimal flaps or pseudoaneurysms, initially producing few or no clinical findings, then resulting in subacute vessel rupture or occlusion.

As a consequence, physical examination was discarded in favor of emergency arteriographic imaging of actually or potentially damaged vessels by trauma surgeons in the 1970s and 1980s.[1,2] Contrast arteriography was used not only to identify and localize arterial injuries, but also was soon promoted as a screening study for occult arterial trauma in clinical settings with a significant risk of underlying vascular trauma (e.g., knee dislocation) or in which a missed diagnosis might be catastrophic (e.g., deceleration trauma to the thoracic aorta). The use of contrast arteriography became routine in trauma victims manifesting "soft" signs of arterial injury, or even in those in whom proximity of the wounding mechanism to a nearby artery raised the specter of occult vascular injury. Numerous studies demonstrated the excellent sensitivity and specificity of contrast arteriography for arterial trauma, and through the early 1980s this approach served as the "gold standard" for the diagnosis of arterial trauma.[1,2]

However, several shortcomings of contrast arteriography as an all-purpose vascular diagnostic procedure in trauma patients became clear. First and most important, contrast arteriography takes time: in one trauma center an average of 2.4 h for examination of an extremity.[3] In the presence of acute arterial insufficiency (which generally must be relieved within 6 h of onset), such a delay risks irretrievable tissue ischemia. Second, especially in polytrauma victims, transfer to the angiography suite may not be appropriate in the context of patient resuscitation and the identification and management of other major injuries. Third, complications associated with arteriography such as reactions to contrast dye and puncture site problems, although uncommon, are not rare. Fourth, contrast arteriography has become extremely expensive, with hospital charges currently approaching $5000 for a single-limb diagnostic arteriogram in many institutions.

Most significantly, longitudinal studies of the overall accuracy of contrast arteriography in the trauma setting began to demonstrate several small but important limitations. These included the occasional failure to diagnose potential important vascular defects such as large intimal flaps, arteriography's inability to assess venous injuries, and the "over-identification" of several types of arterial injury—small intimal flaps, pseudoaneurysms, arteriovenous fistulae, and areas of spasm—that are generally benign but, once discovered, eventuated in operative exploration when, in fact, no such intervention is actually required. Thus, for numerous reasons the availability of a rapid, noninvasive, accurate, and inexpensive vascular diagnostic tool as an alternative to contrast arteriography in the trauma patient was timely.

DOPPLER ARTERIAL PRESSURE MEASUREMENT

The Doppler principle, which correlates changes in wave frequency and velocity, has long been utilized as an investigative tool in physics. Beginning in the 1960s, work by Strandness and coworkers[4] developed the concept of digital strain–gauge plethysmography; simultaneous studies evaluated the use of back-scattered Doppler ultrasound[5] as blood flow velocity detectors. A series of human experiments correlated such examinations with states of normal and abnormal arterial perfusion in the extremities. Now widely used as a screening tool for quantitating chronic arterial occlusive disease, Doppler arterial pressure measurements are accurate, noninvasive, and reproducible.

Doppler Technology in the Assessment of Arterial Trauma

In the early 1980s, impressed by the demonstrated accuracy and simplicity of Doppler arterial pressure measurements for the evaluation of chronic arterial occlusive disease, the author of this chapter[3,6] and other clinicians[7,8] began to examine the possibility that this simple and rapid bedside examination might act as a useful screening test for arterial damage secondary to blunt or penetrating trauma to the arms or legs. Several different arteriography-controlled trials were conducted, notably at Harborview Medical Center in Seattle and at L.A. County–USC Medical Center in Los Angeles.

These studies, in which arterial pressure indices were calculated by dividing systemic blood pressure in the injured limb by that in an uninjured arm, confirmed that such arterial pressure indices are a highly sensitive and specific screen for occult extremity arterial occlusion. Lynch and Johansen,[3] using a Doppler arterial pressure index threshold of less than 0.90 as "abnormal," demonstrated a sensitivity of 95% and specificity of 97% for arteriographically proved arterial injury; overall accuracy was 95%. Weaver and colleagues[7] used a higher arterial pressure index of 1.00 and achieved 100% sensitivity for arterial injury at the cost of a substantially lower specificity (i.e., a higher likelihood of unproductive arteriographic results). Acceptance of the validity of Doppler arterial pressure indices and a reborn willingness to accept the validity of serial physical examinations[9] has enabled clinicians to substitute the much more rapid, safe, and noninvasive method of Doppler arterial pressure measurement for arteriography as a screening tool for occult arterial occlusion following blunt or penetrating trauma in the extremities.

Notwithstanding this significant opportunity to change clinicians' approach to the initial vascular assessment of the trauma victim, the limitations of physical examination (even when augmented by Doppler arterial pressure measurements) are clear. This technique is useful only for identifying significant arterial stenosis or occlusion; that is, it cannot identify, effectively localize, or show the extent of arterial damage. Furthermore, it is not useful or accurate for truncal or cervical vascular injury, or for damage to nonaxial arteries such as the profunda femoris artery, and it cannot assess the presence or extent of venous injury. Clearly a further and more accurate noninvasive diagnostic evaluation would be optimal.

THE DEVELOPMENT OF DUPLEX ULTRASONOGRAPHY

Conceptually, duplex sonography arose from pioneering developmental work in medical ultrasound in the 1970s by Strandness and Bell,[4] Hokanson et al.,[10] and Blackshear et al.[11] Combining B-mode ultrasound and vascular Doppler into the same device, thereby making available both a vascular image and a blood flow waveform, was a seminal advance in the evaluation of blood vessel disease. Duplex scanning was initially validated against contrast arteriography, flowmeter measurements, and pathological specimens, both experimentally and in the clinical setting.[10] Because the initial duplex scanners worked best with interrogation of vessels relatively close to the skin, early clinical trials evaluated atherosclerotic stenoses at the carotid bifurcation.[11] Multiple validation trials carried out in patients undergoing carotid duplex sonography and contrast arteriography clearly affirmed the equivalence (if not the superiority) of duplex scanning to arteriography in the assessment and grading of degree of carotid stenosis.[12] (For example, this author has performed carotid endarterectomy since the late 1980s based solely on duplex scans performed by one of three different accredited vascular laboratories.)

Duplex sonography has become increasingly useful in the assessment of a number of other sites in the arterial tree; in addition, acute and chronic venous disease, arteriovenous dialysis access conduits, microvascular free-flap reconstructions, and shunting procedures in the portal venous system are all readily accessible to, and accurately assessed by, duplex sonography.

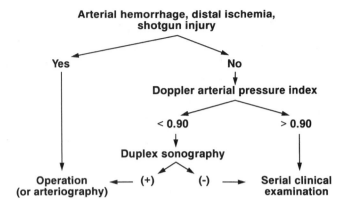

Figure 31–1. Diagnostic algorithm used for penetrating or blunt extremity trauma.[3,5] Weaver et al.[7] utilize a threshold arterial pressure index (API) of 1.00, which produces a higher sensitivity but a substantially lower specificity.[7]

Duplex Ultrasonography for Vascular Trauma

The primary role of duplex sonography in interrogating traumatized blood vessels is to demonstrate the presence or absence of hemodynamically normal arterial flow patterns. Flow disturbances resulting from areas of spasm, thrombus, or extrinsic pressure by hematoma or fracture fragments are thus readily demonstrable. Arteriovenous fistulae are readily identified, and flow arrest secondary to complete vessel occlusion should be apparent. Duplex scan also provides an ultrasonic image of the vessel in question, which may identify intraluminal defects such as intimal flaps, mural lesions such as pseudoaneurysms, and extra- or intramural hematoma.

Experimental studies by Panetta et al.[13] comparing duplex scan and contrast arteriography have been illuminating in this context. In various types of experimental canine arterial defects, duplex scan was found to be significantly more accurate than arteriography at demonstrating arterial injuries in general ($p < .02$), and particularly arterial lacerations ($p < .01$).[13]

Duplex scan has been assessed as a screening tool in trauma victims in whom concerns about extremity vascular trauma exist. In retrospective series by Bynoe and colleagues[14] at South Carolina and Meissner et al.[15] at Harborview Medical Center in Seattle, sensitivity and specificity for arterial injury exceeded 90%. Our current approach in Seattle for patients presenting with knee dislocation, for example, is to perform emergency duplex sonography of the popliteal artery, performing arteriography only if the duplex scan is clearly abnormal.

The validation of Doppler arterial pressure measurement and duplex ultrasonography has revolutionized the vascular diagnostic assessment of patients with extremity trauma. Equivalent or greater diagnostic accuracy has resulted, with dramatic decreases in diagnostic time and resource expenditures. Utilization of the arteriography suite for extremity trauma has been reduced by more than 80%.[6] Our current algorithm for evaluation of patients potentially harboring extremity vascular trauma is shown in Fig. 31–1.

EXTRACRANIAL CAROTID AND VERTEBRAL ARTERY TRAUMA

Controversies abound in the management of penetrating or blunt extracranial vascular trauma—specifically related to continuing uncertainty (despite multiple analyses) about the appropriate role for carotid artery reconstruction in the presence of partial or completed central neurological deficits. Although resolution of these management controversies is outside the scope of the current discussion, the diagnostic accuracy of several noninvasive techniques—specifically carotid duplex scan and contrast-enhanced cerebral computerized tomographic (CT) scanning—offers the real possibility of clarifying the natural history of these complex patients, thereby hopefully improving patient selection and optimizing clinical outcomes.

Few diagnostic arenas have been changed so remarkably as has cerebral CT scan for various cerebral lesions including stroke. High-resolution CT scan has enabled definition not only of the presence of cerebral infarction, but also roentgenographic signs of an unstable cerebral blood–brain barrier such as peri-infarct hemorrhage or hypodensity.[16] These determinations are valuable in the trauma setting because increasingly compelling evidence confirms that, in the absence of CT scan evidence of an unstable blood–brain barrier, cerebral reperfusion is safe and does not risk extension or hemorrhagic conversion of an infarct. However, cerebral revascularization in the presence of an unstable blood–brain barrier clearly has morbid consequences and should be performed only in very unusual circumstances. Data from the carotid atherosclerosis literature suggests that basing a decision-making algorithm for urgent revascularization on cerebral CT scan evidence for a stable blood–brain barrier is safe *and* effective (i.e., patients who would benefit from operation do well, and those in whom no benefit or actual damage might result are spared operation[17]).

Previously, determination of whether penetrating or blunt cervical trauma had resulted in carotid injury depended on the performance of emergency four-vessel contrast arteriography. The time taken to perform this invasive procedure and the necessity to move the patient to a hospital site relatively unfriendly to aggressive resuscitation and serial physical examination frequently nullified the value of these studies; by the time damage to the carotid artery was diagnosed, an established cerebral infarction had often already occurred.

The advent of ultrasonic duplex scanning for the assessment of chronic carotid atherosclerotic occlusive disease[11] provided a novel means for rapid bedside assessment of the extracranial carotid circulation. At the same time comparative studies of arteriography and duplex scanning for chronic carotid disease were demonstrating equivalent accuracy,[12] we[15] and others[18,19] were validating emergency carotid duplex scanning as a highly accurate means of screening trauma victims for evidence for extracranial carotid artery injury.

Limitations of duplex scanning as a screening technique for carotid artery trauma include those associated with the technique in general (availablity of equipment, vascular technologists on call, technologist and interpreting physician expertise), with the evaluation of vascular trauma in general (examination incomplete due to proximity of the wound, hematomas, or dressings) and of trauma specific to evaluation of the cerebral vasculature (relative inability to interrogate the innominate and common carotid arteries in zone I, concerns that extrinsic probe pressure might disrupt thrombus within the damaged carotid artery, relatively lesser success at evaluating the extracranial internal carotid artery in zone III).

Numerous reports have described assessment of the intracranial cerebral circulation by means of transcranial Doppler—a technique of potentially significant value in the trauma setting because it enables accurate determination of the normalcy of direction and velocity of flow in the cerebral circulation.[20] Anecdotal reports of the use of transcranial Doppler in trauma victims have suggested its significant potential value in such a setting; however, its limitations include an even greater "learning curve" for technologists and physicians, longer time required with more unwieldy and obtrusive equipment, and the lack of temporal bone "windows" for interrogation of the intracranial circulation in up to 20% of patients. Demonstration of flow arrest in the intracranial circulation by transcranial Doppler is indicative of brain death.[21]

NONINVASIVE TESTS FOR COMPARTMENT SYNDROME

Compartment syndrome—pathologically elevated skeletal muscle pressures within a noncompliant fascial envelope, usually in the leg or forearm—continues to result in unacceptably high rates of neuromuscular dysfunction, tissue loss, and amputation. When appropriately diagnosed, management of the syndrome by fasciotomy is relatively straightforward; instead, problems arise with timely recogition that compartmental hypertension is present.

Demonstration of increased turgor of the calf or forearm, pain on passive stretch of the affected muscles, and dysfunction of nerves passing through the compartments facilitate the diagnosis of compartment syndrome in the awake and, alert trauma victim with extremity trauma or ischemia. However, when the diagnosis is equivocal or the patient cannot respond appropriately because of intoxication, spinal cord injury, anesthesia, or coma, an objective means of diagnosing compartment syndrome or ruling it out is desirable.

Since 1975, tissue manometry by direct needle puncture or catheter insertion has been practiced.[22,23] Although this technique can be quite accurate, it is both invasive and subject to mechanical failure and observer error. More importantly, conventional tissue pressure thresholds greater than 40 mm Hg (or sustained pressures >30 mm Hg)[22,23] have been shown to be less than totally predictive of the presence or absence of compartment syndrome. Because the critical issue is the gradient between tissue and arterial pressure, whether neuromuscular damage will occur depends to a substantial degree on systemic hemodynamics: recommendations that critical tissue pressure thresholds are reached at 10 to 30 mm Hg less than systemic diastolic[24] or mean[25] arterial pressures have further complicated the interpretation of tissue manometry results.

Once again, noninvasive physiological vascular testing may offer a straightforward solution to this diagnostic dilemma. Jones et al.[26] pointed out that, because thin-walled calf veins necessarily must collapse when tissue pressure exceeds calf venous pressure, duplex scan assessment of tibial vein hemodynamics should be predictive of the presence or absence of compartmental hypertension. Indeed, calf-vein duplex scanning of patients in their series correlated well with the development of compartment syndrome. Experimental studies performed by Ombrellaro and colleagues[27] confirmed the clinical findings of Jones et al.,[26] and documented that loss of lower extremity venous respiratory phasicity is a function of pathologically elevated compartment pressures in the canine hindlimb. Thus, although the diagnosis of compartment syndrome remains a clinical one (the author of this chapter encourages a liberal attitude toward preemptive fasciotomy in the trauma victim), tibial vein duplex scanning appears to offer a useful adjunctive means for provision of objective data about the presence of compartmental hypertension in equivocal or confusing circumstances.

SUMMARY

Noninvasive vascular diagnostic modalities, based primarily on advances in medical ultrasound initially validated for chronic arterial occlusive diseases, have revolutionized screening and early diagnosis in vascular trauma. These techniques, primarily Doppler-derived arterial blood pressure measurement and duplex sonography, are rapid, portable, noninvasive, inexpensive, and reproducibly accurate. Their accuracy in assessing extremity and extracranial cervical arteries and veins has been demonstrated to be equivalent to that of contrast angiography in several prospective observational trials. Duplex scan evaluation of tibial (or forearm) veins may provide highly accurate evidence for the presence of compartmental hypertension.

REFERENCES

1. Snyder WH, Thal ER, Bridges RA, et al. The validity of normal arteriography in penetrating trauma. *Arch Surg.* 1978;113:424–428.
2. Sirinek K, Levine BA, Gaskill HV, et al. Reassessment of the role of routine operative exploration in vascular trauma. *J Trauma.* 1981;21:339–344.
3. Lynch K, Johansen K. Can Doppler pressure measurement replace "exclusion" arteriography in the diagnosis of occult extremity arterial trauma? *Ann Surg.* 1991;214:737–741.
4. Strandness DE Jr, Bell JW. Peripheral vascular disease: diagnosis and objective evaluation using a mercury strain gauge. *Ann Surg.* 1965;161(Suppl):1–12.
5. Strandess DE Jr, McCutcheon EP, Rushmer RF. Application of a transcutaneous Doppler flowmeter in evaluation of occlusive arterial disease. *Surg Gynecol Obstet.* 1966;122:1039–1044.
6. Johansen K, Lynch K, Paun P, Copass M. Non-invasive vascular tests reliably exclude occcult arterial trauma in injured extremities. *J Trauma.* 1991;31:515–522.
7. Weaver FA, Yellin AE, Bauer MAP, et al. Is arterial proximity a valid indication for arteriography in penetrating extremity trauma? A prospective analysis. *Arch Surg.* 1990;125:1256–1260.
8. Anderson RJ, Hobson RW, Padberg FT, et al. Penetrating extremity trauma: identification of patients at high risk requiring arteriography. *J Vasc Surg.* 1990;1:544–548.
9. Francis H, Thal ER, Weigelt JA, et al. Vascular proximity: is it a valid indication for arteriography in the asymptomatic patient? *J Trauma.* 1991;31:512–514.
10. Hokanson DE, Mozersky DJ, Sumner DS, McLeod FD Jr, et al. Ultrasonic arteriography: a noninvasive method of arterial visualization. *Radiology.* 1972;102:435–436.
11. Blackshear WM, Philips DJ, Chikos P, et al. Carotid artery velocity patterns in normal and stenotic vessels. *Stroke.* 1980;11:67–71.
12. Dawson DL, Zierler RE, Kohler TR. Role of arteriography in the preoperative evaluation of carotid artery disease. *Am J Surg.* 1991;161:619–623.
13. Panetta TF, Sales CM, Marin M, et al. Natural history, duplex characteristics, and histopathologic correlation of arterial injuries in a canine model. *J Vasc Surg.* 1992;16:867–874.
14. Bynoe RP, Miles WS, Bell RM, et al. Noninvasive diagnosis of vascular trauma by duplex ultrasonography *J Vasc Surg.* 1991;14:346–352.
15. Meissner M, Paun M, Johansen K. Duplex scanning for arterial trauma. *Am J Surg.* 1991;161:552–555.
16. Moulin T, Catlin F, Crepin-Leblond T, et al. Early CT signs in acute middle cerebral artery infarction: predictive value for subsequent infarct locations and outcome. *Neurology.* 1996;47:366–375.
17. Schneider C, Johansen, K, Konigstein R, et al. Emergency carotid thromboendarterectomy: safe and effective. *World J Surg.* in press.
18. Fry WR, Dort JA, Smith RS, et al. Duplex scanning replaces arteriography and operative exploration in the diagnosis of potential cervical vascular injury. *Am J Surg.* 1994;168:693–695.
19. Montalvo BM, Le Blang SD, Nunez DB Jr, et al. Color Doppler sonography in penetrating injuries of the neck. *Am J Neuroradiol.* 1997;17:943–951.
20. Newell DW, Aaslid R, Stooss R, et al. Evaluation of hemodynamic responses in head injury patients with transcranial Doppler monitoring. *Acta Neurochirurgica.* 1997;139:804–817.
21. Manno EM. Transcranial Doppler ultrasonography in the neurocritical care unit. *Crit Care Clin.* 1997;13:79–104.

22. Matsen FA, III. Compartmental syndrome: a unified concept. *Clin Orthop.* 1975;113:8–13.

23. Whitesides TE Jr, Haney TC, Morimoto K, Harada H. Tissue pressure measurements as a determinant for the need of fasciotomy. *Clin Orthop.* 1975;113:43–51.

24. Matava MJ, Whitesides TE Jr, Seiler JG III, Hewan-Lowe K, et al. Determination of the compartment pressure threshold of muscle ischemia in a canine model. *J Trauma.* 1994;37:50–58.

25. Mabee JR, Bostwick TL. Pathophysiology and mechanisms of compartment syndrome. *Ortho Rev.* 1993;22(2):175–181.

26. Jones WG II, Perry MO, Bush HL Jr. Changes in tibial venous blood flow in the evolving compartment syndrome. *Arch Surg.* 1989;124:801–804.

27. Ombrellaro MP, Stevens SL, Freeman M, Walker E, et al. Ultrasound characteristics of lower extremity venous flow for the early diagnosis of compartment syndrome: an experimental study. *J Vasc Technol.* 1996;20:71–75.

32

Endovascular Techniques in the Treatment of Penetrating Arterial Trauma

Takao Ohki, MD and Frank J. Veith, MD

INTRODUCTION

The first use of an endovascular graft (EVG) in humans was reported by Parodi et al.[1] to treat an abdominal aortic aneurysm (AAA). Following this landmark work, the indications for EVGs have expanded to include arterial occlusive disease,[2,3] occluded grafts,[4] peripheral aneurysms,[5,6] and traumatic arterial lesions. Although the treatment of AAAs with EVGs seems to hold the major interest for both physicians and manufacturers, the validity of EVG for AAA remains to be proved. This is due to the technical difficulty in EVG repair of AAA, which has resulted in the occurrence of complications including endoleaks, arterial injury, and embolization. In addition, the availability of standard aneurysm repair techniques that have been proved safe and durable gives rise to questions concerning the true value of EVG repair at this point in time.

However, based on the reported results of our and other groups, the use of EVG already seems to be justified for the treatment of some traumatic arterial injuries, especially injuries that involve large central vessels. This is particularly true in patients who are critically ill from other injuries or medical comorbidities.

Surgical repair of vascular injuries may be complicated by the inaccessibility of the vascular lesion when trauma occurs to a vessel within the thorax or abdomen, by distorted anatomy due to a large hematoma or a false aneurysm, and by venous hypertension when an arteriovenous fistula is present. These conditions make the use of endovascular techniques appealing because repair can be performed from a remote access site, obviating the need for direct surgical exposure of the injury site, thus reducing the morbidity and mortality rates of the repair. Endovascular techniques for the treatment of vascular trauma include the use of coil embolization, intravascular stents, and the use of stented grafts or covered stents.

Furthermore, when an EVG is used for traumatic lesions, there are usually normal, healthy, proximal and distal arterial segments or graft-fixation zones, which is not always the case with aortic aneurysms. This contributes to the high technical success rate and a low rate of EVG migration or leakage.

This chapter describes various endovascular treatment techniques and reviews our experience with EVGs for traumatic vascular lesions at Montefiore Medical Center in New York. It also reviews the literature on the use of endovascular stented grafts for vascular trauma.

PLACEMENT OF EMBOLIZATION COILS AND INTRAVASCULAR STENTS

Coil embolization has been used to treat relatively small traumatic arteriovenous fistulas and pseudoaneurysms involving nonessential vessels, such as a lumbar artery, the internal mammary artery, or the branches of the hypogastric or deep femoral arteries[7,8] (Fig. 32–1). Long-term follow-up of these coil-treated lesions has proved them to be favorable. Placement of intravascular stents are useful for the repair of intimal flaps. However, due to their porous nature, stents are not indicated for treating arteriovenous fistulas or pseudoaneurysms. Although these endovascular techniques proved to be effective in selected cases, the majority of the patients with vascular trauma were not amenable to such therapy.

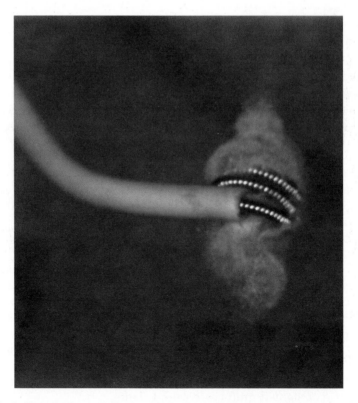

Figure 32–1. Embolization coil (Cook embolization coil, Cook Inc., Bloomington, IN). These coils are delivered through a catheter and have synthetic fibers attached in order to induce thrombosis and hemostasis of the bleeding site. (*Reprinted with permission from: Ohki T, Veith FJ, Kraas C, et al. Endovascular therapy for upper extremity injury. Semin Vasc Surg. 1998; 11:106–115.*)

REVIEW OF THE LITERATURE ON ENDOVASCULAR STENTED GRAFTS FOR ARTERIAL TRAUMA

Endovascular grafts have extended the potential of endovascular therapy for vascular trauma significantly. These grafts have been used to treat almost every kind of injury at various locations in the body, and were used in circumstances in which coil embolization or stent placement was deemed inappropriate.[1,9-25] Although vast majority of the cases that were treated with an EVG were hemodynamically stable, in some instances, it has been used to treat life-threatening acute hemorrhage.[24] The types of devices that have been reported are predominantly a combination of a Palmaz stent and an expanded polytetrafluoroethylene (ePTFE) graft (Fig. 32–2A). Because the traumatized field is often contaminated, the use of a vein graft in combination with a Palmaz stent has also been reported (Fig. 32–2B).[12,17] The different types of stented grafts that have been reported are summarized in Table 32–1 and shown in Fig. 32–2.

The characteristics of lesions, site of arterial access, technical success rate, and the outcome of endovascular stented grafts in the treatment of vascular trauma have been summarized in Table 32–2. These results have been encouraging with a high technical

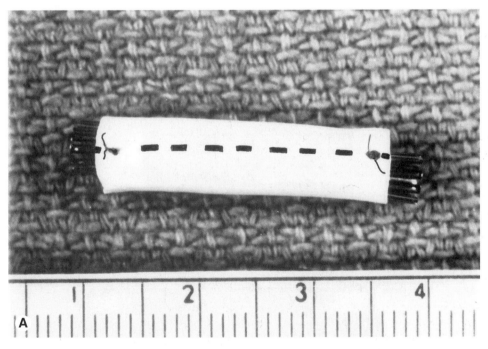

Figure 32–2. Endovascular stented grafts. (**A**) A Palmaz stent is sewn to an ePTFE graft. (**B**) Autologous vein can be used to cover the stents, creating biological stented grafts. The collapsed stent–graft assumes a small profile that effectively covers the struts S of the stent following deployment (*inset*). (**C**) Dacron graft material may be used to cover the balloon-expandable stents. Polyurethane can be fabricated directly onto a stent. This material has "elastic" properties, permitting a closed stent to remain well covered following deployment. (**D**) Corvita endovascular graft. This polycarbonate elastimer fiber–covered stent structurally resembles the Wallstent. A Corvita graft is manually crimped into a 9- or 10-Fr delivery sheath. (*Reprinted with permission from: Ohki T, Veith FJ, Marin ML, et al. Endovascular approaches to vascular injuries. Semin Vasc Surg. 1997;10:272–285.*)

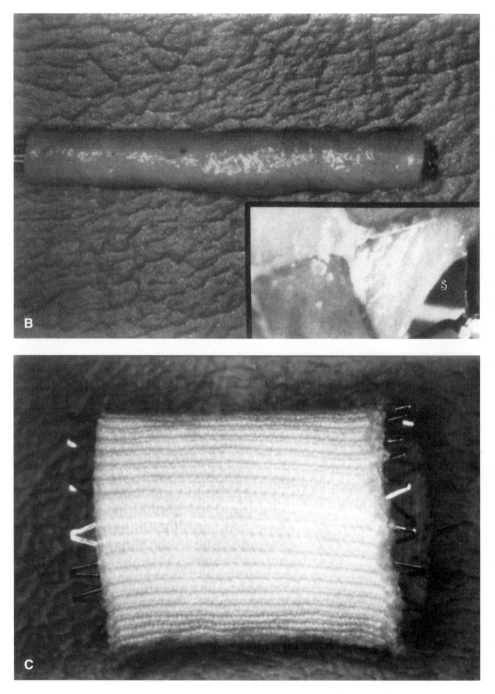

Figure 32–2. (*Continued*)

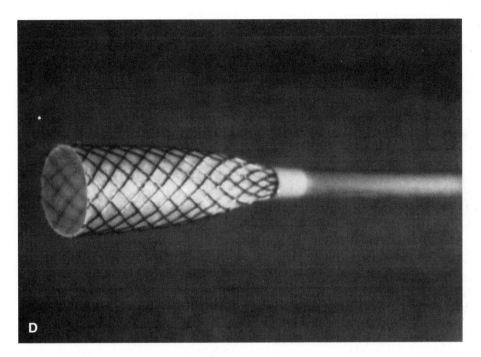

Figure 32–2. (*Continued*)

success rate (94% to 100%) and a complication rate of 0% to 7%, especially when one considers the difficulties that could be encountered in treating these lesions by a direct surgical repair. In addition, the minimal invasiveness and the potential for cost-effectiveness of such endovascular techniques are apparent from the short length of stay (3.3 to 5.3 days) in patients so treated (Table 32–2). Because these EVGs were mainly inserted in nonatherosclerotic, central vessels of a large caliber, it is not surprising that the grafts used to treat traumatic arterial injuries have proved to be durable, with a mean follow-up of 16 months, as shown by the excellent midterm patency rates ranging from 85% to 100%, depending on the location in which they were inserted.

TABLE 32–1. DESCRIPTION OF DEVICE FOR ARTERIAL TRAUMA

Type	Combination of Palmaz Stent and Various Grafts				Cragg Endopro	Corvita Graft
Stent	**Palmaz Stent**				**Nitinol**	**Self-Expanding Braided Stent**
Graft material	PTFE	Dacron	Vein	Silicone	Ultrathin woven polyester fabric	Polycarbonate fibers
Arterial access	1 or 2	2	2	1 or 2	2	2
Reference	11–18, 24	12	14, 19	15, 20	21	12, 22

1, open arteriotomy; 2, percutaneous.
(Reprinted in part from: Ohki T, Marin ML, Veith FJ. Use of endovascular grafts to treat non-aneurysmal arterial disease. *Ann Vasc Surg.* 1997;11:200–205.)

TABLE 32–2. CHARACTERISTICS OF LESION AND OUTCOME BY LOCATION OF INJURY

Location of trauma	Axillary–subclavian artery	Aorta or iliac artery	Femoral artery
Number of cases	18	15	5
Cause of injury	Bullet: 55%; catheterization: 28%; others: 17%	Surgical: 36%; catheterization: 18%; bullet: 9%; others: 36%	Bullet: 60%; catheterization: 40%
Presence of pseudoaneurysm	61%	67%	80%
Presence of AV fistula	44%	73%	40%
Arterial access	Brachial arteriotomy: 39% Brachial percutaneous: 39% Femoral percutaneous: 22%	Femoral arteriotomy: 64% Femoral percutaneous: 36%	Femoral arteriotomy: 80% Femoral percutaneous: 20%
Technical success rate	94% (17/18)[a]	100%	100%
Complication			
Minor	0%	7%	0%
Major	6%[b]	7%[c]	0%
Mean length of stay	3.3 days	4 days	5.3 days
Mean follow-up	18 months	10.5 months	17.4 months
Primary patency	85%[d]	100%	100%
References	11, 12, 14, 16, 17, 20, 22, 24	11, 12, 14, 15, 18, 21, 23	11, 12, 14, 19

[a] One failure due to misdiagnosis.
[b] Brachial artery injury during device insertion.
[c] Distal embolization requiring thrombectomy.
[d] Two failures due to stent deformity.
(Reprinted with permission from: Ohki T, Marin ML, Veith FJ. Use of endovascular grafts to treat non-aneurysmal arterial disease. *Ann Vasc Surg.* 1997;11:200–205.)

MONTEFIORE EXPERIENCE WITH ENDOVASCULAR GRAFTS FOR ARTERIAL TRAUMA

Technique and Devices

We have predominantly used the Palmaz stent [Cordis (Johnson and Johnson Company, Warren, NJ)] in combination with a thin-walled ePTFE graft covering to perform arterial repairs of pseudoaneurysms and arteriovenous fistulas. Depending on the length of the lesion, either a single stent device or a doubly stented device was used (Figs. 32–3 and 32–4). The stents varied between 2 and 3 cm in length (Palmaz P-204, 294, 308) and were fixed inside 6-mm Gore-tex grafts (W.L. Gore and Associates, Flagstaff, AZ) by 2 U stitches (Fig. 32–3A). The stented graft was then mounted on a balloon angioplasty catheter that had a tapered dilator tip firmly attached to its end. The entire device was contained within a 12-Fr delivery system for over-the-wire insertion either percutaneously or through an open arteriotomy.

An alternative device included the Corvita stent–graft (Corvita Corporation, Miami, FL), which is fabricated from a self-expanding stent of braided wire. The stent is covered with polycarbonate elastimer fibers (Figs. 32–2D, 32–5, and 32–6). The stent–graft may be cut to the desired length in the operating room using wire-cutting scissors and then loaded into a specially designed delivery sheath. This sheath has a central

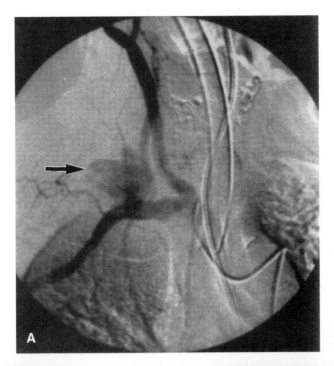

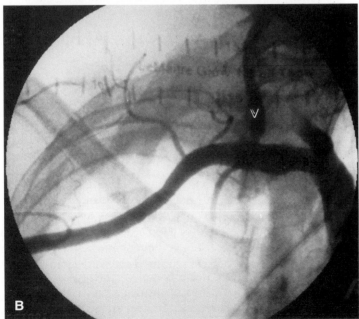

Figure 32–3. (A) This arteriogram shows a large pseudoaneurysm of the subclavian artery (*arrow*) just distal to the right vertebral artery that occurred after an attempted subclavian vein catheter insertion. **(B)** Following stented graft (ePTFE and Palmaz stent) placement through the right brachial artery, the pseudoaneurysm was excluded. Vertebral artery flow was maintained (V). (*Reprinted with permission from: Marin ML, Veith FJ, Panetta TF, et al. Transluminally placed endovascular stented graft repair for arterial trauma.* J Vasc Surg. *1994;20:466–473.*)

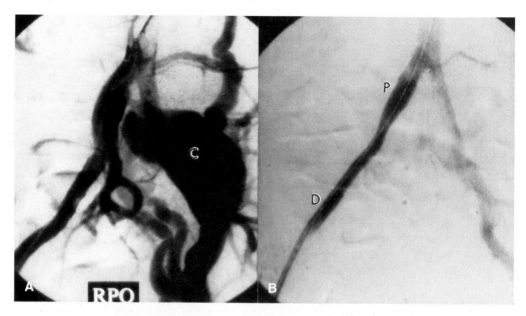

Figure 32–4. (**A**) Preoperative angiogram of an iatrogenic arteriovenous fistula (AVF) following lumbar disc surgery. The patient presented with severe swelling of the left lower extremity. The left common iliac vein (C) is dilated secondary to the fistula. (**B**) Completion angiogram. A PTFE graft was fixed proximally (P) and distally (D) with a Palmaz stent to exclude the fistula from the arterial circulation. Coil embolization of the internal iliac artery was performed prior to stent–graft insertion.

"pusher" catheter, which is used for maintaining the graft in position while the outer sheath is being retrieved.

Results

All procedures but one were performed in the operating room under fluoroscopic (Philips, BV 212, Netherlands) and intravascular ultrasonographic control (Hewlett Packard Company, Paramus, NJ). One Corvita graft was inserted in the angiography suite. A total of 17 stented grafts or covered stents have been used to treat 17 patients with traumatic arterial lesions (Table 32–3). Seven injuries occurred as a result of gunshot wounds; one as a result of a knife wound; four were iatrogenic catheterization injuries; two were iatrogenic arterial trauma (gynecologic or lumbar disk surgery); and three occurred as a result of arterial graft disruptions possibly associated with infection.

All injuries except for one were associated with an adjacent pseudoaneurysm. In five instances the arterial injury formed a fistula to an injured adjacent vein. Associated injuries were present in eight patients with arterial trauma (Table 32–3). The majority of the cases were performed under either local or epidural anesthesia. One patient who had an axillary pseudoaneurysm repaired with a stented graft required a vein patch to close a small brachial artery insertion site. Procedural complications were limited to one distal embolus, which was treated with suction embolectomy, and one wound hematoma, which resolved without further intervention. Graft patency was 100% with no early or late graft occlusions (mean follow-up 30 months; range 6 to 46 months). One patient with a left axillary–subclavian stent–graft developed compression of the

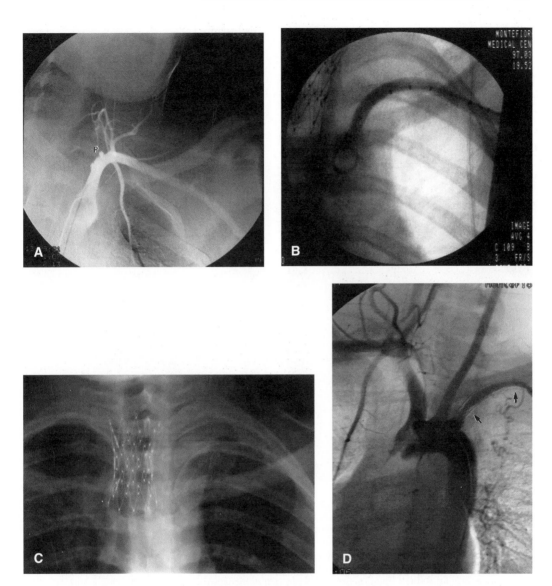

Figure 32–5. The patient is a 19-year-old male status post a gunshot wound to the chest that traversed the mediastinum from right to left, injuring his esophagus, trachea, and left subclavian artery. (**A**) The initial arteriogram shows occlusion of the left vertebral artery and a small pseudo-aneurysm (P) at that site. He was transferred to our institution for endovascular treatment following placement of a covered esophageal stent to repair his tracheoesophageal fistula. (**B**) A Corvita endoluminal graft was placed across the lesion and there was excellent flow through it. (**C**) A plain x-ray film demonstrates the esophageal stent and the Corvita graft in the left subclavian artery. (**D**) At 4 months post–graft insertion, his left radial pulse was diminished although he remained asymptomatic. An angiogram was taken that revealed stenosis at either ends of the graft (*arrows*). These lesions were angioplastied and a Palmaz stent was placed. After the procedure the patient had a strong radial pulse. (*Reprinted with permission from: Ohki T, Veith FJ, Kraas C, et al. Endovascular therapy for upper extremity injury. Semin Vasc Surg. 1998;11:106–115.*)

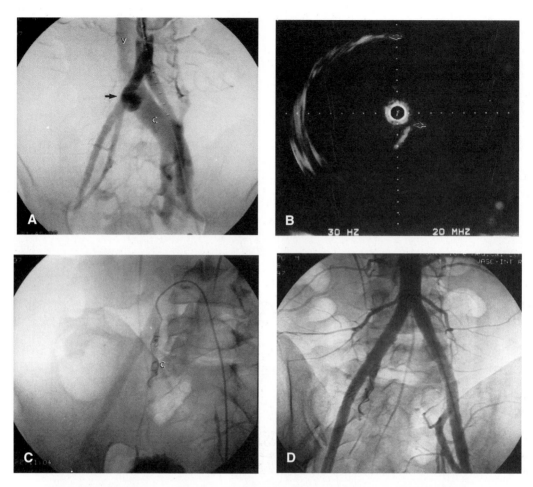

Figure 32–6. (A) Preinterventional angiogram of an iatrogenic arteriovenous fistula (AVF) involving the right common iliac artery due to lumbar disc surgery. The left common iliac vein (C) and the inferior vena cava (V) is visualized by the contrast flowing through the AVF (*arrow*). However, the exact location of the AVF relative to the internal iliac artery and the precise size of the fistula are not clearly shown. **(B)** Intravascular ultrasound (IVUS) image taken at the time of angiography. The amount of substance loss and the location [by identifying the location of the probe (P) of the IVUS under fluoroscopy] are well demonstrated (*arrow* denotes the extent of the fistula). **(C)** Coil embolization of the right internal iliac artery. Because the location of the fistula was 0.5 cm from the origin of the internal iliac artery measured by the technique described previously, the internal iliac artery was embolized with embolization coils (C) at the time of angiogram. **(D)** Completion angiogram. A Corvita graft (10 mm × 6 cm) was used to repair the AVF. Note the preservation of iliac flow and the obliteration of the AVF. (*Reprinted with permission from Ohki T, Veith FJ, Marin, ML, Cynamon J, Sanchez LA. Diagnostic and therapeutic strategies for vascular injuries. In: Baert AL, ed. Medical Radiology—Diagnostic Imaging and Radiation Oncology. Heidelberg: Springer-Verlag Co., Ltd; 1997;235–243.*)

stent at 12 months (Fig. 32–7) that was treated with balloon angioplasty. The problem recurred 3 months later and no intervention was required. This device has not thrombosed with follow-up over 3 years. Another patient developed stenosis at either end of his stent–graft (Corvita) that was treated percutaneously with additional balloon dilatation and Palmaz stent placement (Fig. 32–5D).

TABLE 32–3. STENTED GRAFTS FOR TRAUMATIC ARTERIAL LESIONS: MONTEFIORE EXPERIENCE

Sex/Age	Mechanism of Injury	Vessel(s) Involved	PA	AVF	Anesthesia	Associated Injuries	Injury to Repair Time Interval	Stent Graft Length (cm)	Access	Hospital Stay (days)	Patency (months)	Complications
F/80	Catheterization	RASA	No	No	Local	None	2 days	4[a]	Right brachial artery	2	1	—
M/21	Surgical trauma	RCIA LCIV	Yes	Yes	Local	None	4 weeks	6[a]	RCFA percutaneous	4	6	—
M/22	Bullet	LSFA	Yes	No	Local	Soft tissue injury; left DVT	12 h	3	LSFA arteriotomy	6	9[b]	—
F/85	Surgical trauma	RCIA	Yes	Yes	Local	None	8 yrs	5[a]	LCFA percutaneous	4	11	Distal emboli[c]
M/49	Catheterization	RCIA	Yes	Yes	Epidural	None	18 months	5	RCFA arteriotomy	5	11	Wound hematoma
M/68	Iliac graft disruption	LCIA	Yes	No	Epidural	None	1 month	9	LCFA arteriotomy	5	9	—
M/66	Aortic graft disruption	Aorta	Yes	No	Epidural	None	1 week	10	LCFA arteriotomy	5	18	—
M/76	Aortic disruption	Aorta	Yes	No	Epidural	None	3 days	7	LCFA arteriotomy	7	20	—
M/18	Bullet	RASA	Yes	No	Local	None	6 h	3	Right brachial artery	3	21	—
M/22	Bullet	RASA	Yes	No	Local	Hemothorax	3 h	3	Right brachial artery	6	21	—

(continues)

419

TABLE 32–3. STENTED GRAFTS FOR TRAUMATIC ARTERIAL LESIONS: MONTEFIORE EXPERIENCE (*Continued*)

Sex/ Age	Mechanism of Injury	Vessel(s) Involved	PA	AVF	Anesthesia	Associated Injuries	Injury to Repair Time Interval	Stent Graft Length (cm)	Access	Hospital Stay (days)	Patency (months)	Complications
M/18	Bullet	RSA	Yes	Yes	Local	Hemothorax	48 h	3	Right brachial artery	4	30	—
F/78	Catheterization	RSA	Yes	No	Local	Hemothorax	24 h	3	Right brachial arteriotomy	8 wks[d]	37	—
M/78	Catheterization	LCIA	Yes	No	Epidural	None	4 mos	2	LCFA arteriotomy	2	37	—
M/35	Bullet	RASA	Yes	No	Local	Brachial plexus	3 wks	3	Right brachial arteriotomy	4	38	—
M/24	Knife	LASA	Yes	No	General	Pneumothorax; hemothorax	4 h	3	Left brachial arteriotomy	7	42	Stent compression
M/28	Bullet	RSFA	Yes	No	Local	Left open femur fracture	12 h	3	RSFA arteriotomy	9	45	—
M/20	Bullet	LSFA LSFV	Yes	Yes	General	Soft tissue, buttock	36 h	3	LSFA percutaneous	5	47	—

[a] Corvita stent–graft.
[b] Died 2 months postprocedure (homicide).
[c] Treated with catheter-suction thrombectomy.
[d] Hospitalized for multiple medical problems.

AVF, arteriovenous fistula; DVT, deep venous thrombosis; LCFA, left common femoral artery; LCIA, left common iliac artery; LCIV, left common iliac vein; LSFA, left superficial femoral artery; LSFV, left superficial femoral vein; PA, pseudoaneurysm; RASA, right axillary subclavian artery; RCFA, right common femoral artery; RCIA, right common iliac artery; RSA, right subclavian artery; RSFA, right superficial femoral artery.

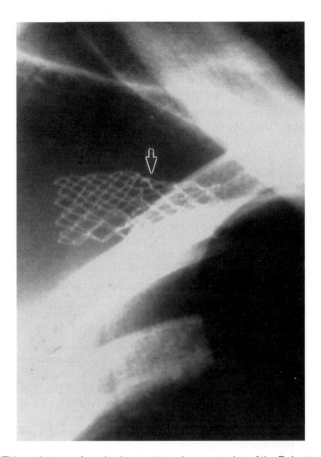

Figure 32–7. This patient was found to have external compression of the Palmaz stent 8 months after stent–graft repair of a left subclavian injury. Plain roentgenogram revealed a stent fracture (*arrow*). Balloon dilatation resulted in protracted patency. (*Reprinted with permission from: Patel AV, Marin ML, Veith FJ, et al. Endovascular graft repair of penetrating subclavian artery injuries. J Endovasc Surg. 1996;3:382–388.*)

DISCUSSION

Surgical repair of vascular injuries may be challenging due to the inaccessibility of the vascular lesion when trauma occurs to a vessel within the thorax or abdomen, by distorted anatomy due to a large hematoma or a false aneurysm, and by venous hypertension when an arteriovenous fistula is present. These conditions make the use of endovascular techniques appealing because repair can be performed from a remote access site, obviating the need for direct surgical exposure of the injury site, thus reducing the morbidity and mortality rates of the repair. Endovascular treatment for vascular injury, including the placement of embolization coils, intravascular stents, and the use of stented grafts, has been reviewed.

Coil embolization and stent placement seem to be effective in a limited number of cases. EVGs have greatly extended the potential of endovascular therapy for vascular trauma. These grafts have been used to treat almost every kind of injury at various locations in the body. Intravascular ultrasound provides certain details that are otherwise difficult to obtain, including the exact location and size of the injury or fistula. These details are especially important when a coexisting arteriovenous fistula makes the angiographic interpretation difficult, and may be essential when performing an endovascular repair. Regardless of the type of the device used, stented grafts appear to be associated with a low morbidity rate, high success rate, less invasive insertion procedure, reduced requirements for anesthesia, and a limited need for an extensive dissection in the traumatized field. These advantages are especially important in patients with central arteriovenous fistulas or false aneurysms, particularly patients who are critically ill from other coexisting injuries or medical comorbidities. In such instances, the use of stented grafts already seems to be justified. EVG is an important tool for the treatment of vascular trauma and should be included in the armamentarium of the vascular surgeon.

REFERENCES

1. Parodi JC, Palmaz JC, Barone HD. Transfemoral intraluminal graft implantation for abdominal aortic aneurysms. *Ann Vasc Surg.* 1991;5:491–499.
2. Marin ML, Veith FJ, Cynamon J, et al. Transfemoral endovascular stented graft treatment of aorto-iliac and femoropopliteal occlusive disease for limb salvage. *Am J Surg.* 1994;168:154–162.
3. Ohki T, Marin ML, Veith FJ, et al. Endovascular aorto–uni-femoral grafts and femorofemoral bypass for bilateral limb-threatening ischemia. *J Vasc Surg.* 1996;24:984–997.
4. Sanchez LA, Marin ML, Veith FJ, et al. Placement of endovascular stented grafts via remote access sites: a new approach to the treatment of failed aortoiliofemoral reconstructions. *Ann Vasc Surg.* 1995;9:1–8.
5. Marin ML, Veith FJ, Lyon RT, et al. Transfemoral endovascular repair of iliac artery aneurysms. *Am J Surg.* 1995;170:179–182.
6. Marin ML, Veith FJ, Panetta TF, et al. Transfemoral endoluminal stented graft repair of a popliteal artery aneurysm. *J Vasc Surg.* 1994;19:754–757.
7. Rosch J, Dotter CT, Brown MJ. Selective arterial embolization. A new method for control of acute gastrointestinal bleeding. *Radiology.* 1972;102:303–306.
8. Panetta TF, Sclafani SJA, Goldstein AS, et al. Percutaneous transcatheter embolization for arterial trauma. *J Vasc Surg.* 1985;2:54–64.
9. Marin ML, Veith FJ, Cynamon J, et al. Initial experience with transluminally placed endovascular grafts for the treatment of complex vascular lesions. *Ann Surg.* 1955;222:449–469.
10. Marin ML, Veith FJ, Ohki T. Endovascular stent–grafts for treatment of traumatic pseudoaneurysms and arteriovenous fistulas. In: Yao JST, Pearce WH, eds. *Vascular Surgery: 20 Years of Progress.* Stamford, CT: Appleton & Lange; 1996;315–327.
11. Marin ML, Veith FJ, Panetta TF, et al. Transluminally placed endovascular stented graft repair for arterial trauma. *J Vasc Surg.* 1994;20:466–473.
12. Parodi JC. Endovascular repair of abdominal aortic aneurysms and other arterial lesions. *J Vasc Surg.* 1995;21:549–557.
13. Becker GJ, Katzen BT, Benenati JF, et al. Endografts for the treatment of aneurysm and traumatic vascular lesions: MVI experience. *J Endovasc Surg.* 1995;2:380–382. (Abstract)
14. Schmitter SP, Marx M, Bernstein R, et al. Angioplasty-induced subclavian artery dissection in a patient with internal mammary artery graft: treatment with endovascular stent and stent–graft. *Am J Radiol.* 1995;165:449–451.
15. Marston WA, Criado E, Mauro M, et al. Transbrachial endovascular exclusion of an axillary artery pseudoaneurysm with PTFE-covered stents. *J Endovasc Surg.* 1995;2:172–176.
16. Zajiko AB, Little AF, Steed DL, et al. Endovascular stent–graft repair of common iliac artery-to-inferior vena cava fistula. *JVIR.* 1995;6:803–806.
17. Dorros G, Joseph G. Closure of a popliteal arteriovenous fistula using an autologous vein–covered Palmaz stent. *J Endovasc Surg.* 1995;2:177–181.

18. Becker GJ, Benenatl JF, Zemel G, et al. Percutaneous placement of a balloon-expandable intraluminal graft for life-threatening subclavian arterial hemorrhage. *JVIR.* 1991;2:225–229.
19. Allgayer B, Theiss W, Naundorf M. Percutaneous closure of an arteriovenous fistula with a Cragg endoluminal graft. *Am J Radiol.* 1996;166:673–674.
20. Gomez-Jorge JT, Guerra JJ, Scagnelli T, et al. Endovascular management of a traumatic subclavian arteriovenous fistula. *JVIR.* 1996;7:599–602.
21. Terry PJ, Houser EE, Rivera FJ, et al. Percutaneous aortic stent placement for life threatening aortic rupture due to metastatic germ cell tumor. *J Urol.* 1995;153:1631–1634.
22. Criado E, Marston WA, Ligush J, Mauro MA, et al. Endovascular repair of peripheral aneurysms, pseudoaneurysms, and arteriovenous fistulas. *Ann Vasc Surg.* 1997;11:256–263.
23. Ohki T, Marin ML, Veith FJ. Use of endovascular grafts to treat non-aneurysmal arterial disease. *Ann Vasc Surg.* 1997;11:200–205.
24. Patel AV, Marin ML, Veith FJ, et al. Endovascular graft repair of penetrating subclavian artery injuries. *J Endovasc Surg.* 1996;3:382–388.
25. Ohki T, Veith FJ, Marin ML, et al. Endovascular approaches for traumatic arterial lesions. *Semin Vasc Surg.* 1997;10:272–285.

IX

Venous Problems

33

Understanding and Managing Thromboembolism in Patients with Malignancy

Mary C. Proctor, MS and Lazar J. Greenfield, MD

INTRODUCTION

The high prevalence of thromboembolism among patients with malignancy has long been recognized. In as many as 10% of cases, the presence of idiopathic deep venous thrombosis (DVT) is the initial step in the recognition of an occult malignancy.[1] Trousseau[2] first identified the association between these two conditions in 1865, and others have gone on to elucidate the potential mechanisms.

Surprisingly, thromboembolism is the second leading cause of death among cancer patients.[3] The prevalence of pulmonary embolism (PE) among patients with malignancy in a large autopsy study was 10.5%, but ranged as high as 34% among females with ovarian cancer.[4] Random testing of cancer patients with metastatic disease demonstrated that 90% had at least one abnormal coagulation test. These abnormalities included thrombocytosis, thrombocytopenia, elevated fibrin–fibrinogen degradation products, or altered clotting factors, all of which placed the patient at risk for either thrombosis or hemorrhage.[5]

Because patients with malignancy are experiencing higher rates of remission and longer survival, physicians from many specialties are becoming involved in their care. In order to provide optimal management, it is necessary to be aware of the factors that place these patients at increased risk of DVT and to appreciate the need for adequate thromboembolism prophylaxis when undergoing hospitalization and medical interventions. It is also necessary to have a clear understanding of the risks and benefits of parenteral and oral anticoagulants and vena caval filters in treating thromboembolism. Finally, knowing that idiopathic DVT may be a harbinger of cancer, the physician must understand the cost-effectiveness of screening protocols when thromboembolism cannot be explained.

PATHOPHYSIOLOGY

The three arms of Virchow's triad provide an inclusive structure for studying the association between cancer and DVT. He postulated that stasis, endothelial damage, and presence of a procoagulant state were the necessary factors for developing thromboembolism. Examining these elements with respect to cancer patients makes the increased incidence easy to understand (Table 33–1).

Stasis, or reduced venous flow, is a major contributing factor to developing DVT. In this situation, blood pools in the lower extremities and activated coagulation factors are prevented from being cleared from the low-flow segments. The effect of stasis is both mechanical and biochemical. Patients with cancer may have prolonged immobility due to anergy or as a result of medical treatments.[6] Patients with massive tumors of the abdomen or pelvis or who have non-Hodgkin's lymphoma may experience extrinsic compression of the major veins draining the lower extremities, including the inferior vena cava. These patients present with bilateral lower extremity edema, sometimes extending to the lower abdomen. In extreme cases, collateral vein formation may be evident on the abdomen. The incidence of DVT among patients with non-Hodgkin's lymphoma is 6.6%, and three-quarters of the cases present prior to or during the early stages of therapy.[5,7] Patients with renal cell carcinoma may have tumor extension into the renal vein and vena cava, resulting in intraluminal obstruction. When stasis is associated with an operation, the risk is increased as blood pools in the venous sinuses.[8] Stasis may also be due to hyperviscosity, which may result from increased red cells as in polycythemia rubra vera, increased white blood cells as in leukemia, thrombocytosis, or increased paraproteins. The result may be organ dysfunction secondary to obstructed or impaired capillary function.[5]

Regardless of the cause, stasis may result in prolonged hypoxemia and damage to the venous endothelium. An intact endothelial lining is the best protection against venous thrombosis. Any insult that damages this surface exposes a highly thrombogenic basement membrane. When platelets become adherent to this surface, the nidus for DVT is established. The platelets of cancer patients are often altered. Thrombocytosis is associated with many solid tumors and results in increased platelet activation and adhesiveness. Thrombocytopenia is frequent in patients undergoing irradiation or chemotherapy from increased platelet consumption or accelerated destruction.[8]

Damage to the endothelium may result from direct invasion of malignant cells. Tumor cells are also capable of activating platelets, which in turn release factors that injure the endothelium while at the same time attracting more platelets. With loss of the endothelium, the ability to release vasodilators, platelet antiaggregants, and anticoagulants is lost, which can result in vasospasm and thrombosis.[9]

Finally, mechanical damage to the venous endothelium is frequently associated with treatment of the underlying disease. Several chemotherapeutic agents cause damage to the endothelium. These drugs can be categorized by the timing of their effects (Table 33–2). The presence of central venous catheters is also responsible for a significant number of DVT among patients receiving chemotherapy, total parenteral nutrition

TABLE 33–1. FACTORS ASSOCIATED WITH INCREASED RISK OF THROMBOEMBOLISM IN CANCER PATIENTS AS RELATED TO VIRCHOW'S TRIAD

Stasis	Endothelial Damage	Procoagulopathy
Tumor compression	Central venous catheter	Tissue factor
Immobility	Chemotherapy	Cancer procoagulant
Reduced venous flow	Tumor invasion of vessel	ACLA[a]
		Decreased clotting factor inhibitors
		Disturbed hemostasis

[a] Anticardiolipin antibodies.

TABLE 33–2. CHEMOTHERAPEUTIC AGENTS AND CARDIOVASCULAR DAMAGE BASED ON THE TIMING OF TOXICITY

Timing	Agent
Immediate effect	Bleomycin
	Carmustine
	Vincristine
Delayed effect	Adriamycin
No effect	Fluorouridine

(TPN), or antibiotic therapy. The characteristics of the catheter material, the difficulty of insertion, and properties of the perfusate such as pH and osmolality are all implicated.[3] De Cicco et al.[10] have demonstrated that thrombus is most often found at the site of catheter insertion or points at which the catheter is in close proximity to the venous wall. They also found that the risk is higher when there is a low level of antithrombin III (AT III) compared to when the level is normal. They demonstrated a venographically verified thrombotic incidence of 66% in patients with malignancy. However, the incidence of PE was only 2.8%.[11]

The existence of a procoagulant state in cancer patients is common, but the underlying mechanisms are difficult to define. It may result from either direct or indirect activation of the clotting system. Membrane-bound tissue factor released from some types of tumor cells may bind factor VII and activate the extrinsic clotting pathway. Other types of tumor cells release a cysteine protease that directly activates factor X. Monocyte–macrophages may become activated in cancer patients due to stimulation by specific antigens, immune complexes, or proteases. These activated cells then initiate coagulation.[12] Cancer can also disrupt the homeostatic balance of coagulation. Clotting factors may be increased although coagulation inhibitors are low.

Several potential procoagulant factors have been recognized although two deserve special attention; tissue factor (TF) and cancer procoagulant (CP). TF is a glycoprotein that is the usual initiator of coagulation. When complexed with factor VIIa, it activates factors IX and X. Cancer procoagulant is a proteinase that activates factor X directly bypassing the factor VII pathway. It is found in the serum of patients with malignancies but not in normal serum.[3]

Chemotherapy is implicated in the deficiency of the naturally occurring anticoagulants proteins C and S as well as AT III.[3] Patients with liver cancer develop deficiencies in the vitamin K dependent clotting factors VII, II, IX, and X, whereas factor VIII may be elevated. Fibrinogen is also elevated.[5]

Zuckerman et al.[13] have studied the incidence of thromboembolic events in cancer patients with anticardiolipin antibodies (ACLA) and found that 22% of the cancer patients were positive for ACLA as compared to only 3% of patients without malignancy. This difference was statistically significant. The incidence of thromboembolic events among cancer patients with positive ACLA was twice that of the ACLA negative cancer patients (28% vs 14%).

PROPHYLAXIS

Having reviewed the coagulation abnormalities that are found in as many as 50% of cancer patients and 90% of patients with metastatic disease, it is appropriate to examine methods of preventing DVT and PE in this high-risk population.

It is the physician's responsibility to maintain a high level of suspicion for thromboembolism when dealing with cancer patients. In general the presence of active malignancy doubles the risk of thromboembolism as compared to patients without this risk. Whenever cancer patients are admitted to the hospital, the issue of prophylaxis must be addressed. When admitted for chemotherapy, especially with agents associated with a high degree of risk for thrombosis (Table 33–2), effective prophylaxis should be administered. In addition, the patient should be kept in optimal condition; fully hydrated, mobile as soon as possible, and receiving adequate nutrition, especially protein.

Patients undergoing surgery are at the highest risk of DVT and treatment should be comparable to that of patients undergoing elective orthopedic surgery. The statement on DVT prophylaxis published by the American College of Chest Physicians provides excellent guidelines based on the patient's level of risk.[14] This may include the use of multiple measures such as intermittent compression devices to overcome stasis combined with heparin to treat the procoagulant state. There is a great need for further research to address the issue of appropriate prophylaxis in prospective, randomized studies. Cohen et al.[15] studied risk factors for bleeding in major abdominal surgery when heparin was used for prophylaxis and identified four independent risk factors: male gender, malignancy, gynecologic surgery, and complex surgery. They ascertained that even though many cancer operations were also complex, these two factors were independent of each other. Possible etiologic factors for excess bleeding included chronic disseminated intravascular coagulation, abnormal platelet function, and enhanced fibrinolysis. These factors may also be related to an increased risk of DVT. This dual risk requires careful perioperative patient management.

Thromboembolism during or following chemotherapy is a well-recognized phenomenon. Gabazza et al.[16] reported a clinical study to determine the alterations in coagulation, fibrinolysis, and other hemostatic parameters when patients with lung cancer received chemotherapy. During the first 2 weeks, the researchers found a higher level of coagulation activation and lower fibrinolytic activity compared to baseline values.

A randomized study of the effect of low-dose warfarin on hypercoagulation in women with metastatic breast cancer undergoing chemotherapy demonstrated a significant reduction in the laboratory markers of hypercoagulability among patients treated with 1 mg of warfarin compared to patients who received placebo. There were two DVT among participants, both in the placebo arm.

Patients with prostate cancer undergoing radical prostatectomy have an incidence of asymptomatic DVT in the range of 28% to 51%. In a clinical trial, patients received combined thromboprophylaxis consisting of intermittent pneumatic compression and warfarin adjusted to maintain the INR at 1.5 or higher. The incidence of DVT among these asymptomatic patients undergoing duplex ultrasound screening was only 2.8%. The authors concluded that this combined regimen contributed to a relatively low incidence of DVT.[17]

Patients with central venous catheters have also been treated with very low-dose warfarin to prevent thrombosis with good results. Bern et al.[18] demonstrated a significant reduction in venous thrombosis when patients received 1 mg of warfarin daily. This regimen required no laboratory monitoring and was not associated with increased hemorrhagic complications. Monreal et al.[19] randomized patients with malignancy who had central venous access catheters to receive 2500 IU fragmin or no prophylaxis, and studied them with venography at 8 and 30 days while they had the access device in place. The study was terminated by the oversight committee due to the highly significant advantage of fragmin prophylaxis. The incidence of venous thrombosis was 6% in the fragmin group vs 62% among the untreated group. There were no bleeding complications with this therapy.

Low molecular weight heparin (LMWH) has been approved for prophylaxis in patients undergoing major abdominal surgery. Bergqvist[46] reported outcomes for patients receiving either 2500 or 5000 IU of fragmin. He was able to demonstrate an advantage in patients receiving the higher dose with respect to DVT. However, there was also a higher incidence of bleeding complications in this group. It is of interest to note that none of the hemorrhagic complications occurred in the 62% of patients with malignancy.

TREATMENT OF THROMBOEMBOLISM

Decisions regarding treatment of thromboembolism are difficult and the physician must weigh the risk of a hemorrhagic complication with the opposing risk of extension or recurrence of DVT or pulmonary embolism. One of the major concerns arises from the belief that patients with cancer have a higher risk of bleeding in response to anticoagulation than other patients. It is also believed that they are more likely to have recurrence or extension of DVT during or following anticoagulation (Fig. 33–1).

Standard therapy for thromboembolism includes an initial period of anticoagulation with intravenous heparin while warfarin is begun concurrently. Once the INR has reached a therapeutic range of 2.0 to 3.0 and there has been an overlap of at least 4 days with heparin, it can be discontinued. The patient should be followed closely while on warfarin. In the majority of cases, cancer patients are candidates for this treatment; however, in situations in which the patient has such a high risk of bleeding that no anticoagulant can be administered or when a bleeding complication has occurred on anticoagulants, insertion of a vena caval filter is an appropriate alternative.

Diagnosis

The initial step in successful treatment of thromboembolism is early and accurate diagnosis. Physicians should maintain a low threshold of suspicion for DVT and PE

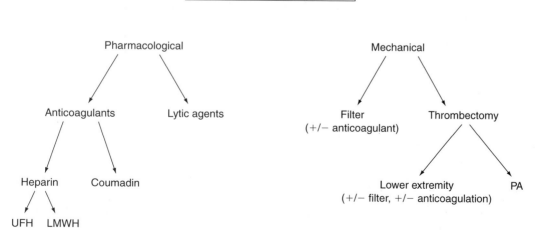

Figure 33–1. Treatment options for patients with diagnosed thromboembolism and malignancy. PA, pulmonary artery; UFH, unfractionated heparin; LMWH, low molecular weight heparin.

when treating patients with malignancy, especially during hospitalization for chemotherapy or surgery. In the vast majority of medical centers, DVT is diagnosed by means of ultrasonography. This technology is rapidly replacing the earlier gold standard of venography as it is noninvasive, requires no contrast agents, and may be repeated as necessary. In symptomatic patients, the sensitivity and specificity of ultrasound using color-flow Doppler is comparable to venography. When PE is suspected, the standard diagnostic method depends on the status of the patient. In cases in which the patient is hemodynamically stable, the lung scan is an appropriate screening test. It is possible to make the diagnosis on the basis of a high probability lung scan, but this can be misleading in the presence of pulmonary malignancies. In some centers, spiral CT, magnetic resonance imaging (MRI), and echocardiography are also used in the diagnosis. The timeliness and the accuracy of the diagnosis are extremely important in this patient population as the failure to make the diagnosis may result in premature or unnecessary mortality, whereas unnecessary anticoagulation may result in significant morbidity from hemorrhage. For the patient who is hemodynamically unstable, pulmonary angiography is the most expeditious and definitive diagnostic study.

Treatment

Decisions regarding treatment of DVT and PE are complex. The risk of thrombus extension or recurrence must be weighed against the risk of a major bleeding complication. Initially, the decision between pharmacologic and mechanical treatment usually must be made based on the presence of ischemia (phlegmasia cerulea dolens), which may require operative thrombectomy. Then each of these subgroups require further decisions (Fig. 33–1). Pharmacological therapy includes both oral and parenteral anticoagulants and thrombolytic therapy. Patients who present with DVT and have no major contraindication to anticoagulation should be given a bolus of IV heparin and begun on a continuous heparin infusion with a target activated partial thromboplastin time (aPTT) of 1.5 to 2.5 times the control.[20] Concurrently, coumadin can be begun to maintain the INR between 2.0 and 3.0.[21]

Many physicians have adopted alternative treatment regimens as they feel that standard therapy may leave the patient at risk of extension of thrombosis or hemorrhage.[22] In the view of many, these risks are more closely associated with coumadin, and so they manage patients on subcutaneous heparin. There has been great interest in using LMWH to treat DVT based on several factors that appear to make it more attractive. Subcutaneous injections of LMWH are better absorbed than unfractionated heparin (UFH) with predictive bioavailability because of less binding to proteins and macrophages. There is no need for laboratory monitoring as LMWH has a predictable dose response curve. Some physicians believe there is less risk of bleeding complications at the microvascular level because there is less binding to platelets and von Willebrand factor, and less direct effect on thrombin.[23] LMWH does not bind to endothelial cells and appears to inhibit the growth of these cells. Finally, there is accumulating evidence that LMWH has a positive effect on mortality in studies in which it is compared to UFH. The effect appears to be statistically independent of the risk of bleeding or recurrent embolism [OR (odds ratio) = 1.5 95% CI (0.92, 2.5)].[23]

There is ongoing controversy regarding the risk of bleeding in cancer patients taking oral anticoagulants. The concept that cancer patients on coumadin bleed more than those on heparin is based on two factors: the high intensity therapy used prior to common acceptance of the INR for prothrombin time reporting and the lack of a consistently applied standard for reporting major bleeding.[22] With oral anticoagulation being monitored more closely by anticoagulation clinics, the risk of bleeding complications has been reduced. Studies have failed to establish a relationship between the presence of cancer and the risk of major bleeding. The reports by Bona et al.[22] and Prandoni et al.[24] support this position. However, in a retrospective report by Gitter et al.[25] from the Mayo Clinic, there was significant association between the presence of cancer at the initiation of oral anticoagulation and an increased risk of both bleeding and thromboembolism. Although these data are contradictory, the Gitter study may suffer from ascertainment bias as the outcomes were obtained from chart review, only 39% of the patients in the cohort had thromboembolism and 61% were at least 65 years of age. Bleeding complications occurred most often when the INR was greater than 4. It appears that the extraneous factors of INR, age, and nutritional status have a greater association with bleeding complications than the malignancy.

Patients should be monitored carefully when oral anticoagulants are discontinued because there is a significant risk of recurrent thromboembolism. Most recommend that anticoagulation should be continued while the cancer is present or during the course of chemotherapy.[6,22,23] In approximately 8.6% of patients with malignancy who are adequately anticoagulated with coumadin, there is recurrence or extension of thrombosis.[6] In these cases, additional treatment may be attempted. Reheparinization and increased coumadin to obtain an INR of 3 to 4.5 has been suggested, but this is associated with an increased bleeding risk. Subcutaneous injections of UFH provide alternative treatment, but thrombocytopenia, osteoporosis, alopecia, and hypoaldosteronism may develop and the aPTT or total clotting time (TCT) must be monitored to prevent toxicity. The use of LMWH offers two major advantages: it does not require laboratory monitoring due to its predictable bioavailability and it may be associated with a lower mortality rate due to its antineoplastic effect; however, this is not fully proved. Hull and others[26] were able to demonstrate a 50% difference favoring LMWH as compared to UFH. It also allows patients to receive treatment in the outpatient setting.

In a subset of cancer patients with malignancy and thromboembolism, the use of anticoagulation has been proved either ineffective or associated with bleeding, and mechanical alternatives are necessary. Although infrequent, when DVT progresses to phlegmasia cerulea dolens and lytic therapy is contraindicated, a venous thrombectomy may be the only means of limb salvage. Although early results have not always been encouraging, the addition of an arteriovenous fistula has helped to prolong patency.[27] In cases in which the patient develops PE and becomes hemodynamically unstable, transvenous pulmonary embolectomy offers a successful alternative therapy. It has the advantage of avoiding general anesthesia and a major procedure associated with open embolectomy, and offers improved mortality rates.[28,29]

Vena caval filters provide long-term mechanical protection from PE. Indications for filter placement do not differ for patients with malignancy but there have been several reports suggesting that filters be used as an alternative to anticoagulation.[30–33] In two publications, Cohen and associates[31,32] reported outcomes for a total of 41 patients who had Greenfield filters placed as the primary therapy for DVT. In the first study,[31] they demonstrated fewer complications, 0/18 vs. 4/11, among patients with filters than among patients treated with anticoagulation. In the second study,[32] they reported on outcomes for 90% of the 41 patients. Although mortality was high, as would be expected, only 5% of patients had developed worsening or new symptoms of DVT. Cantelmo and coworkers[34] advised a more liberal indication for caval interruption among high-risk patients with advanced malignancy based on low procedural morbidity (7%) and stasis sequelae in 14%. Calligaro and associates[30] reported on 30 patients with advanced malignancy, 20 of whom were anticoagulated while 10 received vena caval filters as primary therapy for venous thromboembolism. Three-quarters of the patients treated with anticoagulation had bleeding or rethrombosis, and 10 of the 15 subsequently had Greenfield filters placed. They concluded that placement of a Greenfield filter appeared to be the preferred treatment and reserved anticoagulation for patients with progressive DVT after filter placement. Lossef and Barth[35] studied outcomes for 34 patients with advanced malignancies and thromboembolism. The hospital-related mortality was 18%, and the remaining patients had a mean survival of 6.6 months with no filter-related complications or recurrent PE. Invasive or palliative procedures were made possible due to the presence of the filter in 14% of patients. One of the most comprehensive reports was by Schwarz et al.,[33] who studied 182 patients with cancer and thromboembolism; 170 had a contraindication to anticoagulation and 12 had a failure of anticoagulation. The incidence of filter complications was 3% and the rate of recurrent PE was 2%. There were no postthrombotic complications. In addressing the ethical dilemma of placing filters in patients with terminal cancer, the authors of this study recommended placement based on their ability to discharge 90% of these patients home.

Sarasin and Eckman[36] did a Markov decision and cost-effectiveness analysis factoring in bleeding and thrombotic consequences, filter complications, and excess mortality using quality adjusted life years (QALY) expectancy and total average costs. They compared no therapy to anticoagulation or filter placement, and concluded that if patients were to be treated actively, vena caval filters should be the primary therapy because they resulted in an 11% to 18% increase in QALYs. However, they cautioned against the use of vena caval filters in the absence of thromboembolic disease as this demonstrated no cost savings.

Not all investigators believe that filters should be the primary therapy for thromboembolism in patients with cancer. Magnant and associates[47] studied outcomes for 84 patients who had filters placed for standard indications and one-half had died within the first year, with 27% of the deaths occurring prior to discharge. When the cancer was advanced, 43% did not survive the hospitalization. They suggested that patient selection must be improved to prevent nonbeneficial filter placement.

Rosen et al.[37] conducted a study in 137 patients to identify risk factors that might help prevent placement in patients with a high risk of early mortality. They stratified patients according to the presence of malignancy or suprainguinal DVT, and demonstrated a significantly higher risk of death when either was present vs patients without these factors and a higher risk when both were present. Although survival is an important outcome in these patients, it is not the indication for filter placement. In many cases, a filter allows patients to undergo palliative procedures that could not be done under anticoagulation and facilitates the return home of patients who would otherwise have to remain hospitalized. When used instead of anticoagulation, it may also prove cost-effective as it eliminates the need for serial laboratory studies. In our own experience, we have data on 166 patients treated for cancer who have received a Greenfield filter over a 6-year period.[38] In 72% of cases, distant metastases were present at the time of filter placement. Mean survival in this group was 10 months, which compares favorably to reports of others, but less favorably to survival for other patients in our database ($p = .001$). Interestingly, more than 50% of filters were placed at the time of cancer recurrence, which took place on average 20 months following the first diagnosis and strongly suggests a temporal association between recurrent malignancy and DVT.

A final issue that requires consideration is the role for cancer screening in patients who present with idiopathic thromboembolism. Prandoni and coworkers[39] reported a study in 250 patients with symptomatic DVT followed for 2 years. The difference in the incidence of overt cancer during follow-up was 1.9% in patients with secondary

DVT vs 7.6% among patients with idiopathic DVT.[39] Thromboembolism recurred in 35 of 145 with idiopathic DVT and 17% of this subgroup developed overt cancer. This report provides statistically significant confirmation of an association between idiopathic DVT and future malignancy. Griffin et al.[40] reported results from a study in Olmsted county of patients with objectively documented DVT or PE. They found twice the incidence of future malignancies as would be expected (9 vs 4.5) with a relative risk of two.

Conversely, Rajan and others[41] failed to find a statistical association between idiopathic DVT and future malignancy ($p = .7$). The timing of patient entry to this study may have affected the outcome as there was a 4-week gap between the diagnosis of DVT and inclusion into the cohort, and the authors acknowledged that many cancers were detected during this interval. Because of the association between idiopathic DVT and subsequent malignancy, there has been much discussion of the value of cancer screening in cases of idiopathic DVT. The ultimate goal of a screening program is to change the prognosis of the underlying disease. Prins and associates[42] identify five criteria for a screening program: a serious, common disease; a well-understood natural history; an accurate test; a treatable disease; and an acceptable treatment. As with any screening program, the subsequent diagnostic tests, the economic costs and physical risks must all be weighed against the potential outcome of therapy. For many, the balance is very delicate as the potential for improved mortality is low due to the type of cancer and the stage of the disease. Prins et al.[42] suggest that a screening program in patients with idiopathic DVT may not be effective in extending survival because the cancer is already having a systemic effect. They concluded that the use of expensive screening with CT, gastroscopy, and detection of tumor markers is not justified if there is no expectation of improved survival. However, they caution that the physician should maintain a low threshold of suspicion when the patient presents with symptoms.

In a retrospective cohort study, the incidence of malignancy in patients with idiopathic DVT was 12%.[43] The investigators followed 142 patients who had a history and physical examination, laboratory studies, and chest x-ray. The 12% of patients with cancer had positive findings on at least one of these evaluations and the incidence increased with the number of abnormalities. No patient with normal findings on all tests developed cancer. The most common laboratory findings were increased alkaline phosphatase in 58% and decreased albumin in 81%.[43] The majority of cancers were found during the first 12 months.

When CT scans were added to the screening steps already mentioned, Bastounis et al.[44] found twice the incidence of cancer (25%) compared to Cornuz et al.[43] Seventy percent of cases were found during the initial admission, and half of the cases were asymptomatic. The addition of CT added 25% to the number of cases.[44] Barosi et al.[45] point out that CT may be impractical due to the large number of potential sites and also raise the issue of prolonged survival with diagnosis. Using an incidence of cancer among patients with idiopathic DVT of 2.7 times the general population, they performed a decision-analysis model using the costs and utilities involved in screening for various types of malignancy. For men, screening for colon and prostate cancer was effective, and for women, screening for colon, breast, cervical, and ovarian cancer prolonged life and conserved resources. The consensus of opinion favors simple screening (history, physical, chest x-ray, and blood work) in asymptomatic patients with idiopathic DVT.

SUMMARY

The observations by Trusseau[2] regarding the association between thromboembolism and malignancy have withstood the scrutiny of time. Using Virchow's model of causative factors, this relationship has become better understood. The role of disease-related procoagulant factors, the multiple causes of stasis, and the potential for endothelial damage can be readily identified.

Prophylaxis for DVT among cancer patients remains a challenge. Determining the level of risk and then identifying whether the patient will benefit most from mechanical, pharmacological, or combined therapy is difficult. Unfortunately, there are no good randomized studies on which to base decisions. The one clear fact is that any patient with cancer who is hospitalized for surgery, chemotherapy, or other disease-related factors must receive thromboprophylaxis. When the patient is found to have DVT or PE, the plan for treatment must be individualized. Heparin is effective in controlling DVT when it is not contraindicated. The fact that a large number of patients develop recurrent disease when heparin is discontinued is evidence of its efficacy. In addition, LMWH has been shown to improve long-term mortality in these patients, whereas warfarin is more problematic. There is a frequently noted incidence of recurrent thrombosis and bleeding complications with warfarin despite appropriate levels of anticoagulation (INR 2.0–3.0). In these cases, because therapy must extend over the period when the cancer is present, some physicians have opted to place a Greenfield filter either in addition to or instead of anticoagulation. When patients develop idiopathic DVT, there is an increased risk of developing cancer during the next 6 to 12 months. A simple gender-specific screening protocol allows early detection and treatment of the malignancy that in some cases may result in improved survival. In our own experience, we found that the presence of thromboembolism in patients with known localized cancer was often associated with metastatic recurrence.[38] When treated effectively with adequate anticoagulation or a Greenfield filter, morbidity and mortality specific to thromboembolism can be reduced. Both cancer and thromboembolism are potentially fatal conditions, and the combination decreases the probability of long-term survival. Maintaining a high suspicion for one in the presence of the other provides the best level of protection for the unfortunate patient.

REFERENCES

1. Agnelli G. Venous thromboembolism and cancer: a two-way clinical association. *Thromb Haemost.* 1997;78:117–120.
2. Trousseau A. Phlegmasia alba dolens. *Clin Med Hotel Dieu de Paris.* 1865;3:94
3. Shlebak AA, Smith DB. Incidence of objectively diagnosed thromboembolic disease in cancer patients undergoing cytotoxic chemotherapy and/or hormonal therapy. *Cancer Chemother Pharmacol.* 1997;39:462–466.
4. Svendsen E, Karwinski B. Prevalence of pulmonary embolism at necropsy in patients with cancer. *J Clin Pathol.* 1989;42:805–809.
5. Schwartzberg LS, Holbert JM. Hemorrhagic and thrombtic abnormalities of cancer. *Crit Care Clin.* 1988;4(1):107–128.
6. Prandoni P. Antithrombin strategies in patients with cancer. *Thromb Haemost.* 1997;78:141–144.
7. Ottinger H, Belka C, Kozole G, et al. Deep venous thrombosis and pulmonary artery embolism in high-grade non-Hodgkins's lymphoma: incidence, causes and prognostic relevance. *Eur J Haematol.* 1995;54:186–194.
8. Piccioli A, Prandoni P, Ewenstein BM, et al. Cancer and venous thromboembolism. *Am Heart J.* 1996;132(4):850–855.
9. Naschitz J, Yeshurun D, Lev L. Thromboembolism in cancer. *Cancer.* 1993;71:1384–1390.
10. De Cicco M, Matovic M, Balestreri L, et al. Central venous thrombosis: an early and frequent complication in cancer patients bearing long-term silastic catheter. A prospective study. *Thromb Res.* 1997;86:101–113.

11. De Cicco M, Matovic M, Balestreri L, et al. Antithrombin III deficiency as a risk factor for catheter-related central vein thrombosis in cancer patients. *Thromb Res.* 1995;78:127–137.
12. Goldhaber SZ, Haire WD, Feldstein ML, et al. Alteplase versus heparin in acute pulmlnary embolism: randomized trial assessing right-ventricular function and pulmonary perfusion. *Lancet.* 1993;341:507–511.
13. Zuckerman E, Toubi E, Golan TD, et al. Increased thromboembolic incidence in anticardiolipin-positive patients with malignancy. *Br J Cancer.* 1995;72:447–451.
14. ACCP Consensus Group. Opinions regarding the diagnosis and management of venous thromboembolic disease. *Chest.* 1996;109(1):233–237.
15. Cohen AT, Wagner MB, Mohamed MS. Risk factors for bleeding in major abdominal surgery using heparin thromboprophylaxis. *Am J Surg.* 1997;174:1–5.
16. Gabazza EC, Taguchi O, Yamakami T, et al. Alteration of coagulation and fibrinolysis systems after multidrug anticancer therapy for lung cancer. *Eur J Cancer.* [A] 1994;30A:1276–1281.
17. Kibel AS, Creager MA, Goldhaber SZ, et al. Late venous thromboembolic disease after radical prostatectomy: effect of risk factors, warfarin and early discharge. *J Urol.* 1997;158:2211–2215.
18. Bern M, Lokich J, Wallach S, et al. Very low doses of warfarin can prevent thrombosis in central venous catheters. *Ann Intern Med.* 1990;112:423–428.
19. Monreal M, Alastrue A, Rull M, et al. Upper extremity deep venous thrombosis in cancer patients with venous access devices—prophylaxis with a low molecular weight heparin (Fragmin). *Thromb Haemost.* 1996;75:251–253.
20. Hirsh J. Heparin. *N Engl J Med.* 1991;324(22):1565–1574.
21. Hirsh J. Oral anticoagulant drugs. *N Engl J Med.* 1991;324(26):1865–1875.
22. Bona RD, Hickey AD, Wallace DM. Efficacy and safety of oral anticoagulation in patients with cancer. *Thromb Haemost.* 1997;78:137–140.
23. Walsh-McMonagie D, Green D. Low-molecular-weight heparin in the management of Trousseau's Syndrome. *Cancer.* 1997;80:649–655.
24. Prandoni P, Lensing AW, Cogo A, et al. The long-term clinical course of acute deep venous thrombosis. *Ann Intern Med.* 1996;125(1):1–7.
25. Gitter MJ, Jaeger TM, Peterson TM, et al. Bleeding and thromboembolism during anticoagulant therapy: a population-based study in Rochester, Minnesota. *Mayo Clin Proc.* 1995;70:725–733.
26. Hull RD, Raskob G, Pineo GF, et al. Subcutaneous low-molecular-weight heparin compared with continuous intravenous heparin in the treatment of proximal-vein thrombosis. *N Engl J Med.* 1992;326(15):975–981.
27. Neglen P, al-Hassan HK, Endrys J, et al. Iliofemoral venous thrombectomy followed by percutaneous closure of the temporary arteriovenous fistula. *Surgery.* 1991;110:493–499.
28. Greenfield LJ. Catheter pulmonary embolectomy. *Chest.* 1991;100(3):593–594.
29. Greenfield LJ, Proctor MC, Williams D, et al. Long-term experience with transvenous catheter pulmonary embolectomy. *J Vasc Surg.* 1993;18:450–458.
30. Calligaro K, Bergen W, Haut M, et al. Thromboembolic complications in patients with advanced cancer: anticoagulation versus Greenfield filter placement. *Ann Vasc Surg.* 1991;5(2):186–198.
31. Cohen J, Tenenbaum M, Citron M. Greenfield filter as primary therapy for deep venous thrombosis and/or pulmonary embolism in patients with cancer. *Surgery.* 1991;109(1):12–15.
32. Cohen J, Grella L, Citron M. Greenfield filter instead of heparin as primary treatment for deep venous thrombosis or pulmonary embolism in patients with cancer. *Cancer.* 1992;70:1993–1996.
33. Schwarz RE, Marrero AM, Conlon KC, et al. Inferior vena cava filters in cancer patients: indications and outcome. *J Clin Oncol.* 1996;14:652–657.
34. Cantelmo N, Menzoian J, Logerfo FW, et al. Clinical experience with vena caval filters in high-risk cancer patients. *Cancer.* 1982;50:341–344.
35. Lossef SV, Barth K. Outcome of patients with advanced neoplastic disease receiving vena caval filters. *JVIR.* 1995;6(2):273–277.
36. Sarasin FP, Eckman MH. Management and prevention of thromboembolic events in patients with cancer-related hypercoagulable states: a risky business. *J Gen Intern Med.* 1993;8(9):476–486.

37. Rosen M, Porter DH, Kim D. Reassessment of vena caval filter use in patients with cancer. *JVIR*. 1994;5:501–506.

38. Greenfield LJ, Proctor MC, Saluja A. Clinical results of Greenfield filter use in patients with cancer. *Cardiovasc Surg*. 1997;5:145–149.

39. Prandoni P, Lensing AW, Buller HR, et al. Deep-vein thrombosis and the incidence of subsequent symptomatic cancer. *N Engl J Med*. 1992;327:1128–1133.

40. Griffin MR, Stanson AW, Brown ML, et al. Deep venous thrombosis and pulmonary embolism. Risk of subsequent malignant neoplasms. *Arch Intern Med*. 1987;147:1907–1911.

41. Rajan R, Levine M, Gent M, et al. The occurrence of subsequent malignancy in patients presenting with deep vein thrombosis: results from a historical cohort study. *Thromb Haemost*. 1998;79:19–22.

42. Prins MH, Hettiarachchi RJK, Lensing AW, et al. Newly diagnosed malignancy in patients with venous thromboembolism, search or wait and see? *Thromb Haemost*. 1997;78:121–125.

43. Cornuz J, Pearson SD, Creager MA, et al. Importance of findings on the intital evaluation for cancer in patients with symptomatic idiopathic deep venous thrombosis. *Ann Intern Med*. 1996;125(10):785–793.

44. Bastounis EA, Karayiannakis AJ, Makri GG, et al. The incidence of occult cancer in patients with deep venous thrombosis: a prospective study. *J Intern Med*. 1996;239:153–156.

45. Barosi G, Marchetti M, Piovella F, et al. Cost effectiveness of post routine screening for an occult cancer in patients with idiopathic venous thromboembolism. *Haematologica*. 1995;80(2):61–65.

46. Bengquist D, Burmark US, Flordal PA, et al. Low molecular weight heparin started before surgery as prophylaxis against deep vein thrombosis: 2500 versus 5000 XaI units in 2070 patients. *BJS* 1995;82:496–501.

47. Magnant JG, Walsh DB, Juravsky LI, et al. Current use of inferior vena caval filters. *J Vasc Surg*. 1992;16:701–706.

34

Acute Deep Vein Thrombosis

Outpatient Treatment

David Green, MD, PhD

INTRODUCTION

Acute deep vein thrombosis is a disease associated with considerable morbidity, and when complicated by pulmonary emboli, may cause ventilatory insufficiency, circulatory collapse, and death. Thrombi may embolize to the lungs soon after they appear in the legs, or may become adherent to the venous endothelium of the deep veins, producing acute venous hypertension. The venous occlusion is accompanied by pain, swelling, and erythema of the affected extremity.

The treatment of this disorder has traditionally relied on the intravenous administration of heparin.[1] A bolus dose is followed by a continuous infusion of the drug. Treatment with heparin is continued until effective levels of oral anticoagulation are achieved, which usually takes a minimum of 4 to 5 days. Frequent laboratory monitoring is required to ensure appropriate drug dosing and to avoid inadequate treatment and extension of thrombi or overdosage and bleeding.

However, even with this approach, there may be a poor outcome. This may be due to heparin resistance caused by elevated levels of circulating heparin-binding proteins,[2] resulting in inadequate free drug. Conversely, high levels of heparin may unexpectedly be encountered in elderly patients or patients with renal failure.[3] Another problem is variability in the reagents of the partial thromboplastin time test, which is used to monitor heparin treatment.[4] Increased sensitivity of these reagents to heparin may convey the impression that adequate heparin is being given when in fact the patient is being underdosed.

Because of these problems with heparin, efforts began in the late 1970s to fractionate heparin into smaller molecules, which might be more uniform in their chemical and biological properties.[5] The goals of this work were to develop heparin preparations with high bioavailability following subcutaneous injection; predictable plasma levels so that monitoring would not be required; and a half-life that would allow once or, at most, twice daily dosing. It was also necessary to conduct clinical trials in patients with thromboembolism to demonstrate the safety and efficacy of the preparations. If the heparins met these criteria, they could then be considered for use in the outpatient setting. In this chapter, the characteristics of the low molecular weight heparins are described, the results of clinical trials of thrombosis treatment are reviewed, and the initial experience with outpatient management is examined.

LOW MOLECULAR WEIGHT HEPARIN

Low molecular weight heparin (LMWH) is prepared by the depolymerization of porcine heparin.[6] A variety of methods are used to generate a number of unique products, and each is patented by a different manufacturer. Their molecular weights range from 4000 to 6000, and the number of constituent saccharide units from 13 to 22, in contrast to unfractionated heparin (UH), the molecular weight of which is 12,000 to 15,000, with up to 50 saccharide units.

Heparins exert their anticoagulant effects by binding and activating antithrombin.[7] Heparins with 18 or more saccharide units bind thrombin as well as antithrombin, enhancing thrombin inactivation.[8] Because it has more molecules with 18 or more saccharide units, UH is a better inhibitor of thrombin than is LMWH. However, LMWH is as effective an inactivator of factor Xa as is UH. The ratio of anti-Xa activity to antithrombin activity for LMWHs varies from 2 : 1 to 4 : 1.[6]

When given by subcutaneous injections, the bioavailability of the various LMWHs ranges from 90% to 99%[9]; this is in contrast to UH, whose absorption is dose dependent.[10] For example, the recovery of UH after subcutaneous doses of 5,000 U, 12,500 U, and 17,500 U is 30%, 50%, and 90%, respectively.[1] However, these figures are variable because of the propensity of UH to bind to plasma proteins such as fibrinogen, fibronectin, vitronectin, and von Willebrand factor. Many of these are acute-phase reactants, and therefore the binding of UH and its effective levels vary in disease.[11] LMWHs show much less plasma protein binding, and plasma levels are quite predictable.[12] The half-life of LMWH is about 4 h independent of the dose; the half-life of UH is 56 min after 100 U/kg and 152 min after 400 U/kg.[1]

Monitoring of LMWHs is usually unnecessary because absorption after injection is almost complete and plasma protein binding is minimal.[13] However, there are a few situations when monitoring is required. Children and very obese adults may have greater or lesser responses to the drugs, respectively, and therefore monitoring of doses is appropriate.[14] Renal failure may also affect blood levels, because LMWHs are exclusively eliminated by the kidney.[15] Monitoring should be performed in patients with kidney disease. The laboratory test that best reflects the activity of LMWH is the anti-Xa assay[16]; values of 0.4 to 1.1 U/ml have been considered therapeutic.[17]

LMWHs approved by the US Food and Drug Administration are shown in Table 34–1.

Note that the doses shown in Table 34–1 all refer to the use of LMWH in the prevention of thrombosis; when the drugs are used for treatment of thromboembolism, the doses are at least twofold higher. For example, in the treatment trials evaluating enoxaparin, once-daily doses were 1.5 mg/kg body weight and twice-daily doses were 1 mg/kg.[18] Other LMWHs have been used in once-daily doses of 175[19] to 200[20] anti-Xa U/kg, and twice-daily doses of 100 anti-Xa U/kg.[21]

To summarize, LMWHs have many advantages over UH, not only in terms of their biochemical and pharmacological properties, but also because they have fewer adverse reactions. The most important of these is heparin-induced thrombocytopenia (HIT), which occurs in up to 3% of patients receiving UH[22] but fewer than 1% of those

TABLE 34–1. LOW MOLECULAR WEIGHT HEPARINS APPROVED BY THE US FOOD AND DRUG ADMINISTRATION

Agent (Trade Name)	Manufacturer	Dose (Prophylaxis)	Indication (Surgical Site)
Enoxaparin (Lovenox)	Rhone-Poulenc-Rorer	30 mg q12h 40 mg daily	Hip/knee abdominal
Dalteparin (Fragmin)	Pharmacia-Upjohn	2500 U q12h 5000 U daily	Abdominal
Ardeparin (Normiflo)	Wyeth/Ayerst	50 U/kg q12h	Knee
Danaparoid (Orgaran)	Organon	750 U q12h	Hip

treated with LMWH.[23] The reason for this difference is related to heparin-binding to platelet factor 4, which is much more prevalent with UH.[24] Present understanding of the pathogenesis of HIT suggests that in some persons, the heparin–platelet factor 4 complex elicits antibodies that bind to the complex on the platelet surface.[25] These antibodies also bind and cross-link platelet Fc-receptors, which results in platelet activation, release of thrombogenic platelet microparticles, thrombosis, and thrombocytopenia. A similar reaction involving heparin sulfate on the surface of endothelial cells may lead to vessel injury, enhancing thrombogenesis.

However, in patients who have developed antibodies to UH, cross-reactivity with LMWH is common; therefore, LMWHs should be avoided in such patients. Danaparoid (see Table 34–1) may be given safely to these patients because it has a low degree of cross-reactivity with heparin antibodies.[26] This is because danaparoid does not contain heparin as such, but rather a mixture of glycosaminoglycans, including heparan sulfate, dermatan sulfate, and chondroitin sulfate. When danaparoid is used for the treatment of patients with HIT, the doses given are higher than the doses used for prophylaxis.[27] A typical regimen would consist of a bolus of 2500 U IV, then 400 U/h for 4 h, 300 U/h for 4 h, and 200 U/h as a continuous infusion. These doses apply to average weight patients; doses may be adjusted based on the anti–factor Xa assay in very small or large patients. Platelet counts should be monitored on the infrequent chance that the HIT antibodies will react adversely to the danaparoid. Warfarin should not be started until the patient is stable and the platelet count is recovering. Venous limb gangrene has been associated with warfarin given during acute episodes of heparin-induced thrombocytopenia.[28]

The adverse effects of LMWH include bleeding, HIT, skin necrosis at injection sites, and the current high-costs of the drugs as compared to UH. Preliminary data suggest that the frequency and severity of osteoporosis are less with LMWH than with UH,[29] but large clinical trials to confirm this are still pending.

The antidote for bleeding due to LMWH is protamine.[30] This is because the antithrombin activity of LMWH probably accounts for most bleeding and this can be neutralized by protamine.

CLINICAL TRIALS OF OUTPATIENT MANAGEMENT OF DEEP VEIN THROMBOSIS

The earliest trials of LMWH evaluated the safety and efficacy of these drugs in comparison with UH in inpatients. A meta-analysis of these trials was published in 1995.[31] Ten trials, performed between 1985 and 1994, were analyzed. Five different LMWHs were studied. Doses were given subcutaneously in all but one trial, and twice daily in all but two trials. Thromboembolic complications were significantly lower in patients given LMWH as compared with UH (3.1% vs 6.6%, $p < 0.01$), major bleeding complications less frequent (0.8% vs 2.8%, $p < .005$), and there was lower mortality (3.9% vs 7.1%, $p < .04$). Subsequently, a trial using danaparoid reported that this drug, a heparinoid, was also more effective than UH for the treatment of venous thromboembolism.[32]

Based on these studies demonstrating that LMWH was at least as safe and effective as UH, even when given only once or twice daily by the subcutaneous route, investigators began examining the feasibility of outpatient treatment. Two reports of successful outpatient management using LMWH were published in the *New England Journal of Medicine* on March 14, 1996.[33,34] These two studies are reviewed in some detail.

The trial conducted by Levine et al.[6] recruited patients with acute proximal deep vein thrombosis (DVT), but excluded patients with a history of two or more prior episodes of thromboembolism; concurrent symptomatic pulmonary embolism (PE); likelihood of noncompliance with an outpatient regimen; pregnancy; or known deficiencies of antithrombin III, protein C, or protein S. These exclusions accounted for a third of the patients initially screened for the study. This is important, because such patients might be considered for outpatient treatment under less rigorous circumstances. Patients were randomized to either enoxaparin, 1 mg/kg subcutaneous twice daily, or intravenous UH. Patients received treatment for 5 to 6 days; of patients randomized to LMWH, half were never hospitalized and the rest were in hospital an average of 2.2 days, as compared with 6.5 days for those assigned to UH. The frequency of recurrent thromboembolism and bleeding was no different in the two groups, and the authors concluded that LMWH can be used safely and effectively at home to treat patients with proximal DVT.

Koopman et al.[7] had similar recruitment criteria, but did not consider a patient's ability to be treated at home in the assessment of eligibility. Otherwise, the exclusion criteria were similar to those of Levine et al.,[33] and a similar percentage (31%) were excluded. Patients were randomized to receive either intravenous UH or nadroparin in subcutaneous doses adjusted for body weight; patients weighing less than 50 kg received a total daily dose of 8200 U; patients weighing between 50 and 70 kg received 12,300 U; and patients weighing more than 70 kg received 18,400 U. One-third of patients assigned to the LMWH group were never hospitalized, and of those admitted, 60% stayed less than 48 h. Treatment with LMWH was as safe and effective as treatment with intravenous UH. In addition, the authors assessed physical activity and social functioning; these were better in patients assigned to LMWH.

Because these two trials excluded patients with prior DVT or symptomatic PE, the Columbus Investigators[35] conducted a trial that did not exclude such patients. More than 1000 patients were randomized; 219 had previous thromboembolism and 271 presented with PE. Participants received either intravenous UH in the hospital or subcutaneous reviparin LMWH in doses adjusted to body weight; 27% of the LMWH patients were not hospitalized, and 15% were discharged during the first 3 days. No significant differences were observed in the frequency of recurrent thromboembolism (about 5% in each group), major bleeding (3%), and death (7%). The authors concluded that PE or a history of venous thromboembolism did not preclude the use of LMWH as initial treatment for venous thrombosis, and that suitable patients could be treated outside the hospital.

Table 34–2 lists some of the LMWHs used for the outpatient management of venous thromboembolism, the doses for the specific agents, and if treatment was once or twice daily.

TABLE 34–2. LOW MOLECULAR WEIGHT HEPARINS USED IN THE TREATMENT OF VENOUS THROMBOEMBOLISM

LMWH	Dose (subcutaneous)	
	Once Daily	*Twice Daily*
Dalteparin	200 U/kg	100 U/kg
Enoxaparin	1.5 mg/kg	1.0 mg/kg
Nadroparin	—	100 U/kg
Reviparin	—	6300 U[a]
Tinzaparin	175 U/kg	—
Heparinoid		
Danaparoid	—	2000 U[b]

LMWH, low molecular weight heparin.
[a] Stratified by body weight; average dose shown.
[b] Initial bolus of 2000 U given intravenously.

GUIDELINES FOR THE OUTPATIENT MANAGEMENT OF DEEP VEIN THROMBOSIS

There are a number of important considerations that determine whether a patient is suitable for outpatient management of thromboembolism. These include the location and extent of thrombosis, the willingness of the patient or caregiver to undertake responsibility for home treatment, and the financial aspects of outpatient management (Table 34–3).

With regard to the location of thrombi, iliac vein or vena cava clots may be the source of massive PE. Should such embolization occur, patients are in need of immediate and intensive supportive care and often interventions such as thrombolysis or embolectomy. Thus, close observation in the hospital for at least 72 h is required for patients with thrombi in these locations. By that time, clots should be firmly adherent to the vein wall, permitting antithrombotic treatment to be continued safely at home.

Multiple PE or large pulmonary infarctions require hospital treatment for several reasons including symptoms of shortness of breath due to impaired oxygenation and chest pain when there is pleural involvement. Severe pain and discomfort caused by large thrombi completely obstructing the venous outflow from the lower extremity is another reason for hospitalization. Treatment with leg elevation, elastic wraps, and analgesics is best accomplished under close medical supervision.

Patients should be assessed carefully for disorders that may increase the risk of bleeding. An evaluation for liver disease, cancer, gastritis, thrombocytopenia, or other

TABLE 34–3. APPROPRIATENESS FOR OUTPATIENT MANAGEMENT OF DEEP VEIN THROMBOSIS

1. Thrombus is distal to iliac vein
2. Pulmonary emboli, if present, are minimally impairing ventilation/perfusion
3. Bleeding risks are no more than average
4. Pain and swelling of extremity are not severe
5. Patient is geographically accessible
6. Patient/caregiver is reliable
7. Daily prothrombin times are feasible
8. There are no financial constraints on outpatient treatment

coagulopathies should be performed. A complete history and physical examination are required, and laboratory tests should include a complete blood count with platelet enumeration, partial thromboplastin time and prothrombin time, and liver profile. If these studies are abnormal, anticoagulation should be initiated in the hospital, and possibly at reduced dosage depending on the perceived bleeding risk.

Almost all of the clinical trials of outpatient management of venous thromboembolism required that the patient be geographically accessible to the treating physicians and hospital. There was concern that the patient be able to return promptly if complications occurred, such as new PE, extension of thrombus, or bleeding. Before the patient leaves the outpatient area, one should make sure that a quick return is possible should the need arise. Furthermore, oral anticoagulation will have to be initiated at home and frequent prothrombin times will be necessary to adjust doses. Arrangements for daily prothrombin times should be made, and the communication network between the laboratory, medical service, and patient firmly established so that dosing decisions regarding oral anticoagulants are not delayed.

Home treatment of venous thromboembolism requires that LMWH be injected subcutaneously at specified times, usually every 12 h. When patients first present with thromboembolism, they should be taught proper injection technique by appropriately trained medical personnel. The patient or caregiver must be capable of learning the injection technique, and must be reliable and responsible. Medical personnel should make a judgment as to the suitability of the patient for out-of-hospital treatment during the initial teaching session.

Outpatient management places a considerable financial burden on patients and family. The patient with an acute DVT usually needs to keep the leg elevated almost continually for the first 48 h; a family member may need to remain at home during this period to assist with the activities of daily living as well as help with the administration of medications. Insurance does not reimburse for this time, and also may not pay for the LMWH or other drugs the patient requires. If family members cannot take time off from work, or ready monies are not available to pay for laboratory tests and medications, a short period of hospitalization may be appropriate.

Embarking on outpatient management of venous thromboembolism requires close cooperation between patient and physician. Although some effort must be taken to organize the care, there are many benefits. In addition to the obvious advantage that the patient need spend little or no time in the hospital, there is the less easily characterized improvement in "quality of life." In the study by Koopman et al,[34] this was measured by a questionnaire sensitive to the patient's mental health, perception of health, degree of pain, physical activity, role fulfillment, and social functioning. The investigators found that patients treated with LMWH had better scores for physical activity and social functioning as compared to patients receiving UH in hospital. However, Schafer[36] noted that the instrument used to assess quality of life was constructed to favor an outpatient perspective and therefore would be biased toward the LMWH group. Nevertheless, one could assume that unless considerable discomfort was associated with a DVT, most patients would prefer to remain at home rather than be in a hospital. Also recognized is the cost savings associated with outpatient management; in one study of resource utilization directly related to DVT treatment, a cost reduction of 64% was recorded.[37] However, this may, in part, be due to shifting of costs from the health care industry to the patient or the patient's family.[38] Lastly, the outpatient management of DVT is consistent with the current impetus to move care from hospital to home, and if patients are carefully selected using the guidelines shown in Table 34–3, such treatment should be safe, efficacious, and convenient.

REFERENCES

1. Hirsh J. Heparin. *N Engl J Med.* 1991;324:1565–1574.

2. Manson L, Weitz JI, Podor TH, et al. The variable anticoagulant response to unfractionated heparin *in vivo* reflects binding to plasma proteins rather than clearance. *J Lab Clin Med.* 1997;130:649–655.

3. Freedman JE, Adelman B. Pharmacology of heparin and oral anticoagulants. In: Loscalzo J and Schafer AI, eds. *Thrombosis and Hemorrhage.* Boston: Blackwell Scientific Publications; 1994;1161.

4. Brill-Edwards P, Ginsberg JS, Johnston M, Hirsh J. Establishing a therapeutic range for heparin therapy. *Ann Intern Med.* 1993;119:104–109.

5. Johnson EA. Historical Note. In: Barrowcliffe TW, Johnson EA, Thomas DP, eds. *Low Molecular Weight Heparin,* New York: John Wiley & Sons; 1992;xi–xii.

6. Hirsh J, Levine MN. Low molecular weight heparin. *Blood.* 1992;79:1–17.

7. Rosenberg RD, Bauer KA. The heparin–antithrombin system: a natural anticoagulant mechanism. In: Colman RW, Hirsh J, Marder VJ, Salzman EW, eds. *Hemostasis and Thrombosis: Basic Principles and Clinical Practice,* 3rd ed. Philadelphia: Lippincott; 1994;837–860.

8. Danielsson A, Raub E, Lindahl U, Bjork I. Role of ternary complexes in which heparin binds both antithrombin and proteinase, in the acceleration of the reactions between antithrombin and thrombin or factor Xa. *J Biol Chem.* 1986;261:15467–15473.

9. Barrowcliffe TW, Johnson EA, Thomas DP. In: *Low Molecular Weight Heparin.* Chapter 5. Pharamacology in animals and humans. New York: John Wiley & Sons; 1992;101–123.

10. Bara L, Bilaud E, Gramond G, et al. Comparative pharmacokinetics of low molecular weight heparin (PK 10169) and unfractionated heparin after intravenous and subcutaneous administration. *Thromb Res.* 1985;39:631–636.

11. Young E, Wells P, Holloway S, et al. *Ex-vivo* and *in-vitro* evidence that low molecular weight heparins exhibit less binding to plasma proteins than unfractionated heparin. *Thromb Haemost.* 1994;71:300–304.

12. Frydman A, Bara I, Leroux Y, et al. The antithrombotic activity and pharmacokinetics of enoxaparin, a low molecular weight heparin, in humans given single subcutaneous doses of 20 to 80 mg. *J Clin Pharmacol.* 1988;28:609–618.

13. Boneu B. Low molecular weight heparin therapy: is monitoring needed? *Thromb Haemost.* 1994;72:330–334.

14. Massicotte P, Adams M, Marzinotto V, et al. Low-molecular-weight heparin in pediatric patients with thrombotic disease: a dose finding study. *J Pediatr.* 1996;128:313–318.

15. Cadroy Y, Pourrat J, Baladre MF, et al. Delayed elimination of enoxaparin in patients with chronic renal insufficiency. *Thromb Haemost.* 1991;63:385–390.

16. Samama MM. Contemporary laboratory monitoring of low molecular weight heparins. *Clin Lab Med.* 1995;15:119–123.

17. Laposata M, Green D, Van Cott EM, et al. The clinical use and laboratory monitoring of low molecular weight heparin, danaparoid, hirudin and related compounds, and argatroban. *Arch Pathol. Lab Med.* 1998;122:799–807.

18. The Enoxaparin Clinical Trial Group. A multicenter clinical trial comparing once and twice-daily subcutaneous enoxaparin and intravenous heparin in the treatment of acute deep vein thrombosis. *Blood.* 1997;90(Suppl 1):295a.

19. Hull RD, Raskob GE, Pineo GF, et al. Subcutaneous low-molecular-weight heparin compared with continuous intravenous heparin in the treatment of proximal-vein thrombosis. *N Engl J Med.* 1992;326:975–982.

20. Fiessinger JN, Lopez-Fernandez M, Gatterer E, et al. Once-daily subcutaneous dalteparin, a low molecular weight heparin, for the initial treatment of acute deep vein thrombosis. *Thromb Haemost.* 1996;76:195–199.

21. Prandoni P, Lensing AWA, Buller HR, et al. Comparison of subcutaneous low-molecular-weight heparin with intravenous standard heparin in proximal deep-vein thrombosis. *Lancet.* 1992;339:441–445.

22. George J. Heparin-associated thrombocytopenia. In: Hull R, Pineo GF, eds. *Disorders of Thrombosis*. Philadelphia: WB Saunders; 1996:359–373.

23. Warkentin TE, Levine MN, Hirsh J, et al. Heparin-induced thrombocytopenia in patients treated with low-molecular-weight heparin or unfractionated heparin. *N Engl J Med*. 1995;332:1330–1335.

24. Kelton JG, Smith JW, Warkentin TE, et al. Immunoglobulin G from patients with heparin-induced thrombocytopenia binds to a complex of heparin and platelet factor 4. *Blood*. 1994;83:3232–3239.

25. Warkentin TE, Chong BH, Greinacher A. Heparin-induced thrombocytopenia: towards concensus. *Thromb Haemost*. 1998;79:1–7.

26. Magnani HN. Heparin-induced thrombocytopenia (HIT): an overview of 230 patients treated with Orgaran (ORG 10172). *Thromb Haemost*. 1993;70:554–561.

27. Greinacher A, Alban S. Heparinoids as alternative for parenteral anticoagulation therapy in patients with heparin-induced thrombocytopenia. *Hamostaseologie*. 1996;16:41–49.

28. Warkentin TE, Elavathil LJ, Hayward CPM, et al. The pathogenesis of venous limb gangrene associated with heparin-induced thrombocytopenia. *Ann Intern Med*. 1997;127:804–812.

29. Monreal M, Lafoz E, Olive A, et al. Comparison of subcutaneous unfractionated heparin with a low molecular weight heparin (Fragmin) in patients with venous thromboembolism and contraindications to coumarin. *Thromb Haemost*. 1994;71:7–11.

30. Weitz JI. Low-molecular-weight heparins. *N Engl J Med*. 1997;337:688–698.

31. Lensing AWA, Prins MH, Davidson BL, Hirsh J. Treatment of deep venous thrombosis with low-molecular-weight heparins. *Arch Intern Med*. 1995;155:601–607.

32. de Valk HW, Banga JD, Wester JWJ, et al. Comparing subcutaneous danaparoid with intravenous unfractionated heparin for the treatment of venous thromboembolism. *Ann Intern Med*. 1995;123:1–9.

33. Levine M, Gent M, Hirsh J, et al. A comparison of low-molecular-weight heparin administered primarily at home with unfractionated heparin administered in the hospital for proximal deep-vein thrombosis. *N Engl J Med*. 1996;334:677–681.

34. Koopman MMW, Prandoni P, Piovella F, et al. Treatment of venous thrombosis with intravenous unfractionated heparin administered in the hospital as compared with subcutaneous low-molecular-weight heparin administered at home. *N Engl J Med*. 1996;334:682–687.

35. Columbus Investigators. Low-molecular-weight heparin in the treatment of patients with venous thromboembolism. *N Engl J Med*. 1997;337:657–662.

36. Schafer AI. Low-molecular-weight heparin—an opportunity for home treatment of venous thrombosis. *N Engl J Med*. 1996;334:724–725.

37. van den Belt AGM, Bossuyt PMM, Prins MH, et al. Replacing inpatient care by outpatient care in the treatment of deep venous thrombosis—an economic evaluation. *Thromb Haemost*. 1998;79:259–263.

38. Ancona-Berk VA, Chalmers TC. An analysis of the costs of ambulatory and inpatient care. *Am J Pub Health*. 1986;76:1102–1104.

35

Hematologic Factors in Recurrent Venous Thrombosis

Thomas W. Wakefield, MD and Alvin H. Schmaier, MD

INTRODUCTION

Venous thromboembolism continues to occur with a frequency of approximately 250,000 cases per year. Estimates suggest that despite adequate initial anticoagulation with heparin followed by 3 months of warfarin and the use of surgical support stockings, recurrent venous thromboembolism occurs in 17.5% over 2 years, 24.6% over 5 years, and 30.3% over 8 years.[1] This chapter focuses on the plasma proteins that increase the risk to develop recurrent venous thrombosis. The conditions that contribute to a hypercoagulable state and recurrent venous thrombosis are listed according to their severity (Table 35–1).

ANTITHROMBIN III DEFICIENCY

Antithrombin III deficiency accounts for approximately 1% to 2% of episodes of venous thromboses. The syndrome usually occurs by age 50. Antithrombin III, a serine protease inhibitor (SERPIN), is produced in the liver. It inhibits thrombin and factors Xa, IXa, VIIa, kallikrein, and XIa. In a quiescent state, it has a half-life of 2.8 days; however, in disseminated intravascular coagulation (DIC) or inflammatory states, its half-life is shortened. Heparin works as an anticoagulant by potentiating the anticoagulant effects of antithrombin III. Patients with antithrombin III deficiency present with an inability to be anticoagulated adequately with heparin or with recurrent thrombosis on heparin. If one suspects the diagnosis, it is confirmed by measuring antithrombin III levels of anticoagulants. Heparin administration itself lowers antithrombin III values not only while receiving the drug, but also for a week after discontinuing the agent. Both congenital states and acquired deficiencies have been described. In addition to DIC, the nephrotic syndrome has also been reported to result in a relative antithrombin III deficiency due to the loss of proteins less than 68 kDa into the urine, such as albumin and antithrombin III. In addition, any condition that impairs liver synthetic function can lead to an antithrombin III deficiency.[2] Patients homozygous for antithrombin III deficiency usually die *in utero,* whereas heterozygous patients usually have antithrom-

TABLE 35–1. SPECIFIC PROTEINS AND PROTHROMBOTIC STATES MOST LIKELY TO LEAD TO RECURRENT VENOUS THROMBOSIS, LISTED IN ORDER OF SEVERITY[a]

1. Antithrombin III deficiency (1% to 2%)
2. Protein C and S deficiency (3% to 5%)
3. Resistance to activated protein C (factor V Leiden) (20% to 40%)
4. Hyperhomocystinemia (10%)
5. Prothrombin 20210 polymorphism (4% to 6%)
6. Defective fibrinolysis (1% to 3%)
7. Heparin-induced thrombocytopenia (HIT) and HITTS
8. Lupus anticoagulant/antiphospholipid syndrome
9. Abnormal platelet aggregation

[a] Numbers in parenthesis represent the percentage of patients presenting with this condition.

bin III levels less than 70%. Treatment for a patient with antithrombin III deficiency and venous thrombotic events involves administration of antithrombin III concentrate or fresh-frozen plasma followed by heparin anticoagulation.

DEFICIENCY OF PROTEINS C AND S

Protein C and its cofactor, protein S, are made in the liver. Protein C is activated by thrombin after binding to its endothelial receptor, thrombomodulin. Activated protein C with free protein S inactivates the activated forms of factor VIII:C and factor V:C in the coagulation tenase and prothrombinase complexes, respectively. These activities decrease clot formation.[3] The protein C and S system is the major anticoagulant mechanism. In addition to its direct anticoagulant effects, protein C also affects the fibrinolytic system by inhibiting plasminogen activator inhibitor, thus increasing plasma fibrinolysis. Both protein C and protein S have relatively short half-lives and can be inhibited rapidly on the administration of oral anticoagulation. Protein C deficiency can present as both a homozygous and heterozygous form. When homozygous protein C deficiency presents, the patient dies in infancy if not recognized early from purpura fulminans, a condition that results in unrestricted clotting and secondary clot lysis. Acquired deficiency states also include any condition that impairs hepatic synthetic function, DIC, or any condition in which there are large losses of proteins into the urine, such as the nephrotic syndrome. The diagnosis of protein C or protein S deficiency states is made by measuring either a functional or an antigenic level of protein C or an antigenic level of protein S. Protein S as a protector from thrombosis is best measured as free protein S antigen; that is, protein S that is not bound to C4b binding protein. However, not all patients with low levels of these factors have thrombotic episodes and large populations of asymptomatic blood donors have been described in which low protein C levels were found. In addition, heterozygous family members of homozygous protein C–deficient infants have been reported to be unaffected.[4]

It is essential that all physicians know that patients with protein C and protein S deficiencies may become transiently hypercoagulable when beginning warfarin anticoagulation. Warfarin inhibits the vitamin K–dependent factors protein C, protein S, and factors II, VII, IX, and X. Because protein C and protein S have short half-lives of approximately 4 to 6 h, their levels are lowered faster on warfarin administration. Even though factor VII also has a short 6 to 7 h half-life, factors II, IX, and X have longer half-lives of between 2 and 5 days. Thus, a heterozygous patient who already has a lowered level of protein C and protein S will get a more extensive lowering of these proteins on the initiation of warfarin therapy and induce a "hypercoagulable" state before they are anticoagulated by the lowering of factors II, IX, and X. This situation leads to a prothrombotic state, thrombosis in the microcirculation, and the syndrome of warfarin-induced skin necrosis.[5] This syndrome results in thrombosis of the microcirculation and full-thickness skin loss, especially over fatty areas of the buttock and breast where the blood supply is already poor. In order to prevent this complication from occurring, oral anticoagulation should be begun only when the patient is fully anticoagulated with systemic standard heparin or low molecular weight heparin.

RESISTANCE TO ACTIVATED PROTEIN C (FACTOR V LEIDEN)

Resistance to activated protein C (factor V Leiden) represents perhaps one of the most important advances in the history of the identification of hypercoagulable states. Resistance to activated protein C has been reported to be present in between 20% and 40% of all cases of venous thrombosis. When thrombin binds to thrombomodulin, protein C is activated and, with its cofactor protein S, inhibits the coagulation system. Patients with resistance to activated protein C have a decrease in the anticoagulant function of activated protein C. The most common mutation associated with activated protein C resistance is the substitution of a single amino acid, glutamine for arginine, at position 506 in factor V.[6] This defect (factor V Leiden) accounts for 92% of patients with activated protein C resistance. Other mutations in factor V, such as a substitution for an arginine at position 306, have been reported to cause activated protein C resistance in two patients. Thrombotic manifestations have been found in both the arterial and venous systems with the venous system predominating. Patients may be either heterozygous or homozygous for this mutation. The thrombotic risk is worsened by the presence of other hypercoagulable states such as protein C and S deficiencies. In addition to the large number of cases of venous thrombosis associated with this defect, recurrent venous thrombosis is much more common in patients with this syndrome, and a relative risk increase of 2.4× over an 8-year follow-up has been reported.[7] The diagnosis of this hypercoagulable state is made by both a functional assay involving the activated partial thromboplastin time (aPTT) and also a genetic analysis for the abnormal factor V gene. In the functional assay, activated protein C is added to plasma along with calcium chloride. The presence of a normal factor V in conjunction with activated protein C and calcium results in a prolongation of the aPTT, whereas if factor V has the Leiden mutation, the aPTT is not prolonged appropriately by the addition of activated protein C.

Treatment for this disorder has not been as well defined as other hypercoagulable states, most likely because of its newly described nature. The relative risk for thrombosis in patients heterozygous for the factor V Leiden mutation is 7×, although for those patients homozygous for factor V Leiden the relative risk is 80×.[8] Treatment options include anticoagulation, initially with heparin followed by oral anticoagulation.

HYPERHOMOCYSTINEMIA

Hyperhomocystinemia, a risk factor for atherosclerosis and vascular disease, has been found to increase the risk for venous thrombosis in individuals younger than 40 years of age[9] and for recurrent venous thrombosis in patients between 20 and 70 years of age.[10] In addition, high plasma homocystine levels have been found to be a risk factor for deep venous thrombosis in the general population, with an especially strong association in older women.[11] As in many of the hypercoagulable states, the combination of homocystinuria with other hypercoagulable markers such as factor V Leiden has been suggested to result in an increased risk of thrombosis. The mechanism of thrombosis is not entirely clear. Suggested mechanisms range from an impairment in endothelium-dependent vasodilation from decreased bioavailability of nitric oxide, a decreased production of nitric oxide due to lipid peroxidation, a toxic effect on vascular endothelium and the clotting cascade, to abnormal methionine metabolism affecting the methylation of DNA and cell membranes. Elevated levels of homocysteine may also reduce the activation of protein C on thrombomodulin and increase thromboxane production. Furthermore, it has been shown to decrease tissue plasminogen binding and plasmin formation. The association between hyperhomocystinemia and venous thrombosis has been strongly established. Additional evidence suggests that treatment to specifically lower homocysteine levels such as vitamin B_6, vitamin B_{12}, or folic acid is salutory. Evidence suggest that moderate folate ingestion lowers plasma homocysteine levels. The importance of homocysteine to the venous thrombotic process, both idiopathic and recurrent, has been definitely established and homocysteine levels should be part of the routine hypercoagulable work-up.

PROTHROMBIN 20210 POLYMORPHISM

A new syndrome has been described in which the prothrombin gene has been found to have a polymorphism at position 20210 where a glutamine substitues for an arginine. This variation has been found to increase the risk for venous thrombosis by $5.4\times$.[12] In a total of 219 patients with confirmed venous thrombosis, 12 (5.5%) were heterozygous for this allele, whereas the incidence in a corresponding group of healthy controls was only 1.2%. There is synergistic interaction between this prothrombin gene variant and factor V Leiden.[13]

DEFECTIVE FIBRINOLYSIS

Another cause of a hypercoagulable state is defective fibrinolytic activity. An abnormal plasminogen (dysplasminogenemia), although quite rare (<1%), has been described in cases of spontaneous arterial and venous thrombosis.[14] Abnormal fibrinogens (dysfibrinogenemias) are other causes of venous thrombosis. Abnormal fibrinogens may account for 1% to 3% of patients with thrombosis. Most of these conditions are congenital. Defective fibrinolysis can occur with either a decreased content of plasminogen activators, decreased release of these activators, or an increase of their inhibitors. In the postoperative period, there is temporary fibrinolytic shut-down that results in an altered relationship between tissue plasminogen activator and its inhibitors. Impaired postoperative fibrinolysis may be contributory to the high risk of venous thrombosis seen in surgery patients.[15]

HEPARIN-INDUCED THROMBOCYTOPENIA AND HEPARIN-INDUCED THROMBOCYTOPENIA AND THROMBOSIS SYNDROME

Although strictly not a hypercoagulable state, heparin-induced thrombocytopenia (HIT) occurs in approximately 1% to 30% of patients in whom heparin is administered. Severe thrombocytopenia associated with thrombosis [heparin-induced thrombocytopenia and thrombosis syndrome (HITTS)] is seen much less frequently. In an analysis of 11 prospective studies, the incidence was reported to be 3%, with thrombosis in 0.9%.[16] This syndrome is caused by a heparin-dependent antibody (IgG) that causes platelet aggregation when exposed to heparin. The antibody is directed against the heparin/ platelet factor 4 (PF4) complex and activates platelets by binding to their FcγRIIA receptor. Although both arterial and venous thrombosis have been reported, this condition often manifests itself in a patient who develops further thrombosis while being treated for venous thrombosis with heparin or when there is a fall in platelet count below 100,000/μl (or a 50% or greater decline from the baseline preheparin platelet count).[17]

The pathophysiology for thrombosis has been summarized involving: (1) heparin combines with PF4; (2) at the platelet and endothelial cell surface, IgG forms to the heparin-PF4 complex; (3) the antibody then binds by the FcγRIIA platelet receptor; (4) platelet activation occurs, proaggregatory substances are released, and platelet aggregation occurs; (5) microparticles are released from activated platelets; (6) mediators such as cytokines enhance platelet aggregation; and (7) immunoglobulins and complement are deposited on the surface of endothelial cells and tissue factor is released.[18] Venous thrombosis is especially prominent due to the microparticle release from platelets, the production of tissue factor, and the accelerated rate of thrombin formation.

Both bovine and porcine standard unfractionated heparin (UFH) have been found to cause the syndrome and low molecular weight heparin (LMWH) can also produce it, although perhaps at a lower incidence. The diagnosis is made by either performing platelet aggregation or ^{14}C serotonin release assay on platelets with donor platelets and known concentrations of heparin added to patient plasma. In the latter assay, donor platelets are radiolabeled with ^{14}C-5-hydroxytryptamine. The serotonin assay has a sensitivity up to 94% and a specificity up to 100%.[19] A new enzyme linked immunosorbent assay (ELISA) test also is being developed to detect the antibody. Treatment consists of stopping heparin and protecting the patient from thrombosis associated with activated microparticles by using a second anticoagulant. Antiplatelet agents have met with only limited success. Iloprost, a prostacyclin analog, has been found useful but it is no longer recommended because it is so strongly vasodilatory and produces hypotension. New compounds that have been suggested include: Orgaran (danaparoid sodium), a synthetic heparin preparation made from porcine intestinal mucosa with a low number of sulfur groups, which has shown a 24% level of cross-reactivity with the heparin antibody[20]; a platelet IIb/IIIa receptor antagonist C7E3[21]; the defibrinating agent ancrod[22]; and agents with direct action against thrombin such as argatroban.[23] In our experience, Orgaran or argatroban are the preferred anticoagulants for HIT or HITTS. There is a suggestion that if one is able to test LMWH *in vitro* with the patient's serum and there is no cross-reactivity, LMWH may be substituted in this syndrome,[24] although cross-reactivity with enoxaparin and dalteparin is 92% in our laboratory. Coumadin should be given only after full anticoagulation has been achieved with one of these alternative agents.[25] Although the initial reported morbidity and mortality with this syndrome was quite high, with morbidities of more than 60% and mortalities of more than 20%, morbidity and mortality rates have declined to 6% and 0%, respectively, with early diagnosis and appropriate anticoagulant treatment.[26]

LUPUS ANTICOAGULANT/ANTIPHOSPHOLIPID SYNDROME

This entity is perhaps one of the most difficult abnormalities to relate to the venous thrombotic process. It is unfortunate that this syndrome has been called "anticoagulant" because it is associated with or results in a hypercoagulable state. Antiphospholipid antibodies, usually IgG, participate in the thrombotic process.[27] The antiphospholipid syndrome is associated with the presence of these antibodies and clinical manifestations include episodes of thrombosis, recurrent fetal loss, thrombocytopenia, livido reticularis, strokes, myocardial infarctions, visceral infarctions, and extremity gangrene. The diagnosis is suspected in a patient who has a prolonged aPTT with other standard coagulation tests showing no abnormality. This prolonged aPTT is a laboratory artifact. In the presence of an antiphospholipid antibody, the phospholipid is antagonized and the aPTT is prolonged because less is available to shorten the clotting time. The diagnosis is confirmed either with the prolongation of confirmatory tests such as the dilute Russell viper venom time or tissue thromboplastin inhibition time or with the detection of an antiphospholipid antibody by ELISA, the most common being an anticardiolipin antibody. There is imperfect agreement between diagnostic tests for this abnormality; approximately 80% of patients with a positive aPTT test (lupus anticoagulant) have a positive ELISA antiphospholipid antibody, but only 10% to 50% of patients with a positive ELISA antiphospholipid antibody have a positive lupus anticoagulant. It is suggested that if both tests are positive, the thrombotic risk is the same as if the tests are separately positive. It has also been suggested that the lupus anticoagulant test is a better predictor for thrombotic events, whereas the high-titer ELISA antiphospholipid antibody (especially an IgG anticardiolipin antibody) is more predictive of recurrent fetal loss.[28] Although the mechanisms responsible for fetal loss are unknown, it has been suggested that fetal loss occurs because of thrombosis of the microcirculation in the uterus, and new data demonstrates that levels of annexin V on trophoblasts and endothelial cells are reduced in the presence of antiphospholipid antibodies.[29]

Although the lupus anticoagulant was initially discovered in patients with systemic lupus erythematosus (SLE), it can exist in patients without this disorder. Possible mechanisms for thrombosis with these antibodies include inhibition of prostacyclin synthesis or release from endothelial cells, inhibition of protein C activation by thrombin/thrombomodulin, raised plasminogen activator inhibitor levels, direct platelet activation, and the coexistence of endothelial cell activation. In addition, tissue factor expression has been suggested to be increased on monocytes and free protein S levels have been noted to be lower in patients with antiphospholipid syndrome who have evidence of thrombosis. Although each of the mechanisms mentioned has its proponents in the literature, no dominant theme has emerged. Although thrombosis has been noted in the arterial and venous circulation, at least one-third of patients with a lupus anticoagulant have a history of one or more thrombotic events, with more than 70% in the venous circulation.[27] Treatment for this syndrome in the face of thrombotic events includes anticoagulation. For patients with the antiphospholipid syndrome, a higher level of oral anticoagulation has been suggested to be necessary with an INR greater than 3.0.[30] One of the most difficult aspects in the diagnosis of a hypercoagulable state associated with venous thrombosis is when the presence of an antiphospholipid antibody is the only abnormality noted and then only at an intermediate titer. In these situations, one is not certain that the antibody caused the thrombosis or is present because the thrombotic process releases phospholipids into the circulation and antibodies form to these phospholipids. In situations such as this when all other tests are negative, the usual recommendation is to treat the patient with oral anticoagulation for 3 to 6 months, stop the anticoagulation, and then retest to determine if the antibody persists. If the antibody does persist, then long-term oral anticoagulation becomes necessary.

ABNORMAL PLATELET AGGREGATION

Abnormal platelet aggregation has been associated with thrombosis in the face of malignancy, especially advanced malignancy of the lung and uterus. Moreover, high platelet counts as seen in essential thrombocythemia or other myeloproliferative disorders are associated with venous thrombosis. Although platelets do play a role in thrombosis, in general they are felt to play less of a role in venous thrombosis. In addition, platelet function is probably more dependent on external factors rather than internal factors of platelets themselves.

REFERENCES

1. Prandoni P, Lensing AW, Cogo A, et al. The long-term clinical course of acute deep venous thrombosis. *Ann Intern Med.* 1996;125:1–7.
2. Flinn WR, McDaniel MD, Yao JS, Fahey VA, et al. Antithrombin III deficiency as a reflection of dynamic protein metabolism in patients undergoing vascular reconstruction. *J Vasc Surg.* 1984;1:888–895.
3. Clouse LH, Comp PC. The regulation of hemostasis: the protein C system. *N Engl J Med.* 1986;314:1298–1304.
4. Esmon CT. The regulation of natural anticoagulant pathways. *Science.* 1987;235:1348–1352.
5. Cole MS, Minifee PK, Wolma FJ. Coumadin necrosis—a review of the literature. *Surgery.* 1988;103:271–277.
6. Kalafatis M, Mann KG. Factor V Leiden and thrombophilia. *Arterioscler Thromb Vasc Biol.* 1997;17:620–627.
7. Simioni P, Prandoni P, Lensing AW, et al. The risk of recurrent venous thromboembolism in patients with an Arg506 → Gln mutation in the gene for factor V (factor V Leiden). *N Engl J Med.* 1997;336:399–403.
8. Rosendaal FR, Koster T, Vandenbroucke JP, Reitsma PH. High risk of thrombosis in patients homozygous for factor V Leiden (activated protein C resistance). *Blood.* 1995;85:1504–1508.
9. Falcon CR, Cattaneo M, Panzeri D, Martinelli I, et al. High prevalence of hyperhomocyst(e)inemia in patients with juvenile venous thrombosis. *Arterioscler Thromb.* 1994;14:1080–1083.
10. den Heijer M, Blom HJ, Gerrits WB, et al. Is hyperhomocysteinaemia a risk factor for recurrent venous thrombosis? *Lancet.* 1995;345:882–885.
11. den Heijer M, Koster T, Blom HJ, et al. Hyperhomocysteinemia as a risk factor for deep-vein thrombosis. *N Engl J Med.* 1996;334:759–762.
12. Cumming AM, Keeney S, Salden A, Bhavnani M, et al. The prothrombin gene G20210A variant: prevalence in a U.K. anticoagulant clinic population. *Br J Haematol.* 1997;98:353–355.
13. Ferraresi P, Marchetti G, Legnani C, et al. The heterozygous 20210 G/A prothrombin genotype is associated with early venous thrombosis in inherited thrombophilias and is not increased in frequency in artery disease. *Arterioscler Thromb Vasc Biol.* 1997;17:2418–2422.
14. Towne JB, Bandyk DF, Hussey CV, Tollack VT. Abnormal plasminogen: a genetically determined cause of hypercoagulability. *J Vasc Surg.* 1984;1:896–902.
15. Prins MH, Hirsh J. A clinical review of the evidence supporting a relationship between impaired fibrinolytic activity and venous thromboembolism. *Arch Intern Med.* 1991;151:1721–1731.
16. Hirsh J, Raschke R, Warkentin TE, Dalen JE, et al. Heparin: mechanism of action, pharmacokinetic, dosing considerations, monitoring, efficacy, and safety. *Chest.* 1995;108:258S–275S.
17. George JN, Alving B, Ballem P. Platelets. In: McArthur JR, Benz EJ eds. *Hematology—1994: The Educational Program of the American Society of Hematology.* Washington, DC: The American Society of Hematology; 1994;66.
18. Cancio LC, Cohen DJ. Heparin-induced thrombocytopenia and thrombosis. *J Am Coll Surg.* 1998;186:76–91.

19. Sheridan D, Carter C, Kelton JG. A diagnostic test for heparin-induced thrombocypenia. *Blood.* 1986;67:27–30.

20. Magnani HN. Heparin-induced thrombocytopenia (HIT): an overview of 230 patients treated with orgaran (Org 10172). *Thromb Haemost.* 1993;70:554–561.

21. Liem TK, Teel R, Shukla S, Silver D. The glycoprotein IIb/IIIa antagonist c7E3 inhibits platelet aggregation in the presence of heparin-associated antibodies. *J Vasc Surg.* 1997;25:124–130.

22. Cole CW, Fournier LM, Bormanis J. Heparin-associated thrombocytopenia and thrombosis: optimal therapy with ancrod. *Can J Surg.* 1990;33:207–210.

23. Lewis BE, Iaffaldano R, McKiernan TL, Rao L, et al. Report of successful use of argatroban as an alternative anticoagulant during coronary stent implantation in a patient with heparin-induced thrombocytopenia and thrombosis syndrome. *Cathet Cardiovasc Diag.* 1996;38:206–209.

24. Slocum MM, Adams JG Jr, Teel R, Spadone DP, et al. Use of enoxaparin in patients with heparin-induced thrombocytopenia syndrome. *J Vasc Surg.* 1996;23:839–843.

25. Warkentin TE, Elavathil LJ, Hayward CP, Johnston MA, et al. The pathogenesis of venous limb gangrene associated with heparin-induced thrombocytopenia. *Ann Int Med.* 1997;127:804–812.

26. Almeida JI, Coats R, Liem TK, Silver D. Reduced morbidity and mortality rates of the heparin-induced thrombocytopenia syndrome. *J Vasc Surg.* 1998;27:309–316.

27. Greenfield LJ. Lupus-like anticoagulants and thrombosis (editorial). *J Vasc Surg.* 1988;7:818–819.

28. Lynch A, Marlar R, Murphy J, et al. Antiphospholipid antibodies in predicting adverse pregnancy outcome. A prospective study. *Ann Intern Med.* 1994;120:470–475.

29. Rand JH, Wu XX, Andree HA, et al. Pregnancy loss in the antiphospholipid–antibody syndrome—a possible thrombogenic mechanism. *N Engl J Med.* 1997;337:154–160.

30. Khamashta MA, Cuadrado MJ, Mujic F, Taub NA, et al. The management of thrombosis in the antiphospholipid–antibody syndrome. *N Engl J Med.* 1995;332:993–997.

36

The Fate of Calf Vein Thrombosis

Mark H. Meissner, MD

Based on perceived differences in the incidence of pulmonary embolism (PE) and the postthrombotic syndrome, acute deep venous thrombosis (DVT) is often defined as involving either the proximal veins or the calf veins.[1,2] Proximal venous thrombi involve segments from the popliteal vein to the inferior vena cava, whereas isolated calf vein thrombi may involve any of the paired tibial veins or the soleal–gastrocnemial veins. The incidence of complications following acute proximal venous thrombosis has been well defined. Without treatment, PE may complicate up to 50% of proximal thrombi,[3] whereas 29% to 79% of patients[4-6] may develop long-term manifestations of pain, edema, hyperpigmentation, or ulceration. Accordingly, the treatment of acute proximal venous thrombosis has been well defined by randomized clinical trials. Although the availability of low molecular weight heparins (LMWH) is likely to change treatment algorithms, the importance of early therapeutic anticoagulation with heparin followed by warfarin has been well established.[7,8] In contrast, the natural history of DVT confined to the tibial veins is substantially less well documented and appropriate treatment poorly defined.

DIAGNOSIS OF ISOLATED CALF VEIN THROMBOSIS

Controversies regarding the clinical relevance of calf vein thrombosis (CVT) may in part arise from differences in populations studied and diagnostic tests utilized. Many reports concerning the incidence and outcome of CVT have employed serial ^{125}I-labeled fibrinogen uptake studies in the evaluation of asymptomatic postoperative patients. Such studies are sensitive to small tibial thrombi that have been described as minimal CVT.[3] These asymptomatic thrombi are often smaller, more often confined to the tibial veins, and more frequently nonocclusive than symptomatic thrombi.[3,9] The natural history of these thrombi may differ from the larger, occlusive thrombi commonly present in symptomatic patients. Evidence suggests that such minimal calf vein thrombi have a strong tendency to undergo early lysis and are associated with a low incidence of complications.[2,10,11] Among 176 limbs with DVT detected using ^{125}I-labeled fibrinogen after general or hip surgery, Doouss[11] found that 84% had resolved by the time of hospital discharge, whereas propagation and symptomatic PE were noted in only 6% and 2% of patients, respectively. Kakkar et al.[2] similarly found that 35% of thrombi detected with fibrinogen leg scanning spontaneously resolved within 72 h. All resolved thrombi were less than 5 cm long, localized to the tibial or soleal veins, and unassociated with symptomatic PE. It is also often assumed that minimal calf thrombosis is associated with a low incidence of late postthrombotic manifestations. Follow-up of postoperative screening studies has demonstrated no difference in the prevalence of postthrombotic symptoms among extremities with above-knee thrombosis, below-knee thrombosis, or no thrombosis as detected by radiolabeled fibrinogen scanning.[12,13] Given the questionable clinical relevance of minimal CVT in asymptomatic patients, many clinicians adopted a policy of treating only those thrombi extending above the knee on ^{125}I-labeled fibrinogen studies.

The natural history of symptomatic CVT may differ from that of asymptomatic postoperative thrombosis. Duplex ultrasonography is currently the most widely used clinical diagnostic test, although it does have limitations relevant to the natural history of CVT. The accuracy of duplex scanning in detecting asymptomatic isolated CVT is particularly controversial, with limited data from the literature suggesting a sensitivity as low as 48%.[14] The natural history of thrombi overlooked by duplex screening is likely similar to that of the radiolabeled fibrinogen–detected minimal CVT. Although the accuracy of duplex ultrasonography for the detection of symptomatic CVT is substantially better, sensitivity in this region is dependent on the technical adequacy of the study. Inadequate visualization of the tibial veins most commonly results from marked edema, large calf size, multiple collateral veins, or anatomic inaccessibility.[15,16] Sensitivity and specificity for CVT have been reported to be as high as 95% and 100%, respectively, for technically adequate studies in comparison to 30% and 70%, respectively, for technically limited studies.[16] Using color-flow Doppler with slow flow capabilities, adequate visualization of all three paired tibial veins may be achieved in up to 94% of symptomatic extremities.[15]

In clinical series of largely symptomatic patients, approximately 12% to 33% of DVT detected by duplex ultrasonography are confined to the calf veins.[15,17] This compares with a 9% to 46% incidence of isolated CVT in venographic series.[4,18,19] Isolated CVT most often involves the peroneal veins followed by the posterior tibial veins; isolated anterior tibial thrombosis is distinctly unusual.[15,16,20,21] The data suggests that visualization of both the posterior tibial and peroneal veins is required to achieve acceptable sensitivity, although routine scanning of the anterior tibial veins may be unnecessary.

THE NATURAL HISTORY OF CALF VEIN THROMBOSIS

Although most proximal venous thrombi appear to originate in the calf veins, the natural history of isolated CVT does appear to differ from that of proximal DVT. In comparison to patients with proximal DVT, patients in whom thrombosis remains localized to the calf tend to have fewer thrombotic risk factors and a lower prevalence of concurrent malignancy.[17] The prevalence of thrombotic risk factors among patients with proximal and CVT is illustrated in Table 36–1. Following the acute event, thrombus fragmentation appears to proceed more efficiently in the smaller calf veins.[22] As might be expected, the tibial vein segments recanalize more rapidly than the proximal venous segments when followed with serial duplex ultrasonography.[23] Among limbs with isolated tibial vein thrombosis, 50% recanalization most often occurs within 1 month and complete recanalization within 1 year of the acute event[17] (Fig. 36–1). However, recurrent thrombotic events compete with recanalization and may occur in as many

TABLE 36–1. RISK FACTORS: PROXIMAL DEEP VENOUS THROMBOSIS VERSUS CALF VEIN THROMBOSIS

Risk Factor	Percent with Risk Factor		p
	Proximal DVT	Isolated Calf Vein Thrombosis	
Malignancy	35.3% (416)[a]	19.1% (47)	.03
Bedrest	35.2% (418)	23.4% (47)	.11
Recent surgery	32% (416)	36.2% (47)	.56
Previous venous disease	27.2% (452)	17% (47)	.13
Recent trauma	13.5% (378)	13.3% (45)	.98
Remote trauma	13.3% (375)	8.9% (45)	.40
Family history	9.1% (407)	6.4% (47)	.79
Congestive heart failure	4.1% (411)	2.1% (47)	1.0
Pregnancy	1.9% (417)	2.1% (47)	1.0
Oral contraceptives	1% (417)	0% (47)	1.0

[a] Numbers in parentheses represent the total number of patients assessed for individual risk factor.
From Meissner MH, Caps MT, Bergelin RO, et al. Early outcome after isolated calf vein thrombosis. *J Vasc Surg.* 1997;26:749–756, with permission.

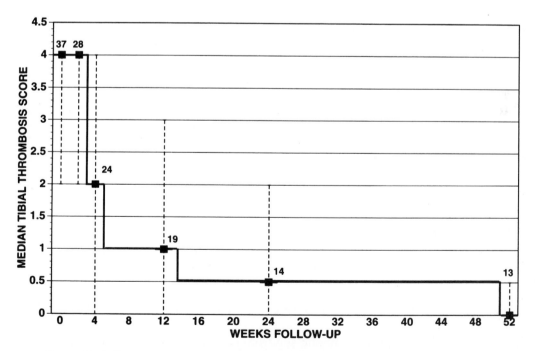

Figure 36–1. The rate of recanalization in isolated calf vein thrombosis as reflected by the median thrombosis score. For each calf vein, including the sural veins, the thrombus load was scored as 2 if completely occluded, 1 if partially occluded, and 0 if patent. Individual calf vein scores were then added to give a total thrombosis score for the limb. Error bars denote the interquartile range (25th to 75th percentile). Numbers represent the number of patients evaluated at each follow-up interval. (*From Meissner MH, Caps MT, Bergelin RO, et al. Early outcome after isolated calf vein thrombosis.* J Vasc Surg. *1997;26:749–756, with permission.*)

as 29% of inadequately treated isolated CVT.[24] This includes propagation to more proximal segments, both contiguous and noncontiguous, in 15% to 23% of limbs.[2,17,24,25] Although propagation to more proximal segments increases the risk of PE, both propagation and rethrombosis of previously involved segments increase the risk of valvular incompetence.[26]

CALF VEIN THROMBOSIS AND PULMONARY EMBOLISM

There is a remarkable paucity of methodologically sound data regarding the relationship between isolated CVT and PE.[27] Venographically controlled studies have suggested that, at the time of presentation, PE is associated with isolated CVT at least as frequently as thigh or pelvic thrombosis.[18] PE has been noted to accompany the presentation of 9% to 33% of patients with CVT.[17,19,20,28] The incidence of concurrent embolism varies from approximately 10% in series using clinical suspicion supplemented by objective tests[17,19,20] to 33% in series employing routine ventilation/perfusion lung scans.[28,29] Routine lung scanning has shown that 56% of calf vein–associated emboli are asymptomatic and that 55% involve less than 15% of total lung volume.[28] Although such emboli tend to be smaller than emboli associated with proximal DVT, not all are clinically insignificant. Despite raising the possibility that calf vein thrombi may embolize, these observations cannot exclude embolization of a more proximal thrombus prior to presentation. The absence of an identifiable lower extremity thrombus in up to 28% of patients with clinically suspected PE suggests that the presenting venogram does not always reflect the distribution of thrombus prior to embolization.[18]

Demonstration of a clear relationship between isolated CVT and PE would require that an initially negative ventilation/perfusion lung scan or pulmonary angiogram become positive in association with serial lower extremity studies showing no evidence of propagation. Although not strictly meeting these criteria, some case reports suggest that this does occasionally occur. Among 79 patients presenting with leg symptoms due to isolated CVT, Passman et al.[20] reported the subsequent development of objectively documented symptomatic PE without proximal propagation on duplex examination in five (6.3%) patients. However, the limited data available from studies with reasonably strong methodology suggests that most symptomatic pulmonary emboli in this setting occur in association with proximal thrombus propagation.[27] Based on a 20% risk of proximal propagation, a 20% to 50% risk of recurrent thromboembolism, and 10% risk of fatal PE for untreated proximal thrombi, the theoretical risk of fatal PE and symptomatic recurrent thromboembolism associated with isolated CVT is 2% and 5% to 10%, respectively.[30] This figure is remarkably similar to the 10% incidence of PE occurring in association with CVT reported by Menzoin et al.[19]

CALF VEIN THROMBOSIS AND THE POSTTHROMBOTIC SYNDROME

Manifestations of the postthrombotic syndrome are secondary to ambulatory venous hypertension, which in turn results from the combined effects of valvular incompetence and residual venous obstruction.[31] The severity of postthrombotic manifestations within an extremity is determined by the extent of reflux and the presence of persistent popliteal obstruction.[32] Determinants of valvular incompetence in individual venous segments include the time required for recanalization[23] and the development of recurrent thrombosis.[26] Although posterior tibial vein incompetence may be particularly important in the development of postthrombotic skin changes,[33,34] these considerations suggest that the incidence and severity of long-term sequelae might be less after CVT than proximal DVT. Not only do isolated calf vein thrombi recanalize faster, they are also associated with fewer risk factors favoring recurrent thrombosis and there is no associated proximal obstruction. Although reflux does appear to develop less frequently in the posterior tibial veins than in the proximal venous segments,[23] there is little long-term data validating such theoretical considerations.

Early follow-up reports suggest that outcome after isolated CVT may be better than after proximal DVT, but that a significant number of patients have mild postthrombotic sequelae. One year after presentation, persistent symptoms have been noted in 54% of limbs with proximal involvement as compared to 23% of limbs with isolated CVT.[17] In contrast, only 9% of uninvolved contralateral extremities were symptomatic after this interval (Fig. 36–2). Manifestations at 1 year were limited to pain and swelling in limbs with isolated CVT, although 3% of extremities with proximal thrombosis developed hyperpigmentation. Other series with longer follow-up suggest a similar prevalence of mild postthrombotic manifestations. Approximately 3.5 years after presentation, McLafferty et al.[21] noted mild to moderate (able to work with compression stockings) symptoms in 38% of patients, whereas Browse and Clemenson[35] reported persistent pain and swelling are in 50% and 75%, respectively, of initially symptomatic patients. In contrast, Prandoni et al.[4] reported mild and severe postthrombotic sequelae

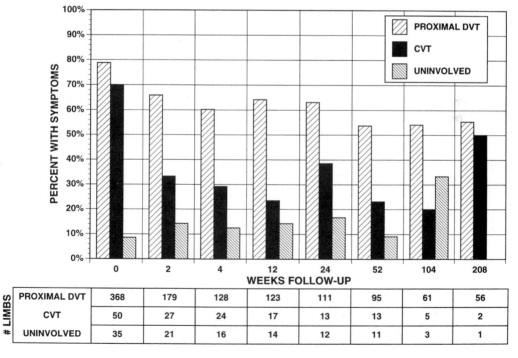

# LIMBS	0	2	4	12	24	52	104	208
PROXIMAL DVT	368	179	128	123	111	95	61	56
CVT	50	27	24	17	13	13	5	2
UNINVOLVED	35	21	16	14	12	11	3	1

Figure 36–2. Prevalence of lower extremity manifestations (edema, pain, hyperpigmentation, or ulceration) during follow-up among extremities with proximal DVT, isolated calf vein thrombosis (CVT), and uninvolved limbs contralateral to an isolated CVT. Differences among the three groups are statistically significant at 12 months (p = .004). The table shows total number of extremities within each group evaluated at each follow-up interval. (*From Meissner MH, Caps MT, Bergelin RO, et al. Early outcome after isolated calf vein thrombosis. J Vasc Surg. 1997;26:749–756, with permission.*)

in 21% and 5%, respectively, of patients after a mean of 45 months, an incidence identical to patients with proximal vein thrombosis. Notably, all patients in this trial were instructed to wear compression stockings and the incidence of postthrombotic syndrome associated with proximal vein thrombosis was quite low. The frequency of late manifestations is greater in the few series with long term follow-up. After 5 to 10 years, Lindner et al.[6] found postthrombotic symptoms in 47% of patients with isolated calf vein thrombosis in comparison to 100% of patients with proximal venous thrombosis.

This limited data suggests that, although postthrombotic manifestations are less frequent after isolated CVT, at least one-quarter of patients have persistent symptoms. Such symptoms are generally limited to pain and swelling over the first 4 years of follow-up, although there are some reports of skin changes and ulceration in association with CVT. Notably, the frequency of venous hemodynamic abnormalities after isolated CVT is strikingly similar to the prevalence of clinical symptoms. At 1 year, valvular incompetence was detected by duplex ultrasonography in 24% of initially involved tibial veins, but no uninvolved contralateral tibial veins[17] (Fig. 36–3). Abnormal photoplethysmographic venous recovery times have similarly been reported in 23% of involved extremities.[21] The prevalence of these hemodynamic abnormalities suggests that more severe clinical manifestations might be seen with a longer duration of follow-up.

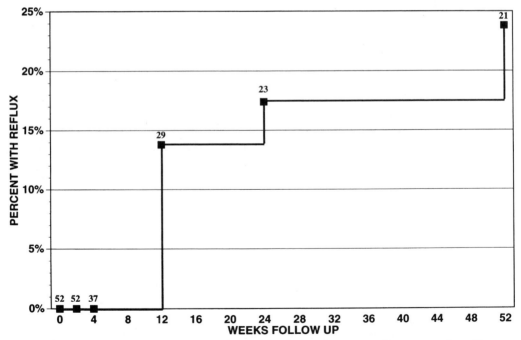

Figure 36–3. Prevalence of reflux as detected by duplex ultrasonography among veins with isolated CVT. Numbers represent the number of initially involved calf vein segments (posterior tibial, peroneal, sural) evaluated at each follow-up interval. (*From Meissner MH, Caps MT, Bergelin RO, et al. Early outcome after isolated calf vein thrombosis. J Vasc Surg. 1997;26:749–756, with permission.*)

MANAGEMENT OF SYMPTOMATIC CALF VEIN THROMBOSIS

Options for the management of symptomatic CVT include no intervention; standard anticoagulation with heparin followed by warfarin; and serial noninvasive follow-up with treatment in the event of proximal extension.[3,36] Therapeutic anticoagulation with heparin followed by warfarin is expensive, inconvenient, and associated with some risk of hemorrhage and heparin-induced thrombocytopenia. However, even accepting the relative lack of data regarding symptomatic thrombosis that remains confined to the calf, proximal propagation and the associated risk of PE and the postthrombotic syndrome complicates approximately 20% of such thromboses. These risks alone should preclude withholding anticoagulation without serial noninvasive follow-up studies. Furthermore, a significant proportion of patients presenting with isolated CVT either have a firm indication for anticoagulation at presentation or develop an indication during follow-up. Among 35 patients followed after an episode of isolated calf vein thrombosis, 54% warranted anticoagulation because of a previous DVT, proximal propagation, or PE at some time during their course.[17] Based largely on the risk of proximal propagation, many have concluded that the benefits of treatment exceed the risk and inconvenience of anticoagulation in most patients.[3,30,36] Such an approach clearly minimizes the risks associated with symptomatic CVT. In one small randomized study, a 3-month course of warfarin after initial heparin treatment reduced the rates of recurrent thrombosis and PE from 29% and 4%, respectively, to 0 at 90 days.[24] Furthermore, the availability of LMWH for the outpatient treatment of DVT may significantly lessen the cost and inconvenience of treatment. It is, however, important to tailor treatment to the individual patient, and serial noninvasive studies may be a reasonable alternative in some patients. The latter may an option in patients with contraindications to anticoagulation who can be followed reliably, particularly ambulatory patients with resolved and reversible risk factors. Current recommendations include follow-up testing at 2- to 3-day intervals for 10 to 14 days after presentation.[30] If serial examinations are also not possible because of anatomic inaccessibility or inability of the patient to return for follow-up, anticoagulation is probably warranted. Serial follow-up without anticoagulation is probably also inappropriate for patients at significant risk for propagation or recurrent thrombosis. Such patients would include those with a previous history of DVT, in whom recurrence rates of 50% have been documented,[24] as well patients with malignancy or multiple thrombotic risk factors in whom the risk of proximal thrombosis is higher.[17]

CONCLUSIONS

The natural history of DVT confined to the calf veins does appear to be different from that of proximal venous thrombosis and may vary according to whether the patient is symptomatic or asymptomatic and identified by postoperative surveillance. Calf vein thrombi recanalize more rapidly and completely than proximal venous thrombi and appear to be associated with a lower incidence of PE and the postthrombotic syndrome. However, this does not imply that isolated calf vein thrombi are entirely benign. There is at least suggestive evidence that calf vein thrombi may embolize, although such emboli appear smaller and more often asymptomatic. Perhaps more importantly, approximately 20% of such thrombi propagate to a more proximal level with an associated increase in the risk of symptomatic PE. Approximately one-quarter of patients have persistent symptoms of pain and edema during the early years of follow-up, although the frequency and severity of early postthrombotic manifestations appear to less than after proximal venous thrombosis. However, the prevalence of venous hemodynamic abnormalities suggests the possibility of more severe manifestations with longer follow-up. Treatment options for symptomatic isolated CVT include standard anticoagulation and serial noninvasive studies to exclude propagation. Although treatment should be individualized to the patient's underlying thrombotic risk factors and risk of anticoagulation, the relative risks and benefits favor anticoagulation in most patients.

REFERENCES

1. Moser KM, LeMoine JR. Is embolic risk conditioned by the location of deep venous thrombosis? *Ann Int Med.* 1981;94:439–444.
2. Kakkar VV, Flanc C, Howe CT, Clarke MB. Natural history of post-operative deep-vein thrombosis. *Lancet.* 1969;2:230–232.
3. Hirsh J, Lensing AWA. Natural history of minimal calf vein deep venous thrombosis. In: Bernstien EF, ed. *Vascular Diagnosis*, 4th ed. St. Louis: Mosby; 1993:779–781.
4. Prandoni P, Villalta S, Polistena P, Bernardi E, et al. Symptomatic deep-vein thrombosis and the post-thrombotic syndrome. *Haematologica.* 1995;80(Suppl 2):42–48.
5. Strandness DE, Langlois Y, Cramer M, Randlett A, et al. Long-term sequelae of acute venous thrombosis. *JAMA.* 1983;250:1289–1292.
6. Lindner DJ, Edwards JM, Phinney ES, Taylor LM, et al. Long-term hemodynamic and clinical sequelae of lower extremity deep vein thrombosis. *J Vasc Surg.* 1986;4:436–442.
7. Hull RD, Raskob GE, Hirsh J, et al. Continuous intravenous heparin compared with intermittent subcutaneous heparin in the initial treatment of proximal-vein thrombosis. *N Engl J Med.* 1986;315:1109–1114.
8. Raschke RA, Reilly BM, Guidry JR, Fontana JR, et al. The weight-based heparin dosing nomogram compared with a "standard care" nomogram. *Ann Intern Med.* 1993;119:874–881.
9. Mattos MA, Londrey GL, Leutz DW, et al. Color-flow duplex scanning for the surveillance and diagnosis of acute deep venous thrombosis. *J Vasc Surg.* 1992;15:366–376.
10. Solis MM, Ranval TJ, Nix ML, et al. Is anticoagulation indicated for asymptomatic postoperative calf vein thrombosis? *J Vasc Surg.* 1992;16:414–419.
11. Doouss TW. The clinical significance of venous thrombosis of the calf. *Br J Surg.* 1976;63:377–378.
12. Francis CW, Ricotta JJ, Evarts CM, Marder VJ. Long-term clinical observations and venous functional abnormalities after asymptomatic venous thrombosis following total hip or knee arthroplasty. *Clin Orthop.* 1988;232:271–278.
13. Lindhagen A, Bergqvist D, Hallbook T. Deep venous insufficiency after postoperative thrombosis diagnosed with ^{125}I-labelled fibrinogen uptake test. *Br J Surg.* 1984;71:511–515.
14. Wells PS, Lensing AWA, Davidson BL, Prins MH, et al. Accuracy of ultrasound for the diagnosis of deep venous thrombosis in asymptomatic patients after orthopedic surgery: a meta-analysis. *Ann Intern Med.* 1995;122:47–53.
15. Mattos MA, Melendres G, Sumner DS, et al. Prevalence and distribution of calf vein thrombosis in patients with symptomatic deep venous thrombosis: a color-flow duplex study. *J Vasc Surg.* 1996;24:738–744.
16. Rose SA, Zwiebel WJ, Nelson BD, et al. Symptomatic lower extremity deep venous thrombosis: accuracy, limitations, and role of color duplex flow imaging in diagnosis. *Radiology.* 1990;175:639–644.
17. Meissner MH, Caps MT, Bergelin RO, Manzo RA, et al. Early outcome after isolated calf vein thrombosis. *J Vasc Surg.* 1997;26:749–756.
18. Browse NL, Lea Thomas M. Source of non-lethal pulmonary emboli. *Lancet.* 1974;1:258–259.
19. Menzoin JO, Sequeira JC, Doyle JE, et al. Therapeutic and clincial course of deep venous thrombosis. *Am J Surg.* 1983;146:581–585.

20. Passman MA, Moneta GL, Taylor LT, et al. Pulmonary embolism is associated with the combination of isolated calf vein thrombosis and respiratory symptoms. *J Vasc Surgery.* 1997;25:39–45.
21. McLafferty RB, Moneta GL, Passman MA, Brant BM, et al. Late clinical and hemodynamic sequelae of isolated calf vein thrombosis. *J Vasc Surg.* 1998;27:50–57.
22. Sevitt S. The mechanisms of canalisation in deep vein thrombosis. *J Path.* 1973;110:153–165.
23. Meissner MH, Manzo RA, Bergelin RO, Markel A, et al. Deep venous insufficiency: the relationship between lysis and subsequent reflux. *J Vasc Surg.* 1993;18:596–608.
24. Langerstedt CI, Olsson C, Fagher BO, Oqvist BW, et al. Need for long-term anticoagulant treatment in symptomatic calf vein thrombosis. *Lancet.* 1985;2:515–518.
25. Lohr JM, Kerr TM, Lutter KS, Cranley RD, et al. Lower extremity calf thrombosis: to treat or not to treat? *J Vasc Surg.* 1991;14:618.
26. Meissner MH, Caps MT, Bergelin RO, Manzo RA, et al. Propagation, rethrombosis, and new thrombus formation after acute deep venous thrombosis. *J Vasc Surg.* 1995;22:558–567.
27. Philbrick JT, Becker DM. Calf deep venous thrombosis. A wolf in sheep's clothing? *Arch Intern Med.* 1988;148:2131–2138.
28. Moreno-Cabral R, Kistner RL, Nordyke RA. Importance of calf vein thrombophlebitis. *Surgery.* 1976;80:735–742.
29. Kistner RL, Ball JJ, Nordyke RA, Freeman GC. Incidence of pulmonary embolism in the course of thrombophlebitis of the lower extremities. *Am J Surg.* 1972;124:169–176.
30. Raskob GE. Calf-vein thrombosis. In: Hull R, Raskob G, Pineo G, ed. *Venous Thromboembolism: An Evidence-Based Atlas.* Armonk, NY: Futura Publishing Co.; 1996:307–313.
31. Johnson BF, Manzo RA, Bergelin RO, Strandness DE. Relationship between changes in the deep venous system and the development of the postthrombotic syndrome after an acute episode of lower limb deep vein thrombosis: a one- to six-year follow-up. *J Vasc Surg.* 1995;21:307–313.
32. Meissner MH, Caps MT, Zierler BK, et al. Determinants of chronic venous disease after deep venous thrombosis. *J Vasc Surg.* 1998. (in press).
33. Gooley NA, Sumner DS. Relationship of venous reflux to the site of venous valvular incompetence: implications for venous reconstructive surgery. *J Vasc Surg.* 1988;7:50–59.
34. van Bemmelen PS, Bedford G, Beach K, Strandness DE. Status of the valves in the superficial and deep venous system in chronic venous disease. *Surgery.* 1990;109:730–734.
35. Browse NL, Clemenson G. Sequelae of an ^{125}I-fibrinogen detected thrombus. *Br Med J.* 1974;2:468–470.
36. Hyers TM, Hull RD, Weg JG. Antithrombotic therapy for venous thromboembolic disease. *Chest.* 1995;108(Suppl):335S–351S.

37

Primary Varicose Veins and Their Treatment

John H. Scurr, BSc, MBBS, FRCS

INTRODUCTION

Primary varicose veins represent one of the most common medical conditions, with up to 30% of the adult population complaining of symptoms. The true number of patients presenting for treatment could exceed this, given that many patients present with cosmetic problems only. Despite the frequency of this condition, there is no consensus on the best way to manage these patients. Management varies from country to country and often within a country, with different specialities getting involved in their management.[1] Varicose veins are treated by dermatologists, physicians, and surgeons. The results of treatment including the initial outcome, the long-term recurrence and subsequent complications also varies. Some doctors advocate one form of treatment with little regard for alternative approaches. Treatment is often dictated by physician's preference, rather than any logical or scientific basis.[2] Studies on treatment of varicose veins are often uncontrolled and take little account of the long-term recurrence.[3] A more scientific approach to the investigation and management of these patients will lead to improved functional and cosmetic results.

PRESENTATION OF PRIMARY VARICOSE VEINS

Varicose veins are tortuous dilated surface veins that may be visible and may be associated with a variety of symptoms. The size of the veins range from under a millimeter (dermal flares) to large dilated truncal varicosities measuring up to 1.5 cm in size. Symptoms include aching, swelling, pain, restlessness, cramps, and tenderness. Veins may be associated with areas of superficial thrombophlebitis (localized or generalized leg swelling). Primary varicose veins are rarely associated with any deep vein problems or any other underlying medical conditions.

Varicose veins are extremely common and, although a family history is commonly elicited, the frequency of this condition means that a family history can almost always be expected.

Studies looking at the constitution of the vein wall, an underlying abnormality of collagen, or a genetic disorder have failed to identify a specific reason why patients develop varicosities. Although varicose veins get worse during pregnancy, a combination of the effects of pressure and hormones, they often improve following the delivery. Occupational factors, standing, or prolonged sitting may affect the presentation.

History and Examination

When a patient presents with varicose veins it is important to obtain a proper history. Patient satisfaction following treatment is the most important outcome measurement. Although many patients in the United Kingdom present with symptoms, it is the underlying appearance of the veins that in fact causes patients greater distress. It is a commonly held view that only patients with symptoms can receive treatment on the National Health Service.

When obtaining a history, it is important to enquire about previous treatment for varicose veins, the presence or absence of venous thromboses, and a family history of varicose veins or of thrombotic tendencies.

When examining a patient with varicose veins it is important to examine them standing with their legs fully exposed, having removed their socks and shoes. The appearance of the leg and the distribution of the veins on the leg should be noted. If a patient has been sitting for any period of time, and in particular if they have been sitting with their legs up, it can take 20 to 40 sec before the veins will refill. If the socks are not removed, areas of skin change around the ankles may be missed. The distribution of the veins within the long saphenous system and the short saphenous system are noted. The presence or absence of scars that may indicate previous surgery are also noted. Gentle palpation along the vein reveals the presence of the varicosities, in particular a saphenofemoral varix or saphenopopliteal varix. Very prominent varicose veins may be associated with a venous hum and perhaps an underlying arteriovenous fistula. These veins would not be considered primary varicosities. By applying a tourniquet to the leg after first elevating the leg and then having the patient stand up again, the site from which the veins fill can be identified. By moving the tourniquet from the midthigh to above the knee and then to below the knee, repeating the exercise of lying the patient down, applying the tourniquet, and having the patient stand up, perforating veins can be identified and a clinical estimation of whether the patient has junctional incompetence made.

These tests, the Trendelenburg test, are widely taught and students are still examined on them. However, the tests have largely been replaced in clinical practice by noninvasive venous assessments.

NONINVASIVE VENOUS ASSESSMENT

A simple hand-held Doppler, the minimum investigation required by all patients with varicose veins, demonstrates forward and reverse flows. A Doppler applied over the groin when the leg is compressed first demonstrates forward flow, followed by reverse flow if there is reflux within the veins. A Doppler probe can be placed in the groin over the long saphenous vein and over the saphenopopliteal junction. Although reflux can be detected, the Doppler probe gives no indication as to which vein is being examined.

Failure to use a noninvasive test results in a large number of patients with saphenopopliteal junction incompetence going unrecognized.

Photoplethysmology provides a useful screening test differentiating patients with superficial venous insufficiency from patients with deep vein problems. The application of the probe in combination with a tourniquet demonstrates refilling times that correct when the tourniquet is placed below the perforating vein.

Duplex ultrasound imaging, a combination of B-mode ultrasound with a Doppler probe, provides the most effective and reliable method of venous assessment. If all patients with a primary diagnosis of varicose veins are assessed using duplex ultrasound imaging, a significant number will be noted to have abnormalities in both the long and short saphenous systems and a number of patients will be detected who have had previous problems with their deep veins.

Prior to the introduction of routine duplex ultrasound imaging of patients with primary varicose veins, the incidence of patients undergoing saphenopopliteal junction ligation less than 10%. Following the introduction of duplex ultrasound imaging for patients with primary varicose veins, up to 30% have abnormalities in their saphenopopliteal junction or reflux in the short saphenous system. In the past, a number of these patients would have re-presented with recurrent varicosities. Imaging of both the long and short saphenous systems is carried out and the presence or absence of reflux at the saphenopopliteal or saphenofemoral junction recorded. Blood refluxing from the long saphenous system via the Giacomini vein into the short saphenous system should also be noted. The presence of significant perforators both above and below the knee are identified and located by reference to either the medial malleolus or the knee itself. A systematic examination of the deep veins including the iliac, femoral, popliteal and calf veins should also be carried out. The presence of previous thrombosis, partial occlusion of the veins, scarring, and deep venous insufficiency should be recorded.

Following a noninvasive venous assessment patients can be divided into patients with superficial venous insufficiency alone or patients with junctional incompetence and reflux in the short saphenous system, the long saphenous system, or both. A subgroup of patients can be divided with reflux in either the long or short saphenous veins. The last group of patients consists of patients who have dilated superficial veins without junctional or truncal incompetence. On the basis of a full noninvasive venous assessment, treatment of primary varicose veins can be undertaken.

TREATMENT

Background

Varicose veins have been treated by a combination of surgery, sclerotherapy, and, more recently, laser and high intensity light treatment. Surgical treatment involves ligation of junctions with or without removal of truncal varicosities. Sclerotherapy involves injection of an irritant material into a vein, producing at best endothelial disobliteration and at worst thrombosis. Laser treatment is really reserved for the smaller vessels and relies on thermal destruction. High intensity light treatment (photoderm) produces a similar effect, but with minimal scarring. In the past, the treatment a patient received was often determined by the abilities of the first doctor the patient visited. More recently, the use of noninvasive venous testing a more rational approach to the treatment of varicose veins has been established. The principle of treating varicose veins is to remove or destroy the superficial veins. The more complete the removal and destruction, the smaller the chance of recurrence, the better the resolution of symptoms, and the better the cosmetic appearance.

Surgical Treatment of Varicose Veins

Patients with junctional incompetence or long segments of superficial vein reflux respond well to surgical treatment. Surgery involves a careful dissection of the saphenofemoral junction, taking care to identify all branches arising from the common and superficial femoral vein in the vicinity of the saphenofemoral junction. Once all the branches have been identified, they are divided.[1] A debate as to whether to remove or to leave the long saphenous vein has in part been answered by Sarin et al.,[5] who showed a much higher recurrence rate if the long saphenous vein is left *in situ*.[4]

PIN stripping (Oesch)   (Perforate - INvaginate)

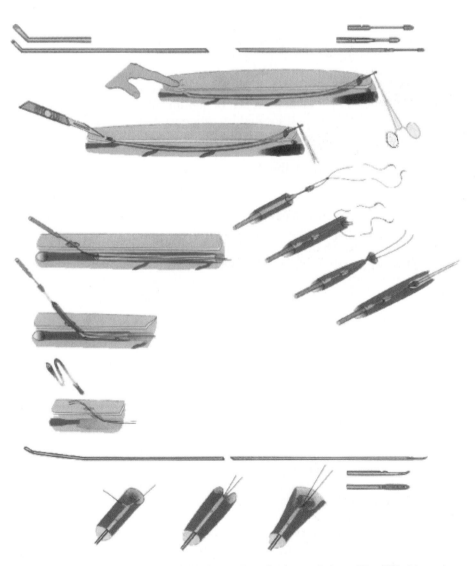

Figure 37–1. Varicose vein stripping using an invagination technique. The PIN stripper is a rigid device that can be steered through the venous system and which can easily be felt below the skin. The vein is then avulsed from proximal to distal.

Removal of the long saphenous vein to the ankle is associated with a very high incidence of saphenous nerve injury. Removing the long saphenous vein to the upper or midcalf avoids this complication. Various stripping techniques have been described, some using a flexible stripper and others using a rigid (PIN) stripper[6] (Fig. 37–1). The PIN stripper offers the advantage that the end can be steered along the vein, carefully negotiating any residual valves. The end can be felt beneath the skin and retrieved by making a small (1.5 mm) incision. The top end of the vein is then tied on to the PIN stripper and the PIN stripper is removed, inverting the vein and delivering the vein through the small incision just below the knee.[7]

The saphenopopliteal junction can be identified using duplex ultrasound imaging. Although 80% of short saphenous veins enter the popliteal fossa within 4 cm of the popliteal skin crease, the actual size of entry remains variable. The saphenopopliteal

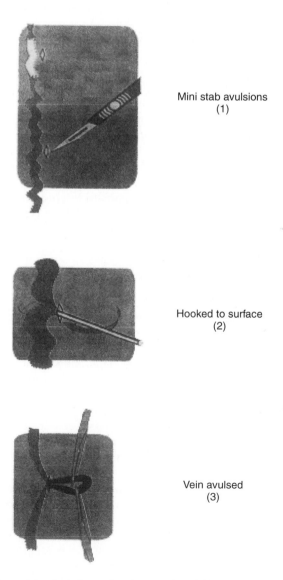

Mini stab avulsions
(1)

Hooked to surface
(2)

Vein avulsed
(3)

Figure 37–2. Stab avulsion technique of varicose veins. (1) Demonstrates minimal incision using a 15 blade scalpel. (2) Modified crochet hook to snare varix. (3) Avulsion of varix.

junction can be identified easily prior to surgery using duplex ultrasound imaging. Some surgeons still rely on on-table venography to identify the junctions.[8]

The importance of identifying the junction cannot be overemphasized and is associated with a much lower incidence of popliteal nerve damage. The saphenopopliteal junction is deep to the fascia and, having made an incision behind the knee, the incision is deepened to beneath the fascia. The short saphenous vein can be identified and then traced until its origin with the popliteal vein. The presence of a Giacomini vein ascending in the posterior thigh is often noted.

Having identified the saphenopopliteal junction, it can be clipped and divided. The Giacomini vein can usually be avulsed with gentle traction. The short saphenous vein can safely be removed to the midcalf. Removal of the short saphenous vein to the ankle is again associated with a significant incidence of sural nerve injury, often resulting in numbness, followed by pain and tingling over the lateral aspect of the foot. If the vein is only stripped to the midcalf, this complication is almost completely avoided. The PIN stripper is ideally suited to remove the upper portion of the short saphenous vein. If the vein is removed by an invagination technique the risk of damage to the sural nerve is decreased still further (Fig. 37–1).

Having removed truncal varicosities and controlled junctional leaks, residual veins can be removed through multiple ministab avulsions. Using Oesch hooks and 1.5 mm incisions, the residual veins can be removed (Fig. 37–2). If the incisions are placed carefully there is no need to suture them, and they heal without leaving any scars. The best results are achieved by careful preoperative marking to make sure that all the varicosities are identified so that they can be removed.

Following surgery, compression is applied to the limbs. Bandages or elastic compression stockings are then worn for up to 10 days. These operations are always associated with considerable bruising. The pain following surgery is often minimal, but increases on the third or fourth day due to a phlebitic type of reaction. This pain responds to nonsteroidal anti-inflammatory drugs.

Complications of Surgery

Neurological Complications

Damage to major nerves should not occur following varicose vein surgery. Using careful techniques, the femoral and popliteal nerves should be preserved.

Damage to the lateral popliteal nerve resulting in foot drop is reported following varicose vein surgery. The incidence of this complication should be less than 1 in 1000 cases and probably less than 1 in 5000 cases. This is an avoidable complication, and usually represents an error in surgical technique. Areas of numbness following ministab avulsions, however, are quite common. Each area of numbness can extend from a centimeter squared to several centimeters squared. The numbness almost certainly results from direct damage to cutaneous nerves as a result of the ministab avulsions. When carrying out ministab avulsions, if the tissue being avulsed is not elastic, then it may well be nervous. This should be left and a further incision made in an attempt to extract the vein at a different site.

Large areas of numbness usually represent damage to the sural nerve. Sometimes the damage is a direct result of the actual stripping technique or ministab avulsions, but sometimes the numbness occurs as a result of bruising within the tissues. Where the numbness is related to the bruising in subcutaneous tissues, the prognosis is good. The numbness eventually settles leaving an area of hypersensitivity that also will settle.

Damage to Main Veins and Arteries

Damage to main vessels following varicose vein surgery almost always represents poor surgical technique. Either the surgeon has failed to identify the anatomy properly or, during the course of the procedure, has damaged a vessel through surgical carelessness.

Each year, cases of femoral artery and femoral vein damage are reported. Damage to the femoral artery may go unnoticed. Having damaged or ligated the femoral artery, the operative field may improve such that the surgeon is totally unaware of any damage. However if the femoral vein is ligated, the surgeon is usually aware of the problem because the ministab avulsions turn into small fountains. Immediate vascular reconstruction produces the best result. Where there is a delay in making the diagnosis, particularly in the case of the femoral artery, compromise to the circulation may be permanent. Damage to the popliteal artery and popliteal vein may also occur. These are avoidable complications given a good surgical technique.

If a surgeon does encounter bleeding from the popliteal vein, gentle pressure usually causes the bleeding to stop. Attempts at trying to control the bleeding by inserting sutures or by trying to ligate the popliteal vein are associated with increased bleeding. Direct surgical intervention is rarely necessary, unless there has been very extensive trauma.

SCLEROTHERAPY

Sclerotherapy involves the injection of an irritant solution designed to destroy the intimal lining of the vein. The primary indication for sclerotherapy is varicose veins not associated with junctional or truncal reflux.[2] It can be used as an adjuvant treatment following surgery to treat any residual varicosities. Sclerotherapy is injection treatment of large veins and microsclerotherapy is injection treatment of the dermal flares, telangectasia, and spider veins. Both are very effective.

Although three schools of sclerotherapy have been described, Fegan[9] (the Irish school), Sigg[10] (the Swiss school), and Tournay[11] (the French school), most surgeons and physicians carrying out sclerotherapy have modified the techniques.[12] Fegan[9] established clear principles of sclerotherapy, namely the use of an effective sclerosant, injection into an empty vein to produce endothelial disobliteration rather than thrombosis, and adequate compression to allow the epithelial disobliteration to become effective. Compression and exercise were two important aspects of his treatment. Injection into a full vein is more likely to cause a thrombophlebitis, with subsequent recanalization and recurrence. Inadvertent injection into the deep veins may cause thrombosis. Fegan[9] argued strongly that the injection should be given beside a perforating vein, which he readily identified with his finger. Subsequent ultrasound examination of these sites suggest that many "perforating vein sites" do not in fact have perforating veins beneath them. The principle of his treatment, however, remains sound, and it is a very effective way of treating patients with varicose veins who have had junctional ligation and truncal varicosities removed. Sclerotherapy enthusiasts will treat some patients with extensive varicosities. The use of ultrasound-guided sclerotherapy (echosclerotherapy) to achieve injections at the site of junctions has been advocated. My own personal practice, however, is to use surgery in these indications, leaving sclerotherapy to treat the residual varicosities.

Technique

Although every physician/surgeon carrying out sclerotherapy will have developed his own technique, the principles remain the same (Fig. 37–3). With the leg dependent, injection sites can be identified, an appropriate sclerosant should be selected, and a needle inserted into the vein. Once the needle is within the vein, the leg can be elevated

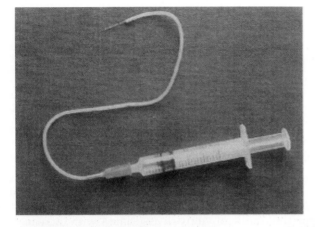

Syringe and
needle

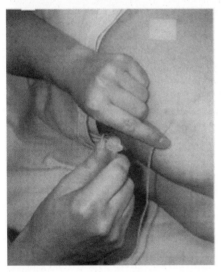

Needle inserted into
vein by transfixing
view and then
pulling back.

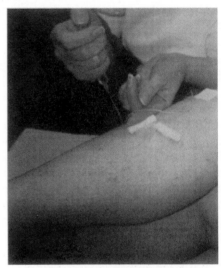

Slow injection until
large area of veins
disappears

Figure 37–3. Technique to perform sclerotherapy using a butterfly syringe. The butterfly syringe is inserted into the varix and the vein is injected until a large area of the varix disappears.

such that the vein empties. Once the vein is emptied, a suitable quantity of sclerosant can be injected. The amount of sclerosant depends on the size of the vein, but should not exceed 1 ml. The concentration of sclerosant should be sufficient to produce a brisk reaction within the lumen, but not a reaction that produces severe changes. Once the injection has been completed, pressure should be applied to the vein and a bandage applied.[13–15] Multiple injections can be carried out in any one session until segments or a number segments of vein have been obliterated.

Microsclerotherapy

Many patients who have undergone varicose vein surgery complain of dermal flares. Indeed, dermal flares may be the presenting sign in many patients, and 30% of patients presenting with dermal flares have underlying superficial venous insufficiency. If the underlying superficial venous insufficiency is not corrected before starting treatment, the results are unlikely to be successful.

Following surgery, some of the ministab avulsions may lead to the development of dermal flares. If a patient is warned about this beforehand, they accept it and can then undergo a course of microsclerotherapy to remove these flares after surgical treatment.

The purposes of microsclerotherapy is to remove the dermal flares and to achieve a satisfactory cosmetic result. Patients' expectations change during the course of treatment, and at the end of treatment they are extremely critical of any residual flares. Treatment can be continued until the patient is entirely satisfied.

The principle of microsclerotherapy is to inject a vein with a dilute sclerosant solution.[16] Although some clinicians use a trial-and-error technique, injecting slowly until the contrast material is seen to spread through the vein, this author prefers a different technique that involves a needle attached to a fine plastic tube. This ensures that the needle can be inserted into the vein before an injection takes place. As soon as blood comes back into the tube, the injection is commenced and a large area of superficial flares disappear. If the pressure is maintained, inflammation occurs in the vein wall with surrounding redness, and the veins then become permanently obstructed. In some patients the blood will leak back into the veins, but the walls are damaged such that the veins disappear over a 3-month period.

Complications of Sclerotherapy

Failure to Achieve a Good Cosmetic Result

Despite fairly extensive sclerotherapy or microsclerotherapy, some patients have residual veins. No patient should ever be guaranteed a good outcome, although in practice more than 70% of the veins treated by sclerotherapy disappear on a permanent basis.

Injection Ulcers

Large ulcers following injection treatment occur because a significant quantity of sclerosant is injected outside the vein and close to the skin. The amount of sclerosant required to produce an ulcer depends on the concentration and the depth from the skin surface.

Although pain is an indication to stop injecting, many of the sclerosant solutions have been buffered such that the pain is not felt. If there is any doubt about the position of the needle, the injection should be stopped and the needle should be reinserted.

Mini Ulcers

Occasionally following sclerotherapy the bandages rub, and local infection gets into the injection site, which initially goes red. If it is recognized and treated with antibiotics the area settles without any further problems. If no treatment is given, the redness may extend, forming a small necrotic ulcer of up to 4 mm across. These ulcers usually heal without any specific treatment apart from antibiotics and leave a minimal white scar.

Pigmentation

If a surgeon injects into a full vein and produces a thrombosis, the thrombosis resolves but often leaves an area of pigmentation. A brown streak may appear over the vein. This produces an unsightly cosmetic result and is one of the principle indications for removing rather than injecting large varicosities.

LASER/PHOTODERM

Laser and high intensity light (photoderm) are used for the treatment of residual flares. Reticular veins and dermal flares respond nicely to thermocoagulation produced either by the laser or by photoderm. The principle is that light of the correct frequency is absorbed by red blood, producing a heating effect that destroys the blood and the vein wall.

CONCLUSIONS

With proper assessment and appropriate treatment, all patients presenting with primary varicose veins can achieve a very good functional and cosmetic result. Recurrence rates following primary varicose vein surgery remain high, but with careful assessment and good operative technique followed by sclerotherapy, the recurrence rates are falling.

REFERENCES

1. Scurr J, Tibbs D, Sabiston D, Davies M, et al. *Varicose Veins, Venous Disorders, and Lymphatic Problems in the Lower Limbs.* Oxford: Oxford University Press; 1997.
2. Ad Hoc Committee of the American Venous Forum. Classification and grading of chronic venous disease in the lower limbs: a consensus statement, 1994. In: Gloviczki P, Yao JST, eds. *Handbook of venous disorders.* London: Chapman & Hall; 1996.
3. Loftgren K. Management of varicose veins: Mayo Clinic experience. In: Bergan J, Yao JST, eds. *Venous problems.* Chicago: Mosby Year Book; 1978.
4. McMullin G, Coleridge-Smith P, Scurr J. Objective assessment of high ligation without stripping the long saphenous vein. *Br J Surg.* 1991;78:1139–1142.
5. Sarin S, Scurr J, Coleridge-Smith P. Assessment of stripping the long saphenous vein in the treatment of primary varicose veins. *Br J Surg.* 1992;79:889–893.
6. Oesch A. Pin-stripping: a novel method of atraumatic stripping. *Phlebology.* 1993;8:171–173.
7. Goren G, Yellin A. Minimally invasive surgery for primary varicose veins: limited invaginated axial stripping and tributary. *Ann Vasc Surg.* 1995;9:401–414.
8. Hobbs J. Pre-operative venography to ensure accurate sapheno-popliteal ligation. *Br Med J.* 1980;ii:1578.
9. Fegan W. Continuous compression technique for injecting varicose veins. *Lancet.* 1963;2:109.
10. Sigg K. Treatment of varicose veins by injection sclerotherapy as practised in Basle. In: Hobbs JT, ed. *Treatment of Venous Disorders in the Lower Limb.* MTP Press; 1976.
11. Tournay R. *La Sclérose des Varices,* 4th ed., Paris: Expansion Scientific Francaise; 1985.
12. Conrad P. Continuous compression techniques of injecting varicose veins. *Med J Aust.* 1967;1(20):1011–1014.
13. Dormandy J. A randomized trial of bandaging after sclerotherapy for varicose veins. *Phlebologie.* 1982;35(1):125–131.
14. Fraser I, Perry E, Hatton M, Watkin D. Prolonged bandaging is not required following sclerotherapy of varicose veins. *Br J Surg.* 1985;75(6):488–490.
15. Scurr J, Coleridge-Smith P, Cutting P. Varicose veins: optimum compression following sclerotherapy. *Ann R Coll Surg Engl.* 1985;67(2):109–111.
16. Goldman M. Sclerotherapy for superficial venules and telangiectasias of the lower extremities. *Dermatol Clin.* 1987;5(2):369–379.

38

Venous Reflux and Chronic Venous Insufficiency

Andrew W. Bradbury, BSc, MD, FRCSEd and
C. Vaughan Ruckley, ChM, FRCSEd

INTRODUCTION

Although, taken literally, the term *chronic venous insufficiency* (CVI) can be used to describe the full spectrum of venous disease affecting the legs, it is used conventionally to describe the stage of venous disease in which there are visible pathological changes in the skin and subcutaneous tissues of the gaiter area; for example, corona phlebectatica, lipodermatosclerosis (LDS), and chronic venous ulceration (CVU). These changes are the consequence of sustained venous hypertension acting on a superficial venous system whose macro- and microcirculatory structure is designed to function optimally in the presence of a low ambulatory venous pressure (AVP). Failure to lower venous pressure in the erect position is due primarily to venous reflux, which in turn is a consequence of primary or secondary valve failure in the deep or superficial veins. In approximately 10% of patients with CVI there is also a significant degree of obstruction to venous outflow from the leg, which may further increase venous pressure on ambulation. Although the relationship between reflux and CVI is now well established, it is still not understood why some patients with reflux and raised AVP develop severe and refractory CVI whereas other patients with apparently similar levels of macrovascular derangement do not. One possible explanation is that individuals respond differently at the microcirculatory level to a given level of venous hypertension and that there is an as yet poorly defined genetically determined susceptibility or resistance to the condition. Alternatively, it may be that, to date, investigators have simply failed to define and quantify reflux with sufficient precision to allow the complete separation of patients with venous disease of different clinical severities on the basis of macrovascular hemodynamic abnormalities alone.

The aim of this chapter is to examine the relationship between the distribution and magnitude of venous reflux and the development of CVI. Not only is this relationship of academic interest, it is also of direct clinical importance to the surgeon when decisions are being made regarding if, when, in whom, and how surgical resources should be directed toward this potentially difficult patient population.

INVESTIGATION OF PATIENTS WITH VENOUS DISEASE

Virtually every patient with CVI referred to a vascular surgeon undergoes some form of investigation as history and examination alone are inadequate and may even be potentially misleading in the evaluation of CVI. However, the relationships between the results of various venous investigations and clinical status are the subject of a large and confusing literature in which the conclusions drawn are often conflicting.[1,2] Some observers have reported a reasonable degree of agreement between the extent and duration of venous reflux as defined duplex ultrasonography (US) and the results of air plethysmography (APG), photoplethysmography (PPG), and foot volumetry (FV).[3–5] Other researchers have been less impressed by their concordance and advocate that most, if not all, patients should have both duplex US and a plethysmographic test as part of their venous assessment.[6,7] Invasive studies such as various forms of phlebography and direct AVP measurements, long thought to represent the standards by which all other tests should be compared, are now rarely employed even for research purposes. Although understandable for reasons of convenience and patient comfort, in scientific terms this is perhaps a regrettable development, as (1) noninvasive studies, including duplex US, may not be able to characterize patients with CVI[8] with the same precision as, for example, direct AVP measurements[9]; (2) there is not always a good level of agreement between the results of noninvasive studies and AVP[10,11]; and (3) duplex US may not be able to distinguish post-thrombotic from so-called primary deep venous incompetence as accurately as phlebography.[12] As these two disease processes may differ significantly in terms of prognosis, natural history, and response to surgical intervention, this may be a serious deficiency of duplex US.[13–15]

Nevertheless, in day-to-day clinical practice, duplex US has virtually replaced all other forms of noninvasive venous assessment, with plethysmographic tests being reserved for research purposes in most hospitals in the United Kingdom. For these reasons as well as constraints on space, this chapter focuses on the relationship between the anatomic and functional information provided by duplex US regarding venous reflux and the clinical status of the patient with CVI.

METHODOLOGY OF THE EDINBURGH VEIN STUDY

Much of the data presented in this chapter originates from a preliminary analysis of the results of the Edinburgh Vein Study (EVS) performed by Dr. A.J. Lee, study statistician. For that reason, the EVS methodology is now briefly described. The EVS is a cross-sectional population survey of an age-stratified random sample of men and women aged 18 to 64 years selected from the computerized age–sex registers of 12 general practices, the catchment areas of which were geographically and socioeconomically distributed throughout Edinburgh. Subjects were examined clinically, completed a self-administered questionnaire, and underwent duplex US examination of both legs. Venous disease was classified and graded according to the Basel Study.[16] A total of 1566 subjects attended for examination, 867 women and 699 men. The mean age of participants was 44.8 years for women and 45.8 years for men ($p > .05$). There was no significant difference between right and left legs with regard to any of the variables described in this chapter.

NORMAL VENOUS DUPLEX ULTRASOUND EXAMINATION

Before considering the relationship between reflux and the presence of CVI, it is first necessary to define what constitutes a normal duplex US examination. As most duplex

Subjects with CVI (%)

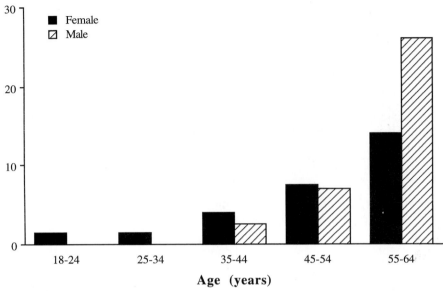

Figure 38–1. Prevalence (in percent) of chronic venous insufficiency (CVI) on clinical examination in male and female subjects in the Edinburgh Vein Study.

US–based studies have involved the examination of patients, there is a lack of data describing patterns and duration of reflux in normal subjects.

EVS is the first study to have examined a randomly selected cross-section of the adult population both clinically and with duplex US and has demonstrated the prevalence of CVI and reflux to be high (Fig. 38–1). Thus, superficial and deep venous reflux of 0.5 sec or more was found in up to 18.6% and 12.3% of limbs, respectively, with reflux exceeding 1.0 s being found in 17.7% and 5% (Table 38–1). However, when subjects with and without clinically apparent venous disease were separated, it became

TABLE 38–1. PREVALENCE OF REFLUX IN THE LEGS OF SUBJECTS IN THE EDINBURGH VEIN STUDY

Venous Segment	Right Leg		Left Leg		Both Legs	
	≥ *0.5 sec* (%)	> *1.0 sec* (%)	≥ *0.5 sec* (%)	> *1.0 sec* (%)	≥ *0.5 sec* (%)	> *1.0 sec* (%)
Superficial system						
LSV upper thigh	10.0	9.6	10.8	10.1	4.8	4.6
LSV lower thigh	18.6	17.7	17.5	16.7	8.0	7.5
SSV	4.6	3.7	5.6	4.2	1.6	1.1
Deep system						
CFV	7.8	2.1	8.0	2.1	2.5	0.6
SFV upper thigh	5.2	1.2	4.7	1.3	1.7	0.3
SFV lower thigh	6.6	2.5	6.4	2.7	2.2	0.8
PV above-the-knee	12.3	5.0	11.0	5.3	3.9	1.3
PV below-the-knee	11.3	4.7	9.5	4.6	3.3	1.0

CFV, common femoral vein; SFV, superficial femoral vein; PV, popliteal vein; LSV long saphenous vein; SSV, short saphenous vein.

apparent that relatively few subjects without signs of venous disease had superficial (or deep) reflux of 0.5 sec or more (Table 38–2). It would seem, therefore, that in this nonpatient population there is reasonably good agreement between a duplex US scan that fails to demonstrate reflux of 0.5 sec or more in any superficial or deep venous segment and a normal clinical appearance of the leg.

This does not, of course, mean that subjects with reflux exceeding 0.5 sec necessarily have symptoms or signs of venous disease. For example, in the study reported by Labropoulos et al.[17] from St. Mary's Hospital in London, duplex US was used to examine of the legs of 28 vascular surgeons and 25 normal volunteers who had no clinical signs or symptoms suggestive of venous disease, no history of deep or superficial venous thrombosis, and who had not undergone any venous operation or injection sclerotherapy. The authors defined pathological reflux as that which exceeded 1 sec. Venous reflux was found in 52% of vascular surgeons and in 32% of controls ($p = .04$, χ^2 test). In the group of surgeons, pathological reflux was present in the superficial veins only in 22/56 (39%), in deep or perforating veins only in 4/56 (7%), and in the superficial and deep systems in 3/56 (5%). In the control group, superficial reflux was found in 9/50 (18%), deep or perforator reflux in 3/50 (6%), and superficial and deep venous reflux in 4/50 (8%). Superficial reflux was thus present in 45% (25/56) of limbs of vascular surgeons compared with 13/50 controls (26%) ($p = .05$, χ^2 test). Long saphenous vein (LSV) reflux in the lower thigh accounted for 48% of superficial reflux in vascular surgeons and 39% in control subjects. The authors concluded that venous reflux is found more frequently in symptom-free vascular surgeons than in symptom-free age- and sex-matched controls. Perhaps more importantly, the study also demonstrates that, although deep venous reflux exceeding 1.0 sec is unusual in symptom-free adult males, superficial reflux, predominantly in the lower LSV, is frequently present.

Lagatolla et al.[18] at St. Thomas' Hospital, London, who had performed a duplex US assessment of the deep veins of 61 subjects who had normal venous function. Their subjects had no history of venous thromboembolic disease, significant lower limb trauma, abdominal surgery, or symptoms or signs of venous disease. Furthermore, they had normal venous function on FV. Subjects were examined in three positions:

TABLE 38–2. DURATION OF REFLUX IN SUBJECTS WITH AND WITHOUT CLINICALLY APPARENT VENOUS DISEASE IN THE EDINBURGH VEIN STUDY[a]

Venous Segment	No Venous Disease[b] (n = 861)			Venous Disease[c] (n = 579)		
	Median	*IQR*	*95th Centile*	*Median*	*IQR*	*95th Centile*
Superficial system						
LSV upper thigh	0.00	0.00–0.10	0.29	0.15	0.00–4.3	8.00
LSV lower thigh	0.11	0.05–0.16	6.46	2.30	0.10–6.97	8.00
SSV	0.10	0.00–0.14	0.27	0.13	0.10–0.24	4.08
Deep system						
CFV	0.09	0.00–0.26	0.54	0.18	0.00–0.48	1.63
SFV upper thigh	0.11	0.00–0.25	0.52	0.15	0.00–0.33	1.14
SFV lower thigh	0.13	0.04–0.25	0.53	0.18	0.06–0.40	2.88
PV above-the-knee	0.17	0.10–0.32	0.84	0.25	0.13–0.68	2.63
PV below-the-knee	0.14	0.10–0.28	0.88	0.20	0.12–0.53	2.30

IQR, interquartile range; CFV, common femoral vein, SFV, superficial femoral vein; PV, popliteal vein; LSV, long saphenous vein; SSV, short saphenous vein.
[a] Duration of reflux is measured in seconds.
[b] No venous disease—no clinically apparent trunk varices, perforators or skin changes of CVI and a maximum of grade I hyphen-web and/or reticular varices.
[c] Venous disease—patients with clinically apparent trunk varices and/or skin changes of CVI.

10° and 45° of head-up tilt and standing. The duration of reverse flow was recorded following sudden release of cuff compression and during a Valsalva maneuver. Ninety-five percent of all reverse flow was less than 0.65 sec and 93% was within the 0.5 sec cut off. Importantly, reverse flow of more than 0.5 sec was never observed in the posterior tibial veins of standing subjects, nor was it observed in the popliteal vein of any subject during a Valsalva maneuver. The authors of this study concluded that reverse flow exceeding 0.5 sec cannot be used as a marker of deep venous disease in the superficial femoral vein when a cut off of 1.0 sec may be more informative, but that in the popliteal and posterior tibial veins they could support the use of a 0.5 sec cut off provided that the patient is examined in the erect position and that a Valsalva maneuver is used to elicit reverse flow. Other workers have suggested 0.3 sec[19] and 0.5 sec[20-22] to be reliable cut-off points for defining abnormality, and have also stressed the influence of the subjects' position and how the reverse flow is elicited on the duration of reflux observed.

CHRONIC VENOUS INSUFFICIENCY AND VENOUS REFLUX

Several studies have examined patterns of venous reflux by means of duplex US in patients with CVU (Table 38–3).[23-31] These series indicate that, although more than half of such patients have deep venous disease, this is associated with superficial reflux in the majority of cases. Furthermore, up to a third of patients have isolated superficial venous reflux. The patterns of deep and superficial reflux are examined in more detail next.

Superficial Reflux

Labropoulos and colleagues[32] used color-flow duplex US to define the pattern of venous reflux in 255 limbs (217 patients) with superficial venous reflux but who had normal deep and perforating veins. In 123 limbs (48.2%), reflux was confined to the LSV; in 83 limbs (32.6%) to the short saphenous vein (SSV), and in 49 limbs there was reflux exceeding 1 sec in both systems. The authors conducted a careful study of the relation-

TABLE 38–3. PREVALENCE OF DEEP AND SUPERFICIAL REFLUX IN PATIENTS WITH CHRONIC VENOUS ULCERATION

Authors	Year	Limbs	Superficial Reflux Detected (%)	Deep Reflux Detected (%)	Superficial Reflux Only Detected (%)
van Bemmelen et al.[23]	1990	25	92	92	8
Hanrahan et al.[24]	1991	95	79	50	17
Mastroroberto et al.[25]	1992	51	76	47	4
Shami et al.[26]	1993	79	75	47	53
Lees et al.[27]	1993	25	88	48[a]	52[a]
van Rij et al.[28]	1994	120	—	—	40
Myers et al.[29]	1995	95	86	56	36
Labropoulos et al.[30]	1996	120	90	58	37[a]
Scriven et al.[31]	1997	95	88	43	57[a]

[a] Includes incompetent perforating veins.

ship between the presence of CVI and the pattern of superficial reflux (Table 38–4). Skin changes appeared to be related to below-the-knee LSV reflux, regardless of whether the LSV in the thigh was affected. CVI was also common in patients with reflux limited to the SSV. Perhaps surprisingly, the prevalence of CVI was not increased by the presence of coexisting reflux in the gastrocnemius veins. The highest incidence of CVI was found in patients with full-length LSV and SSV reflux. However, even in the group with maximal superficial venous incompetence, the prevalence of ulceration was only 14%, and one in five patients had normal skin.

Deep Reflux

Labropoulos et al.[30] produced similar data with respect to the relationship between deep venous disease and CVI (Table 38–5). The development of skin changes and ulceration was associated with an increasing prevalence of mixed superficial and deep venous reflux. With respect to the deep system, skin changes and ulceration appear to be associated with popliteal and crural, particularly posterior tibial vein, reflux. Other researchers have reported similar results.[24,27,29] However, one must again note that, even in patients with apparently maximal superficial and deep venous reflux on duplex scanning, less than half had any evidence of skin changes. This may be because severity of reflux is only one of many factors that determine whether skin changes and ulceration develop. Alternatively, it could be argued that reflux is important, but that duplex US is not the best way of quantifying it. Thus, the risk of future skin changes in patients with simple varicose veins (VVs) may be better defined by the venous filling index as determined by plethysmography than the anatomic pattern of reflux as shown by duplex US.[33,34]

TABLE 38–4. RELATIONSHIP BETWEEN CHRONIC VENOUS INSUFFICIENCY AND THE PATTERN OF SUPERFICIAL REFLUX IN PATIENTS WITH NO REFLUX IN THE DEEP VENOUS SYSTEM

Pattern of Reflux	Total	Skin Changes n (%)	Ulceration n (%)
Reflux confined to the LSV			
LSV–AK only	24	1 (4)	0
LSV–BK only	21	10 (48)	0
LSV full length	78	42 (58)	6 (8)
TOTAL	123	53 (43)	6 (5)
Reflux confined to SSV			
Giacomini vein only	2	0	0
SSV only	46	24 (52)	0
MGV or LGV only	9	0	0
SSV + Giacomini	11	2 (18)	1 (9)
SSV + MGV or LGV	13	5 (38)	1 (8)
TOTAL	83	31 (37)	2 (2)
Reflux in LSV and SSV			
SFJ + SSV	1	0	0
LSV–AK + SSV	5	1	0
LSV–BK + SSV	16	7 (44)	0
LSV–AK + BK + SSV	3	1	0
SFJ + LSV–AK + LSV	2	1	0
SFJ + LSV–AK + BK + SSV	22	16 (73)	3 (14)
TOTAL	49	26 (53)	3 (6)

LSV, long saphenous vein; SFJ, saphenofemoral junction; AK above knee; BK, below knee; SSV, short saphenous vein; MGV, medial gastrocnemius vein; LGV, lateral gastrocnemius vein.

TABLE 30–5. SITE AND EXTENT OF REFLUX IN THE DEEP VEINS OF PATIENTS WITH CHRONIC VENOUS INSUFFICIENCY

Site of Reflux	Skin Changes (%) (n = 155)	Ulcer (%) (n = 120)	Total (%) (n = 594)
Superficial only	23	18	31
Perforator only	1	1	1
Deep only	5	4	3
Superficial and perforator	12	19	8
Superficial and deep	21	13	10
Perforator and deep	1	2	1
Superficial and perforator and deep	34	39	17
Normal	4	3	30
Extent of deep reflux (where present)	(n = 109)	(n = 89)	(n = 219)
CFV	16	12	15
SFV	9	8	8
PV	31	36	32
CV	44	44	45

CFV, common femoral vein; SFV, superficial femoral vein; PV, popliteal vein; CV, crural veins.

Payne et al.[35] also used duplex US to determine the pattern of venous reflux in 274 limbs and then employed multivariate logistic regression analysis to relate these findings to the clinical status of the leg in terms of the presence of ulceration. Superficial femoral, profunda femoris, and short saphenous reflux was not related to the presence of CVI, whereas reflux in the common femoral, popliteal, and LSV was. The adverse clinical impact of popliteal vein reflux was particularly apparent; the tibial veins were not specifically examined.

In one study, Sakurai and colleagues[36] from Japan used duplex scanning and PPG to correlate the anatomic distribution of venous reflux with clinical status and venous hemodynamics in a consecutive series of 191 patients (266 legs) presenting with "obvious" VV [43 men (61 legs); 148 women (205 legs), mean age 52.6 (range 17 to 80) years]. Patients with a clear history of previous deep venous thrombosis (DVT) and duplex US evidence of postthrombotic deep venous disease were excluded. According to the CEAP classification, 192 limbs were class 2 (VV only), 14 limbs were class 3 (VV and edema), 54 limbs were class 4 (skin changes), and 6 limbs were class 6 (active ulceration). They discovered that 219 legs (82%) exhibited reflux (> 0.5 sec) in the LSV and 69 legs (26%) in the SSV; 164 legs (62%) had incompetent medial calf perforating veins (IPV); and 128 legs (48%) had reflux in the deep venous system. Superficial venous reflux was thus detected on duplex US in 253 limbs (95%); surprisingly, in 13 limbs no main stem reflux was detected. Patients with both LSV and SSV reflux, with or without IPV, had reduced refilling times on PPG when compared with patients with incompetence in a single system. Of the 60 limbs with class 4 and 6 disease, the pattern of superficial reflux was LSV 57 (95%), SSV 19 (32%), and IPV 45 (75%). Skin changes and ulceration were strongly associated with the presence of femoropopliteal deep venous reflux and markedly reduced refilling times on PPG.

POPLITEAL VEIN REFLUX

As well as allowing the surgeon to tailor the operation to the patients' needs, there are data to suggest that defining the pattern of disease by means of duplex US may provide important prognostic information with regard to the patient's response to both medical and surgical intervention.

In one study, the relationship between deep and superficial reflux and healing of venous ulceration in 155 patients treated nonoperatively with compression bandaging was studied. At 24 weeks, 104 (67%) of ulcers had healed. There was no significant difference in the patterns of either deep or superficial reflux between healed and nonhealed ulcers except with respect to the popliteal vein. In ulcers that healed, 39 (38%) duplex scans indicated competence (reflux $<$ 0.5 sec) of the above-the-knee popliteal vein compared with 5 (10%) in the nonhealing group ($p <$ .001, χ^2 test). Similarly, 43 scans (42%) demonstrated below-the-knee popliteal vein competence in the ulcers that subsequently healed compared with only 5 (10%) in the legs that did not heal ($p <$ .001, χ^2 test).[37] These data suggest that the presence of popliteal vein reflux is a useful adverse prognostic factor in patients with venous ulceration being treated nonoperatively. Such information is of immediate relevance to the surgeon when making judgments about whether a particular patient may be managed entirely in the community or in a shared-care environment.

Popliteal vein reflux also appears to affect the outcome after surgical intervention for venous ulceration.[38] In the Edinburgh series of 43 patients undergoing superficial venous surgery and open perforating vein ligation (Linton's procedure) for chronic venous ulceration, 9 developed recurrent ulceration during a median follow-up of 66 (range 18 to 144) months. Of these, 6 had femoral vein incompetence and all had popliteal vein incompetence on duplex examination. By contrast, of the 34 patients

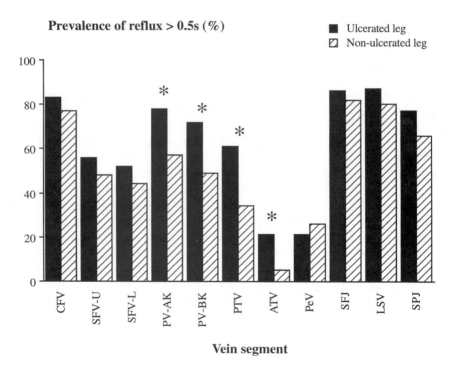

Figure 38–2. Prevalence (in percent) of reflux ($>$ 0.5 sec) in the ulcerated and nonulcerated legs of patients with unilateral venous ulceration. CFV, common femoral vein; SFV, superficial femoral vein, upper (U) and lower (L); PV, popliteal vein, above knee (AK) and below knee (BK); PTV, posterior tibial vein; ATV, anterior tibial vein; PeV, peroneal vein; SFJ, saphenofemoral junction; LSV, long saphenous vein; SPJ, saphenopopliteal junction (* $p <$ .05 by χ^2 test with Yates' correction).

who remained ulcer-free, 5 had femoral vein and only 1 had popliteal vein reflux. This provides popliteal vein reflux with a positive predictive value for recurrent ulceration of 90%.

The importance of popliteal vein reflux in the development and chronicity of venous ulceration is demonstrated by a further study in which the duplex-defined pattern of venous reflux was compared in the affected and nonaffected legs of patients with unilateral ulceration.[39] In 54 patients with unilateral ulceration of "pure" venous etiology, the only difference between the affected and nonaffected legs was with respect to the popliteal segment (Fig. 38–2).

Lastly, these data also underline how important it is that, when contemplating trials comparing nonoperative and operative interventions for venous ulceration, the randomization process must ensure that equal numbers of high-risk and low-risk patients are entered into each group. Stratifying on the basis of popliteal vein reflux appears to be one means of achieving this.

PERFORATING VEIN REFLUX

The physiological significance of reflux within IPV and role of subfascial endoscopic perforator surgery (SEPS) in the surgical management of CVI remain controversial.[31,40,41] Although several groups have reported encouraging results with the SEPS procedure in terms of feasibility, safety, and efficacy,[42-45] there are no randomized controlled data to support its widespread use.

As isolated perforator incompetence is unusual (< 5%) in patients with CVI, and most IPV are seen in conjunction with superficial and particularly deep venous reflux, the question remains as to whether IPV is merely associated with the presence of skin changes or whether it plays a role in their causation.[46,47] Although several authors have reported low recurrence rates following perforator ligation performed at the same time as standard saphenous surgery,[38] others report no further hemodynamic[40] or clinical benefit from the addition of perforator ligation.[13] Furthermore, it has been suggested that eradication of superficial reflux alone may restore competence to IPV.[48] Two studies from the Edinburgh unit have provided new data that address some of these issues. The aim of the first study was to determine the relationship between the number, diameter, and flow characteristics of medial calf perforating veins and the clinical and hemodynamic status of the leg affected by CVI. Three groups of patients were examined clinically, by means of PPG and by duplex scanning (Table 38–6). These data indicate that deteriorating clinical status is associated with an increase in the total number of medial calf perforators detectable by duplex US and an increase in the proportion of those perforators that permit pathological (> 0.5 sec) outward or bidirectional flow on foot squeeze. With respect to maximal perforator diameter, perforators allowing bidirectional flow were significantly wider than those permitting only unidirectional inward flow. However, perforators permitting unidirectional flow were significantly wider in patients with venous disease when compared to normal controls. In summary, therefore, CVI is associated with an increased number and diameter of medial calf perforating veins permitting bidirectional flow.

The aim of the second study was to determine which patients, if any, require SEPS in addition to standard saphenous surgery in order to correct pathological flow within medial calf perforating veins. Forty-seven patients (18 male, 29 female; median age 58, range 35 to 77 years) (62 limbs) who underwent saphenofemoral ligation, stripping of the LSV in the thigh and multiple phlebectomies ($n = 51$), or saphenopopliteal ligation

TABLE 38–6. RELATIONSHIP BETWEEN NUMBER, DIAMETER, AND FLOW CHARACTERISTICS OF MEDIAL CALF PERFORATING VEINS AND THE CLINICAL AND HEMODYNAMIC STATUS OF THE LEG AFFECTED BY CHRONIC VENOUS INSUFFICIENCY

	Group I Normal (CEAP Class 0)	Group II Varicose Veins (CEAP Class 2)	Group III CVI (CEAP Classes 4–6)
Number of subjects	17	34	28
Number of limbs	31	48	34
Median (range) age (years)	29 (23–79)	55 (30–77)	264 (38–83)
VRT 50 on PPG (sec)	11.7	5.3	2.2
Number of perforators permitting			
Only inward flow	40	50	16
Only outward flow	1	2	5
Bidirectional flow (incompetence)	1	51	64
Any flow	42	103	85
Number of medial calf perforators per leg	1.3	2.1	2.7
Number of incompetent medial calf perforators per leg	0.03	0.97	2.11
Mean (range) diameter of medial calf perforators	1.7 (1.0–3.0)	3.7 (1.0–8.0)	4.5 (2.5–8.3)

VRT, venous refilling time.

and multiple phlebectomies ($n = 10$) or both ($n = 1$) were studied. When performing phlebectomies, the surgeon avoided avulsing superficial varices in the immediate vicinity of the medial calf perforating veins that had been marked preoperatively on the leg by duplex US. The indications for surgery were varicose veins ($n = 47$, CEAP classes 2 and 3), skin changes of CVI ($n = 5$, CEAP class 4), and ulceration ($n = 10$, CEAP class 5). Patients were examined with duplex US to ascertain the presence of reflux (> 0.5 sec) in the superficial and deep systems as well as in medial calf perforating veins. Three patients had a clearly documented history of previous DVT. A further 10 patients had deep venous reflux (> 0.5 sec) but had no history of DVT. The examination was performed immediately before surgery and a median of 14 (range 6 to 26) weeks postoperatively.

The pattern of pre- and postoperative deep and superficial main stem venous reflux is shown in Table 38–7. Medial calf perforators, competent or incompetent, were imaged in 60 limbs both pre- and postoperatively. In two limbs perforators were not imaged either before or after surgery. Surgery was associated with a small reduction in the total number of perforators, competent or incompetent, imaged (preoperatively, $n = 130$; vs. postoperatively, $n = 120$); a significant reduction in the total number of limbs in which incompetent perforators were imaged (preoperatively, 40/62, 65%; vs. postoperatively 23/72, 37%; $p < .01$, χ^2 test); a significant reduction in the proportion of perforators imaged that were incompetent (preoperatively, 68/130, 52%; vs. postoperatively, 34/120, 28%; $p < .01$, χ^2 test) and a reduction in the median diameter of all perforators imaged [preoperatively, 4 mm (range 1 to 11 mm); vs. postoperatively, 3 (range 1 to 8 mm); $p < .01$, Mann-Whitney U test]. IPV was detected postoperatively in only 8 of 41 (20%) limbs in which main stem venous reflux was abolished by surgery and deep venous reflux was absent. By comparison, IPV was imaged in 15 of 21 (72%) limbs in which deep venous reflux was present or surgery failed to eradicate reflux completely in the main stem or major tributaries of the LSV or the SSV ($p < .01$, χ^2

TABLE 38–7. SITES OF REFLUX BEFORE AND AFTER SUPERFICIAL VENOUS SURGERY

Site of Reflux	Preoperative n (%)	Postoperative n (%)
Long saphenous vein	55 (89)	4 (6)
Short saphenous vein	12 (19)	3 (5)
Common femoral vein	36 (58)	26 (58)
Superficial femoral vein	8 (13)	7 (11)
Popliteal vein	6 (10)	6 (10)
Posterior tibial vein	6 (10)	6 (10)
Superficial reflux only	49 (79)	5 (8)
Deep reflux only	—	14 (23)
Deep and superficial reflux	13 (21)	2 (3)

test). IPV was imaged postoperatively in 14 of 47 limbs (30%) operated for uncomplicated varicose veins, compared with 9 of 15 limbs (60%) operated for CVI ($p < 0.05$, χ^2 test). The relationship between the postoperative distribution of main stem deep or superficial reflux and the presence of IPV is shown in Fig. 38–3.

The first main conclusion to be drawn from this study is that, in patients undergoing saphenous surgery in the absence of significant reflux in the deep venous system, complete eradication of main stem superficial reflux leads to correction of pathological outward flow in medial calf perforating veins in most (33 of 41) but not all cases. In those cases in which outward reflux was abolished by superficial surgery, one might

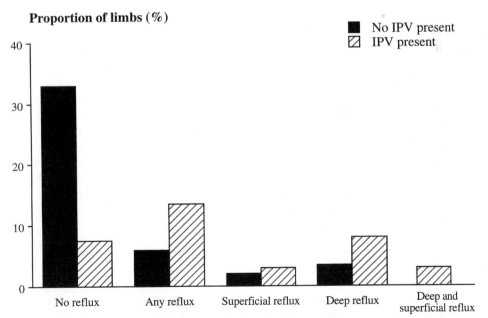

Figure 38–3. The relationship between superficial or deep main stem reflux and the prevalence (in percent) of incompetent medial calf perforating vein (IPV) reflux in patients following superficial venous surgery.

hypothesize that medial calf perforators have been rendered incompetent preoperatively due to (reversible) dilatation occurring as a result of excessive filling of the deep venous system from a refluxing saphenous system during calf muscle pump diastole. Eradication of superficial reflux allows perforating veins to return toward their normal diameter and regain competence. That superficial venous reflux may overload the deep venous system leading to "secondary" deep venous reflux is supported by two previous studies showing that surgical eradication of superficial venous reflux can correct reflux in the femoral vein, presumably due to the removal of thigh perforators at the time of superficial stripping.[49,50] In the Edinburgh study a similar effect of superficial surgery has been observed on femoral and calf perforating vein incompetence, but not on popliteal or tibial vein reflux, possibly because the calf perforating veins were purposely left undisturbed.

These and previous observations have led the Edinburgh group to develop a perforator classification based on the distribution of reflux feeding the IPVs and the type of venous surgery required to correct bidirectional perforator flow.

> Type I IPV: Fed by a refluxing saphenous vein (long or short) in the presence of a normal deep system. In majority of such cases (80%), saphenous surgery alone corrects bidirectional perforator flow.
>
> Type II IPV: Found in association with isolated deep venous reflux. That is, there is no significant saphenous reflux. In these circumstances correction of IPV requires direct surgical interruption.
>
> Type III IPV: Found in association with mixed superficial and deep venous reflux and are the commonest group in patients with CVI . In these circumstances saphenous surgery alone does not affect IPV, and SEPS is required to correct bidirectional flow.
>
> Type IV IPV: Acts as part of the collateral circulation bypassing an occluded deep venous system. It is important that such IPVs are clearly identified because perforator interruption, with or without saphenous extirpation, could be detrimental to these patients.

Widely disparate results have been reported following perforator surgery leading to continued controversy regarding the appropriateness of perforator ligation in the management of venous disease. This may be due to differences in case mix and selection. For example, with regard to the Edinburgh classification, one might not expect patients with type I IPV to gain any additional hemodynamic or clinical benefit from perforator ligation performed in addition to standard saphenous surgery in the great majority of cases. Perforator ligation in patients with type IV IPV is likely to be detrimental and may be contraindicated. By contrast, patients with type III perforators will not be corrected by superficial surgery alone, leaving a route for the transmission of raised deep venous pressure to the vulnerable skin of the gaiter area.

SUMMARY

The term *chronic venous insufficiency* (CVI) is applied indiscriminately in the literature. For the purposes of this chapter, CVI is defined as the stage of venous disease at which there are visible pathological changes of lipodermatosclerosis, with or without ulceration, as a consequence of chronic ambulatory venous hypertension.

Duplex scanning has become the universally popular method of assessment, although the correlation between symptoms, signs, the results of functional tests, and ultrasound imaging is not yet sufficiently consistent or precise for any noninvasive investigation to be regarded as the sole reference standard.

In the popliteal and posterior tibial veins (probably the critical segments in relation to the development of, and prognosis for, skin changes) reflux of more than 0.5 sec in the erect posture separates pathological from normal venous function.

The Edinburgh Vein Study (EVS) investigated 1566 subjects, aged 18 to 64 years, selected randomly from the normal population. A close association was found between clinical normality and absence of reflux of more than 0.5 sec in either the superficial or deep veins.

Overview of studies of duplex scanning in patients with CVI and ulceration shows that although around half have reflux in the deep system, three-quarters have superficial reflux, and a third of such cases the deep system is apparently normal. In patients with superficial reflux only, CVI is associated with multilevel, below-the-knee, and two-system (long and short saphenous) disease.

Where reflux affects the deep system, the segment that carries the worst prognosis in terms of healing with conservative methods, or in response to surgery of the superficial and perforating veins, is the popliteal and posterior tibial veins.

CVI is associated with an increase in the number of medial calf perforating veins, particularly veins permitting bidirectional flow.

Surgery to the saphenous systems, without any attempt to remove perforators, in the absence of deep venous reflux, results in the restoration of perforator competence in the majority of cases.

A classification of calf perforating veins is proposed based on the distribution of the reflux "feeding" the perforators, and on the type of surgery require to correct bidirectional perforator flow.

CONCLUSIONS

The studies reviewed in this chapter are leading to a rapidly growing understanding of the relationship between patterns of reflux on duplex scanning, the clinical manifestations, and the response to therapy. However, the fact that the relationship between the development of CVI and patterns of reflux is not entirely consistent and predictable suggests that other as yet ill-defined factors remain to be elucidated.

REFERENCES

1. Moulton S, Bergan JJ, Beeman S. Gravitational reflux does not correlate with clinical status of venous stasis. *Phlebology.* 1993;8:2–6.
2. McMullen GM, Scott HJ, Coleridge-Smith PD. A comparison of photoplethysmography, Doppler ultrasound and duplex scanning in the assessment of venous insufficiency. *Phlebology.* 1989;4:75–82.
3. Neglen P, Raju S. A rational approach to detection of significant reflux with duplex Doppler scanning and air plethysmography. *J Vasc Surg.* 1993;17:590–595.
4. Bays RA, Healy DA, Atnip RG, Neumyer M, et al. Validation of air plethysmography, photoplethysmography, and duplex ultrasonography in the evaluation of severe venous stasis. *J Vasc Surg.* 1994;20:721–727.
5. Weingarten MS, Czeredarczuk M, Scovell S, Branas CC, et al. A correlation of air plethysmography and colour-flow assisted duplex scanning in the quantification of chronic venous insufficiency. *J Vasc Surg.* 1996;24:750–754.

6. van Bemmelen PS, van Ramshorst B, Eikleboom BC. Photoplethysmography re-examined: lack of correlation with duplex scanning. *Surgery.* 1992;112:544–548.

7. van Bemmelen PS, Mattos MA, Hodgson KJ, Barkmeier DE, et al. Does air plethysmography correlate with duplex scanning in patients with chronic venous insufficiency. *J Vasc Surg.* 1993;18:796–807.

8. Iafrati MD, Welch H, O'Donnell TF, Belkin M, et al. Correlation of venous non-invasive tests with the Society for Vascular Surgery/International Society for Cardiovascular Surgery clinical classification of chronic venous insufficiency. *J Vasc Surg.* 1994;19:1001–1007.

9. Nicolaides AN, Hussein MK, Szendro G, Christopoulos D, et al. The relation of venous ulceration with ambulatory venous pressure measurements. *J Vasc Surg.* 1993;17:414–419.

10. Rosfors S. A methodological study of venous valvular insufficiency and musculovenous pump function of the lower leg. *Phlebology.* 1992;7:12–19.

11. Payne SPK, Thrush AJ, London NJM, Bell PRF, et al. Venous assessment using air plethysmography: a comparison with clinical examination, ambulatory venous pressure measurement and duplex scanning. *Br J Surg.* 1993;80:967–970.

12. Baker SR, Burnand KG, Sommerville KM, Lea Thomas M, et al. Comparison of venous reflux assessed by duplex scanning and descending phlebography in chronic venous disease. *Lancet.* 1993;341:400–403.

13. Darke SG, Penfold C. Venous ulceration and saphenous ligation. *Eur J Vasc Surg.* 1992;6:4–9.

14. Janssen MCH, Wollersheim H, van Austen WNJC, de Rooij MJM, et al. The post-thrombotic syndrome: a review. *Phlebology.* 1996;11:86–94.

15. Burnand KG, Lea Thomas M, O'Donnell T, Browse NL. Relation between post-phlebitic changes in the deep veins and results of surgical treatment of venous ulcers. *Lancet.* 1976;i:936–938.

16. Widmer LK (ed). *Peripheral Venous Disorders—Prevalence and Socio-Medical Importance.* Bern: Hans Gruber; 1978;1–90.

17. Labropoulos N, Delis KT, Nicolaides AN. Venous reflux in symptom-free vascular surgeons. *J Vasc Surg.* 1995;22:150–154.

18. Lagatolla NRF, Donald A, Lockhart S, Burnand KG. Retrograde flow in the deep veins of subjects with normal venous function. *Br J Surg.* 1997;84:36–39.

19. Araki CT, Back TL, Padberg FT, Thompson PN, et al. Refinements in the ultrasonic detection of popliteal vein reflux. *J Vasc Surg.* 1993;18:742–748.

20. van Bemmelen PS, Bedford G, Beach K, Strandness DE. Quantitative segmental evaluation of venous valvular reflux with duplex ultrasound scanning. *J Vasc Surg.* 1989;10:425–431.

21. Sarin S, Sommerville K, Farrah J, Scurr JH, et al. Duplex ultrasonography for the assessment of venous valvular function of the lower limb. *Br J Surg.* 1994;81:1591–1595.

22. Masuda EM, Kistner RL, Eklof B. Prospective study of duplex scanning for venous reflux: comparison of Valsalva and pneumatic cuff techniques in the reverse Trendelenberg and standing positions. *J Vasc Surg.* 1994;20:711–720.

23. van Bemmelen PS, Bedford G, Beach K, Strandness DE. Status of the valves in the superficial and deep venous system in chronic venous disease. *Surgery.* 1990;109:730–734.

24. Hanrahan LM, Araki CT, Rodriguez AA, Kechejian GJ, et al. Distribution of valvular incompetence in patients with venous stasis ulceration. *J Vasc Surg.* 1991;13:805–812.

25. Mastroroberto P, Chello M, Marchese A. Distribution of valvular incompetence in patients with venous stasis ulceration. *J Vasc Surg.* 1992;16:307 [Letter].

26. Shami SK, Sarin S, Cheatle TR, Scurr JH, et al. Venous ulcers and the superficial venous system. *J Vasc Surg.* 1993;17:487–490.

27. Lees TA, Lambert D. Patterns of venous reflux in limbs with skin changes associated with chronic venous insufficiency. *Br J Surg.* 1993;80:725–728.

28. van Rij AM, Solomon C, Christie R. Anatomic and physiologic characteritics of venous ulceration. *J Vasc Surg.* 1994;20:759–764.

29. Myers KA, Ziegenbein RW, Zeng GH, Matthews PG. Duplex ultrasonography scanning for chronic venous disease. Patterns of reflux. *J Vasc Surg.* 1995;21:605–612.

30. Labropoulos N, Delis K, Nicolaides AN, Leon M, et al. The role of the distribution and anatomic extent of reflux in the development of signs and symptoms in chronic venous insufficiency. *J Vasc Surg.* 1996;23:504–510.

31. Scriven JM, Hartshorne T, Bell PRF, Naylor AR, et al. Single-visit venous ulcer assessment clinic: the first year. *Br J Surg.* 1997;84:334–336.

32. Labropoulos N, Leon M, Nicolaides AN, Giannoukas AD, et al. Superficial venous insufficiency: correlation of anatomic extent of reflux with clinical symptoms amd signs. *J Vasc Surg.* 1994;20:953–958.

33. Vasdekis SN, Clarke GH, Nicolaides AN. Quantification of venous reflux by means of duplex scanning. *J Vasc Surg.* 1989;10:670–677.

34. Nicolaides AN, Sumner DS. *Investigation of Patients with Deep Venous Thrombosis and Chronic Venous Insufficiency.* London: Med-Orion; 1991.

35. Payne SPK, London NJM, Jagger C, Newland CJ, et al. Clinical significance of venous reflux detected by duplex scanning. *Br J Surg.* 1994;81:39–41.

36. Sakurai T, Gupta PC, Matsushita M, Nishikimi N, et al. Correlation of the anatomic distribution of venous reflux with clinical symptoms and venous haemodynamics in primary varicose veins. *Br J Surg.* 1998;85:213–216.

37. Brittenden J, Bradbury AW, Allan PL, Prescott RJ, et al. Popliteal vein reflux reduces the healing of chronic venous ulceration. *Br J Surg.* 1998;85:60–62.

38. Bradbury AW, Stonebridge PA, Callam ML, Ruckley CV, et al. Foot volumetry and duplex ultrasonography after saphenous and sub-fascial perforating vein ligation for recurrent venous ulceration. *Br J Surg.* 1993;80:845–848.

39. Bradbury AW, Brittenden J, Allan PL, Ruckley CV. Comparison of venous reflux in the affected and non-affected leg in patients with unilateral venous ulceration. *Br J Surg.* 1996;83:5135.

40. Akesson H, Bridin L, Cwikile W, Ohlin P, et al. Does the correction of insufficient superficial and perforating veins improve venous function in patients with deep venous insufficiency? *Phlebology.* 1990;5:113–123.

41. Ruckley CV, Makhdoomi KR. The venous perforator. *Br J Surg.* 1996;83:1492–1493.

42. Gloviczki P, Cambria RA, Rhee RY, Canton LG, et al. Surgical technique and preliminary results of endoscopic subfascial division of perforating veins. *J Vasc Surg.* 1996;23:517–523.

43. Pierik EGJM, van Urk H, Wittens CHA. Efficacy of subfascial endoscopy in eradicating perforating veins of the lower leg and its relation with venous ulcer healing. *J Vasc Surg.* 1997;26:255–259.

44. Pierik EGJM, Toonder IM, van Urk H, Wittens CHA. Validation of duplex ultrasonography in detecting competent and incompetent perforating veins in patients with venous ulceration of the lower leg. *J Vasc Surg.* 1997;26:49–52.

45. Stuart WP, Adam DJ, Bradbury AW, Ruckley CV. Sub-fascial endoscopic perforator surgery is associated with significantly less morbidity and shorter hospital stay than open operation (Linton's procedure). *Br J Surg.* 1997;84:1364–1365.

46. Sarin S, Scurr JH, Coleridge Smith PD. Medial calf perforators in venous disease: the significance of outward flow. *J Vasc Surg.* 1992;16:40–46.

47. Stuart WP, Adam DJ, Allan PL, Ruckley CV. What is the relationship between abnormal perforators, venous function and clinical status? *Phlebology.* 1996;11:169–170.

48. Campbell WA, West A. Duplex ultrasound audit of operative treatmentof primary varicose veins. *Phlebology.* 1995;1(Suppl.):407–409.

49. Walsh JC, Bergan JJ, Beeman S, Comer TP. Femoral venous reflux is abolished by greater saphenous stripping. *Ann Vasc Surg.* 1994;8:566–570.

50. Sales CM, Bilof ML, Petrillo KA, Luka NL. Correction of lower extremity deep venous incompetency by ablation of superficial venous reflux. *Ann Vasc Surg.* 1996;10:186–189.

39

Impact of Superficial Venous Reflux in Chronic Venous Insufficiency

Frank T. Padberg, Jr., MD and
Robert W. Hobson II, MD

INTRODUCTION

Symptoms of venous disease may result from abnormalities in one or all of the superficial, deep, or perforating venous systems. Chronic venous insufficiency (CVI) may result from functional abnormalities of each system alone, but usually implies concomitant abnormalities of more than one system. Superficial venous reflux is the most obvious and its treatment is the most familiar. Perforator and deep venous incompetence are more difficult to diagnose and the effects of treatment remain controversial. Although the role of perforator ablation is not clearly established, the endoscopic approach offers reduced morbidity as compared to previous open surgical procedures.

In our experience, ablation of the superficial venous system restored near normal venous hemodynamics and produced significant clinical improvement when combined with correction of perforating veins. Complete and accurate diagnosis is essential and is facilitated by a working knowledge of current clinical classifications, modern diagnostic imaging, plethysmography, and common anatomic variations. Venous insufficiency manifests symptoms that range from cosmetic defects to disabling ulceration, this chapter focuses primarily on the role of superficial venous reflux in CVI.

CLINCAL EVALUATION AND CLASSIFICATION

Patients with venous insufficiency have a wide spectrum of symptoms, the care of which involves many medical and surgical specialties: dermatology, radiology, vascular medicine, general medicine, physical medicine and rehabilitation, phlebology, surgery, plastic surgery, nursing, wound care specialists, and family practice, as well as vascular surgery. Although the interest of each group is focused on its specific areas of expertise, there is substantial overlap in the approach to wound healing, management of noncompliance, utilization of sclerotherapy, and application of external elastic compression therapy. Because the majority of these patients may initially receive care from nonsurgical practitioners, an integrated approach to interdisciplinary management is important. To accomplish this goal, consensus committees of American and European specialists have attempted to standardize the knowledge base and classification of CVI to facilitate communication across specialty and geographic barriers.[1-3] The standards recommended by the American Venous Forum are reviewed in terms of clinical symptoms, etiology, anatomy, and pathophysiology, which are the cardinal features of the clinical evaluation and classification (CEAP).[1,3]

Clinical Classification and Symptoms

The clinical symptoms in the limbs of patients with CVI are classified as 0–6. Limbs with no venous abnormalities are class 0. Class 1 consists of telangectasia and reticular veins. A superficial varix of the saphenous or its tributary veins is clinical class 2. Edema resulting from venous insufficiency is clinical class 3; however, cautious evaluation of the patient is important here, because edema is also a common manifestation of systemic disease (ie, cardiac, hepatic, or renal failure). Clinical class 4 limbs demonstrate the skin changes typically associated with CVI: brawny edema, thickening, pigmentation, and the subdermal scarring termed *lipodermatosclerosis.* A limb may qualify as a class 4 with any of these skin changes or manifest the chronic mature fibrosis typically described by the shape of an inverted champagne bottle. These patients may develop pruritis, weeping skin, and pain before developing ulceration. Ulcers that have the capacity to heal and reepithelialize are denoted class 5, and ulcers that are currently active are denoted class 6 (Fig. 39–1).

The most severe CVI limbs are those with chronic skin abnormalities that have progressed to healed or active ulceration (class 5 or 6). The clinical scoring system weights the size and frequency of ulceration heavily in defining severity; numeric parameters provide an objective means of comparing interval response for a given limb.[1,3] The maximum clinical symptom score is 18 and consists of values from 0–2 for nine complaints. A disability and anatomic score is also described.[1] Hemodynamic improvement is not recognized in the scores, but may be compared objectively using plethysmographic measurements.

Etiology

The Etiology of CVI is characterized as primary, secondary, or congenital. Primary CVI usually indicates valvular degeneration with or without a known initiating factor. Secondary CVI, usually refers to postthrombotic CVI, but includes that related to prior trauma, and accounts for approximately 20% to 30% of most series of limbs with severe CVI.[4-6] A congenital etiology is unusual and generally requires a different approach to management.

Anatomy

Lower extremity veins are distributed between three systems—the superficial, the deep, and the communicating or perforating veins. The superficial system consists of the greater saphenous vein (GSV) and the lesser saphenous vein (LSV) and their tributaries. The infrainguinal deep system includes the common femoral, [superficial] femoral, profunda, popliteal, tibial, peroneal, soleal, and gastrocnemius veins. The saphenofemoral and saphenopopliteal junctions are important anatomic communications between the two major systems, and accurate identification of these "escape points" is the key

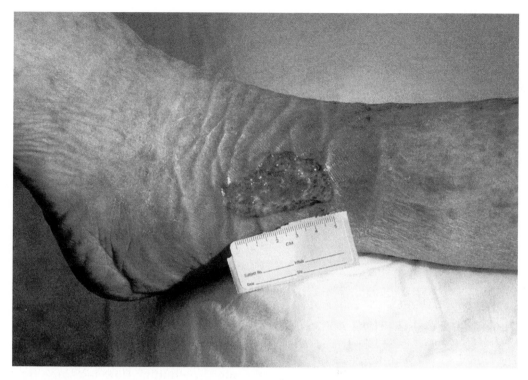

Figure 39–1. A typical ulcer resulting from superficial venous incompetence. The healthy granulating base is encouraging, although epithelial ingrowth is minimal at this time.

to successful understanding and treatment. Severe clinical symptoms resulting from isolated involvement of the superficial or deep venous systems are known to occur, but most individuals with severe CVI have abnormalities of more than one system. [6–11] Perforating veins have several eponyms, are less constant anatomically, and may occur in multiple sites in both the thigh or calf. Isolated perforator vein incompetence is uncommon, and occurs in less than 5% of individuals. [6,8,11–13]

Pathophysiology

Reflux is the most common pathophysiological abnormality in CVI. Obstruction affects a much smaller proportion of limbs with CVI, although it is the predominant factor in acute venous thrombosis. The incidence of limb symptoms resulting from postthrombotic disease remains somewhat controversial. Long-term observation (8 to 13 years) in subjects studied phlebographically and treated with intravenous heparin and oral anticoagulants identified notable skin changes in 16% to 29% and ulcerative venous insufficiency in 3% to 9% [14–17] (Table 39–1). Patients with postthrombotic CVI are younger, tend to be referred to specialty services because of these symptoms, and may respond to conservative or medical management. [18] Patients with superficial reflux are generally older but represent the best surgical candidates. [7,9,19] The clinical evaluation of patients with severe CVI should not be restricted by advanced age. In our own experience, the mean age of 66 years was little different from the 61 years reported by a British investigator. [9] The incidence of severe CVI increases further with increasing age. [2,20]

TABLE 39–1. INCIDENCE OF LIMB SYMPTOMS FOLLOWING PHLEBOGRAPHICALLY CONFIRMED DEEP VENOUS THROMBOSIS

Ref.	Number of Limbs	Mean F/U (years)	Skin Changes (%)	Leg Ulcer (%)
Prandoni et al., 1996[14]	148	8	29	9
Franzeck et al., 1996[15]	39	11.6	28	3
Lindner et al., 1986[16]	24	7.1	16	4
Eichlisberger et al., 1994[17]	223	13	26	
				8
Milne and Ruckley, 1994[18]	86	7	24	15

Subjects treated with intravenous heparin and oral anticoagulants were observed for many years at the same institution. Skin changes consisting of pigmentation and fibrosis, and ankle ulceration represent severe postthrombotic changes. Normal limbs were noted by some, but presence and severity of edema was not recorded consistently. The last study (Milne) included regional referrals from general practitioners for limbs with severe post-thrombotic complaints; substantial improvement in their complaints was achieved by regular use of elastic compression stockings.

CLINICAL EVALUATION AND DIAGNOSTIC IMAGING

The initial focus of examination is to determine whether there is superficial system involvement and subsequently to localize the site(s) permitting flow to escape from the deep to superficial venous systems. The functional abnormality commonly originates from the saphenofemoral or saphenopopliteal junction. However, other communicating veins in the thigh or the calf may also contribute substantial reflux (Figs. 39–2 and 39–3).

The clinical assessment of limbs with CVI is significantly enhanced by the use of noninvasive techniques, particularly Doppler ultrasound.[7,8,21–24] With the patient standing, the saphenous vein trunk and prominent varices are identified. These are then assessed by direct palpation and Doppler insonation. Presence or absence of venous reflux is assessed by Valsalva or coughing maneuvers. In conjunction with Doppler augmentation, percussion of distended veins is useful to determine superficial venous incompetence. By careful observation of the effects of digital control at the escape points, a reasonable clinical localization of these sites can be ascertained.

Duplex ultrasonography characterizes venous reflux and obstruction in each anatomic segment using color- and gray-scale imaging, complemented by directional flow signals. A widely accepted ultrasound criteria for reflux is retrograde venous flow of greater than 0.5 sec following Valsalva or proximal venous compression.[8,9,21–23] Obstruction from prior deep system thrombosis is an important prognostic finding. Mapping communicating veins is a helpful adjunct prior to surgical intervention (Fig. 39–4). A more comprehensive discussion of duplex imaging for CVI can be found in another chapter of this book.

Phlebography, ascending or descending (antegrade or retrograde), may be required to further define the anatomic basis of CVI. However, its importance has declined as the accuracy of noninvasive imaging has improved. It is particularly useful in unusual situations, such as congenital and anatomic variants (see Fig. 39–2). Direct puncture varicography is also useful for evaluation of recurrent variceal disease. Venous applications of magnetic resonance imaging (MRI) and computed tomography (CT) are not well defined at this time.

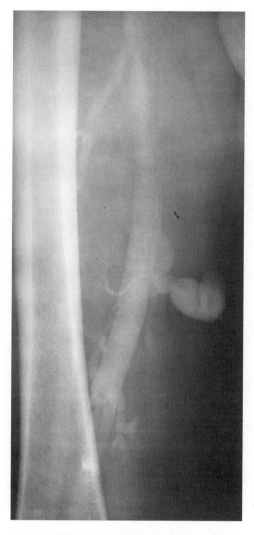

Figure 39–2. This ascending phlebogram demonstrates a large, incompetent perforating vein in the thigh. (*Reprinted from* Cardiovascular Surgery, *(in press), Padberg FT Jr, Surgical intervention in venous ulceration, copyright (1998), with permission from Elsevier Science.*)

PHYSIOLOGICAL EVALUATION—PLETHYSMOGRAPHY

The hemodynamic abnormalities of CVI have been evaluated using plethysmographic and dynamic pressure studies. These include air plethysmography,[25-27] photoplethysmography,[4,5,28,29] and foot volume plethysmography.[19,30,31] Ambulatory venous pressures accurately assess calf pump function, but are cumbersome and invasive.[27,31] The air plethysmograph (APG) measures reflux, calf pump function, and obstruction in a single examination and returns reproducible results on serial examinations.[7,25-27] Foot volume plethysmography, which has been validated and used extensively in Europe, also measures calf pump function and reflux, but requires the patient to perform 20 rapid deep-knee bends and is not used in limbs with open ulcers.[19,30,31] The residual volume

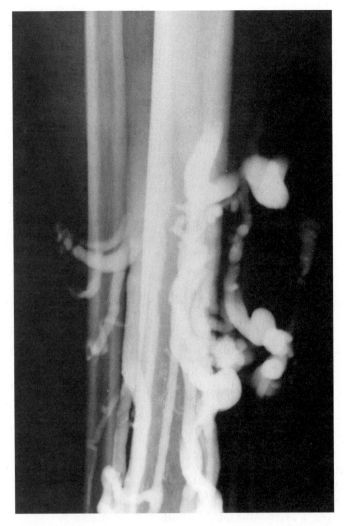

Figure 39–3. This ascending phlebogram demonstrates a pair of calf perforating veins. The perforators are also marked on the skin in Fig. 39–4. (*Reprinted from* Cardiovascular Surgery, *(in press), Padberg FT Jr, Surgical intervention in venous ulceration, copyright (1998), with permission from Elsevier Science.*)

fraction measured by APG compares favorably with ambulatory venous pressure (Fig. 39–5). We currently recommend APG, which contributes multiple physiological measurements from a single noninvasive instrument.

Air plethysmographic examinations are conducted as described by Back et al.[25] and by Christopoulos et al.[26] (APG 1000C; ACI Medical Inc., Sun Valley, CA). Reflux into the calf is determined by measurement of the venous filling index (VFI), which is a measure of the average rate of increase in calf volume that occurs when the subject changes from a supine position with the leg elevated to a standing position. The venous system is tested for obstruction by measurement of outflow fraction (OF), which is measured in the supine position with a thigh-occluding cuff placed on the elevated extremity; OF represents the percentage of venous volume drained from the calf within 1 s of release of the occluding cuff. Calf pump function was

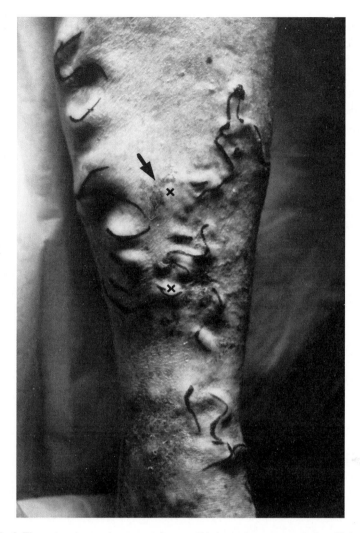

Figure 39–4. The extensive saphenous varices on this lower leg communicate with two marked perforating veins (X) that communicate with the posterior tibial vein. See Fig. 39–3 for venographic correlation.

determined by measurement of ejection fraction (EF), the measure of the percentage of venous volume expelled from the calf with a single tiptoe maneuver; and by residual volume fraction (RVF), a measure of the percentage of venous volume remaining in the calf after a series of 10 tiptoe maneuvers. These maneuvers and a typical tracing are illustrated in Fig. 39–6. Studies may be performed on the ulcerated limb, are obtained prior to surgical intervention, and are repeated at regular postoperative intervals.

TECHNICAL ASPECTS OF THE PROCEDURE

The surgical plan is facilitated by preoperative marking of calf and thigh perforating veins in the vascular laboratory (see Fig. 39–4). Superficial tributaries designated for

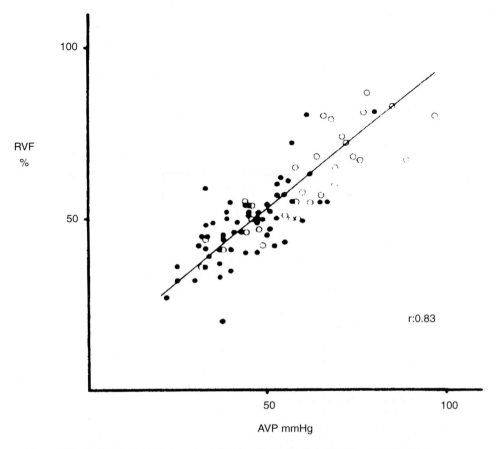

Figure 39–5. Relationship between residual volume fraction (RVF) and ambulatory venous pressure (AVP) at the end of tenth tiptoe movement (solid circles represent limbs with superficial venous incompetence; open circles represent limbs with deep venous disease). (*Reprinted from* Journal of Vascular Surgery, *page 153, volume 5, Christopoulos D et al, Air plethysmography and the effect of elastic compression on venous hemodynamics of the leg, copyright (1987), with permission from Mosby, Inc.*)

ablation are also marked with the patient in the standing position. Cellulitis and inflammation are brought under control; ideally, ulcers are healed prior to surgical intervention.

The saphenofemoral junction is approached via a transverse incision 1 to 2 cm below and parallel to the inguinal ligament. The saphenous trunk is identified and dissection extended proximally into the fossa ovalis. The junction with the common femoral vein is visualized and all tributary branches are ligated as is the saphenous stump. Identification of the main saphenous trunk in the proximal lower leg is facilitated by its anatomic proximity to the saphenous nerve and by intraluminal passage of the obturator from the proximal dissection. More distal stripping of the main venous trunk is not recommended because of its associated higher incidence of saphenous neuritis. When extensive and large variceal tributaries are present in this area, dissection and ligation is facilitated by enlarging the incision. The main saphenous trunk is separated from the nerve and ligated at the distal aspect of the incision. The stripper is visualized

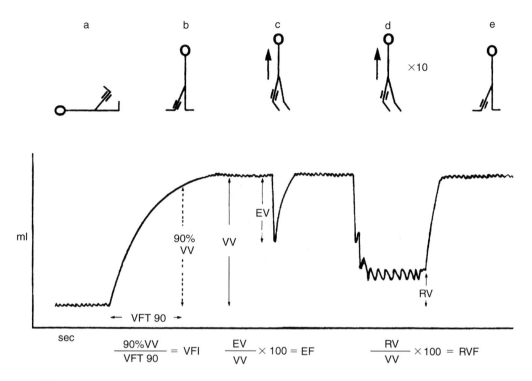

$$\frac{90\%VV}{VFT\ 90} = VFI \qquad \frac{EV}{VV} \times 100 = EF \qquad \frac{RV}{VV} \times 100 = RVF$$

Figure 39–6. This schematic is a diagrammatic representation of a typical recording of volume changes during a standard sequence of postural changes and exercise. (**A**) The patient begins in the supine position with the leg elevated 45°. (**B**) The patient then stands with weight on the nonexamined leg. (**C**) Single tiptoe movement. (**D**) Ten tiptoe movements. (**E**) Same as in (**B**). VV, function venous volume; VFT, venous filling time; VFI, venous filling index; EV, ejected volume; RV, residual volume; EF, ejection fraction; RVF, residual volume fraction. (*Reprinted from Journal of Vascular Surgery, p. 150, vol. 5. Christopoulos D, et al., Air plethysmography and the effect of elastic compression on venous hemodynamics of the leg, copyright (1987), with permission from Mosby, Inc.*)

within the vein, brought out through a small venotomy, and a ligature placed around the vein and the stripper. The removed vein is inspected in its full length on the obturator. This incision is also useful as a trocar insertion site for endoscopic ligation of the perforating veins in the subfascial plane. A second incision is then used for a second port. Using CO_2 insufflation, the subfascial space is dissected. Both the marked and unmarked perforating veins are clipped using a 5 mm or 10 mm clip applier. The endoscopic technique for perforator ligation has proved as effective as the open procedure[12] and reduced the high morbidity from the lengthy incision previously used for open surgical ligation.[32]

Although some have attempted to preserve the saphenous vein by high ligation of the saphenous trunk alone, this has not proved as durable as ligation and stripping.[24,33] Because of its high early recurrence rate, sclerotherapy for perforating veins or saphenofemoral and saphenopopliteal incompetency has been shown to be inferior to surgical treatment.[2,34]

Postoperative clinical evaluation is supplemented by duplex ultrasonography and APG at 1- and 6-month intervals thereafter, thus providing both hemodynamic and anatomic data on the durability of the procedure. Residual symptoms are assessed, as is compliance with compression stockings.

RESULTS

Sustained improvement in hemodynamics and clinical outcome have been demonstrated for combined superficial and perforating vein ligations.[7,10,19,28,29] We combined communicating vein ligations with superficial vein procedures in patients whose saphenous incompetence was accompanied by deep reflux, in the absence of prior thromboses.[7] Thus, mean postoperative hemodynamic parameters were evaluated by serial APG, and returned toward normal (Fig. 39–7).[7,35] Reflux, as determined by VFI, decreased from 12 ± 5 ml/s to 2.6 ± 1.3 ml/s at last follow-up exam. Calf pump function, as determined by EF and RVF, returned to normal values during extended observation. Ejection fraction (EF) 43 ± 11% increased to 65 ± 14%; greater than 60% is considered normal. RVF decreased from 56 ± 15% to 26 ± 14%; greater than 35% is considered abnormal. The continued trend toward normal values for both reflux and calf pump function (Fig. 39–8) has been sustained to date.

Mean clinical symptom scores (CEAP) decreased significantly from 10 ± 1 to 1.45 ± 1.0 ($p < .0001$). These results have remained stable following the procedure, and there has been no recurrent ulceration. A clinical outcome grade of +2.2 was assigned to these individuals on clinical reassessment following surgical intervention. A general sense of improved well-being and improved daily function have been remarked on by the patients, but this has not been subjected to scientific evaluation.

Perforating vein ligations were also combined with superficial vein procedures by Bradbury and associates,[19] who followed a series of patients for a median of 66 months. Superficial incompetence was identified on clinical examination by these experienced British surgeons, and serial hemodynamics evaluated by foot volumetry. Outcome was measured by freedom from ulceration and improved hemodynamics; after 42 months,

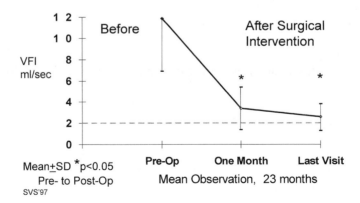

Figure 39–7. Impact of surgical intervention on reflux. Graphic representation of changes in venous filling index (VFI as ml/s) measured before, 1 month after, and 2 years after saphenous and perforating vein ablation. (*Reprinted from* Cardiovascular Surgery, *(in press), Padberg FT Jr, Surgical intervention in venous ulceration, copyright (1998), with permission from Elsevier Science.*)

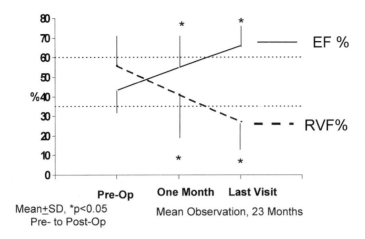

Figure 39–8. Impact of surgical intervention on calf pump function. Graphic representation of changes in ejection fraction (EF) and residual volume fraction (RVF) measured before, 1 month after, and at 2 years after saphenous and perforating vein ablation.

although 79% of limbs remained ulcer-free, hemodynamic deterioration in the remainder heralded recurrence of ulceration. Duplex evaluation became available during later follow-up and was employed to evaluate 9 limbs with recurrent ulceration. Popliteal incompetence was found in 8 of 9 and saphenous incompetence in 6 of 9. This experience demonstrates the value of regular hemodynamic observations in this patient population; foot volume plethysmography, like APG, is an accurate and noninvasive measure readily accepted on a repetitive basis by the CVI patient. A companion report strongly supported the routine use of Doppler investigation in the preoperative evaluation of patients with advanced CVI.[24] Darke and Penfold[10] performed saphenous excision without perforator ligations on 54 patients with combined saphenous and perforator incompetence; at 3 years, 9% of the ulcers recurred in limbs, with Doppler findings of popliteal area and lesser saphenous incompetence. Thus, surgical correction of both saphenous veins and perforator incompetence is appropriate when identified preoperatively.

In our own experience, deep vein valvular incompetence was also present as determined by duplex evaluation. Severity ranged from segmental to extensive. In some limbs, this was completely corrected following superficial and perforator ligations, an observation also noted by Walsh et al.[23] Pearce et al.,[28] using photoplethysmography, and Akesson et al.,[31] using direct venous pressures and foot volumetry, have also demonstrated that superficial ablation improved venous function in the presence of deep venous incompetence. Others have also advocated superficial and perforating vein ablation for ulcerative CVI in limbs with deep venous incompetence; continued use of elastic compression hosiery is recommended to manage the residual deep vein incompetence.[18,29]

Thus, a consensus has developed in which patients with severe CVI have improved clinically and hemodyamically after ablation of incompetent superficial and communicating veins.[2,7,10,19,23,24,28,29,31,33,35] Duplex evaluation adds accuracy to the initial examination.[7,9,19,21] Abnormal hemodynamics or deterioration during observation should stimulate further duplex evaluation, with the goal of identifying correctable sites of reflux.[10,19,24,33]

RECURRENCE

Recurrence of symptoms in patients with chronic venous disease is often expected. However, recurrence of saphenous varices should be evaluated separately from recurrence of ankle ulceration, as different management approaches are generally recommended. In 5-year observation, supervised medical therapy achieves freedom from ulceration in approximately 70% of compliant individuals.[4,5] Zippered stockings, ingenious smooth insertion slippers, and prestretching frames are available to help maintain compliance with external elastic compression. However, despite these mechanical aids, many patients have difficulty with this regimen. Noncompliance with a conservative program of care is a major issue that, if present, increases the likelihood of recurrent symptoms and ulcers. Frequent counseling of patients, recruitment of their families, and home care visits are helpful in reducing the impact of this factor.

Because surgical ablation of the superficial and perforating veins has proved efficacious in maintaining freedom from ulceration, recurrence of superficial venous incompetence becomes a significant issue in management. Although saphenous ligation and stripping has usually been regarded as a straightforward procedure, reports describing recurrence following saphenectomy have emphasized technical considerations at the site of saphenectomy. The cause of recurrence ranges from retention of major venous trunks or branches and neovascularization with enlargement of small venous collaterals to popliteal–lesser saphenous incompetence.[10,24,33,36] It is often unclear whether these findings were missed at the original operation or if they developed during interval follow-up. Postoperative hemodynamic and duplex examinations may identify the cause and define appropriate procedures for revision. Phlebography is particularly useful in the evaluation of recurrent superficial venous incompetence. Operative management of recurrent disease usually involves repeat saphenofemoral ligation or ablation of unusual thigh-perforating veins, saphenous duplications, or other incompetent veins in the region of the popliteal.[10,19,24,33,36] Rivlin,[36] in an experience of more than 2000 procedures, reported a 6% recurrence rate for superficial varicosities in the era that preceded the wide use of duplex evaluation. Of the vein operations performed in the Lothian region, 20% were performed for recurrent disease; the authors specifically addressed the improved preoperative assessment by routine use of Doppler ultrasound.[24] More widespread application of duplex imaging coupled with experienced surgical intervention results in a minimal recurrence rate and improved outcome from these procedures.

NONSURGICAL MANAGEMENT OF CHRONIC VENOUS INSUFFICIENCY

Not all patients with severe CVI are appropriate candidates for surgical intervention. Despite ingenious surgical management, limbs with evidence of prior thrombosis have not responded as favorably as limbs with reflux alone. Although establishing the daily routine can present a clinical challenge, a reasonable outcome is achieved by habitual use of prosthetic external compression hosiery.[4,5,18] With the interrelationship between calf pump function, joint mobility, and muscle strength, there is promise for additional intervention, such as directed physical therapy.[21,25]

Similarly, there is a discrepancy between clinical symptomatology and the physiological abnormalities described with venous insufficiency. Although there is a clear association between the severity of disease and the physiological abnormality, it is not uniform. For example, not all limbs with "severe" reflux develop symptoms of severe CVI.[6,10,18,26] Similarly, there is a question of why more patients do not develop postthrombotic sequelae following deep venous thrombosis (DVT). Something other than the hemodynamic abnormality is necessary to explain the symptoms of severe CVI. Further investigation into microscopic and molecular interactions (i.e., topical growth factors, such as platelet derived growth factor or PDGF) also hold promise for improved therapeutic interventions.[37,38]

SUMMARY AND CONCLUSIONS

The impact of superficial venous ablation on clinical symptoms and hemodynamic outcome is significant and durable. Directed surgical intervention follows accurate diagnosis. Saphenous ligation and superficial vein excision is beneficial for many patients with CVI. Advanced adjunctive procedures involving directed ligation of calf and other perforating veins are indicated for patients with skin and subcutaneous manifestations of CVI (CEAP classes 4, 5, and 6). Accurate diagnosis of recurrent or unusual "escape points" from the deep to the superficial venous systems may require more extensive diagnostic evaluation.

REFERENCES

1. Statement of the International Consensus Committee on Chronic Venous Diseases. Classification and grading of chronic venous disease in the lower limbs. Chap 38 in Handbook of Venous Disorders, Gloviczki P, Yao JST, eds. London: Chapman and Hall; 1996;652–660.
2. Alexander House Group. Consensus statement: consensus paper on venous leg ulcers. *Phlebology*. 1992;7:48–58.
3. Porter J, Moneta G. Reporting standards in venous disease: an update. *J Vasc Surg*. 1995;21:635–645.
4. Mayberry JC, Moneta GL, Taylor LM, Porter JM. Fifteen-year results of ambulatory compression therapy for chronic venous ulcers. *Surgery*. 1991;109:575–581.
5. Erickson CA, Lanza DJ, Karp DL, Edwards JW, et al. Healing of venous ulcers in an ambulatory care program: the roles of chronic venous insufficiency and patient compliance. *J Vasc Surg*. 1995;22:629–636.
6. Labropoulos N, Delis K, Nicolaides AN, Leon M, et al. The role of the distribution and anatomic extent of reflux in the development of signs and symptoms in chronic venous insufficiency. *J Vasc Surg*. 1996;23:504–510.
7. Padberg FT Jr, Pappas PJ, Araki CJ, Back TL, et al. Hemodynamic and clinical improvement after superficial vein ablation in primary combined venous insufficiency with ulceration. *J Vasc Surg*. 1996;24:711–718.
8. Lees TA, Lambert D. Patterns of venous reflux in limbs with skin changes associated with chronic venous insufficiency. *Br J Surg*. 1993;80:725–28.
9. Shami SK, Sarin S, Cheatle TR, Scurr JH, et al. Venous ulcers and the superficial venous system. *J Vasc Surg*. 1993;17:487–490.
10. Darke SG, Penfold C. Venous ulceration and saphenous ligation. *Eur J Vasc Endovasc Surg*. 1992;6:4–9.
11. Kistner RL. Definitive diagnosis and definitive treatment in chronic venous disease: a concept whose time has come. *J Vasc Surg*. 1996;24:703–710.

12. Gloviczki P, Bergan JJ, Menawat SS, et al. Safety, feasibility, and early efficacy of subfascial endoscopic perforator surgery: a preliminary report from the North American registry. *J Vasc Surg*. 1997;25:94–105.

13. Burnand KG, O'Donnell TF, Lea Thomas M, Browse NL. The relative importance of incompetent communicating veins in the production of varicose veins and venous ulcers. *Surgery*. 1977;82:9–14.

14. Prandoni P, Lensing AWA, Cogo A, Cuppini S, et al. The long-term clinical course of acute deep venous thrombosis. *Ann Intern Medicine*. 1996;125:1–7.

15. Franzeck UK, Schalch I, Jager KA, Schneider E, et al. Prospective 12-year follow-up study of clinical and hemodynamic sequelae after deep vein thrombosis in low-risk patients (Zurich study). *Circulation*. 1996;93:74–79.

16. Lindner DJ, Edwards JM, Phinney ES, Taylor LM, et al. Long-term hemodynamic and clinical sequelae of lower extremity deep vein thrombosis. *J Vasc Surg*. 1986;4:436–442.

17. Eichlisberger R, Frauchiger B, Widmer MT, Widmer LK, et al. Spatfolgen der tiefen venenthrombose: ein 13-jahres follow-up von 223 patienten. *VASA*. 1994;23:234–243.

18. Milne AA, Ruckley CV. The clinical course of patients following extensive deep venous thrombosis. *Eur J Vasc Surg*. 1994;8:56–59.

19. Bradbury AW, Stonebridge PA, Callam MJ, Ruckley CV, et al. Foot volumetry and duplex ultrasound after saphenous and perforating vein ligation. *Br J Surg*. 1993;80:845–848.

20. Callam MJ, Harper DR, Dale JJ, Ruckley CV. Chronic ulcer of the leg: clincal history. *Brit Med J*. 1987;294:1389–1391.

21. Araki CT, Back TL, Padberg FT, Thompson PN, et al. Refinements in the detection of popliteal vein reflux. *J Vasc Surg*. 1993;18:742–748.

22. vanBemellen PS, Bedford G, Beach K, Strandness DE. Quantitative segmental evaluation of venous valvular reflux with duplex ultrasound scanning. *J Vasc Surg*. 1989;10:425–431.

23. Walsh JC, Bergan JJ, Beeman S, Comer T. Femoral venous reflux is abolished by greater saphenous stripping. *Ann Vasc Surg*. 1994;8:566–570.

24. Bradbury AW, Stonebridge PA, Ruckley CV, Beggs I. Recurrent varicose veins? Correlation between preoperative clinical and hand-held Doppler ultrasonographic examination and anatomical findings at surgery. *Br J Surg*. 1993;80:849–851.

25. Back TL, Padberg FT, Thompson PN, Hobson RW. Limited range of motion is a significant factor in venous ulceration. *J Vasc Surg*. 1995;22:19–23.

26. Christopoulos DG, Nicolaides AN, Szendro G, Irvine AT, et al. Air plethysmography and the effect of elastic compression on venous hemodynamics of the leg. *J Vasc Surg*. 1987;5;148–159.

27. Nicolaides AN, Christopolous D, Vasdekis S. Progress in the investigation of chronic venous insufficiency. *Ann Vasc Surg*. 1989;3:278–289.

28. Pearce WH, Ricco JB, Queral LA, Flinn WR, et al. Hemodynamic assessment of venous problems. *Surgery*. 1983;93:715–721.

29. Negus D, Friedgood A. The effective management of venous ulceration. *Br J Surg*. 1983;70:623–627.

30. Stacey MC, Burnand KG, Layer GT, Pattison M. Calf pump function in patients with healed venous ulcers is not improved by surgery to the communicating veins or by elastic stockings. *Br J Surg*. 1988;75:436–439.

31. Akesson H, Brudin L, Cwikiel W, Ohlin P, et al. Does the correction of insufficient superficial and perforating veins improve venous function in patients with deep venous insufficiency? *Phlebology*. 1992;5:113–123.

32. Linton R. John Homans' impact on diseases of the veins of the lower extremity, with special references to deep thrombophlebitis and the post-thrombotic syndrome with ulceration. The John Homans Lecture, Society for Vascular Surgery, 1976. *Surgery*. 1977;81:1–11.

33. Darke SG. Recurrent varicose veins and short saphenous insufficiency: evaluation and treatment. Chapter 15. Bergan JJ and Yao JST, eds, *Venous Disorders*. Philadelphia: WB Saunders; 1991;217–232.

34. Hobbs JT. Surgery and sclerotherapy in the treatment of varicose veins: a random trial. *Arch Surg*. 1974;109:793–796.

35. Padberg FT Jr. Surgical intervention in chronic venous ulceration. *Cardiovascular Surgery*. (in press).

36. Rivlin S. The surgical cure of primary varicose veins. *Br J Surg.* 1975;62:913–917.
37. Pappas PJ, DeFouw DO, Venezio LM, Gorti R, et al. Morphometric assessment of the dermal microcirculation in patients with chronic venous insufficiency. *J Vasc Surg.* 1997;26:784–795.
38. Rothe M, Falanga V. Growth factors: their biology and promise in dermatologic diseases and tissue repair. *Arch Dermatol.* 1989;125:1390–1398.

40

Treatment Strategies for Venous Leg Ulcers

Vincent Falanga, MD, FACP

INTRODUCTION

There has been increasing appreciation of the morbidity associated with venous ulcers, including a markedly decreased quality of life and loss of independence.[1] It is also becoming clear that venous ulcers do not heal as readily as individual physicians' experience or retrospective studies might suggest.[2-5] Several large prospective studies indicate that standard compression therapy alone in the ambulatory setting heals about 50% to 60% of patients within a 6 month period of treatment.[3-5] The longer the ulcer remains unhealed, of course, the more likely certain complications become, including the need for frequent surgical debridement and hospitalization for cellulitis or grafting. Other major components of the morbidity and costs associated with nonhealing venous ulcers are specialized dressings and bandages, doctors' visits and the need for home visiting nurses, and the patients' inability to work and loss of productivity.[1,6] Hence, there is a great deal of interest in finding new and effective means of accelerating venous ulcer healing.

The focus of venous ulcer care is to reduce healing time and, ultimately, ulcer recurrence. This article reviews some of the newer approaches and what might be expected in the first decade of the twenty-first century, specifically in the context of venous ulcer pathogenesis.

PATHOPHYSIOLOGY AND TREATMENT IMPLICATIONS

In normal subjects, contraction of the calf muscles causes increased venous return from the foot and lower leg, which leads to a decrease in deep vein pressure and to the development of a pressure differential between the deep and superficial venous systems. As a result, blood flows from the superficial veins through the communicating veins and into the deep venous system. In patients with obstructed deep veins, valvular dysfunction or malformation, or faulty action of the calf muscles, the sequence of events outlined does not occur normally. Thus, pressure fails to fall in the deep veins, resulting in venous hypertension.[7] There are important therapeutic implications to the physiological steps outlined. For example, a patient with venous ulcers would be at a greater disadvantage in performing a job requiring immobile standing—for instance, being a cashier—than a job in which walking is required. This has to be kept in mind when advising patients and disability insurance companies. For similar reasons, inelastic compression bandages (such as the Unna boot), which require muscle pump action for optimal effectiveness, may be a poor choice for a nonambulatory patient confined to a nursing home.[8]

It is common to regard venous hypertension and its associated problems in a global sense; that is, as affecting the entire leg and measurable by air plethysmography or other more direct determinations of vein pressure. However, less is known about "localized" effects of venous hypertension, which are likely to be quite variable in different segments of the leg, and probably dictate where loss of tissue integrity and ulceration occur. For example, Greenberg et al.[9] reported that in early lipodermatosclerosis without ulceration, an underlying incompetent perforator can frequently be found.[9] Advances in the direct (ie, endoscopic) and noninvasive (ie, color duplex scanning) assessment of venous disease and localization of abnormal communicating veins facilitates ulcer treatment based on faulty underlying venous vessels. This may be accomplished by sclerotherapy or by surgical means, depending on the circumstances and the extent of venous disease.

At the tissue and molecular levels there are several abnormalities that might help explain the development of venous ulcers. Proposed by Browse and Burnand in 1982,[10] the first well-articulated hypothesis for the development of venous ulcers suggested that fibrinogen leaks out of distended dermal capillaries (thought to be increased in number at that time), polymerizes to fibrin cuffs around the capillaries, and leads to the formation of a barrier to the diffusion of oxygen and other nutrients. A different view of the significance of fibrin deposition in venous disease was expressed by Falanga and Eaglstein in 1993,[11] who proposed that fibrinogen deposition is but one of the many macromolecules that leak into the dermis and suggested that such leaked macromolecules, including albumin and α2-macroglobulin, bind to or trap growth factors and matrix materials and make them unavailable to the repair process or for overall tissue integrity. Evidence for and against these two hypotheses has been reviewed.[7] From the therapeutic standpoint, the notion that fibrin deposition and fibrin cuffs play a key pathogenic role suggests that fibrin removal may be beneficial. Indeed, Falango and coworkers[12] showed that the topical application of tissue plasminogen activator (tPA), which is able to break down fibrin, may accelerate ulcer healing. Also, if trapping of growth factors by fibrin and other macromolecules does take place, there might be ways to block this process pharmacologically.

Clear therapeutic implications also underlie the hypothesis of lymphocyte trapping, where leukocytes are thought to adhere to the endothelium and cause vascular damage by the release of certain mediators.[7,13] Reports of the effectiveness in venous ulcers of pentoxifylline, a drug interfering with the activity of tumor necrosis factor α and with lymphocyte adherence to endothelial cells, fit nicely with the lymphocyte trapping hypothesis.[4]

Other useful hypotheses are emerging that also provide direct links to therapeutic intervention. For example, there is increasing evidence that the wound fluid from venous ulcers contains proteases capable of digesting extracellular matrix components, such as fibronectin and vitronectin.[14] These studies point to control of this highly proteolytic environment as a possible treatment. There have also been reports that wound fluid collected from venous ulcers, in contrast to fluid obtained from acute wounds,[15] inhibits proliferation of keratinocytes, fibroblasts, and endothelial cells.[16]

Whether removing possible inhibitors of cell growth that accumulate in wound fluid would enhance even further the positive effects of occlusion is a tantalizing thought. Perhaps there are ways to modify wound dressings so as to remove such inhibitors selectively.

More recently, Hasan et al.[17] showed that fibroblast cultures derived from venous ulcers and surrounding skin are unresponsive to the stimulatory action on collagen synthesis of certain growth factors, such as transforming growth factor $\beta 1$. These findings of phenotypic alteration of resident cells from within the wound have a number of therapeutic implications, including the possible need for more extensive debridement than is presently being done. Also, the findings of altered cells would argue for thorough debridement followed by greater use of grafting with either autologous or cultured skin. Autologous grafts and bioengineered skin may work by providing, at least for a critical period of time, new cells capable of producing the proper matrix material or growth factors.

CURRENT MANAGEMENT OF VENOUS ULCERS

The previous section serves the dual purpose of describing some of the main concepts regarding the pathogenesis of venous ulcers and linking them to present and future therapeutic strategies. This section describes what is presently available to treat venous ulcers and highlights new therapeutic interventions.

Compression Therapy

The mainstay of treatment of venous disease and ulceration is directed at correcting or improving some of the consequences of venous hypertension. Compression therapy, usually with bandages or graded stockings, or with sequential extremity pumps, achieves that purpose to a reasonable extent, mainly by removing edema. It should be noted that it is unlikely that compression bandages alone, without, for example, surgical procedures, are actually able to correct the venous hypertension. There is a great deal of controversy about what constitutes optimal compression therapy, and here one might point out that this often becomes an emotional issue among investigators, and not one that is always based on experimental and controlled evidence. The first problem encountered is that clinicians do not always recognize the different mechanisms of action of rigid (ie, Unna boot) versus elastic bandages. In reality, the Unna boot is not a true compression bandage, and it is inappropriate to assess or make predictions about its effectiveness based on measurements of the resting pressure it exerts over the leg. Whereas elastic bandages work by exerting pressure over the leg at all times, the mechanism of action of the Unna boot is more complex and is based on pressing of the calf muscles against the bandage's semirigid structure during ambulation.[18] The Unna boot remains a favorite bandage among many clinicians in the United States. It is easy to apply, reasonably effective, and inexpensive. Its major drawbacks are that it generally requires an ambulatory patient in order to be effective (ie, it requires muscle pump action), does not readjust pressure as edema decreases, and has ingredients and preservatives that may exacerbate venous dermatitis. Also, because it is generally changed once a week, the Unna boot becomes soiled with wound exudate and can be quite malodorous. Some of these drawbacks can be dealt with, but it is clear that many clinicians, particularly in Europe, prefer elastic compression for treatment of venous ulcers.

There have been several attempts to classify compression bandages in a more rational manner.[19] There are three major classes of bandages: class 1 (conforming stretch), class 2 (light support), and class 3 (compression). Class 3, or compression bandages, are further classified (classes 3a, 3b, 3c, and 3d) depending on an increasing level of subbandage resting pressure at the ankle. High-compression bandages (3c) are commonly used and produce ankle pressures of 25 to 35 mm Hg. This classification is useful but, for most clinicians, it may be easier to think of bandages as being either short stretch or long stretch. The Unna boot, which one might consider as having no stretch at all, has undergone some modifications (ie, UnnaFlex, Convatec) and can probably be classified as short-stretch bandage (or perhaps as class 2 in the previously mentioned classification). Such short-stretch bandages have a low resting pressure and a high working pressure (ie, during ambulation). The Unna boot and other types of short-stretch bandages are useful and safe in the treatment of edema in the ambulatory patient with venous ulcers. Because their resting pressures are low, short-stretch bandages are less likely to cause edema of the toes, which in this author's experience can be a problem with more aggressive use of compression in patients with venous ulcers and concomitant lymphatic disease. If the patient is nonambulatory or if the clinician wishes to achieve more rapid removal of edema, long-stretch bandages, such as Coban (3M), Co-Plus (Smith & Nephew), and Surepress (Convatec) can be used. In treating patients with long-stretch bandages, it is important to monitor the patient more closely at the beginning to ensure that distal edema does not develop and that there is no vascular compromise.

Treatment with compression bandages can be modified by applying more than one bandage or by first applying nonstretch material to better prepare the leg for a compression bandage. For example, the four-layer bandage system (ie, Profore, Smith & Nephew) has gained some popularity. It consists of a first layer of cotton padding to protect certain vulnerable areas of the leg (malleoli, tibial surface) and to make the leg more uniformly conical in shape. A second crepe-type bandage is used to smooth out the first layer, and is followed by a high (25 to 35 mm Hg) compression bandage applied in a figure of eight. The last, fourth layer consists of a cohesive bandage applied in a spiral fashion.[20]

Studies are needed to compare the efficacy of the different schemes of bandaging outlined previously. For now, our view is that the expertise and experience in applying and managing the problems associated with a particular bandage are probably more important than the bandage category chosen. One published meta-analysis of several venous ulcer trials that used different compression bandages supports this view.[21] True correction of venous hypertension is unlikely to be achieved with any of the compression modality. Also, we may not be paying enough attention to the possibility that certain areas of the leg, including those bearing the ulcer, may be receiving less compression than other areas. Laplace's law states that pressure is directly proportional to bandage tension and inversely proportional to the radius: $P = NT/R$, where P is pressure, N is number of layers, T is tension, and R is radius. Because the leg is not exactly conical, the radius of curvature differs at locations along each horizontal segment. For this reason, some form of padding is commonly used immediately over the ulcer before a bandage is applied. This has the effect of increasing pressure over the ulcer.

Quite reasonable healing rates can be obtained with the combination of proper compression and a moist wound environment. A prospective study showed that up to 55% of venous ulcer patients healed completely and within a very short period of time (12 weeks) when the ulcer was treated with a hydrocolloid followed by a short-stretch bandage and an elastic compression bandage.[5]

Wound Debridement and Topical Therapy

It has already been mentioned that debridement may be an effective way not only of removing necrotic material, treating infection, and stimulating the wound, but also as a method for eliminating cells within and around the wound that have undergone what is termed *phenotypic dysregulation*. Surprisingly, it is not known whether thorough surgical debridement of venous ulcers would result in better healing rates, either when the wound heals primarily or when autologous grafts are used. The impression is that surgeons and other physicians have been much less aggressive in debriding venous ulcers than, for example, pressure ulcers or diabetic neuropathic ulcers. One reason for this is that clear-cut necrotic and nonviable tissue is often present within pressure-induced ulcers, whereas the wound bed of venous ulcers often presents a fibrinous appearance, without eschar; the viability of this tissue is more difficult to interpret.

There is substantial evidence that a first, painless approach to venous ulcer debridement is to rely on the autolytic action of occlusive dressings. Hydrocolloids, films, and gels have been used for this purpose. At this point, there is a large body of information about the unlikelihood that occlusive therapy leads to infection.[22] However, considerable fear of this complication still exists, particularly among surgeons, who have to deal with many different types of wounds and who have generally been taught to leave the wound dry. It is suspected that it will take continued and consistently positive experience with moist wound healing for most surgeons to accept it as a mode of therapy. It also must be recognized that every form of therapy has its complications. For example, it has been reported, and this author has had a similar experience, that the use of occlusive dressings in venous ulcers may lead to a form of wound bed contamination (without obvious clinical signs of infection) manifested by a green–yellow wound base[20]; discontinuation of the occlusive therapy often improves the situation, but surgical debridement may be required. At the moment, it is not possible to predict which venous ulcers will behave this way when treated with occlusion. However, it remains prudent not to occlude wounds that appear infected or in which heavy bacterial contamination is present. It is of great interest that occlusion of wounds has proved safe in the experimental and clinical situation, despite the fact that bacterial wound counts increase under occlusive dressings.[23] It is possible that the pathogenicity of organisms is a function of their growth configuration in addition to their absolute number and type.

Topical debriding enzymes or antibiotics are often used for debridement or treatment of venous ulcers. Their effectiveness is variable and not certain, although in some circumstances the results can be dramatic. It is possible that topical enzymatic treatment requires optimal wound conditions to be effective (ie, pH). Some topically applied antibiotics, such as silver sulfadiazine, appear to be effective. However, in a double-blind randomized study, topically applied mupirocin was not effective in improving many chronic wound parameters, including wound bed appearance.[24] One of the problems with topical antibiotics is that they lead to bacterial resistance and, probably, to the emergence of organisms that are difficult to treat in the wound bed. Cadexomer iodine could be used as an alternative.[25] This effective antimicrobial and debriding agent is probably underutilized, especially in the United States. It is possible that clinicians, including surgeons, have become so very suspicious of antiseptics and their potential to interfere with healing that they are now reluctant to reconsider what appear to be safe versions of antiseptic therapy. Cadexomer iodine is a slow-release preparation of iodine that appears to be highly effective in eliminating bacteria, even methicillin-resistant *Staphylococcus aureus*. There is considerable evidence that cadexomer iodine is effective in stimulating venous ulcer healing, and there is no evidence that it slows down the healing process of this and other chronic exuding wounds.[25,26]

Skin sensitization with the use of cadexomer iodine has not been observed by this author, but this complication has been seen frequently with many other topically applied products, especially neomycin-containing antibiotics. Patients with venous ulcers have a high rate of sensitization to topically applied preparations.[27] The reason for this propensity is unclear, but it is definitely wise to minimize or, preferably, avoid altogether the use of emollients or topical steroids to the affected leg. Indeed, so-called stasis dermatitis is actually contact dermatitis to topical agents. Similarly, soap and other abrasive agents should not be used in and around venous ulcers.

Grafting

Many clinicians believe that autologous grafting of venous ulcers is not effective. However, published reports indicate that grafting of venous ulcers is probably an underutilized and effective treatment, and that the failure rate of split-thickness autologous grafting is overestimated.[28,29] Grafting is particularly helpful in elderly patients, who have substantial problems dealing with a chronic wound and its treatment. Particularly in elderly patients, it has been policy to graft ulcers that do not appear to be healing (or healing fast enough) after about 6 to 8 weeks of optimal conventional treatment. Ulcers that are very large (ie, circumferential) and that would take an inordinate period of time to achieve complete wound closure also respond well to grafting. Whether this surgical approach for difficult to heal venous ulcers is cost-effective is unclear at this time. It may well be cost-effective when the expenses associated with frequent dressing changes, visits to doctors and by visiting nurses, and complications associated with failure to heal (ie, cellulitis) are considered. Recurrence rates after grafting are probably unchanged compared to what is observed after secondary intention healing. However, that too has not been studied and deserves closer attention. It goes without saying that life-long compression therapy remains critical after the procedure. Indeed, it is essential to apply compression immediately after grafting, especially if the patient is not hospitalized. There has also been clinical experience that grafts that take but do not seem to spread fare much better if the level of compression over the ulcer is increased.

Other Surgical Procedures

Other surgical procedures have been reviewed and their evaluation is beyond the scope of this chapter.[30-34] In general, the goal of surgical approaches to the treatment of venous disease and ulceration has been to remove or ligate diseased vessels and to restore the function of malfunctioning valves. In the Linton procedure, subfascial ligation of incompetent perforators has long been used as a successful treatment modality; it can be used to ligate superficial and perforating veins in patients with venous ulcers. Free flaps containing competent valves can also be used to replace excised tissue from the wound bed. Moreover, superficial femoral vein valvuloplasty can be very effective in relieving reflux.

The surgical procedures mentioned previously can be challenging, especially in patients who already have substantial skin changes associated with venous disease. Therefore, the surgical results are not always as good as would be expected from a theoretical standpoint. It is hoped that advances in visualizing the surgical field with less invasive procedures can produce better results. For example, endoscopic subfascial division of perforating veins seems to be very promising in healing ulcers. It remains to be seen whether this procedure can also decrease the recurrence rate.

Pentoxifylline Therapy

There have been several small trials suggesting that pentoxifylline (400 mg three times daily) may be useful in the treatment of venous ulcers.[35-37] However, the optimal effective dose for this indication has not been established. The results from a multicenter double-blind randomized study of 131 patients suggest that higher doses of pentoxifylline (800 mg three times daily) may be more effective.[4] Using this dosage, pentoxifylline was found to heal ulcers faster than placebo. Whereas the placebo group had only achieved complete healing in half of the cases by week 16, all of the subjects remaining in the group receiving the high dose of pentoxifylline had healed completely. It would be invaluable to know whether maintenance doses of pentoxifylline could delay or prevent ulcer recurrence. However, there are not studies that have been done to evaluate this important question.

Bioengineered Skin ("Smart Treatments")

Bioengineered skin products consist of extracellular matrix materials, cells, or both. Such products can be viewed both as a tissue replacement (at least temporarily) or as agents capable of stimulating tissue repair.[6] In the opinion of this author, they represent a totally new class of therapeutic agents for the treatment of wounds and can be thought of as "smart treatments," in that they are capable of adjusting and responding to the wound microenvironment. It this regard, bioengineered skin products have been shown to produce a number of cytokines and mediators in addition to being able to synthesize their own matrix proteins.[3] A number of these products are being evaluated for treatment of burns or chronic wounds. Some consist of keratinocyte sheets (Epicel, Genzyme Corporation, Cambridge, MA) or dermal components (Alloderm, Life Sciences). Other products, like Dermagraft (Advanced Tissue Sciences, La Jolla, CA), are under consideration by the FDA for treatment of diabetic wounds. One product that has been tested specifically in venous ulcers in a large trial is Graftskin (Apligraf).[3] This is a bilayered construct of human neonatal keratinocyte and fibroblasts, the latter forming a contracted dermis-like structure with bovine collagen. Structurally, its gross histology is remarkably similar to that of human skin. However, Apligraf lacks endothelial cells and other professional antigen-presenting cells, which might explain why no obvious clinical or laboratory evidence of rejection have been noted. Although the full data set for the Apligraf clinical trial was published, this chapter considers the revised data that was accepted by the FDA and led to the approval of this product. It was determined that Apligraf treatment is safe and effective and provides significant benefits for patients with venous leg ulcers. Very importantly, when applied to ulcers of more than 1 year in duration, Apligraf achieved complete wound closure in more than twice as many patients as compression therapy alone, and in less time. Thus, in these difficult to heal patients, complete wound closure occurred in 34 (47%) of 72 ulcers treated with Apligraf and in 9 (19%) of 48 ulcers treated with active control (compression alone). Accelerated healing of venous ulcers in response to Apligraf was already statistically significant by week 6 (24% vs. 8%; $p = .048$) and continued through the end of the study at week 24 (47% vs. 19%; $p = .002$). Although the trend favored Apligraf, there were no differences in the recurrence rates of ulcers between the Apligraf and the control groups. However, a much larger trial would be needed to evaluate this endpoint. Therefore, Apligraf is able to make a claim that none of the treatments for acute or chronic wounds can presently make: it performs best when used in ulcers of long duration and that are difficult to heal. It is likely that its use, at least initially, is in ulcers that are of long duration and are more difficult to heal. However, depending on how it fares in socioeconomic analyses, it is possible that Apligraf may become a standard treatment for venous ulcers.

There are many attractive features to the use of Apligraf and other bioengineered products in venous ulcers and other chronic wounds. For one, they may act as temporary replacement of cells; the long-term fate of cells from Apligraf in the wound is not certain at the moment. The keratinocytes and fibroblasts in Apligraf are fetal in origin and much more active in their synthesis of matrix components and autocrine growth factors. Bioengineered products may also provide growth factors in the right concentration and in the right sequence. It is hoped that this "smart" delivery of peptides will overcome the problems associated with exogenous application of growth factors, which have largely failed with the notable exception of platelet-derived growth factor for the treatment of diabetic ulcers.[38] In addition, Apligraf and other bioengineered skin products are only "first generation" and will likely be improved in the way they deliver cells, matrix materials, and possibly transfected or transduced genes.

CONCLUSIONS

After decades of pessimism and frustration, the treatment of venous ulcers has suddenly become very exciting and quite varied. There are now better dressings, compression bandages, and topical and systemic agents. Many of these advances are, at least in part, due to substantial progress in our understanding of the pathogenesis of venous disease. However, new surgical approaches and technological advances are major reasons for this revolution in venous ulcer care. In the opinion of this author, the development of bioengineered skin is likely to redefine venous ulcer care and perhaps the treatment of all cutaneous wounds. As is often the case, the greatest challenge will be to integrate and assess the use of new therapeutic agents with existing therapies in a way that is maximally beneficial and cost-effective.

REFERENCES

1. Phillips T, Stanton B, Provan A, Lew R. A study of the impact of leg ulcers on quality of life: financial, social, and psychological implications. *J Am Acad Dermatol*. 1993;19:764–771.
2. Porter JM, Moneta GL. An international consensus committee on chronic venous disease. Reporting standards in venous disease: an update. *J Vasc Surg*. 1995;21:635–645.
3. Falanga V, Margolis D, Alvarez O, Auletta M, et al. Healing of venous ulcers and lack of clinical rejection with an allogeneic cultured human skin equivalent. *Arch Dermatol*. 1998;134:293–300.
4. Falanga V, for the Trental Collaborative Study Group. Pentoxifylline (Trental) accelerates the healing of venous ulcers in a double blind randomised study. In: Proceedings from the European Tissue Repair Society: August 25, 1997, Cologne, Germany.
5. Phillips TJ, and the Ifetroban Study Group. A standard of care for venous ulcers. In: Proceedings from the Seventh European Conference on Wound Management: November 1997; Harrogate, England. London, England: European Wound Management Association; 1997;19.
6. Phillips T. New skin for old. Developments in biological skin substitutes. *Arch Dermatol*. 1998;134:344–349.
7. Van de Scheur M, Falanga V. Pericapillary fibrin cuffs in venous disease. A reappraisal. *Dermatol Surg*. 1997;23:955–959.
8. Falanga V. Venous ulceration. In: Krasner D, Kane D, eds. *Chronic Wound Care: A Clinical Source Book for Health Care Professionals*. Health Management Publications, Inc. 1997;165–171.
9. Greenberg AS, Hasan T, Montalvo BM, Falabella A, et al. Acute lipodermatosclerosis is associated with venous insufficiency. *J Am Acad Dermatol*. 1996;35:566–568.

10. Browse NL, Buranad KG. The cause of venous ulceration. *Lancet.* 1982;ii:243–245.
11. Falanga V, Eaglstein WH. The trap hypothesis of venus ulceration. *Lancet.* 1993;341:1006–1008.
12. Falanga V, Carson P, Greenberg A, Hasan A, et al. Topically applied tPA for the treatment of venous ulcers. *Dermatol Surg.* 1996;22:643–644.
13. Coleridge Smith PD. The microcirculation in venous hypertension. *Cardiovasc Res.* 1996; 32:769–795.
14. Falanga V, Grinnell F, Gilchrest B, Maddox YT, et al. Experimental approaches to chronic wounds. *Wound Rep Reg.* 1995;3:132–140.
15. Katz MH, Alvarez AF, Kirsner RS, Eaglstein WH, et al. Human wound fluid from acute wounds stimulates fibroblast and endothelial cell growth. *J Am Acad Dermatol.* 1991; 25:1054–1058.
16. Bucalo B, Eaglstein WH, Falanga V. Inhibition of cell proliferation by chronic wound fluid. *Wound Rep Reg.* 1993;1:181–186.
17. Hasan A, Murata H, Falabella A, Ochoa S, et al. Dermal fibroblasts from venous ulcers are unresponsive to the action of transforming growth factor-β 1. *J Dermatol Sci.* 1997;16:59–66.
18. Partsch H. Compression therapy of the legs: a review. *J Dermatol Surg Oncol.* 1991;17:799–808.
19. Nelson EA. Compression bandaging in the treatment of venous leg ulcers. *J Wound Care.* 1996;5:415–418.
20. Falanga V, Eaglstein WH. Leg and foot ulcers: a clinician's guide. London: Martin Dunitz Publisher; 1995;154–155.
21. Fletcher A, Cullum N, Sheldon TA. A systematic review of compression treatment for venous leg ulcers. *Br Med J.* 1997;315:576–580.
22. Helfman T, Ovington L, Falanga V. Occlusive dressings and wound healing. In: Bernstein EF, ed. *Clinics of Dermatology,* vol. 12, Elsevier; 1994;121–127.
23. Mertz PM, Eaglstein WH. The effect of a semiocclusive dressing on the microbial population in superficial wounds. *Arch Dermatol.* 1984;119:287–289.
24. Pardes JB, Carson PA, Eaglstein WH, Falanga V. Empirical mupirocin treatment of exudative venous ulcers. *J Am Acad Dermatol.* 1993;29:497–498.
25. Falanga V. Iodine-containing pharmaceuticals: a reappraisal. In Proceedings of the 6th European Conference on Advances in Wound Management. Amsterdam. October 1–4, 1996, London; Macmillan Magazines Ltd; 1997;191–194.
26. Ormiston MC, Seymour MTJ, Venn GE, Fox JA. Controlled trial of iodosorb in chronic venous ulcers. *Br Med J* 1985;291:308–310.
27. Fraki JE, Peltonen L, Hopsu-Havu VK. Allergy to various components of topical preparations in stasis dermatitis and leg ulcer. *Cont Derm.* 1979;5:97–100.
28. Lofgren KA, Lauvstad WA, Bonnemaison MF. Surgical treatment of large stasis ulcer: review of 129 cases. *Mayo Clin Proc.* 1965:40:560–563.
29. Kirsner RS, Mata SM, Falanga V, Kerdel FA. Split-thickness skin grafting of leg ulcers. The University of Miami's Department of Dermatology Experience. *Dermatol Surg.* 1995; 21:701–703.
30. Hafner J, Boumameaux H, Burg G, Brunner U. Management of venous leg ulcers. *VASA.* 1996;25:161–167.
31. Ruckley CV, Prescott RJ. Treatment of chronic leg ulcers. *Lancet.* 1994;344:1512–1513.
32. Ruckley CV. Does venous reflux matter? *Lancet.* 1993;341:411–412.
33. Goldman MP, Weiss RA, Bergan JJ. Diagnosis and treatment of varicose veins: a review. *J Am Acad Dermatol.* 1994;31:393–413.
34. Lee S, Singh S, Beard J, Spencer P, et al. Prospective audit of surgery for varicose veins. *Br J Surg.* 1997;84:44–46.
35. Colgan M-P, Dormandy JA, Jones PW, Schraibman IG, et al. Oxpentifylline treatment of venous ulcers of the leg. *Br Med J.* 1990;300:972–975.
36. Weitgasser H. The use of pentoxifylline (Trental 400) in the treatment of leg ulcers: results of a double blind trial. *Pharmatherapeutica.* 1983;3(Suppl 1):143–151.
37. Arenas R, Atoche C. Post-thrombotic leg ulcers: safety and efficacy of treatment with pentoxifylline (double blind study in 30 patients). *Dermatol Rev Mex Seg Epoca.* 1988; 32:34–38.
38. Steed DL, and the Diabetic Ulcer Study Group. Clinical evaluation of recombinant human platelet–derived growth factor for the treatment of lower extremity diabetic ulcers. *J Vasc Surg.* 1995;21:71–81.

41

New Techniques for Sclerotherapy of Spider Veins and Small Varicose Veins

John R. Pfeifer, MD, Roger Higgins, PhD, Brian G. Brazzo, MD, and Frank A. Nesi, MD

INTRODUCTION

Although many surgeons inject bulging varicose veins, the authors of this chapter are of the opinion that large, bulging varicose veins are best treated surgically by using small incisions and sparing the great saphenous vein whenever possible. Although injection of cutaneous spider veins or telangiectasia of the lower extremity is often done for cosmetic reasons, most such lesions produce symptoms ranging from numbness or paresthesia to pain (either aching or burning).[1] Sclerotherapy is tedious and time-consuming, with a significant incidence of recurrence. However, because of the unattractive appearance of telangiectasia and the associated symptoms, there is a high patient demand for this form of therapy.[2] Our current cumulative experience includes a total of 132,743 injections in 2681 patients between January 1982 and April 1998. The average injection treatment consists of 11 injections at a single session. The majority of these patients presented with lower extremity lesions, with a limited number in the face, chest wall, and breast. This chapter outlines our current management of these patients and a description of our diagnostic approach and our sclerotherapy technique.

The following is a description of three new techniques utilized in our sclerotherapy practice:

1. The use of diagnostic ultrasound for evaluation prior to sclerotherapy.
2. The use of 6-power loupes and 31-gauge needles to facilitate sclerotherapy of very small spider veins (down to 0.25 mm in size).
3. The use of the potassium–titanyl–phosphate (KTP) laser to facilitate the elimination of spider veins not injectable by usual sclerotherapy techniques (under 0.25 mm).

INITIAL EVALUATION

Our current practice is to perform a complete preliminary history and physical, with special attention to the arterial and venous systems. All patients have one or two noninvasive laboratory studies to complete the assessment of the venous system.

The patient is examined in the erect position (after 5 to 10 min of standing to allow for maximum inflation of bulging varicosities). Bulging varicosities and spider veins are accurately marked on leg diagrams at the time of initial examination (Figs. 41–1 and 41–2). A copy of this diagram is attached to the chart at the time of each injection treatment to facilitate an accurate record of injection locations.

The patient is then measured for custom-fitted support hose by the office staff. (In our clinic, this is performed by a specialized pressure-gradient therapist.) A variety of brands are available. Over-the-counter types are to be discouraged because the patient needs a stocking specific to his or her measurements and the stocking must have an appropriate pressure gradient. The patient brings the compression stocking to each injection appointment.

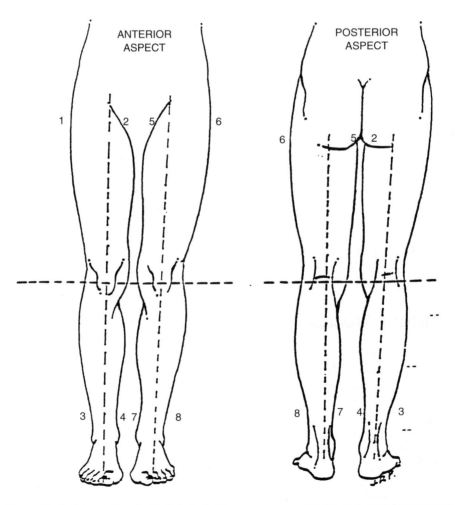

Figure 41–1. Vein marking sheet. Note that all leg areas are numbered; thus, each leg segment has a number identification for purposes of computer analysis. (*Villavicencio, FDA combined study on sclerotherapy.*)

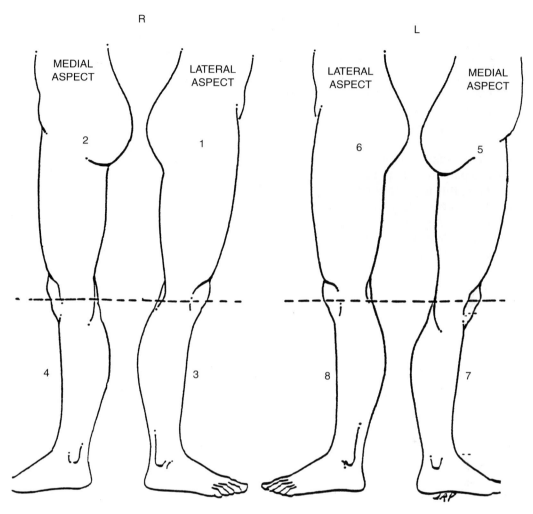

Figure 41–2. Vein marking sheet. Note that all leg areas are numbered. Thus, each leg segment has a number identification for purposes of computer analysis. (*Villavicencio, FDA combined study on sclerotherapy.*)

LABORATORY STUDIES

Sclerotherapy cannot be viewed as injection of small varicose veins and spider veins to the exclusion of other methods of therapy. With appropriate diagnostic techniques, superficial and deep venous insufficiency can be differentiated and managed along with sclerotherapy of surface veins. Initially, photoplethysmography (PPG) is used to evaluate, in a general way, venous valve function and the degree of venous insufficiency.[3,4] In addition, we now use routine duplex examination to determine locations of major venous reflux. Duplex scanning is the guide to appropriate treatment, which ranges from ligation of the greater or lesser saphenous vein, phlebectomy, injection sclerotherapy, or laser therapy.

Duplex Scanning

In the assessment of lower extremity venous change, image is critical. Color is important, but attention to the smallest detail is paramount. Sacrificing detail for color may compro-

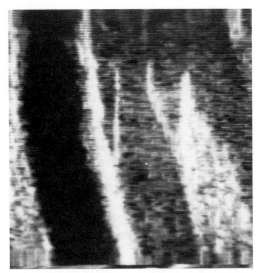 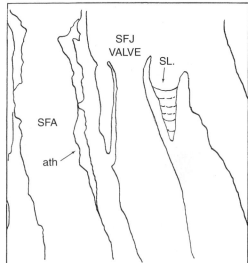

Figure 41–3. A longitudinal view of the saphenofemoral junction area showing a normal pair of valve leaflets (SFJ valve). Some sludging (SL) is seen behind the right valve leaflet. Some modest atherosclerotic (ath) change is also seen in the superficial femoral artery (SFA).

mise the ability of the examiner to detect fine points of reflux. The absence of a color-flow capability can be adequately compensated for by spectrum analysis or hand-held bidirectional Doppler. Inferior image resolution of some color-flow equipment may miss distal incompetent perforators.

Reflux is a result or effect, not the cause. To determine the cause of reflux requires the identification of distal connections between the deep and superficial venous net-

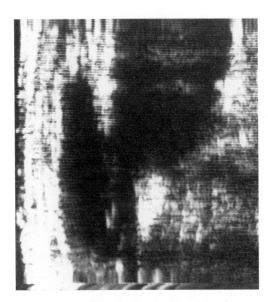 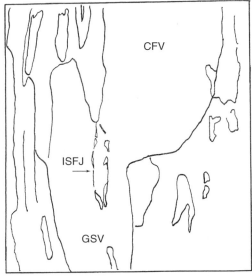

Figure 41–4. A longitudinal view of the saphenofemoral junction area showing an incompetent SFJ valve (ISFJ). GSV, greater saphenous vein; CFV, common femoral vein.

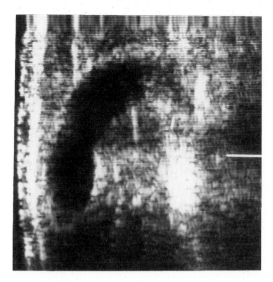 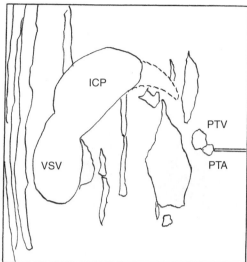

Figure 41–5. A transverse view above the medial malleolus showing an incompetent perforator (ICP) bulging through the fascia. This perforator connects with the posterior tibial vein deep, and with a varicosed superifcial tributary (VSV) of the greater saphenous vein.

works. Flow in these connections may be little to none at rest, making them invisible to some lower-resolution scanners.

Compression and Valsalva maneuvers are helpful once a connection has been localized, but these techniques cannot be used very easily to identify the perforator.

In view of the foregoing, it is our opinion that a high-resolution duplex scanner, not necessarily with color capability, coupled with a high-frequency (8 MHz) probe with limited depth of field (4 cm) allows the most accurate and thorough survey of lower extremity venous systems.[5] Normal (Fig. 41–3) and abnormal (Fig. 41–4) valvular function can often be visualized directly. Venous structures of less than 1.0 mm diameter can be identified (Fig. 41–5). Direction of flow can be assessed by spectrum analysis or by subsequent hand-held bidirectional Doppler probe.

Excellent detail and gray-scale range allow chronic and acute problems to be separated and recanalization to be monitored.

If there is any question of deep vein thrombosis (DVT), duplex scanning is the best method for assessing deep venous occlusion precisely, either acute or chronic.[6] The presence of chronic deep vein occlusion is not a contraindication for sclerotherapy; however, the presence of acute DVT is an absolute contraindication for sclerotherapy. If acute DVT is detected, sclerotherapy should be postponed for 6 months.

PATIENT SELECTION

Our experience utilizing duplex scanning has resulted in several clearly definable patient groups:

- Unexpected saphenofemoral junction incompetence.
- Isolated tributary vein changes with normal greater saphenous vein and lesser saphenous vein.

- Unexpected large incompetent perforators, and incompetent perforators in un-usual locations (likely to be missed by hand-held Doppler examination alone). Such incompetent perforators make successful sclerotherapy unlikely, and may also result in a high incidence of "blush" formation following sclerotherapy.
- Unusual venous anatomy. Variations from the norm invariably perform less well than the normal anatomy.

We also believe that demonstrating the compressibility of the lower extremity veins to the patient helps reinforce the usefulness of compression hose in the control of incompetent perforator function.

Using the duplex scan, the decision of whether to interrupt larger venous communications prior to sclerotherapy of spider veins can be made on a scientific basis.

Patient Support Prior to Injection

It is important to realize that although sclerotherapy is done for symptoms of pain, paresthesia, and so on, the majority of patients have also come for cosmetic concerns. Therefore, results are not based on the usual physician parameters of clinical improvement. Here, the patient's own assessment of results is important. In fact, the patient's decision to proceed with treatment depends on his or her reaction to the degree of pain during the procedure and his or her assessment of the result. In sclerotherapy, patient comfort and patient satisfaction become critical factors in determining whether they will continue with treatment. Thus, the physician's preinjection preparation of the patient becomes an important component of treatment. A supportive physician is important, but supportive and kind office personnel are equally important, as they handle the many questions posed by these patients.

Explanation of Risk

Before injection sclerotherapy is performed, a comprehensive explanation of the procedure, with its attendant risks, is given to the patient (both verbal and written) at the time of preliminary examination (Table 41–1).

Presclerotherapy Photography

Evaluation of results in sclerotherapy is highly subjective. Frequently, as the series of sclerotherapy treatments progresses, patients forget how extensive their veins were prior to injection. Therefore, it is important to photograph all areas of planned injection prior to beginning sclerotherapy.

We use a Minolta-7000 35-mm camera with a macro 35–70 zoom lens. A databack on the camera allows us to protect the identity of the patient by assigning a code number to each patient. Prints are kept in the patient file and are reviewed periodically with the patient. This photographic record also allows the treating physician to evaluate improvement objectively as treatment progresses.

Sclerotherapy (Operative) Permit

A signed permit is obtained, even though this is an office procedure. Written permission to photograph the patient is also obtained. We use a single Consent to Treatment form, which includes both injection and photography (Table 41–2).

Compression Stockings

Faria and Morales[7] pointed out that most spider telangiectasia are related to venous insufficiency and that there is direct communication between telangiectatic channels

TABLE 41–1. COMPREHENSIVE EXPLANATION OF INJECTION SCLEROTHERAPY GIVEN TO PATIENTS BEFORE BEGINNING THE PROCEDURE

INJECTION THERAPY FOR SPIDER VEINS

As you begin a program of sclerotherapy for your spider veins, there are some things that we would like for you to remember:

1. CERTAIN VEINS REQUIRE THREE OR FOUR TREATMENTS BEFORE THEY DISAPPEAR.

   The principle of injection therapy for small skin veins is to inject a sclerosing (scarring) agent into the vein that causes the vein wall to become inflamed and seal together. When the vein can no longer carry blood, it is no longer visible through the skin. Certain veins require three or four treatments before they disappear.

2. THERE IS OCCASIONAL SKIN PIGMENTATION (BROWN SPOTS).

   When the tiny needle is inserted into the vein for injection purposes, as the salt solution is injected, occasionally, the vein ruptures, allowing this solution to leak into the surrounding tissue. This may result in a brown pigmented spot on the skin that is occasionally permanent but usually disappears with time. It is usually small and no more obvious than the vein that was treated initially. However, you should be aware that this is a complication of injection of veins, although it only occurs in approximately 10% of cases.

3. THERE IS A RARE OCCURRENCE OF SMALL SKIN ULCERS FORMING AFTER INJECTION.

   Very rarely, an injection is irritating enough to cause a small area of skin loss (or ulcer). In our experience of more than 70,000 cases of injection, this complication has occurred 37 times. The size of a pencil eraser, these ulcers have healed without incident, leaving a small white scar.

4. YOU WILL BE REQUIRED TO SUPPORT YOUR LEGS AFTER TREATMENT.

   After injection, your legs will be compressed with small gauze pads and a compression stocking (either calf-high or panythose). This compression support stays in place for 3 days and 2 nights, during which time you will not be able to shower or have a complete bath. Then the stocking alone is used for an additional 2 weeks, and daily showers may be resumed.

5. ACTIVITIES AFTER INFECTION.

   During the injection treatments, your daily activities are not restricted. You may continue to work and perform your daily activities. However, aggressive exercising such as jogging, tennis, or high-impact aerobics should be avoided during a period of 1 to 3 weeks following treatment.

6. NEW SPIDER VEINS MAY FORM, REQUIRING SUBSEQUENT TREATMENT.

   Because we function and work in the erect position, extra pressure is placed on the veins of the leg. Thus, there is a tendency for new spider veins to form. Even after the majority of your veins have been removed by sclerotherapy, be aware that *new spider veins could develop.* We ask that all our patients return for periodic reevaluation so that any new veins can be injected before they become too large or too numerous.

7. FLARE FORMATION.

   Occasionally, immediately after injection, a new cluster of veins may form in close proximity to the vein just injected. This has the appearance of a "blush" in the skin, and can usually be controlled by repeated injection.

and the deep venous system or an incompetent superficial venous system. Our observations have supported this finding. A leg that is not supported with a compression stocking following injection has a more rapid rate of recurrence of spider veins.[8,9] Goldman et al.[10] noted improvement in sclerotherapy results when compression was used. In our experience, the use of an adequate compression stocking has reduced recurrence by approximately 50%. Therefore, we maintain a full-time compression therapist on staff in our clinic and all are fitted patients for compression stockings at the time of preliminary evaluation. Patients are carefully instructed in the application of pressure gradient hose using rubber gloves, which prolongs the life of the hose.

If only below-the-knee injections are carried out, then 30 to 40 mm Hg below-the-knee stockings can be used. If thigh injections are performed, a 20 to 30 mm Hg pantyhose or thigh-length stocking is fitted. If large, bulging veins are injected, 4- or

TABLE 41–2. CONSENT TO TREATMENT FORM

CONSENT TO TREATMENT

I have been informed by the doctor of the nature of injection treatment of varicose veins. I understand the possible side effects, which include recurrence, skin pigmentation, skin ulcers, and localized clotted veins.

I authorize the doctor to take photographs of me before and after treatment, and to permit such photographs to be used at the doctor's discretion for purposes of medical lecturing, research, or scientific publication, with the provision that I will not be identified.

FEES AND PAYMENT

Injections are billed individually at $ _____ each. Most treatments will not exceed twenty (20) injections per appointment.

Due to the costs of providing this treatment, payment is expected at the time this service is rendered.

A deposit of $100.00 is required no later than ten (10) days prior to your scheduled appointment. This deposit confirms your appointment time and will be credited to your balance on your treatment day. All future scheduled appointments will also require a deposit in advance.

The balance at the time of treatment will then be that which exceeds the $100.00 deposit.

For your convenience, we do accept payment by cash, check, Visa, or MasterCard.

I understand all terms as written above, and I authorize the doctor to administer such treatment to me.

_____
PATIENT SIGNATURE

_____
DATE

** *Due to the cost of providing these treatments, fees will be subject to change on an annual basis.*

6-inch Ace bandages are applied snugly to the leg and the compression stocking is worn over the Ace bandage for the first 3 days.

The patient is required to wear the compression stocking for 3 days and 2 nights after treatment and is asked to avoid strenuous exercise. For the first 3 days, the injection sites are padded with gauze compression pads underneath the compression hose. After the first 3 days, the patient may take daily showers but must wear the support stocking during the day for 2 weeks, removing it only at night. When breast lesions are treated, they are compressed with elastic bandages overnight only.

On a long-term basis, we recommend that patients wear compression stockings for most of their standing activities. For women patients who are concerned about the appearance of compression stockings, there are several companies that provide relatively sheer hose. Most patients are allowed to put aside the stockings in the hot summer months and for important social occasions. Our recommendation: "Wear them when you can hide them."

PATIENT SYMPTOMS

Weiss and Weiss[1] pointed out that most spider veins are symptomatic (numbness, paresthesia, aching, burning pain, etc). Injection of veins almost always reduces or eliminates cutaneous symptoms, although the generalized aching of incompetent deep veins may persist.

INDICATIONS FOR SCLEROTHERAPY

Vein Size

There are three types of varicose veins, and they are as follows:

1. Small, bulging branch varicose veins, which are 3 to 6 mm
2. Dilated venules (reticular veins), which are 1 to 3 mm
3. Telangiectasia (spider veins), which are less than 1 mm

Although controversial, many sclerotherapists do inject larger veins. However, when injected, large veins are often complicated by skin pigmentation, which can be distressing to patients. We believe that larger varicose veins should be surgically excised using 6-mm phlebectomy incisions. The results are very cosmetic and the recurrence rate is lower with operation. Injection sclerotherapy of reticular veins and spider veins is the treatment of choice.

Treatment of Very Small Spider Veins

Although most patients initially want only larger spider veins injected, our experience is that they ultimately want *all* spider veins injected, down to the smallest visible vein. To facilitate management of these very small veins, we are successfully utilizing 6-power loupes and 31-gauge needles, which has significantly increased our success rate with spider veins as small as 0.25 mm in size.

Effect of Natural Skin Pigment on Injection and Laser Therapy

The concept of skin typing was created in 1975 to classify patients with psoriasis and white skin for ultraviolet A treatment (PUVA).[11] A simple classification system was based on patient reports of their initial response to sun exposure:

SKIN TYPE	ERYTHEMA AND TANNING TO FIRST SUMMER EXPOSURE
I	Always burn, never tan
II	Usually burn, tan less than average
III	Sometimes mild burn, tan about average
IV	Rarely burn, tan more than average

Later, the classification was expanded to include people of brown (type V) and black (type VI) skin colors.[12]

Type I people are typically of Scandinavian ancestry. Types II and III people are commonly of northern European descent. Type IV people are generally of Mediterranean, Hispanic, or Asian descent. People of Middle Eastern and Indian backgrounds are often classified as skin type V. People of African descent usually have type V or VI skin.

Pigmentary disturbances are the most common complication of both laser treatment and sclerotherapy because the peak absorption of hemoglobin is similar to that of melanin. Hemoglobin has absorption peaks at 577 nm and at 585 nm, with a third peak at 532 nm. For this reason, patients with significant skin pigmentation (types IV to VI) must be treated extremely cautiously with sclerotherapy and laser.

New Laser Technology

We previously reported a comparison of injection sclerotherapy using 22% hypertonic saline with carbon dioxide laser ablation of spider veins of the lower extremity.[13]

Patients preferred injection sclerotherapy because laser treatment left scars, was more painful, and had a higher recurrence rate. However, new laser technology with smaller spot size (1 and 2 mm) has suggested that we reevaluate that position.

We now utilize 6-power loupes and 31- and 32-gauge needles to eliminate spider veins down to 0.25 mm in size. We then utilize KTP laser to eliminate the very small but vexing spider veins (under 0.25 mm) that remain.

Although sclerotherapy remains the gold standard for reducing lower extremity veins, treatment of the smallest superficial vessels remains difficult. Treatment of many acquired and congenital vascular lesions has been advanced significantly by laser technology. Nd:YAG, krypton, KTP, long-pulse dye, alexandrite, copper vapor, and copper bromide lasers as well as an intense pulsed light source have been used to treat vascular lesions throughout the body. Although each type of laser has a unique profile of advantages and disadvantages, very few of these applications are uniformly effective and safe in the treatment of leg veins.

The treatment of vascular lesions by laser is based on the concept of selective photothermolysis, in which a target tissue absorbs a wavelength selectively. Sufficient energy must be delivered to the target, but the exposure duration must be less than or equal to the thermal relaxation time of the intended target. Applying high energy of long pulses to the skin may have undesirable side effects, including pain, erythema, blistering, and scarring. Thus, the goal is "cool" skin, "hot" vein.

Although lesions respond better when multiple passes of laser are performed, no more than two passes can be done on most patients due to the cumulative thermal effect. An ideal treatment for the removal of telangiectasias should provide high energy to the vessel over one or multiple passes while limiting cutaneous absorption.

To facilitate higher energy delivery to a target and lessen the risk of epidermal damage, cutaneous cooling is employed, either by contact or spray technique.[14] Cooling the skin immediately before application of the laser protects the epidermis from thermal necrosis and lessens the discomfort of the laser pulse. A temperature gradient between the cooled skin and blood vessel remains, and with higher energy, the laser-treated vessels can be heated to a destructive level faster than the nonvascular tissue.

Two lasers commonly used to treat leg telangiectasias are the KTP laser, at 532 nm, and the long-pulse dye laser, at variable 590 nm and 595 nm. Although the pulse dye appears to be more effective in clinical trials, it is associated with more discomfort and purpura.[15] Whereas both lasers are very effective at treating facial telangiectasias, neither is able to approach similar success rates with leg vessels because of the effect of venous insufficiency and hydraulics on the treated areas.

A frequency-doubled Nd:YAG laser (532 nm) with a cooled contact handpiece showed more favorable efficacy in treating leg telangiectasias.[16] Because of its ability to protect the epidermis and utilize long-pulse duration, multiple passes over a vessel may be performed with minimal discomfort. Although preliminary results are more consistent and encouraging, the treatment of leg telangiectasias remains a challenge for physicians and is probably most effective when performed in conjunction with sclerotherapy. Laser treatment has the same requirement for compression therapy as does sclerotherapy.

CONTRAINDICATIONS TO SCLEROTHERAPY

The multicenter FDA trial on Sotradecol/Aethoxysklerol has established excellent exclusion criteria for the study. A partial list of these exclusion criteria serves as a reference for relative and absolute contraindications to injection.

Absolute Contraindications

There are several absolute contraindications to sclerotherapy, and they are as follows:

- Pregnancy
- Generalized systemic disease (cardiac, renal, hepatic, pulmonary, and collagen diseases and malignancies)
- Advanced rheumatic disease, osteoarthritis, or any disease that interferes with patient mobility
- Acute deep vein thrombophlebitis
- Acute febrile illness
- Patients on anticoagulants

Relative Contraindications

There are several relative contraindications to sclerotherapy, and they are as follows:

- Patients with large varicose veins (more than 6 mm in diameter). These are best treated with surgery because they are often in communication with a source of venous reflux
- Patients who are both elderly (older than 65 years of age) and sedentary
- Arterial insufficiency of lower extremities (depending on location of planned injection)
- Bronchial asthma or demonstrated allergies
- Obesity
- Acute superficial thrombophlebitis

SCLEROSING SOLUTIONS

A variety of solutions are available for injection. Discussion of the advantages and disadvantages of each is beyond the scope of this chapter. Goldman's[2] text on sclerotherapy is highly recommended for the interested reader. Hypertonic saline is recommended here because of the low risk of complication and the generally excellent outcome.

Injection Technique

Our injection technique is as follows:

1. Accuracy of intraluminal injection is enhanced by the use of 3- to 6-power loupes and a variable-intensity lamp.
2. The patient lies flat, in a horizontal position, on the treatment table (either supine or prone, depending on location of venous lesion). A high-intensity light is utilized. Trendelenburg position and tourniquets are not necessary. The Ritter electric table is an excellent table for injection.
3. The legs are photographed and recorded in a log book. Photos may be taken in a standing or a horizontal position.
4. A copy of the initial venous mapping diagram is placed at the patient's bedside to allow accurate charting of all injections.
5. The leg area is prepped with aqueous Zephiran or similar colorless antiseptic solution. Infection after sclerotherapy is rare. One of the principal reasons for prepping the site is to render the skin more transparent so the veins are seen more easily.

6. We use an injection solution of 23.4% saline (0.4 cc) plus 2% plain lidocaine (0.1 cc) mixed in a 1-cc tuberculin syringe. (This solution is prepared in advance by injecting 2 cc of 2% plain xylocaine into a 30-cc multiple dose vial of 23.4% saline. This dilutes the saline to 22%.)

7. *Each injection is limited to 0.5 cc of solution* to minimize the risk of injectant traversing the communicating vein and reaching the deep venous system.

8. *Retraction by assistant.* Retraction of the skin, to make it slightly taut, is helpful in assuring accurate injection.

9. A 30-gauge needle is used to enter the vein. A 3- to 6-power ocular loupe facilitates accurate entry of the vein. *Injection must be intraluminal.* Perivenous injection leads to pigmentation and skin necrosis. We bend the needle to 30° to allow easier entry into the vein.

10. *The injection should be made slowly.* Watch the tip of the needle as you inject. The appearance of a small bubble, suggesting extravasation, means that individual injection should be terminated. If the physician watches carefully and stops immediately when extravasation occurs, these small bubbles subside without leaving a blemish. It is not necessary, and may in fact be harmful, to attempt to dilute small extravasation bubbles.

11. Proper injection results in blanching along the course of the injected vein. Erythema around the injected vein appears immediately after injection, indicating that the saline solution has been injected correctly throughout the distribution of the vein.

12. After injection, withdraw the needle and apply a pressure pad of three 4 × 4 gauze squares folded once. Use paper tape to hold the gauze pad in place.

13. Our sessions average 11 injections per treatment session, and the usual patient has three sessions. We have injected as many as 80 sites in a single session if the patient has constraints of travel distance or time.

14. During the course of the sclerotherapy treatment, the injection sites are compressed with gauze pressure pads secured with paper tape. The compression hose are applied before the patient is allowed to get off the treatment table. Thus, the patient's legs are not permitted to be in the dependent position until the compression stocking is in place.

The office nurse, compression therapist, or trained office assistant should put the stocking on the patient and instruct in the proper application and removal of the hose.

When larger veins are injected, we apply a 4- or 6-inch Ace bandage directly over the compression pads. The stocking is worn over this bandage for the first 3 days. This allows extra compression and reduces the likelihood of painful clot formation.

Patients are given a list of instructions to follow for the first 2 weeks after treatment (Table 41–3).

Postinjection Compression Pads

We utilize a longitudinal pressure pad made of three 4 × 4 gauze squares applied immediately after injection. The *entire* length of injected vein must be compressed, not just the point of needle entry. A 4 × 4 pad allows the clinician to compress the entire length of vein to achieve more effective ablation (Fig. 41–6). If only a cottonball is used at the needle-entry site, the remainder of the injected vein may refill, resulting in persistence of the injected vein and necessitating further injections (Fig. 41–7).

TABLE 41–3. PATIENT INSTRUCTION SHEET

INSTRUCTIONS TO FOLLOW AFTER INJECTION TREATMENT

DAYS 1–3

The stockings should remain in place for 3 days (including wearing them at night). The compression stocking is an important part of the treatment, as it minimizes the blood reentering the injected vein. Elevate your legs as much as possible. Do not participate in jogging or high-impact aerobics at this time. At the end of the 3 days, you may remove the stockings and discard the gauze pads. (You may find that standing in the shower is a convenient way to loosen the tape holding the gauze pads to avoid blistering sensitive skin). Do not be surprised if injected areas appear bruised at this time; that is normal for many skin types.

DAYS 4–14

Continue to wear the compression stockings daily. Remove them at night to sleep. You may resume daily showers. Avoid jogging or high-impact aerobics during this time.

FROM DAY 15 ON

Continue to wear the compression stockings when you can hide them, as this reduces the rate of recurrence of spider varicose veins.

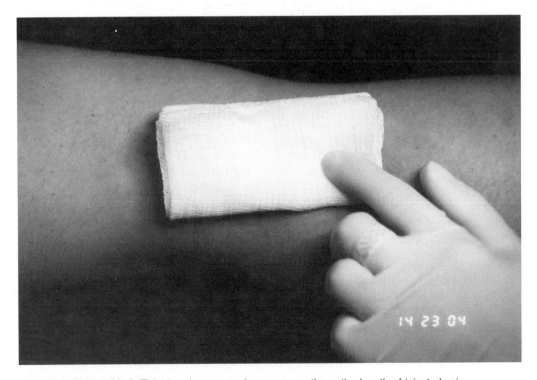

Figure 41–6. This 4 × 4 gauze pad compresses the entire length of injected vein.

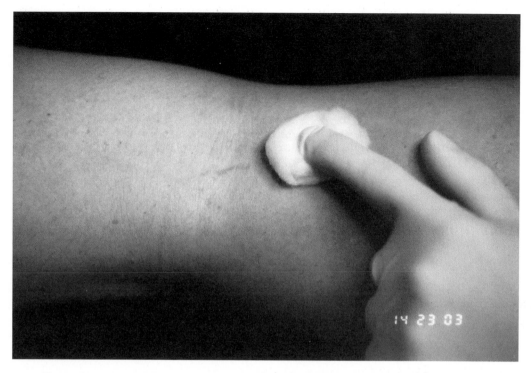

Figure 41–7. Cottonball compresses only needle entry–point and can result in persistence of distal noncompressed vein.

COMPLICATIONS OF SCLEROTHERAPY

Several complications may result from sclerotherapy, and they are as follows:

- Recurrence—Although not a complication of sclerotherapy, patients view recurrence as a complication. Remember, this is a gravity-related disorder and all varicose and spider veins tend to recur. If patients are warned prior to injection, they tend to be less concerned about recurrence and the need for repeat injections.
- Pigmentation (5% to 10% of patients)—This usually disappears in a few months, but may last for as long as a year. Close attention must be paid to skin types so that patients can be prepared in advance for this possibility.
- Telangiectatic matting or flare formation (5% of patients)—These small venous blush formations near the site of injection are very distressing to patients. They can be prevented by injection of dominant veins within the blush formation, and by injection or ligation of large proximal incompetent veins.
- Ulceration (80/132,743 injections, or 1 per 1660 injections)—After hypertonic saline injection, these are usually small, full-thickness ulcers less than 1 cm in diameter. They all heal within a period of 1 to 3 months with minimal scarring. With some undiluted sclerosants, ulcers may be much larger.
- Thrombosis of small veins at injection site—Such clots should be evacuated by small stab wounds, preferably within 2 or 3 weeks, to avoid pain and pigmentation.
- Superficial phlebitis—Occasionally seen in larger veins adjacent to the injection site.

- Deep vein thrombosis—DVT is an occasional complication of large vein sclero-therapy.[17] In our series, it has only occurred in two patients with spider vein injection. Both were treated with anticoagulants and hospitalization and experienced no long-term sequelae. If a patient experiences unusual pain, fullness, or edema in the first few weeks after injection, noninvasive studies to rule out deep vein thrombosis should be carried out.

CONCLUSION

The duplex scan is an invaluable preinjection method of detecting unsuspected larger perforator veins or superficial venous channels prior to injection. such large feeding veins must be dealt with prior to injection sclerotherapy. Injection sclerotherapy using hypertonic saline solution is a safe, relatively painless method of ablating small varicose veins, reticular venules, and spider telangiectasias, with minimal complications. Although spider veins are symptomatic, most patients seek treatment because they are unhappy with the appearance of their legs. Caution should be exercised so that a worse blemish is not created. Sclerotherapy should be viewed as a semicosmetic procedure, and the patient's high degree of expectation must be considered carefully. Careful preinjection discussion of risk must be carried out with patients so they are fully aware of the protracted and tedious nature of sclerotherapy as well as its potential complications. The effect of gravity and incompetent venous valves must always be remembered. Varicose veins and spider veins tend to recur. The wearing of compression hose during the immediate postinjection period is mandatory. On a long-term basis, compression hose reduce recurrence significantly. New methods in the form of 6-power loupes with 31-gauge needles and fine-spot laser technology permit the ablation of the smallest spider vein. With careful and precise technique, the majority of small spider veins and telangiectasias can be eliminated. Patient satisfaction with the procedure is high.

REFERENCES

1. Weiss RA, Weiss MA. Resolution of pain associated with varicose and telangiectatic leg veins after compression sclerotherapy. *J Dermatol Surg Oncol.* 1990;16:333–336.
2. Goldman, MP. *Sclerotherapy.* Chicago: Mosby Year Book, Inc.: 1991.
3. Bergan JT, Yao JST. *Venous Problems.* Chicago: Mosby Year Book; 1978.
4. Browse, Burnard, Thomas. *Diseases of the Veins.* Edward Arnold Pub.; 1988.
5. Georgiev, M. The preoperative duplex examination. *Dermatol Surg.* 1998;24:433–440.
6. Karkow, Baldridge, Cranley, et al. *Atlas of Duplex Scanning.* Philadelphia: WB Saunders; 1992.
7. Faria JL, Morales IN. Histopathology of the telangiectasia associated with varicose veins. *Dermatologica.* 1963;127:321–329.
8. Fegan WG. Continuous compression technique of injecting varicose veins. *Lancet.* 1963;2:109.
9. Hobbs JT. The treatment of varicose veins: a random trial of injection compression therapy versus surgery. *Br J Surg.* 1968;55:777.
10. Goldman MP, Beaudoing D, Marley W, Lopez L, et al. Compression in the treatment of leg telangiectasia: a preliminary report. *J Dermatol Surg Oncol.* 1990;6:4.
11. Fitzpatrick TB. Soleil et peau. *J Med Esthat.* 1975;2:33–34.
12. Fitzpatrick TB. The validity and practicality of sun-reactive skin type I through VI. *Arch Dem.* 1988;124:869–871. [Editorial]

13. Pfeifer JR, Hawtof GD. Injection sclerotherapy and CO_2 laser sclerotherapy in the ablation of cutaneous spider veins of the lower extremity. *Phlebology.* 1989;4:231–240.
14. Chess C, Chess Q. Cool laser optics treatment of large telangiectasia of the lower extremity. *J Dermatol Surg Oncol.* 1993;19:74–80.
15. West TB, Alster TS. Comparison of the long-pulse dye (590–595 nm) and KTP (532 nm) lasers in the treatment of facial and leg telangiectasias. *Dermatol Surg.* 1998;24:221–226.
16. Adrian RM. Treatment of leg telangiectasias using a long-pulse, frequency-doubled Neodynium: YAG laser at 532 nm. *Dermatol Surg.* 1998;24:19–23.
17. Williams RA, Wilson SE. Sclerosant treatment of varicose veins and deep vein thrombosis. *Arch Surg.* 1984;119:1283–1285.

Index

Page numbers followed by *t* and *f* refer to tables
and figures, respectively.

Page numbers followed by *t* and *f* refer to tables
and figures, respectively.

Page numbers followed by *t* and *f* refer to tables and figures, respectively.

Page numbers followed by *t* and *f* refer to tables
and figures, respectively.

Page numbers followed by *t* and *f* refer to tables
and figures, respectively.